New Frontiers in Angiology

Edited by Vince O'Riely

hayle
medical

New York

Hayle Medical,
750 Third Avenue, 9ᵗʰ Floor,
New York, NY 10017, USA

Visit us on the World Wide Web at:
www.haylemedical.com

ISBN: 978-1-63241-443-4

The publisher's policy is to use permanent paper from mills that operate a sustainable forestry policy. Furthermore, the publisher ensures that the text paper and cover boards used have met acceptable environmental accreditation standards.

Trademark Notice: Registered trademark of products or corporate names are used only for explanation and identification without intent to infringe.

Printed in the United States of America.

Cataloging-in-Publication Data

New frontiers in angiology / edited by Vince O'Riely.
  p. cm.
Includes bibliographical references and index.
ISBN 978-1-63241-443-4
1. Blood-vessels. 2. Blood-vessels--Diseases. 3. Blood-vessels--Physiology. 4. Neovascularization.
I. O'Riely, Vince.
RC691 .N49 2017
616.13--dc23

Table of Contents

Permissions

List of Contributors

Index

Preface

The study of physiological process through which new blood vessels are formed from the pre-existing vessels is called angiology. This field is also known as vascular medicine and studies in detail the diseases related to arteries and viens such as aorta, heart attack, etc. This book is a valuable compilation of topics, ranging from the basic to the most complex advancements in the field of angiogenesis. This text on angiology elaborately discusses the application of angiogenesis in medicine. From theories to research to practical applications, case studies related to all contemporary topics of relevance to this field have been included in this book. The topics covered in this book offer the readers new insights in the field of angiology and its varied applications.

All of the data presented henceforth, was collaborated in the wake of recent advancements in the field. The aim of this book is to present the diversified developments from across the globe in a comprehensible manner. The opinions expressed in each chapter belong solely to the contributing authors. Their interpretations of the topics are the integral part of this book, which I have carefully compiled for a better understanding of the readers.

At the end, I would like to thank all those who dedicated their time and efforts for the successful completion of this book. I also wish to convey my gratitude towards my friends and family who supported me at every step.

Editor

MicroRNA-377 Regulates Mesenchymal Stem Cell-Induced Angiogenesis in Ischemic Hearts by Targeting VEGF

Zhili Wen[1,2◑], Wei Huang[2◑], Yuliang Feng[2], Wenfeng Cai[2], Yuhua Wang[2], Xiaohong Wang[3], Jialiang Liang[2], Mashhood Wani[2], Jing Chen[4], Pin Zhu[5], Ji-Mei Chen[5], Ronald W. Millard[3], Guo-Chang Fan[3], Yigang Wang[2]*

1 Department of Infectious Disease, Nanchang University Medical School, Nanchang, Jiangxi, China, 2 Department of Pathology and Lab Medicine, University of Cincinnati Medical Center, Cincinnati, Ohio, United States of America, 3 Department of Pharmacology and Cell Biophysics, University of Cincinnati Medical Center, Cincinnati, Ohio, United States of America, 4 Department of Environmental Health, University of Cincinnati Medical Center, Cincinnati, Ohio, United States of America, 5 Guangdong Cardiovascular Institute, Guangdong Academy of Medical Sciences, Guangzhou, Guandong, People's Republic of China

Abstract

MicroRNAs have been appreciated in various cellular functions, including the regulation of angiogenesis. Mesenchymal-stem-cells (MSCs) transplanted to the MI heart improve cardiac function through paracrine-mediated angiogenesis. However, whether microRNAs regulate MSC induced angiogenesis remains to be clarified. Using microRNA microarray analysis, we identified a microRNA expression profile in hypoxia-treated MSCs and observed that among all dysregulated microRNAs, microRNA-377 was decreased the most significantly. We also validated that vascular endothelial growth factor (VEGF) is a target of microRNA-377 using dual-luciferase reporter assay and Western-blotting. Knockdown of endogenous microRNA-377 promoted tube formation in human umbilical vein endothelial cells. We then engineered rat MSCs with lentiviral vectors to either overexpress microRNA-377 (MSC$^{miR-377}$) or knockdown microRNA-377 (MSC$^{Anti-377}$) to investigate whether microRNA-377 regulated MSC-induced myocardial angiogenesis, using MSCs infected with lentiviral empty vector to serve as controls (MSC^{Null}). Four weeks after implantation of the microRNA-engineered MSCs into the infarcted rat hearts, the vessel density was significantly increased in MSC$^{Anti-377}$-hearts, and this was accompanied by reduced fibrosis and improved myocardial function as compared to controls. Adverse effects were observed in MSC$^{miR-377}$-treated hearts, including reduced vessel density, impaired myocardial function, and increased fibrosis in comparison with MSC^{Null}-group. These findings indicate that hypoxia-responsive microRNA-377 directly targets VEGF in MSCs, and knockdown of endogenous microRNA-377 promotes MSC-induced angiogenesis in the infarcted myocardium. Thus, microRNA-377 may serve as a novel therapeutic target for stem cell-based treatment of ischemic heart disease.

Editor: Yao Liang Tang, Georgia Regents University, United States of America

Funding: This work was funded in part by National Institutes of Health grants HL107957 and HL110740 to Yigang Wang and grant HL-087861 to Guo-Chang Fan. The funders had no role in study design, data collection and analysis, decision to publish, or preparation of the manuscript.

Competing Interests: The authors have declared that no competing interests exist.

* Email: yi-gang.wang@uc.edu

◑ These authors contributed equally to this work.

Introduction

The formation of new blood vessels is critical for the repair of ischemic myocardium, and VEGF is one of the most extensively characterized angiogenic factors [1]. While direct administration of VEGF into the ischemic myocardium has been used successfully to stimulate therapeutic angiogenesis in animal models, clinical trials of VEGF have been largely unsuccessful [2], [3]. These results underscore our incomplete knowledge of myocardial angiogenesis under ischemic conditions.

During the past decade, it has been demonstrated that MSCs can facilitate new blood vessel growth by secretion of pro-angiogenic factors (e.g. VEGF, IGF-1α, HGF, etc.) that contribute to cardiac repair and enhance the reparative process [4–6]. MSCs

are, however, highly sensitive to ischemic conditions, and the majority of injected MSCs die within several hours of delivery *in vivo* [7]. In this regard, multiple approaches (e.g. hypoxic treatment, genetic modification, and pre-conditioning) have been applied to MSCs in an effort to improve their survival and pro-angiogenic capacity both *in vivo* and *in vitro* [8]. Although hypoxia is well recognized to promote MSC-mediated myocardial angiogenesis by induction of VEGF expression [9], [10], the underlying mechanisms underlying these effects have not been delineated.

miRs are a class of 20–24 nt non-coding RNAs that negatively regulate protein-coding gene expression primarily through post-transcriptional repression or mRNA degradation in a sequence-specific manner [11–13]. Recently, miRs regulated by hypoxia

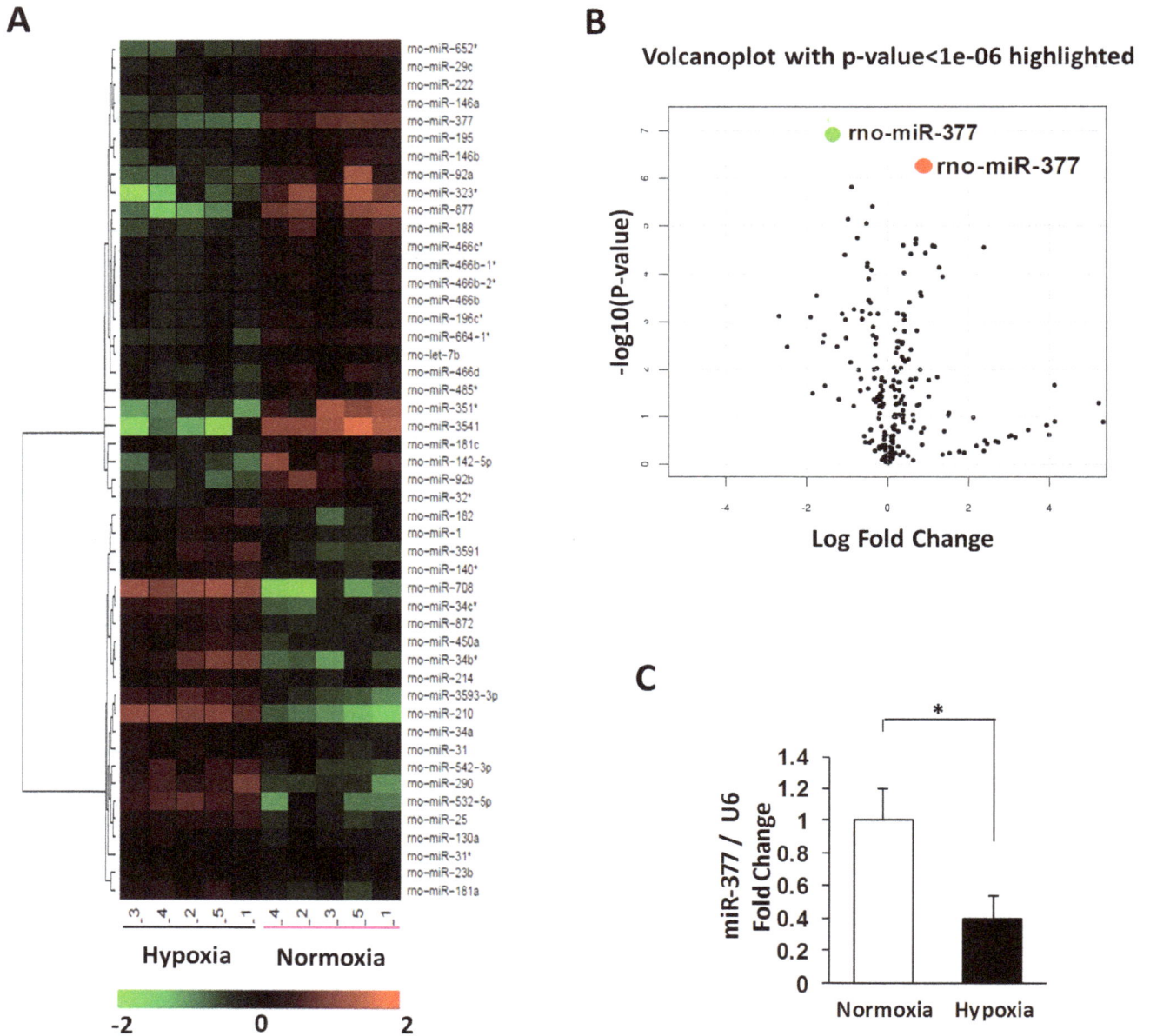

Figure 1. miRNA expression profile is determined in hypoxia-treated mesenchymal stem cells (MSCs). (**A**): A heat map of all dysregulated miRNAs in hypoxia-treated rat MSCs miRNA microarray. All of the miRNA array raw data are available in the online supplemental Table (n = 5 independent experiments). (**B**): Microarray data are summarized by volcano plot graph, which displays both fold-change and t-test criteria (log odds). MiR-377 and miR-210 are the most significantly dysregulated miRs in hypoxia-treated rat MSCs compared to normoxia-treated MSCs (the green stands for down-regulation, and the red stands for upregulation). (**C**): Alterations in expression levels of miR-377 was validated by qPCR (normalized to control U6, n = 5, p<0.05).

have been profiled in endothelial cells (ECs) and cancer cells. For example, Kulshreshtha, *et al.* [14] identified that a set of miRs were consistently up-regulated in breast tumor and colon cancer cells in response to hypoxia. In addition, Fasanaro, *et al.* [15] first reported that hypoxia-driven miR-210 promotes angiogenic response in ECs by down-regulation of EFNA3, an ephrin family member involving vascular development. Recent studies also indicate that a panel of miRNAs (i.e., miR-10, miR-15b, miR-16, miR-20a, miR-20b, miR-27a, miR-126, miR-145, miR-195, miR-205, and miR-210) is involved in the regulation of VEGF expression in ECs and tumor cells [16–26]. Few studies however,

have examined how hypoxia affects the miR expression profile in MSCs. In addition to further investigation of this process, a significant additional question for examination is whether hypoxia-associated miRs regulate MSC-induced myocardial angiogenesis in ischemic hearts.

In this study, we first sought to determine the alterations of miRs in MSCs under hypoxic conditions in rats. We then identified which hypoxia-inducible miRs could directly regulate VEGF expression and tested whether manipulation of such miR in MSCs could affect MSC-induced angiogenesis in ischemic myocardium. Our results show for the first time that miR-377

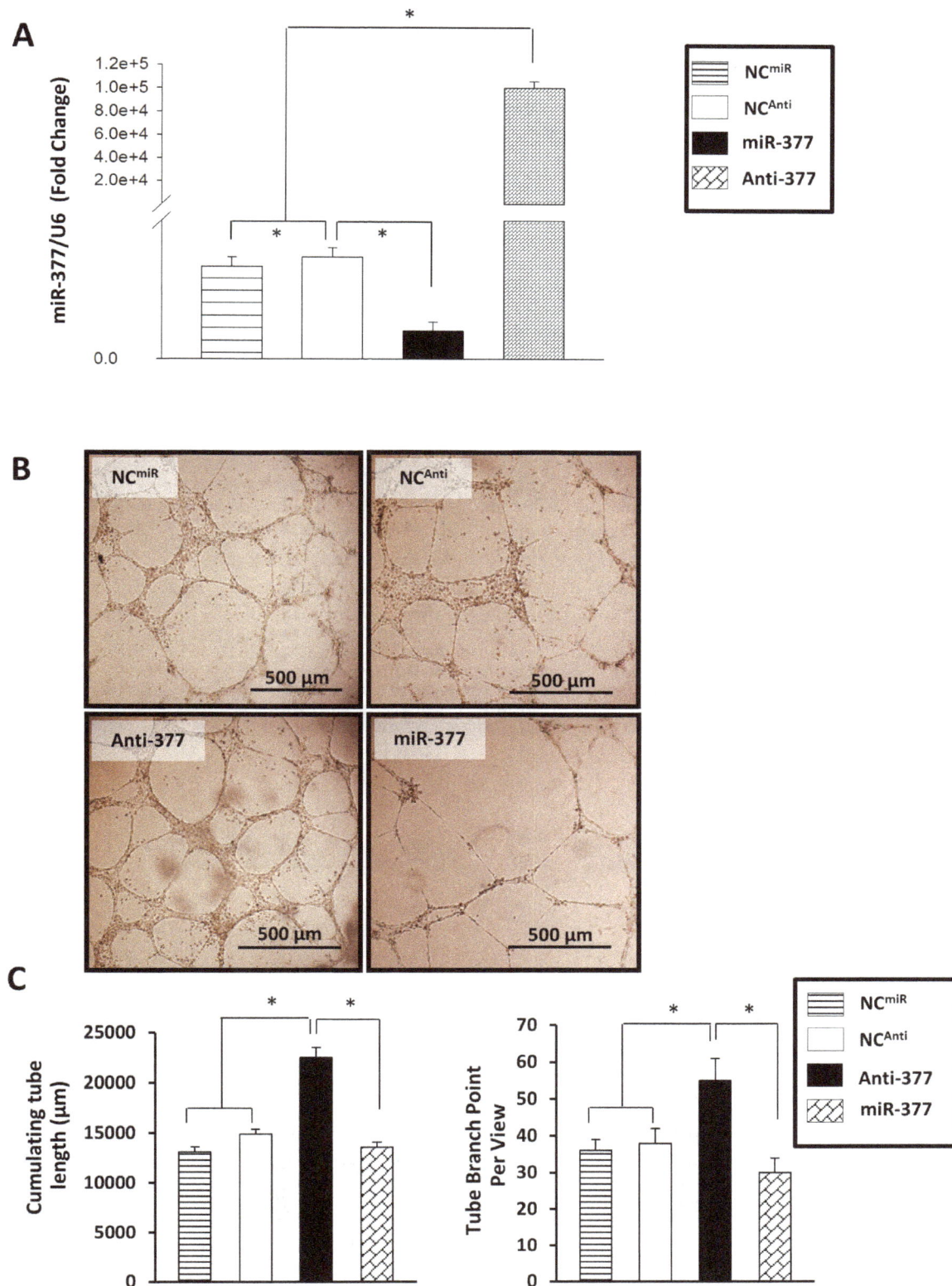

Figure 2. Suppression of miR-377 induced *in vitro* formation of capillary-like structures. (**A**): qPCR analysis after normalization against U6 verified the knockdown of endogenous miR-377 (Anti-377) and overexpression of miR-377 (miR-377) into HUVECs transfected with either miR-377 inhibitor or mimic. (**B**): *In vitro* tube formation assay indicated that knockdown of miR-377 enhanced the formation of capillary-like structures, but this effect was limited by miR-377 overexpression. Scale bars = 500 µm. (**C**): Total capillary tube lengths and tube branch points were measured by analytical software Image-Pro Plus 6.0 (IPP). All values were expressed as means ± SE; n = 6 independent experiments for each group; *P<0.05.

was strongly down-regulated in hypoxia-treated MSCs, which was a major factor contributing to the increased VEGF levels. Thus, injection of miR-377-knockdown MSCs into an infarcted myocardium reduced overall infarction size and improved contractile function by promoting angiogenesis. These findings suggest that miR-377 may serve as a novel potential therapeutic target for treatment of ischemic heart diseases.

Materials and Methods

Animal Experiments

All research protocols conformed to the Guidelines for the Care and Use of Laboratory Animals published by the National Institutes of Health (National Academies Press, 8th edition, 2011). All animal use protocols and methods of euthanasia (pentobarbital overdose followed by thoracotomy) used in this study were approved by the University of Cincinnati Animal Care and Use Committee. The Institutional Biosafety Committee (IBC)

conducted an independent review and approval of our cell and virus methods.

In Vitro Studies

In order to culture MSCs, they were extracted from Sprague-Dawley (SD; 8-wk-old male) rats following previously published procedures from our laboratory [9]. MSCs were then cultured in Dulbecco's Modified Eagle Medium(DMEM) supplemented with 10% (v/v) fetal bovine serum (FBS) and antibiotics (100 U/mL penicillin and 100 μg/mL streptomycin). The cells were kept in a humidified 5% CO_2 incubator at 37°C and culture medium was changed after 3 days. Non-adherent cells were removed by changing the medium and the remaining adherent cells were primary MSCs. Passage 2–4 MSCs were used in this study.

Hypoxic MSCs were cultured in DMEM without glucose and with 1% FBS under hypoxic conditions of 1% O_2, 5% CO_2 and 94% N_2 at 37°C in a hypoxic incubator (O_2/CO_2 incubator-

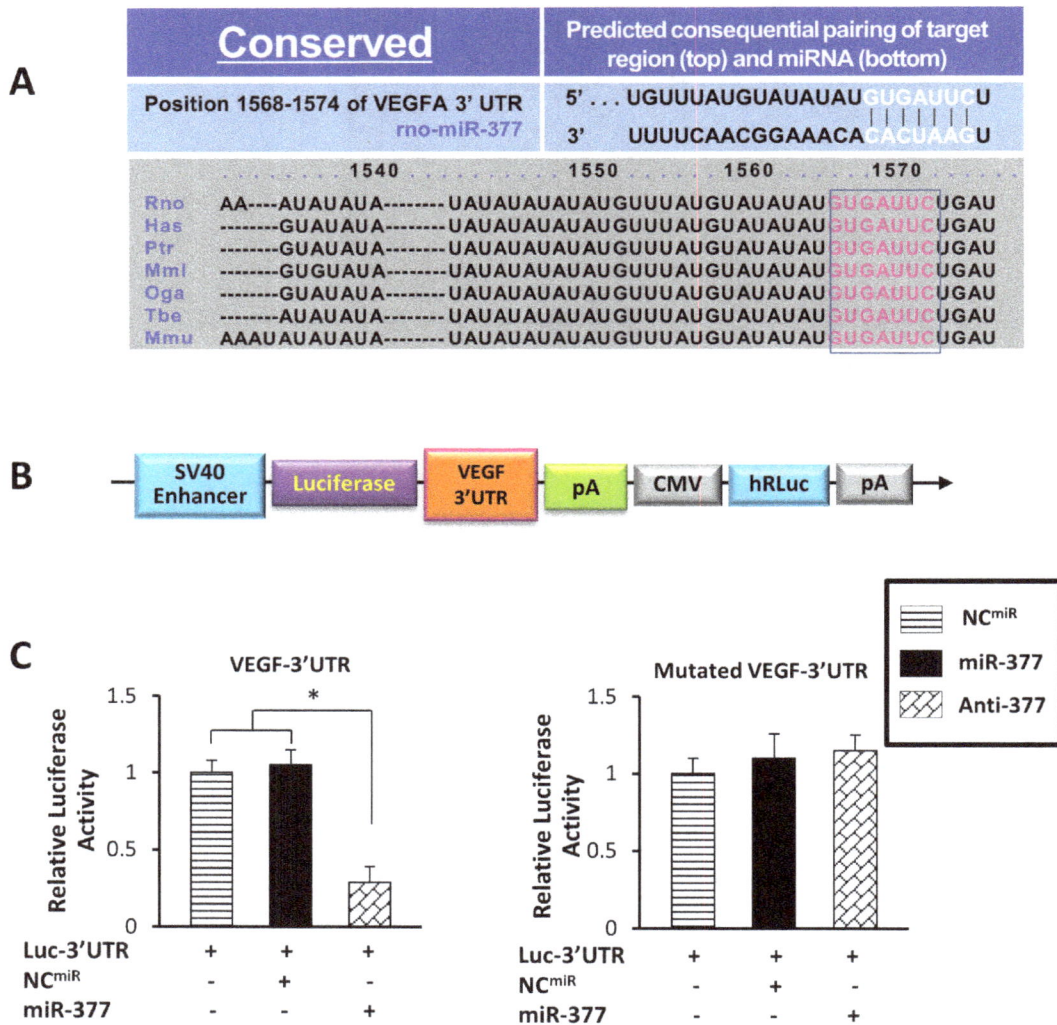

Figure 3. Dual-luciferase reporter assay validates that miR-377 directly targets VEGF. (A): Computational miRNA target prediction analysis coincidentally reveals that the fragment 5'-GAAUCAC-3' of miRNA-377 pairs well with the fragment 5'-GUGAUUC-3' located at the 1568–1574 nt of VEGF 3' UTR, which is a highly conserved site (red fonts) in most of mammals (e.g. rat, human, chimpanzee, rhesus, bushbaby, treeshrew, mouse). **(B):** Schematic diagram of Dual-Luciferase reporter vector (pEZX-MT01) carrying the VEGF3' UTR. **(C):** Quantitative data for dual-luciferase reporter assay results. All values were expressed as means ± SE; n = 6 for each group. *P<0.05 was considered statistically significant.

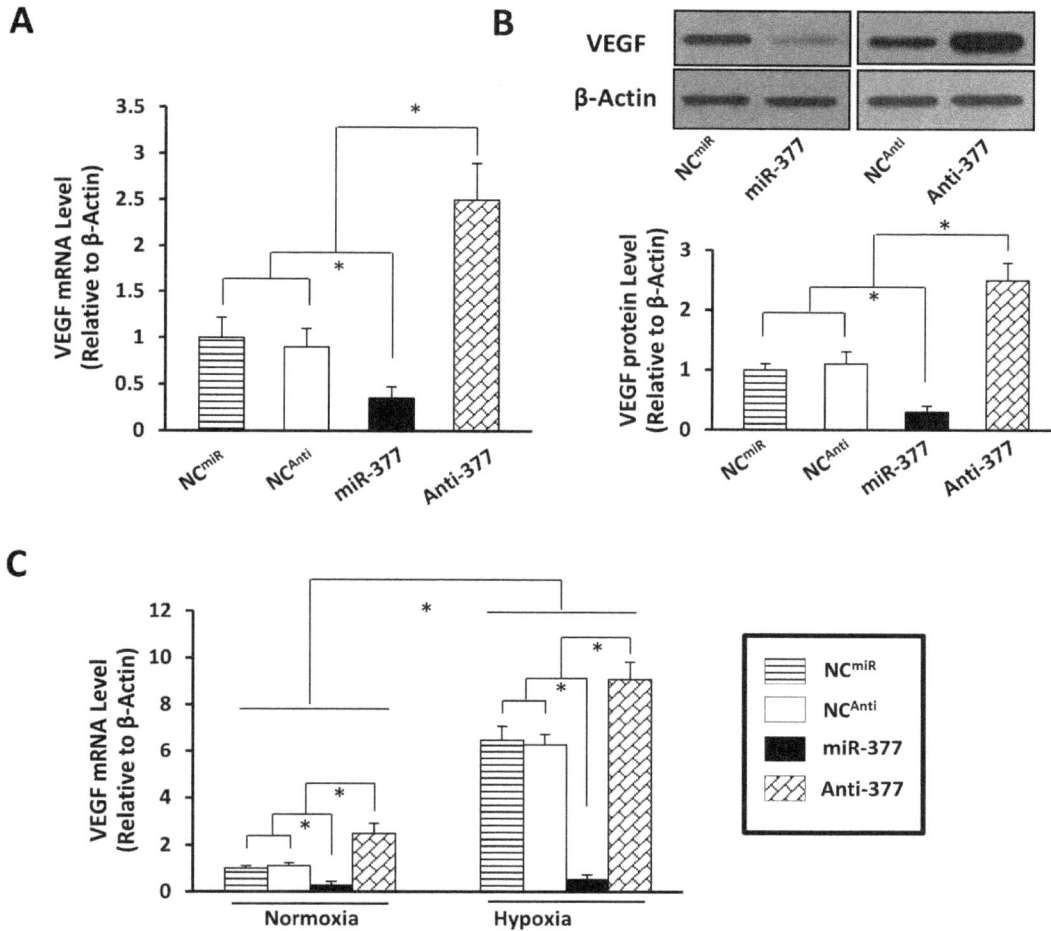

Figure 4. miR-377 directly down regulates the expression of VRGF in MSCs. (A): qPCR analysis after normalization against β-actin showed that miR-377 mimic (miR-377) downregulated VEGF mRNA in MSCs, while miR-377 inhibitor (Anti-377) upregulated VEGF mRNA in MSCs. MSCs transfected with a scrambled sequence according to miR-377 mimic and miR-377 inhibitor as negative control (NC^{miR} and NC^{Anti} respectively). **(B)**: Western blot assay showed protein level changes of VEGF in MSCs induced by miR-377 mimic (miR-377) and miR-377 inhibitor (Anti-377) as well as its quantitative data. All values were expressed as means ± SE; n = 8 for each group; *P<0.05 was considered statistically significant. **(C)**: qPCR analysis after normalization against β-actin showed significant up-regulation of VEGF in hypoxia-treated MSCs in comparison with normoxia-treated MSCs, which was further increased in MSC$^{Anti-377}$, when compared with NC group and miR-377 groups. All values were expressed as means ± SE; n = 8 for each group. *P<0.05 was considered statistically significant.

MCO-18M; Sanyo) for 24 h. MSCs cultured in normal conditions (normoxia) served as a control.

RNA Extraction and RT-PCR

Total RNA from the MSCs was extracted using the Trizol reagent (Invitrogen, Carlsbad, Calif., United States), as recommended by the manufacturer. Total RNA concentrations were determined by NanoVue plus (GE Healthcore, Piscataway, New Jersey, USA). The mRNA levels of VEGF and miRs were examined by reverse transcription-polymerase chain reaction (RT-PCR) or quantitative real-time PCR (qPCR), and β-Actin or U6 was used as an internal reference. The primers for VEGF and β-Actin were designed as follows: **VEGF** forward: 5′-GCAACAC-CAAGTCCGAATGCAGAT-3′, reverse: 5′-TCTGGCTTCA-CAGCACTCTCCTTT-3′; **β-Actin** forward: 5′-TGTGATGGTGGGAAT GGGTCAGAA-3′, reverse: 5′-TGTGGTGCCAGATCTTCTCCATGT-3′. The primers for miRNA and U6 were purchased from QIAGEN. The primers for miRs consisted of a specific primer (Rn_miR-377_2 miScript

Primer Assay) and a universal primer (10× miScript Universal Primer). The amplification profiles for PCR: 94°C 5 min., followed by 30 cycles of 94°C 30 sec., 55°C 30 sec., 72°C 45 sec., and a final 5 min. extend; and for qPCR: 95°C 15 min., followed by 40 cycles of 94°C 15 sec., 55°C 30 sec., 72°C 30 sec. with 0.5°C/15 sec. in 55°C~95°C. PCR products were analyzed with 1.5% agarose gel. The qPCR expression of VEGF mRNA relative to β-Actin under experimental and control conditions was calculated based on the threshold cycle (Ct) as n = $2^{-\Delta\ (\Delta Ct)}$, where $\Delta Ct = Ct\ _{VEGF} - Ct\ _{\beta-Actin}$ and $\Delta\ (\Delta Ct) = \Delta Ct$ experimental $-$ ΔCt control. Individual experiments were repeated at least 3 times, and the n-mean value was calculated.

Western-Blotting Analysis

Protein samples were collected from MSCs treated under different conditions, and 60 μg of protein was loaded and subjected to SDS-PAGE, as described previously [6]. PageRuler^{TM} Plus Prestained Protein Ladder (Thermo Scientific Inc., MA, USA) was loaded as a protein marker to estimate molecular

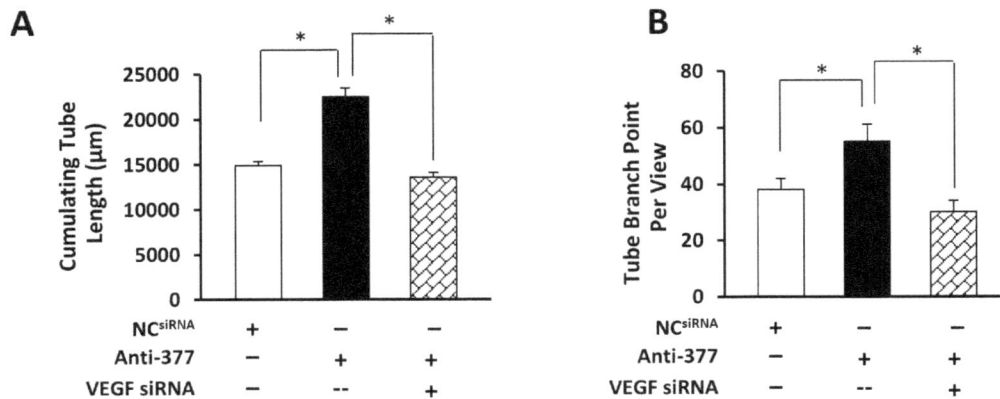

Figure 5. Pro-angiogenic effects elicited by knockdown of miR-377 are largely dependent on VEGF. *In vitro* Tube Formation Assay showed that total capillary tube lengths (**A**) and tube branch points (**B**) were significantly reduced by the VEGF siRNA transfection in miR-377-knockdown HUVECs. All values were expressed as means ± SE; n = 6 for each group; $^{*}P<0.05$ was considered statistically significant.

weight of samples. A VEGF antibody (Rabbit, 1:500) was purchased from Santa Cruz Biotechnology. β-Actin (mouse 1:1000) was purchased from Santa Cruz Biotechnology.

miRNA Array Analysis and Target Prediction

Total RNA samples obtained from MSCs under normoxia or hypoxia were sent to LC Sciences (Houston, TX) for miRNA microarray profiling. Data was analyzed by LC Sciences with in-house developed computer programs. Intensity values were transformed into log2 scale, and fold changes were given in log2 scale. A *t*-test was performed between normoxic MSCs and hypoxic MSCs, and statistical significance was considered at $P<0.01$. The microarray data were confirmed using an miRNA detection protocol with RT^2 miRNA First Strand Kit (SA biosciences). Computational miRNA target prediction analysis was performed with TargetScan (version 6.2) and miRDB to predict potential binding between VEGF 3'UTR and miRNA.

Transient Transfection of MSCs with miRNA Mimic, miRNA Inhibitor or siRNA

miR-377 mimic and its negative control (NC) (miRIDIAN Mimic, Thermo Scientific), miR-377 inhibitor and its negative control (miRCURY LNA microRNA inhibitor, Exiqon), VEGF siRNA and its negative control(ON-TARGET plus SMARTpool, rat VEGF-A, Thermo Scientific) were assigned into 6 groups for transfection as follows: **A**. miR-377 mimic (miR-377); **B**. Negative control (NC)-miR-377-mimic (NC^{miR}); **C**. miR-377 inhibitor (Anti-377); **D**. NC-miR-377-inhibitor (NC$^{Anti-377}$); **E**. VEGF siRNA; **F**. NC-VEGF siRNA (NC^{siRNA}). MSCs were seeded (2.5×10^5) in 6-well plates 24 hours prior to transfection. The NC^{miR}, miR-377, Anti-377, NC$^{Anti-377}$ and VEGF siRNA were added at the final concentration (100 nM for each well) after mixing with DharmaFECT Duo Transfection Reagent (Thermo Scientific) according to the manufacturer's instructions. 48 hours after transfection, the cells of each group were harvested, followed by PCR and Western blot analysis.

Dual-Luciferase Reporter Assay

Rat VEGF 3'-UTR (nt1660–3545) was inserted into the Dual-Luciferase reporter vector (pEZX-MT01, Genecopoeia Corp. MD, USA) downstream from the Firefly luciferase (hLuc) reporter gene, and was driven by SV40 Enhancer promoter. In addition, Renilla luciferase (hRLuc) reporter driven by a CMV promoter

was cloned into the same vector, serving as the tracking gene and internal control. The dual-reporter vector system enabled transfection-normalization for accurate across-sample comparison. The 293TN cells were assigned into three groups to be transfected with **A**. pEZX-MT01 vector; **B**. pEZX-MT01 vector+NC-miR-377 mimic; **C**. pEZX-MT01 vector+miR-377 mimic. Cell lysates were collected and assayed 48 hours after transfection. Firefly and Renilla luciferase activities were measured using a Dual Luciferase Reporter Assay System kit (Promega Corp. WI, USA) and each transfected well was assayed in triplicate as described [27]. The mutated pEZX-MT01 plasmid containing the mutated VEGF-3'UTR with mutation in the seed region was synthesized using Phusion^{TM} site-directed mutagenesis kit (New England Biolabs. MA, USA) with the following primer, mutated VEGF 3'UTR forward primer 5'-AAGGATAAAATAGACATTGC-TATTCTG-3'; reverse primer 5'-AGACTATATACATAAACA-TATATATATATATATACAC-3'.

In Vitro Tube Formation Assay

HUVECs were purchased from American Type Culture Collection (ATCC) and cultured in endothelial cell growth medium (Cell Application). HUVECs were transiently transfected with **A**. negative control (NC^{miR}/NC^{Anti}); **B**. miR-377 mimic; **C**. miR-377 inhibitor; **D**. miR-377 inhibitor+VEGF siRNA. After 48 h, *in vitro* tube formation assay was performed with a tube formation assay kit (Chemicon), per the manufacturer's instructions. Briefly, ECMatrix Solution was thawed on ice for 1~2 hours, then was mixed with 10×ECMatrixdilutent (v: v = 9:1). The mix was added to a 96-well tissue culture plate (50 µl/well) and was placed at 37°C for 1 hour to allow the matrix solution to solidify. HUVECs were digested by 0.125% trypsin and were placed (1×10^4 cells/well) on top of the solidified matrix solution and incubated at 37°C for 18 hours. Cellular network structures were fully developed and photos were taken using an inverted light microscope at 40× magnification. Total capillary tube length and tube branch points were measured using analytical software Image-Pro Plus 6.0 (IPP, Media Cybernetics, Carlsbad, CA). Tube formation was defined as a structure exhibiting a length four times its width. Five independent fields were assessed for each well, and the average number of tubes was calculated [28].

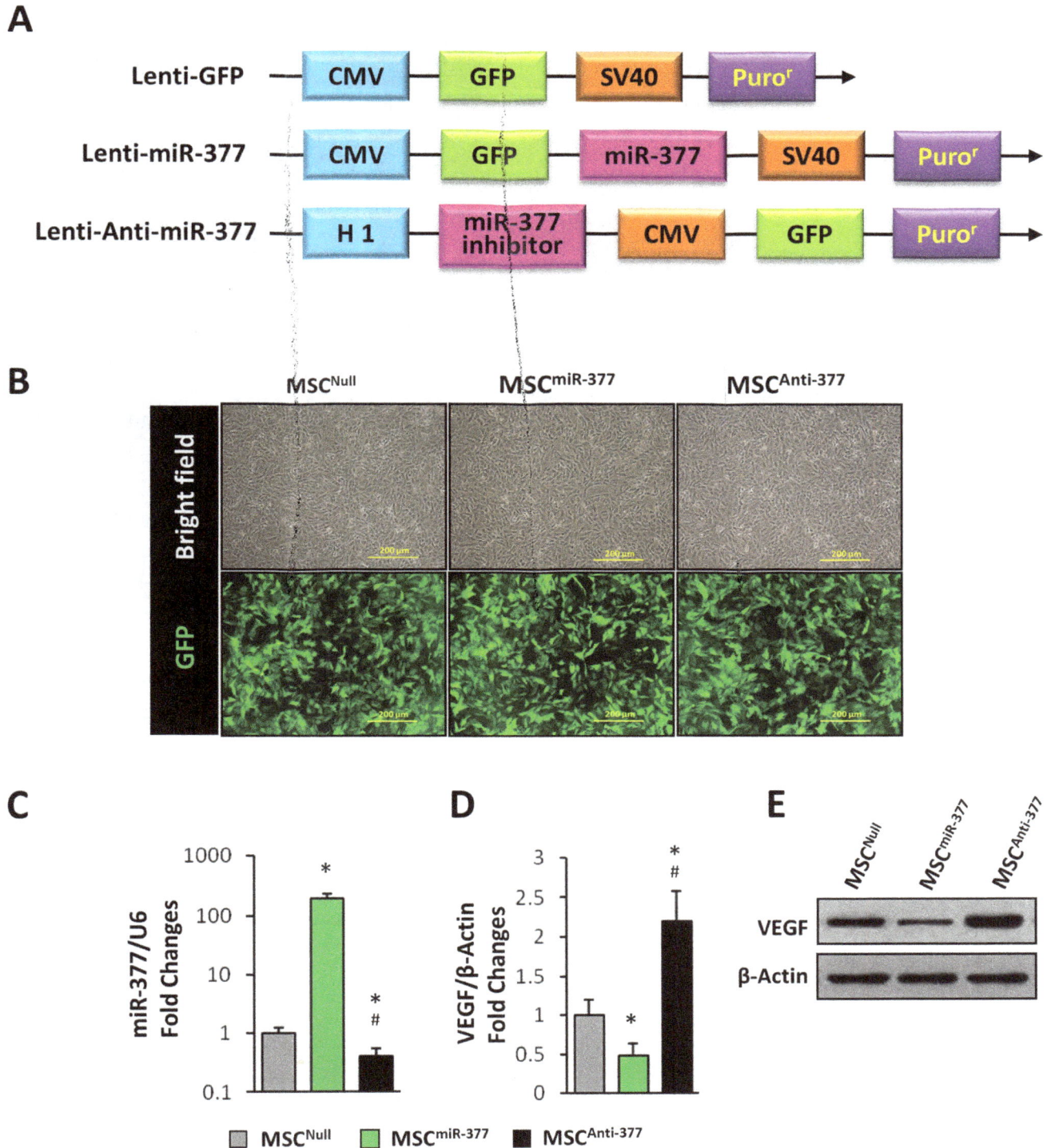

Figure 6. Engineering rat MSCs with lentiviral vectors to overexpress or knockdown of miR-377. (**A**): Schematic diagram of recombinant lentiviral vectors. Lenti-GFP, lentiviral empty vector; Lenti-miR-377, lentiviral miR-377 overexpressing vector; Lenti-Anti-miR-377, lentiviral miR-377 inhibitor expression vector. (**B**): Nearly 100% of MSCs were transfected with Lenti-GFP (MSC^{Null}), Lenti-miR-377 (MSC$^{miR-377}$) or Lenti-Off-miR-377 (MSC$^{Anti-377}$) after 72-hour lentiviral infection, as indicated by GFP fluorescence. No morphological changes were found among MSC^{Null}, MSC$^{miR-377}$, and MSC$^{Anti-377}$. Scale bars = 200 μm. (**C**): qPCR analysis after normalization against U6 showed that the knockdown of miR-377 in MSC$^{Anti-377}$ and the overexpression of miR-377 in MSC$^{miR-377}$. (**D**): qPCR analysis after normalization against β-Actin. (**E**): Western-blot consistently showed that the expression of VEGF was reduced in MSC$^{miR-377}$ while increased in MSC$^{Anti-377}$, compared with that in MSC^{Null}. All values were expressed as means ± SE; n = 6 for each group; $^{*}P<0.05$ vs. MSC^{Null}; $^{#}P<0.05$ vs. MSC$^{miR-377}$.

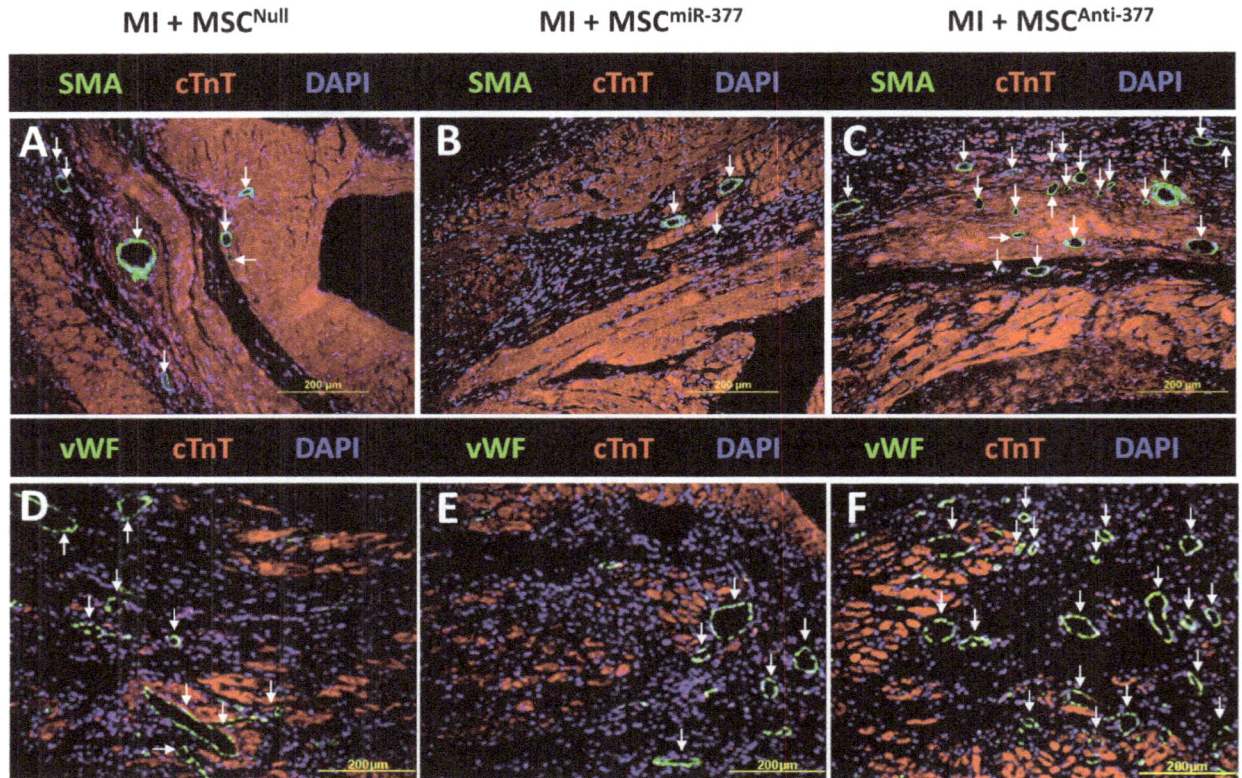

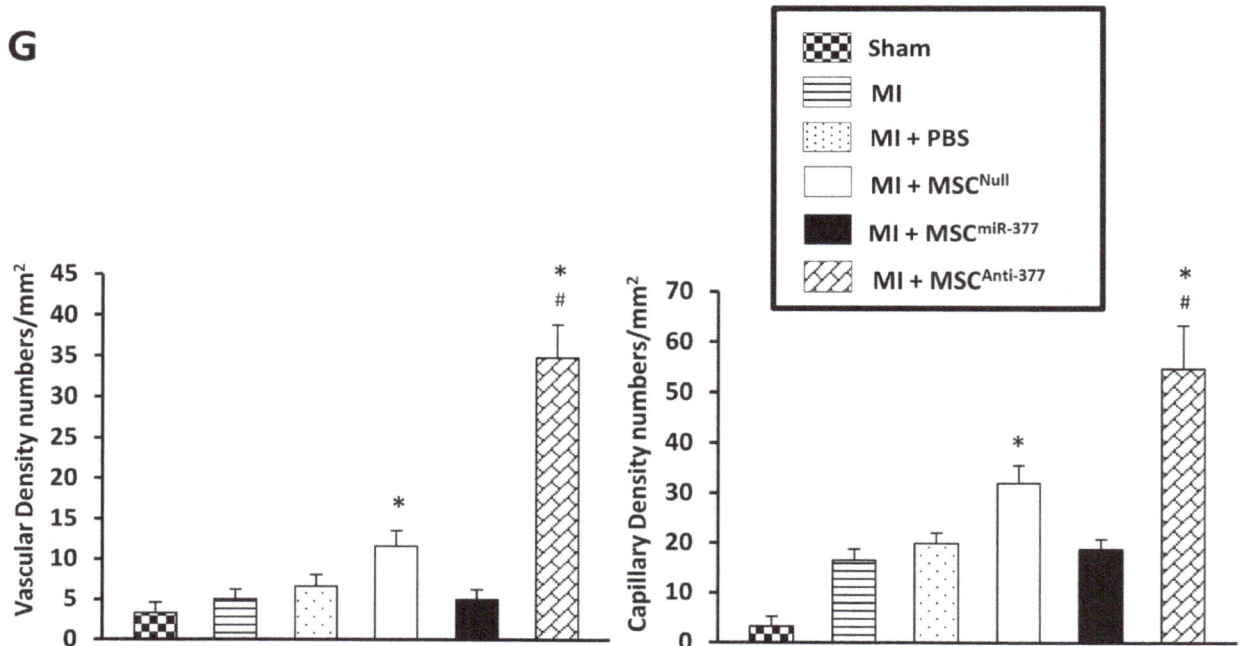

Figure 7. Knockdown of endogenous miR-377 enhances MSC-mediated myocardial angiogenesis in vivo. (**A**): Slice sections of heart samples, collected from MI rats 4 weeks after the injection of miR-engineered MSCs, were triple-stained with troponin I (cTnT) antibody (Ab) (for cardiomyocytes, red), α-smooth muscle actin (SMA) Ab (for vascular cells, green; white arrows) and DAPI (for nuclei, blue). Vascular density was measured in (A) MSC^Null group, (**B**) MSC^miR-377 group, and (**C**) MSC^Anti-377 group. Capillary density was identified by Von Willebrand (vWF) staining (green; white arrows) in (**D**) MSC^Null group, (**E**) MSC^miR-377 group and (**F**) MSC^Anti-377 group. IPP software was used to quantitatively analyze (**G**) vascular density, and capillary density in different treatment groups. All values were expressed as means ± SE; n = 6 for each group. *P<0.05 vs. MI; # P<0.05 vs. MI+MSC^Null.

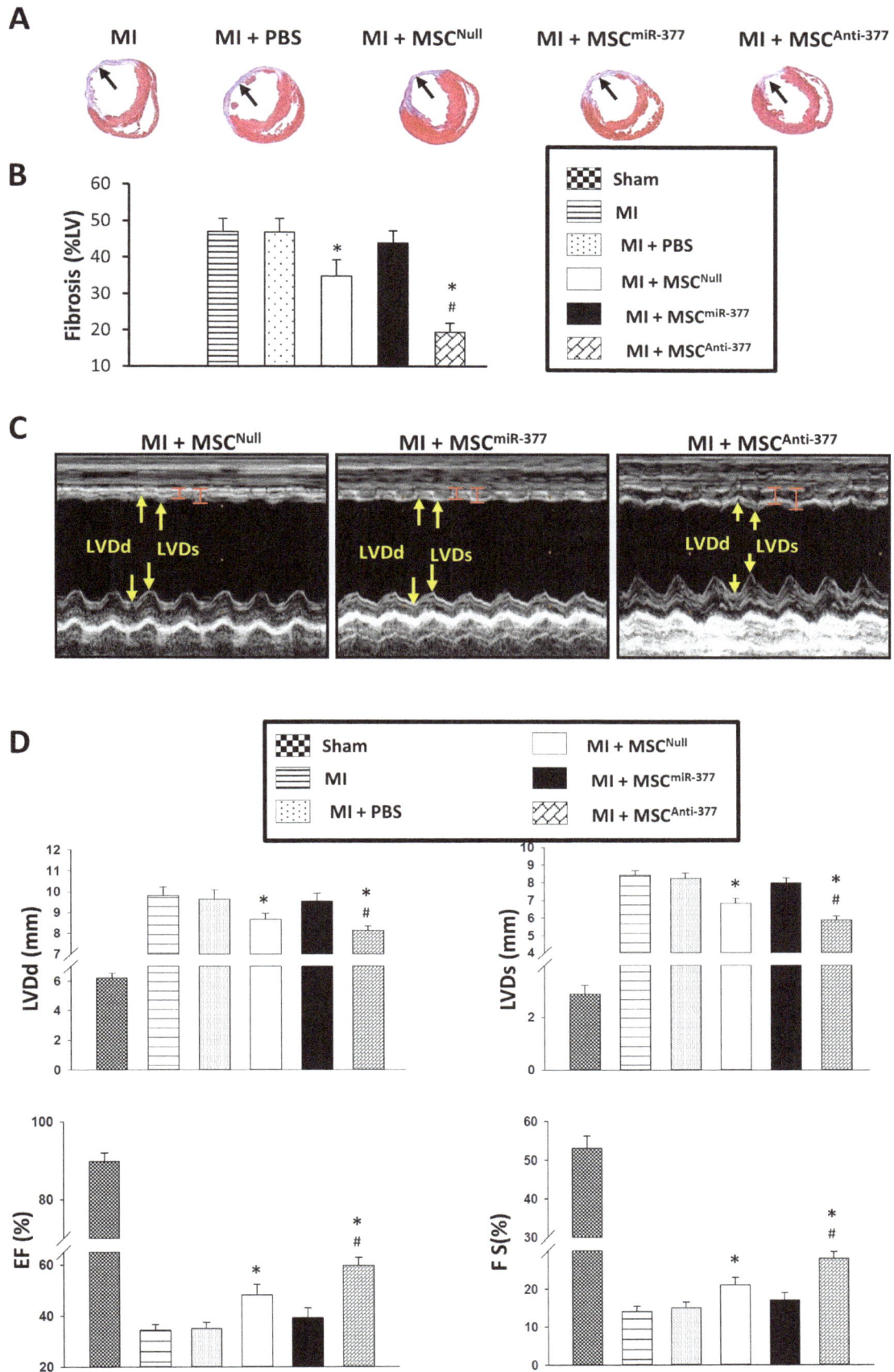

Figure 8. Injection of miR-377-knockdown MSCs into the rat infarcted hearts limits fibrosis and improves cardiac functions. (A): 5-μm sections of heart slices, collected from MI rats 4 weeks after the injection of miR-engineered MSCs, were stained with Masson-Trichome. **(B)**: Percentage of fibrosis in left ventricle (LV) in various treatments determined with Image J software. All values were expressed as means ± SE; n = 6 for each group. *P<0.05 was considered statistically significant. **(C)**: The LV end-diastolic diameters (LVDd, yellow arrow) and LV end-systolic diameters (LVDs, yellow arrow) in MSC^{Null} group, MSC$^{miR-377}$ group and MSC$^{Anti-377}$ group were measured using echocardiographic M-mode recordings. All echocardiographic measurements were averaged from at least 3 separate cardiac cycles. **(D)**: Quantitative data of LVDd, LVDs, LV ejection fraction (EF) and fractional shortening (FS) were analyzed and compared among various groups. All values were expressed as means ± SE; n = 6 for each group. *P<0.05 vs. MI; #P<0.05 vs. MI+MSC^{Null}.

Lentiviral Overexpression and Suppression of miR-377

Lentiviral vectors (pEZX-MR03) for overexpression and suppression of miR-377 (Null, miR-377, and Anti-377) were purchased from Genecopoeia Corp. (MD, USA) and Applied Biological Materials Inc. (ABM, MC, Canada). Lentiviral particles were produced via transfection of the lentiviral vectors into 293T cells per manufacturer's protocol.

In Vivo Studies

SD rats (200–250 g) were randomly divided into the following groups to evaluate the direct effects of miR-377 on angiogenesis of MI model: 1.) Sham operated rats had a loose suture placed around the left anterior descending (LAD) coronary artery (Sham group); 2.) Myocardial infarction alone created by LAD ligation (MI group); 3.) MI plus PBS treatment (MI+PBS group); 4.) MI plus MSC^{Null} transplantation (MI+MSC^{Null} group); 5.) MI plus MSC$^{miR-377}$ transplantation (MI+MSC$^{miR-377}$ group); 6.) MI plus MSC$^{Anti-377}$ (MI+MSC$^{Anti-377}$ group).

Surgical Procedures for the LAD Occlusion and MSC Implantation

An MI model was developed in SD rats (200–250 g), as described previously [29]. Briefly, isofluorane anesthesia was induced by spontaneous inhalation. The animals were mechanically ventilated with room air supplemented with oxygen (1.5 L/min) using a rodent ventilator (Model 683; Harvard Apparatus, South Natick, MA). Body temperature was carefully monitored with a probe (Cole Parmer Instrument, Vernon Hill, IL) and was maintained at 37°C throughout the surgical procedure. The heart was exposed by left side limited thoracotomy, and the left anterior descending coronary artery (LAD) was ligated with a 6-0 polyester suture 1 mm from the tip of the normally positioned left auricle. MSCs (30 μl, 2×10^6) were injected into border area of the left ventricle (LV) wall at 10 minutes after LAD ligation. The chest was closed with 5-0 silk sutures. Approximately 10% of rats succumbed during surgical procedures.

Immunohistochemical Analysis

Immunohistochemical studies were performed on heart tissue at 4 weeks after cell implantation. Heart tissue sections were harvested, fixed in 10% Formalin, and sectioned at 5-μm thickness. The cardiac troponin T (cTnT) antibody (Thermo Scientific) was used to identify cardiomyocytes, while 4′, 6-diamino-2-phenyindole (DAPI, Sigma) was used to identify nuclei. Von Willebrand Factor (vWF, DAKO, Agilent Technologies) rabbit polyclonal antibody (Santa Cruz Biotechnology) and α-smooth muscle actin (SMA) mouse monoclonal antibody (Sigma) were used to assess capillary and vascular density. Fluorescence labeled secondary antibodies (Jackson Immuno Research Laboratories or Molecular Probes) were used following these primary antibodies. Fluorescent imaging was performed with an Olympus BX41 microscope (Olympus America Inc., Melville, NY, U.S.A.) equipped with epiflourescence attachment, and images were recorded using a digital camera with MagnaFire 2.1 software.

Measurement of Infarct Size

Fixed hearts were embedded in paraffin, and sections from apex, mid-LV, and base were stained with Masson's Trichrome. An Olympus BX41 camera was used to obtain images of LV area on each slide using MagnaFire (Olympus) software. Fibrosis and total LV area of each image were measured using Image J software, and the percentage of the fibrotic area was calculated as shown: (fibrosis area/total LV area) ×100, as previously described [9].

Assessment of Heart Function

Heart function was assessed by transthoracic echocardiography, which was performed at 4 weeks after MI using iE33 Ultrasound System (Phillips) with a 15-MHz probe. After rats were anesthetized with pentobarbital sodium (40 mg/kg) by intraperitoneal injection, hearts were imaged two-dimensionally in long-axis view at the level of the greatest LV diameter. This view was used to position the M-mode cursor perpendicular to the LV anterior and posterior walls. The LV end-diastolic diameters (LVDd) and LV end-systolic diameters (LVDs) were measured from M-mode recordings according to the leading-edge method. LV parameters were obtained from two-dimensional images. LV ejection fraction (EF) was calculated as: EF (%) = [(LVDd)^3-(LVDs)^3]/(LVDd)^3×100. Fractional shortening (FS) was measured using the equation FS (%) = [(LVDd − LVDs)/LVDd] ×100. All echocardiographic measurements were averaged from at least three separate cardiac cycles.

Statistical Analysis

Experiments were performed in quadruplicate and repeated at least three times. Data are expressed as means ± SE. Statistical significance was assessed by one-way ANOVA followed by Bonferroni/Dunn testing. P<0.05 was considered statistically significant.

Results

miRNAs Profiling in Rat MSCs under Hypoxia and Normoxia

miR microarray analysis was used to examine the potential mechanisms underlying MSC-induced myocardial angiogenesis in response to hypoxia. Among 679 miR probes, a total of 48 miRs were identified that were differentially expressed in hypoxia-treated MSCs as compared to normoxia-treated samples (n = 5, p<0.01, Fig. 1A). When the signal density of miRs was cut off by a value of 100, a group of 13 miRs were significantly up-regulated including miR-210, -25, -450a, -130a, -3593-3p, -34c*, -214, -181a, -23b, -34a, -31, -31*, and -140*; whereas 20 miRs (miR-377, -146a, -222, -652*, -466b-1*, -664-1*, -196c*, -466c*, -29c, -32*, -195, -466b, -188, -146b, -92a, let-7b, -466b-2*, -466d, -485*, and -181c) were significantly down-regulated in MSCs under hypoxic conditions. miR-210 was the most significantly increased miR in hypoxia-treated MSCs (Fig. 1B), a finding consistent with previous observations in tumor cells, endothelial cells, and cardiomyocytes in responsive to hypoxia [15], [30], [31]. miR-377 was the most down-regulated in MSCs upon hypoxia treatment (Fig. 1B). This finding was further validated by real-time stem-loop PCR (Fig. 1C). While miR-210 is well recognized to have pro-angiogenic property *in vivo* and *in vitro* [15], [17], it is unknown whether hypoxia-responsive miR-377 also regulates angiogenesis. Moreover, it is also unknown whether alteration of miR-377 expression affects MSC-induced angiogenesis in ischemic myocardial tissue. Therefore, determination of the role of miR-377 in myocardial angiogenesis and its associated mechanisms could be of major significance for techniques aimed at regeneration of heart tissue.

Reduced Expression of miR-377 in HUVECs Promotes Angiogenesis

HUVECs were transfected with either miR mimic to overexpress miR-377 or miR inhibitor to specifically knockdown miR-377 (Fig. 2A) in order to determine the significance of miR-377 in angiogenesis, followed by an *in vitro* tube-formation assay using Matrigel-precoated wells. HUVECs transfected with either negative control miR mimic (NC^{miR}) or negative control miR inhibitor (NC^{Anti}) was used as negative control groups. The negative control (NC^{miR} and NC^{Anti}) groups exhibited some tube-like shapes and half-full cellular networks, while the miR-377 mimic group (miR-377 group) revealed less tube-like structures and hardly formed cellular networks (Fig. 2B). However, the miR-377 inhibitor group (Anti-377 group) displayed the formation of full and dense cellular networks (Fig. 2B). The cumulative capillary tube length, measured using IPP software, was reduced by 40±6% in miR-377-HUVECs, whereas it was increased by 54±5% in Anti-377 cells when compared to negative controls (NC^{Anti}) (Fig. 2C). No significance was observed between NC^{miR} group and NC^{Anti} group. In addition, the number of tube branch point in miR-377 group (19.5±2.2) was less than that of negative controls (NC^{miR}36.0±2.9; NC^{Anti}38.0±3.0 respectively), and was significantly increased in Anti-377 group (55.0±3.5) (Fig. 2C).

MiR-377 Acts Directly at the 3′UTR of VEGF

Computational miRNA target prediction analysis was performed to elucidate the potential mechanism of miR-377 in the regulation of angiogenesis, using TargetScan and miRDB. VEGF-A (usually referred to as VEGF) is listed among the top of assumed targets for rno-miR-377 and the seed sequence of VEGF 3′UTR interacting with rno-miR-377 is highly conserved among the species of rat, human, chimpanzee, rhesus, bushbaby, treeshrew, and mouse (Fig. 3A). HEK293TN cells were transfected with a Dual-Luciferase reporter vector containing the 3′-UTR of VEGF or mutated 3′-UTR of VEGF fused downstream to the Luciferase coding sequence (Fig. 3B) along with miR-377 mimic or a NC (NC^{miR}) to validate whether miR-377 directly recognizes the 3′UTR of VEGF. Luciferase activity was repressed by 67% when miR-377 was co-expressed with the VEGF-3′-UTR luciferase reporter vector (Fig. 3C), whereas luciferase activity of mutated VEGF-3′-UTR was not affected. In contrast, transfection with NC did not affect the activity of luciferase.

MiR-377 Negatively Regulates VEGF Expression in MSCs and ECs

MSCs were harvested 48 hours after transfection with either NC-miR (NC^{miR}), NC-Inhibitor (NC^{Anti}), miR-377 mimic (miR-377), or miR-377 inhibitor (Anti-377) to ascertain if miR-377 modulates VEGF expression. Elevation of miR-377 in MSCs suppressed VEGF expression at both mRNA and protein levels (by

~70%) in Fig. 4A and 4B, which conversely were upregulated by ~2.5-fold in miR-377-knockdown MSCs (Anti-377) (Fig. 4Aand 4B). In addition, we observed that VEGF was significantly increased in normoxia-treated Anti-377 group as compared with other groups, which further increased in hypoxia-treated Anti-377 group (Fig. 4C). This was well correlative with the reduced expression of miR-377 (Fig. 1C).

Negative Effects of miR-377 in Angiogenesis are Largely Dependent on VEGF

It is important to determine whether miR-377 reduction-caused angiogenesis is dependent on VEGF given that VEGF is a target for miR-377. The expression of VEGF was knocked down in miR-377-reduced HUVECs by siRNA, followed by *in vitro* tube formation assay. Similar to previous findings (Fig. 2), it was observed that miR-377-inhibitor-transfected HUVECs had well-developed networks of capillary-like tubes, evidenced by a 1.5-fold increase of cumulative tube length and 1.45- fold increase of tube branch points, compared with NC^{miR} cells. In contrast, HUVECs co-transfected with miR-377 inhibitor+VEGF siRNA exhibited sparse capillary-like structures in which the tube length and the number of tube branch points are similar to NC group (Fig. 5A and 5B). These results indicate that enhanced effects in the formation of tube-like structures induced by knockdown of miR-377 were abolished by inhibition of VEGF expression.

Suppression of miR-377 in MSCs Enhances Angiogenesis in Ischemic Hearts

Rat MSCs were genetically engineered to overexpress or suppress miR-377 using lentiviral transduction (Fig. 6A) to investigate the functional significance of miR-377 in MSC-induced angiogenesis in ischemic hearts. Nearly 100% of MSCs were infected with Lenti-GFP (MSC^{Null}), Lenti-miR-377 (MSC$^{miR-377}$), or Lenti-Off-miR-377 (MSC$^{Anti-377}$) after 72-hour transduction, as indicated by GFP fluorescence (Fig. 6B). qPCR confirmed that MSC$^{Anti-377}$ exhibited lower levels of miR-377, whereas MSC$^{miR-377}$ exhibited significantly higher levels of miR-377 than MSC^{Null} (Fig. 6C). Accordingly, qPCR (Fig. 6D) and Western blot (Fig. 6E) showed that VEGF expression was significantly reduced in MSC$^{miR-377}$ when compared with MSC^{Null}, whereas it was significantly increased in the MSC$^{Anti-377}$ group. 2×10^6 MSC^{Null}, MSC$^{miR-377}$, or MSC$^{Anti-377}$ was then injected into the border zone of ischemic left ventricular (LV) wall at 10 min. after LAD ligation. 4 weeks later, myocardial vascular density was evaluated by α-SMA immunofluorescence staining. Compared with MSC^{Null} group (11.6±1.9/mm^2; Fig. 7A and G), the MSC$^{miR-377}$ group exhibited a lower vascular density (4.9±1.2/mm^2; Fig. 7B and G; $p<0.05$), whereas MSC$^{Anti-377}$group displayed a higher vascular density (34.8±4.1/mm^2; Fig. 7C and G; $p<0.05$). Capillary density, as determined by vWF immunofluorescence staining, was significantly decreased in MSC$^{miR-377}$-treated hearts, but was significantly increased in MSC$^{Anti-377}$-treated hearts, compared with MSC^{Null} (Fig. 7D–F, Fig. 7G).

Reduced Expression of MiR-377 in MSCs Limits Fibrosis and Improves Contractile Function in Infarcted Hearts

Fibrosis area was evaluated using Masson's Trichrome staining in which normal myocardium was colored red while fiberized myocardium was blue in color due to its inner collagen. The percentage of fibrosis in the left ventricle wall was significantly reduced in the MSC$^{Anti-377}$group, but was increased in MSC$^{miR-377}$-implanted hearts, as compared with MSC^{Null} (Fig. 8A–B).

Echocardiographic measurements showed that cardiac function was significantly improved in MSC$^{Anti-377}$, as evidenced by a shorter LVDd (7.94±0.2 mm) and LVDs (5.875±0.2 mm), a higher ratio of EF (59. 5±2.2%) and FS (26.0±1.8%), compared with MSC^{Null}-hearts (8.68±0.3 mm; 6.97±0.3 mm; 48.2±1.9%; 20±1.2%; respectively, $p<0.05$) and MSC$^{miR-377}$ group(9.56±0.38 mm; 7.968±0.3 mm; 39.19±3.9%; 17±1.3%; respectively, $p<0.05$) (Fig. 8C–D). However, no significant differences were noted in these parameters between MI and MI+PBS groups.

Discussion

Angiogenesis is a key regenerative event in ischemic injured hearts after MI, and VEGF plays an important role in MSC-induced angiogenesis [1]. Given that miRNAs are endogenous regulators of gene expression, it is reasonable to hypothesize that miRNAs may be involved in the regulation of VEGF expression in MSCs. We therefore employed hypoxia, a well-established VEGF inducer, to pre-treat MSCs and determined the miRNA expression profile. The results showed that miR-377 expression was decreased by more than 2-fold in hypoxia-treated MSCs as compared with normoxic condition. By computational miRNA target prediction analysis, we identified VEGF as a potential target of miR-377. Furthermore, both dual-luciferase reporter assay and Western-blotting verified that miR-377 can directly bind with VEGF 3′UTR leading to negatively regulation of its expression.

Accordingly, *in vivo* by transplanting MSCs with genetic overexpression or knockdown of miR-377 in the rat MI hearts, we observed that myocardial angiogenesis was significantly improved in MSC$^{Anti-377}$-treated hearts, whereas it was poor in MSC$^{miR-377}$-treated hearts when comparable to MSC^{Null}-injected hearts. It is important to note here, while the degree of fibrosis was less in MSC$^{Anti-377}$-treated myocardium than MSC^{Null}-injected group, there were no significant changes in MSC$^{miR-377}$-treated group when compared to controls. Consistent with the alteration of myocardial fibrosis, cardiac function was significantly improved in the MSC$^{Anti-377}$-treatedgroup, but there were no obvious changes in MSC$^{miR-377}$-implanted hearts as compared with MSC^{Null}-injected hearts. This may be interpreted that myocardial angiogenesis is reduced in MSC$^{miR-377}$-treated hearts, but not enough to affect MSC-induced beneficial effects on the reduction of fibrosis and improvement of function in infarcted hearts. However, numerous studies have indicated that an increase in myocardial angiogenesis improves contractile function in the infarcted myocardium [10], [32], [33].

It should be noted that VEGF can be regulated either indirectly or directly by different miRNAs in different cells and different diseases [15–26]. MiR-210 is a key player of cell response to hypoxia [25] and indirectly up-regulates VEGF-mediated angiogenesis by targeting Ephrin-A3 [15], and enhances MSC-mediated angiogenesis [26]. MiR-145 indirectly down-regulates VEGF in cancer cells to inhibit tumor growth and angiogenesis by targeting p70S6K1, an upstream molecule of VEGF [21]. MiR-10 indirectly down-regulates VEGF-mediated angiogenesis in HU-VECs by targeting fms-related tyrosine kinase 1 (FLT1), a cell-surface protein that sequesters VEGF [16]. However, miR-15b, miR-16, miR-20a, miR-20b [17], [18], miR-205 [23] and miR-195 [22] down-regulate angiogenesis by directly targeting VEGF. Such a role has previously only been reported in carcinoma cells, mouse embryonic fibroblast cells, glioma cells, and human hepatocellular carcinoma (HCC) cells. For the first time we demonstrate that miR-377 is responsive to hypoxia and directly targets VEGF in MSCs. Both *in vitro* and *in vivo* evidence presented in this study indicate that knockdown of endogenous miR-377 enhances MSC-mediated angiogenesis and recovery of cardiac function in infarcted myocardium. Therefore, our study indicates that miR-377 may be a novel therapy target for treatment of ischemic heart disease.

Conclusion

In conclusion, our study indicates thathypoxia-reducedmiR-377 directly targets VEGF, and knockdown of endogenous miR-377 promotes MSC transplantation-induced angiogenesis and subsequent heart function improvement post MI. These data may suggest a new therapeutic strategy for ischemic heart disease treatment in the future.

Acknowledgments

The authors wish to recognize Christian Paul for technical assistance.

Author Contributions

Conceived and designed the experiments: ZW WH GF Yigang Wang PZ. Performed the experiments: ZW WH YF WC Yuhua Wang XW JL MW. Analyzed the data: RM GF Yigang Wang JC. Contributed reagents/materials/analysis tools: Yigang Wang JMC. Contributed to the writing of the manuscript: ZW RM GF Yigang Wang.

References

1. Zhao T, Zhao W, Chen Y, Ahokas RA, Sun Y (2010) Vascular endothelial growth factor (VEGF)-A: role on cardiac angiogenesis following myocardial infarction. Microvasc Res 80: 188–194.

2. Stewart DJ, Kutryk MJ, Fitchett D, Freeman M, Camack N, et al. (2009) VEGF gene therapy fails to improve perfusion of ischemic myocardium in patients with advanced coronary disease: results of the NORTHERN trial. Mol Ther 17: 1109–1115.

3. Yla-Herttuala S, Rissanen TT, Vajanto I, Hartikainen J (2007) Vascular endothelial growth factors: biology and current status of clinical applications in cardiovascular medicine. J Am Coll Cardiol 49: 1015–1026.

4. Huang W, Zhang D, Millard RW, Wang T, Zhao T, et al. (2010) Gene manipulated peritoneal cell patch repairs infarcted myocardium. J Mol Cell Cardiol 48: 702–712.

5. Copland IB (2011) Mesenchymal stromal cells for cardiovascular disease. J Cardiovasc Dis Res 2: 3–13.

6. Zhang D, Fan GC, Zhou X, Zhao T, Pasha Z, et al. (2008) Over-expression of CXCR4 on mesenchymal stem cells augments myoangiogenesis in the infarcted myocardium. J Mol Cell Cardiol 44: 281–292.

7. Aicher A, Brenner W, Zuhayra M, Badorff C, Massoudi S, et al. (2003) Assessment of the tissue distribution of transplanted human endothelial progenitor cells by radioactive labeling. Circulation 107: 2134–2139.

8. Samper E, Diez-Juan A, Montero JA, Sepulveda P (2013) Cardiac cell therapy: boosting mesenchymal stem cells effects. Stem Cell Rev 9: 266–280.

9. Wang Y, Zhang D, Ashraf M, Zhao T, Huang W, et al. (2010) Combining neuropeptide Y and mesenchymal stem cells reverses remodeling after myocardial infarction. Am J Physiol Heart Circ Physiol 298: H275–286.

10. Liang J, Huang W, Yu X, Ashraf A, Wary KK, et al. (2012) Suicide gene reveals the myocardial neovascularization role of mesenchymal stem cells overexpressing CXCR4 (MSC(CXCR4)). PLoS One 7: e46158.

11. Hu W, Coller J (2012) What comes first: translational repression or mRNA degradation? The deepening mystery of microRNA function. Cell Res 22: 1322–1324.

12. Jeker LT, Bluestone JA (2013) MicroRNA regulation of T-cell differentiation and function. Immunol Rev 253: 65–81.

13. Zhang Z, Qin YW, Brewer G, Jing Q (2012) MicroRNA degradation and turnover: regulating the regulators. Wiley Interdiscip Rev RNA 3: 593–600.

14. Kulshreshtha R, Ferracin M, Wojcik SE, Garzon R, Alder H, et al. (2007) A microRNA signature of hypoxia. Mol Cell Biol 27: 1859–1867.

15. Fasanaro P, D'Alessandra Y, Di Stefano V, Melchionna R, Romani S, et al. (2008) MicroRNA-210 modulates endothelial cell response to hypoxia and inhibits the receptor tyrosine kinase ligand Ephrin-A3. J Biol Chem 283: 15878–15883.

16. Hassel D, Cheng P, White MP, Ivey KN, Kroll J, et al. (2012) MicroRNA-10 regulates the angiogenic behavior of zebrafish and human endothelial cells by promoting vascular endothelial growth factor signaling. Circ Res 111: 1421–1433.

17. Hua Z, Lv Q, Ye W, Wong CK, Cai G, et al. (2006) MiRNA-directed regulation of VEGF and other angiogenic factors under hypoxia. PLoS One 1: e116.

18. Dejean E, Renalier MH, Foisseau M, Agirre X, Joseph N, et al. (2011) Hypoxia-microRNA-16 downregulation induces VEGF expression in anaplastic lymphoma kinase (ALK)-positive anaplastic large-cell lymphomas. Leukemia 25: 1882–1890.

19. Lai Y, Zhang X, Zhang Z, Shu Y, Luo X, et al. (2013) The microRNA-27a: ZBTB10-specificity protein pathway is involved in follicle stimulating hormone-induced VEGF, Cox2 and survivin expression in ovarian epithelial cancer cells. Int J Oncol 42: 776–784.

20. Sasahira T, Kurihara M, Bhawal UK, Ueda N, Shimomoto T, et al. (2012) Downregulation of miR-126 induces angiogenesis and lymphangiogenesis by activation of VEGF-A in oral cancer. Br J Cancer 107: 700–706.

21. Xu Q, Liu LZ, Qian X, Chen Q, Jiang Y, et al. (2012) MiR-145 directly targets p70S6K1 in cancer cells to inhibit tumor growth and angiogenesis. Nucleic Acids Res 40: 761–774.

22. Wang R, Zhao N, Li S, Fang JH, Chen MX, et al. (2013) MicroRNA-195 suppresses angiogenesis and metastasis of hepatocellular carcinoma by inhibiting the expression of VEGF, VAV2, and CDC42. Hepatology 58: 642–653.

23. Yue X, Wang P, Xu J, Zhu Y, Sun G, et al. (2012) MicroRNA-205 functions as a tumor suppressor in human glioblastoma cells by targeting VEGF-A. Oncol Rep 27: 1200–1206.

24. Liu F, Lou YL, Wu J, Ruan QF, Xie A, et al. (2012) Upregulation of microRNA-210 regulates renal angiogenesis mediated by activation of VEGF signaling pathway under ischemia/perfusion injury in vivo and in vitro. Kidney Blood Press Res 35: 182–191.

25. Fasanaro P, Greco S, Lorenzi M, Pescatori M, Brioschi M, et al. (2009) An integrated approach for experimental target identification of hypoxia-induced miR-210. J Biol Chem 284: 35134–35143.

26. Alaiti MA, Ishikawa M, Masuda H, Simon DI, Jain MK, et al. (2012) Up-regulation of miR-210 by vascular endothelial growth factor in ex vivo expanded CD34+ cells enhances cell-mediated angiogenesis. J Cell Mol Med 16: 2413–2421.

27. Jin Y, Chen Z, Liu X, Zhou X (2013) Evaluating the microRNA targeting sites by luciferase reporter gene assay. Methods Mol Biol 936: 117–127.

28. Arnaoutova I, George J, Kleinman HK, Benton G (2009) The endothelial cell tube formation assay on basement membrane turns 20: state of the science and the art. Angiogenesis 12: 267–274.

29. Huang W, Wang T, Zhang D, Zhao T, Dai B, et al. (2012) Mesenchymal stem cells overexpressing CXCR4 attenuate remodeling of postmyocardial infarction by releasing matrix metalloproteinase-9. Stem Cells Dev 21: 778–789.

30. Mutharasan RK, Nagpal V, Ichikawa Y, Ardehali H (2011) microRNA-210 is upregulated in hypoxic cardiomyocytes through Akt- and p53-dependent pathways and exerts cytoprotective effects. Am J Physiol Heart Circ Physiol 301: H1519–1530.

31. Staszel T, Zapala B, Polus A, Sadakierska-Chudy A, Kiec-Wilk B, et al. (2011) Role of microRNAs in endothelial cell pathophysiology. Pol Arch Med Wewn 121: 361–366.

32. Cochain C, Channon KM, Silvestre JS (2013) Angiogenesis in the infarcted myocardium. Antioxid Redox Signal 18: 1100–1113.

33. Tomita S, Mickle DA, Weisel RD, Jia ZQ, Tumiati LC, et al. (2002) Improved heart function with myogenesis and angiogenesis after autologous porcine bone marrow stromal cell transplantation. J Thorac Cardiovasc Surg 123: 1132–1140.

2

MicroRNA-223-3p Inhibits the Angiogenesis of Ischemic Cardiac Microvascular Endothelial Cells via Affecting RPS6KB1/hif-1a Signal Pathway

Guo-Hua Dai[1]*, Pei-Ze Ma[2], Xian-Bo Song[2], Ning Liu[2], Tong Zhang[1], Bo Wu[1]

1 Affiliated Hospital of Shandong University of Traditional Chinese Medicine, Jinan, China, 2 Shandong University of Traditional Chinese Medicine, Jinan, China

Abstract

Background: MicroRNAs (miRNAs) are a recently discovered class of posttranscriptional regulators of gene expression with critical functions in the angiogenesis and cardiovascular diseases; however, the details of miRNAs regulating mechanism of angiogenesis of ischemic cardiac microvascular endothelial cells (CMECs) are not yet reported.

Methods and Results: This study analyzes the changes of the dynamic expression of miRNAs during the process of angiogenesis of ischemic CMECs by applying miRNA chip and real-time PCR for the first time. Compared with normal CMECs, ischemic CMECs have a specific miRNAs expression profile, in which mir-223-3p has the most significant up-regulation, especially during the process of migration and proliferation, while the up-regulation is the most significant during migration, reaching 11.02 times. Rps6kb1 is identified as a potential direct and functional target of mir-223-3p by applying bioinformatic prediction, real-time PCR and Western blot. Pathway analysis report indicates Rps6kb1 regulates the angiogenesis by participating into hif-1a signal pathway. Further analysis reveals that both the gene and protein expression of the downstream molecules VEGF, MAPK, PI3K and Akt of Rps6kb1/hif-1a signal pathway decrease significantly during the process of migration and proliferation in the ischemic CMECs. Therefore, it is confirmed that mir-223-3p inhibits the angiogenesis of CMECs, at least partly, via intervening RPS6KB1/hif-1a signal pathway and affecting the process of migration and proliferation.

Conclusion: This study elucidates the miRNA regulating law in the angiogenesis of CMECs; mir-223-3p inhibits the process of migration and proliferation of ischemic CMECs probably via affecting RPS6KB1/hif-1a signal pathway, which in turn suppresses the angiogenesis. It is highly possible that mir-223-3p becomes a novel intervention core target in the treatment of angiogenesis of ischemic heart diseases.

Editor: Ingo Ahrens, University Hospital Medical Centre, Germany

Funding: This work was funded by Chinese National Natural Science Foundation #81173441. The funders had no role in study design, data collection and analysis, decision to publish, or preparation of the manuscript.

Competing Interests: The authors have declared that no competing interests exist.

* Email: Daigh2004@163.com

Introduction

Myocardial ischemia and myocardial infarction are the most common and frequently encountered diseases in clinic. Present studies haven't revealed the function and mechanism of endogenous factor in ischemia myocardial. MicroRNAs are a class of recently-discovered endogenous non-coding RNAs (~22 nt), which pair-bond 3′ non-coding region of target gene mRNAs and negatively regulate the expression of target mRNAs post-transcriptionally, in addition to playing a vital role in the cell differentiation, proliferation, apoptosis, individual development and the body metabolism [1–4]. According to the bioinformatics analysis, one miRNA may have hundreds of potential target mRNAs and about 30% of human genes are controlled by the miRNA, which indicates miRNA probably affects the entire signal pathway [5,6]. MiRNA has tissue specificity and time sequence and it expresses on the specific tissues and during the specific development stage, and in this way, it regulates the expression of target genes dynamically [7].

When myocardial ischemia attacks, it is highly possible that the dynamic change of miRNA affects the expression of lots of target protein, which in turn damages the construction and function of the ischemic myocardium. Therefore, to study miRNA that is closely related to the angiogenesis will contribute to the treatment of ischemic diseases by applying newly-discovered ways of regulating angiogenesis. From analyzing the expression of the human umbilical vein endothelial cell (HUVEC) miRNA, Fish, etc. find that miRNA-126 is a specific endothelial cell miRNA out of 15 high-expressed miRNAs, which promotes angiogenesis and the formation of vascular integrity [8]. While Poliseno, etc. identify 27 high-expressed miRNAs in HUVEC, and confirm that miR-221/222 inhibits the angiogenesis via regulating the expression of the C-KIT gene [9]. Currently, there are incongruous reports on the miRNA target related to the angiogenesis, which vary from miR-126 [10], miR-130a [11], miR-378 [12], and miR-27b [13] to miR-210 [14], all of which are regarded as miRNAs which promote the angiogenesis while miR-92a [15], miR-221 [16] and

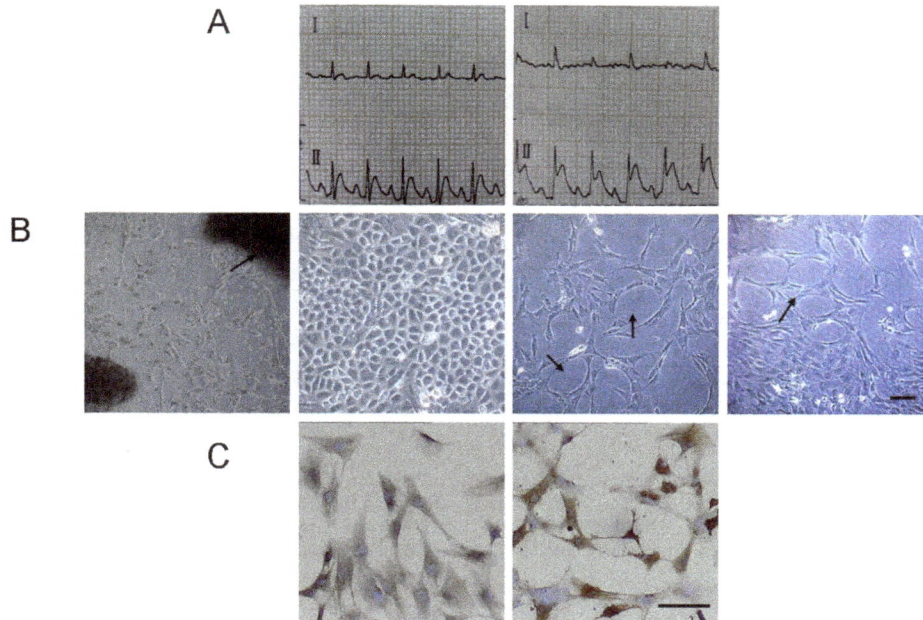

Figure 1. A. Left: a normal electrocardiogram or rat before the model building. Right: After the model building, electrocardiograms lead II indicated ST segment elevated significantly, which indicated ischemia myocardial and proved the artery ligation was successful. B. The cells were in the shape of stars or polygons when they initially disassociated out of the tissue block and had a low density, they were in the shape of paving stones when the cells bespreaded the bottom of the culture flask, in some of which tube structure and vessel network structure could be spotted. C. Immunocytochemical stain revealed that: (left) after the staining of VIII factor, the cytoplasm was brown coloring, the coloring was the most significant in pericaryon; (right) after the staining of CD31, their cell membrane showed yellowish brown particles, which proved that the cultured cells were CMECs.

miR-222 inhibit the migration and proliferation of endothelial cells and the angiogenesis. However, further experiments are needed to confirm which one is at the core or main position, whether it is a kind of miRNA or a group of miRNAs, which will become the therapeutic target in the treatment of ischemic diseases. Only a small proportion of the dynamic expression of miRNA is revealed, thus the discovery of the regulating expression of miRNA during the pathophysiologic process of the vascular diseases and the target genes will contribute to a keener understanding of the function miRNA in the vessels.

When the ischemic vascular diseases attack, the compensation of endogenous collateral circulation in the body is limited, namely, the angiogenesis of endothelial cells is restricted. However, the feature of the angiogenesis of the ischemic CMECs has not been reported yet.

Based on the above mentioned knowledge, this study analyzes the changes of the dynamic expression of miRNAs during the process of angiogenesis of CMECs by applying miRNA chip and real-time PCR for the first time and confirms the key miRNA in three different stages of the ischemic CMECs proliferation, migration and tube formation respectively. It is found in this study that the expression of mir-223-3p in the angiogenesis of the ischemic CMECs increases significantly and Rps6kbl is the target gene of mir-223-3p, it is also revealed that mir-223-3p inhibits the process of migration and proliferation of ischemic CMECs via affecting RPS6KB1/hif-1a signal pathway, which finally suppresses the angiogenesis.

Materials and Methods

Rats myocardial infarction model building and cell culture

The study was approved by the Ethic Committee for the Protection of Animal Care of Shandong University of TCM (Jinan, China). 38 male SD rats (220~280 g) were purchased from Shandong University of TCM Experimental Animal Center (Jinan, China). The rats myocardial infarction models were made as previously described by Drexler H et al. [17]: rats were anesthetized by 10% chloral hydrate, 0.3 mL/100 g and their electrocardiograms were recorded after being fixed, cervical trachea was isolated, breathing machine was connected after the chest was opened and the heart was exposed, left anterior descending coronary artery (LAD) was ligated, ST segment elevation, T wave ascending or inverting in the recorded electrocardiograms proved the ligation was successful. Rats woke up from anesthesia in 1–3 hours after operation. Those survived 24 hs after the operation became models. General characteristics of myocardial infarcted rats, such as body weight, mental condition, respiratory frequency, animal hair, urine, feces and etc., were monitored twice a day before ischemic CMECs were isolated from the apex of myocardial infarction model rats for about 2weeks. The food and water consumption, animal activity, expression in eyes, color of the tails and etc. of myocardial infarction model rats were observed after surgery. The temperature, humidity and ventilation of the feeding chamber were

A

B

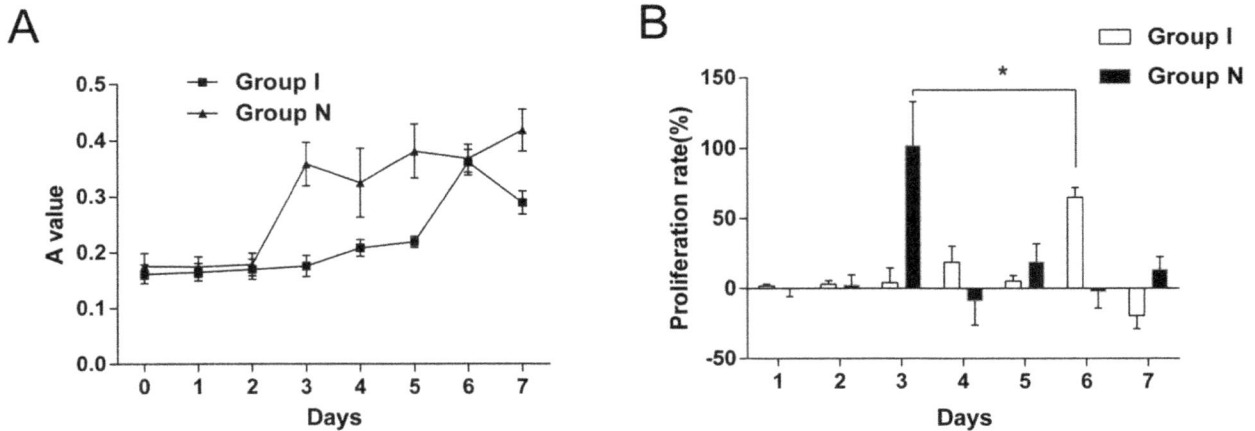

Figure 2. A. The OD value of normal CMECs exceeded that of ischemic CMECs, the normal CMECs proliferated vigorously on the third day while the cell growth curve of ischemic CMECs was even, the OD value reached a peak till the sixth day. B. A dynamic observation revealed that the proliferating phase of the normal CMECs was the third day while the proliferating phase of the ischemic CMECs was the sixth day. The cell proliferation ratio of ischemic CMECs decreased significantly compared with that of the normal CMECs (P<0.05).

regulated timely. Providing the sterilized water and changing the bedding for the rats everyday to ensure animal welfare. Meanwhile, weak rats or rats before recovery after anesthesia were kept separately to prevent them from being attacked. Ischemic CMECs were isolated from the apex of myocardial infarction model rats and cultured using previously reported methods [18] and normal CMECs were isolated from the apex of healthy male SD rats, also cultured as described [18]: rats were anesthetized by 10% chloral hydrate, 0.3 mL/100 g and were sterilized by immersing in 75% ethanol for 8 minutes, then their chests were opened and their hearts were sheared under sterility, and rats were euthanized by overdose anesthesia with 10% chloral hydrate (0.6 mL/100 g) after hearts harvest in the experiment. The hearts were next put in sterile culture medium, their great vessels, both of the atrium cordis, ventriculus dexter and interventricular septum were dislodged, then they were rinsed in PBS repeatedly, the rest of the ventricular muscle was transferred into a beaker and was cut into pieces of 2 mm³ by using ophthalmic scissors, then, they were inoculated evenly into a culture flask with 1 ml fetal bovine serum and cultured statically for 4 hs at 37°C in 5% CO_2 in a humidified incubator, which was followed a continuous culture of 60~70 h in added 2 ml DMEM high glucose medium (Gibco, Carlsbad, CA) containing 20% fetal bovine serum (FBS; Gibco), tissue masses were removed and DMEM high glucose medium was changed per 3 days till the cells reached fusion. VIII factors and CD31 were identified by immunocytochemistry. All the rats involved were euthanized by overdose anesthesia with sodium pentobarbital (80 mg/kg, i.p.) after the experiment.

Cell proliferation

Cell proliferation was detected by using MTT methods as previously described [19–22]. Briefly, the normal CMECs and ischemic CMECs were resuspended in 10% fetal calf serum medium respectively, and then made into single cell suspension, which was inoculated into sixteen 96-well cell culture plates, 4000 cells per well, 8 plates for one group, 200 μ for one well, and 6 duplicate well for every group. 20 μL of a 5 g/L MTT solution was added to each well ten hours, one day, two days, three days, four days, five days, six days, seven days after inoculation respectively and culture was terminated after another incubation of 4 hs at 37°C. Next, the medium was carefully aspirated from each well and 150 μL DMSO was added, absorbance was detected at a wavelength of 490 nm by using microplate reader (Bio-Tek, ELX 800, USA) and the proliferation rate was calculated to find the window phase of proliferation, and the cell growth curve was finally drawn with time as abscissa and observance as ordinate.

Cell migration

Scratch test was applied to detect the migration of cells [23]. When the cell growth reached 80% fusion, two groups of cells digestion were inoculated into 24 well plates, six duplicate wells for each group, a cross was scratched in the middle of the bottom of 24 well plates with steriled 10 μL spear, cultured at 37°C in 5% CO_2 in an incubator and took a picture of the intersection of the scratch zero hour, one day, two days, three days, four days respectively after the scratch to observe the healing power, to count the number of cell migration, to calculate the migration rate and to find the window phase of migration.

Table 1. The window phases of proliferation, migration, tube formation of the two groups.

Group	n	migration	tube formation	proliferation
ischemia	6	The first day	The second day	The sixth day
normal	6	The first day	The second day	The third day

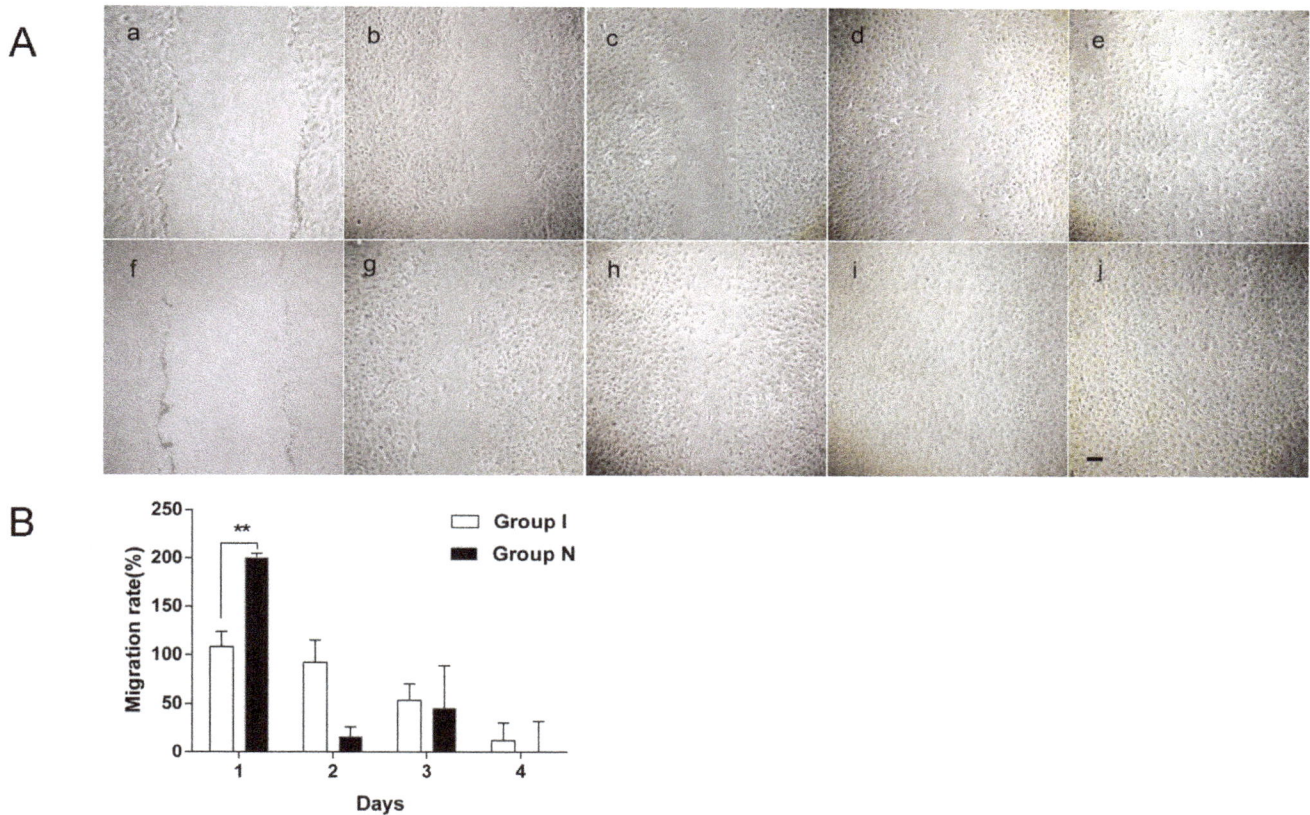

Figure 3. A. Under microscope, for normal CMECs, a clear scratching blank area could be spotted after the scratching test. The blank area decreased significantly with amount of cells crossed the scratching line one day later. The blank area was gradually covered with increasing proliferated cells two days later. The blank area was completely covered with proliferated cells three days later. For ischemic CMECs, a similar scratching blank area could also be spotted after the scratching test. The blank area could still be clearly spotted one day later because there was only a small amount of cell migrated to the blank area. The migrated cells increased two days later, but were still less than that of normal CMECs. The migrated cells increased three days later, but the blank area could still be spotted. B. A dynamic observation revealed that the cell migration ratio of ischemic CMECs decreased significantly compared with that of the normal CMECs ($P<0.01$).

Tube formation

CMECs tube formation was observed by using inverted phase contrast microscope and the formation was counted. When the cell growth reached 80% fusion, two groups of cells digestion were inoculated into two 6 well plates, six duplicate wells for each group, tube formation was observed by using inverted phase contrast microscope ($100\times$) one day, two days, three days, four days respectively after the inoculation, a tube was formed when the connection of endothelial cell showed "C" [24–25]. The number of the tube formation was counted in the amplificated ($100\times$) vision from three most intense tube gathering vision per well. 10 pictures of each group were taken randomly to get the average in order to calculate the tube formation rate to find the window phase of tube formation.

MiRNA gene chip analysis

Based on the "window" feature of normal/ischemic CMECs angiogenesis process, two groups of cells were further divided according to the time of proliferation, migration and tube formation. The total RNA was extracted from the cells of each group (the total number is about 2×10^6). RNA quality was detected by measuring OD260/OD280 ratio and using formaldehyde denaturation agarose gel electrophoresis, the ratio varied from 1.8 to 2.1, which indicated that the quality of RNA was reliable. MiRNA isolation, fluorescence labeling, microarray hybridization experiments and data analysis were made according to manufacturer's instructions. MiRNA was labeled by using miRCURY Array Power Labeling kit. The labeled sample was concentrated by using Rneasy mini kit. MiRNA microarray hybridization was made by using miRCURY Array microarray kit and Hybridization Chamber II kit. Fluorescence excitation was made at 635 nm and the Axon GenePix 4000B microarray scanner (Axon Instruments, Foster City, CA) was used to scan the images, scanned images were then imported into GenePix Pro 6.0 software (Axon) for the digital transformation of the microarray images, the median normalization method was used to calculate the standard value. Firstly, differential expression ≥2times is used as criterion, according to the gene expression, differential expressed miRNA was filtered and given a cluster analysis, which included miRNA that had a more than 2 times up-regulated-expression and miRNA that had a less than 2 times down-regulated-expression, the key of which was to choose miRNA with a significant differential expression. Secondly, major miRNA related to proliferation, miRNA related to migration and miRNA related to tube formation were spotted according to the code of differential expression during stages of miRNA proliferation, migration and tube formation, the core miRNA of ischemic CMECs was worked out. Microarray hybridization experiments

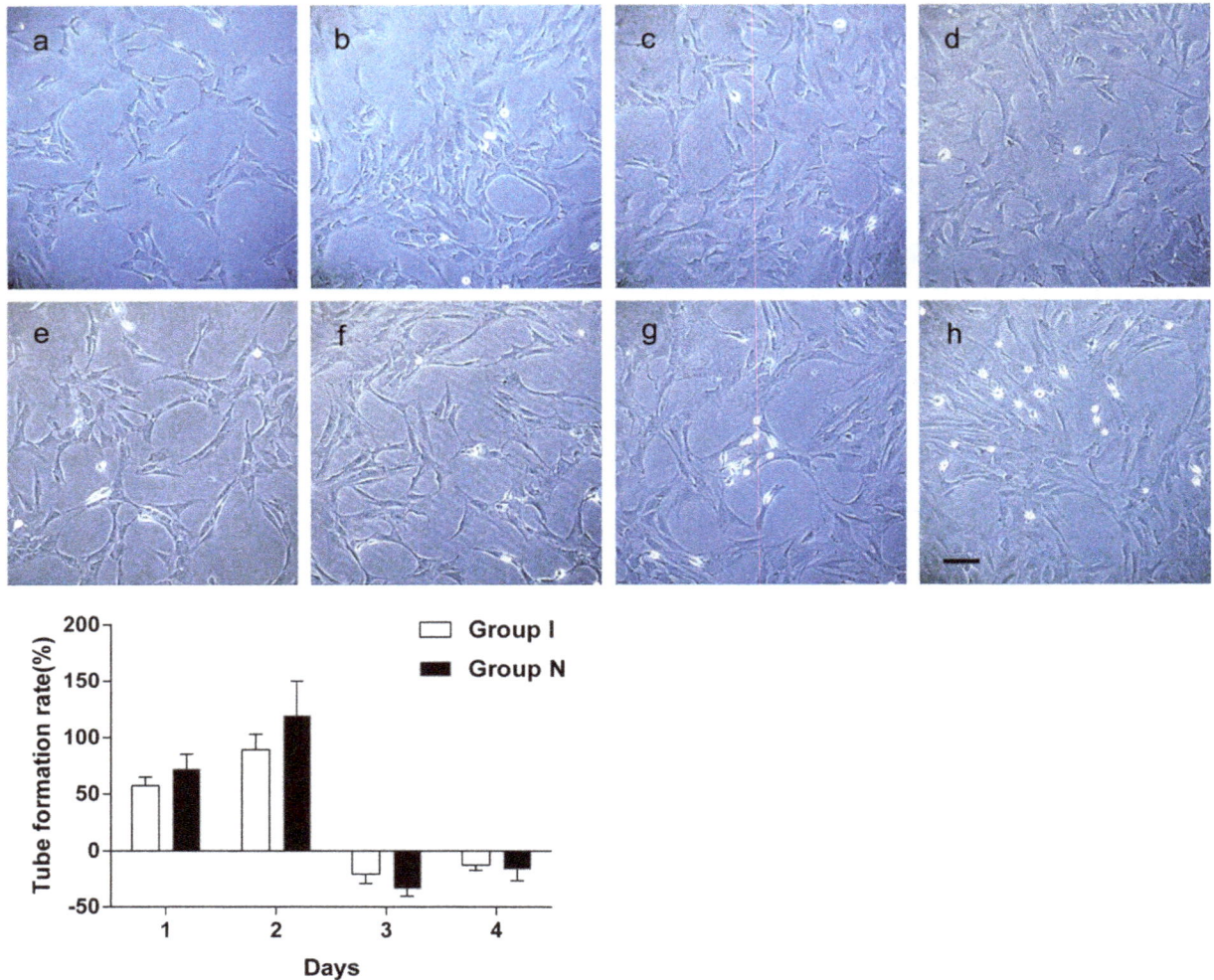

Figure 4. A. For normal CMECs, observation under inverted phase contrast microscope (100×) revealed that amounts of "C"-shaped tube structure were formed one day after inoculation. The "C"-shaped tube structures were clearer and increased significantly two days after inoculation. The "C"-shaped tube structure decreased with an increased cell number three days after inoculation. The "C"-shaped tube structure further decreased four days after inoculation. For ischemic CMECs, there was no obvious tube formation one day after inoculation, only several "C"-shaped structure were spotted under inverted phase contrast microscope (100×). Several tube formations were spotted two days after inoculation, of which the number was less than that of normal CMECs. The tube structure decreased with an increased cell number three days after inoculation. The tube structure disappeared four days after inoculation. B. A dynamic observation revealed that the migration phase of normal/ischemic CMECs was the second day. Tube formation ratio of ischemic CMECs decreased compared with that of the normal CMECs, but that was of no statistical significance.

and consequent data analysis were finished by Shanghai KangCheng Bio-technology.

Real-time PCR testing and verifying core miRNA

As is described in the previous part, two groups of cells were further divided according to the time of proliferation, migration and tube formation to detect the expression of core miRNA in different groups. The total RNA was extracted from the cells of each group and the purity and density of RNA were detected. RNA sample primer was given a reverse transcription into cDNAs according to reverse transcriptase. All cDNA samples were allocated to real-time PCR reaction system respectively, which followed the following procedure: Reactions were incubated at 95°C for 10 minutes, followed by 40 PCR cycles of 95°C for 10 seconds, 60°C for 60 seconds to get the primary curve; after the amplification reaction, reactions were incubated at 95°C for 10 seconds, 60°C for 60 seconds and 95°C for 15 seconds; the temperature increased from 60°C to 99°C gradually (the test system carried it out automatically at a Ramp Rate of 0.05°C/ second) to establish the solubility curve of PCR primer. The data were analyzed by using $2^{-\Delta\Delta Ct}$ method.

MiRNA target prediction

MiRNA target gene wasere predicted by retrieving data bases of mirbase (http://www.ebi.ac.uk/, mirbase(http://www.ebi.ac.uk/) and mirdb (http://mirdb.org/miRD B/), a predictive analysis of the secondary structure and target gene of miRNA was made to spot the gene with a characteristic of a high degree of sequence matching, stable secondary structure and target sequences being highly conserved among species. The gene predicted in this three software simultaneously was given a GO analysis and pathway

Table 2. The differential expression of miRNAs in ICP and in NCP (n = 3 in each group).

Gene	Fold change	P value
Up-regulated miRNA in ICP		
rno-miR-511-3p	7.157	0.007
rno-miR-301b-3p	5.408	0.004
rno-miR-142-5p	5.022	0.00007
rno-miR-142-3p	4.776	0.00001
rno-miR-421-3p	4.346	0.0005
rno-miR-3576	4.213	0.002
rno-miR-203b-5p	3.858	0.037
rno-miR-363-5p	3.855	0.008
rno-miR-10a-5p	3.843	0.001
rno-miR-450a-5p	3.757	0.007
rno-miR-141-5p	3.721	0.007
rno-miR-883-3p	3.711	0.001
rno-miR-223-3p	3.679	0.006
rno-miR-322-5p	3.494	0.019
rno-miR-146a-5p	3.409	0.003
rno-miR-292-5p	3.096	0.003
rno-miR-29c-3p	3.015	0.003
rno-let-7f-5p	2.976	0.0001
rno-miR-26b-5p	2.709	0.018
rno-miR-499-3p	2.652	0.004
rno-miR-32-5p	2.647	0.005
rno-miR-98-5p	2.573	0.002
rno-miR-206-5p	2.453	0.004
rno-miR-145-5p	2.437	0.029
rno-miR-101b-3p	2.409	0.023
rno-miR-187-3p	2.408	0.025
rno-miR-195-5p	2.384	0.033
rno-miR-362-3p	2.381	0.0004
rno-miR-336-5p	2.246	0.006
rno-miR-1-3p	2.193	0.042
rno-miR-30e-5p	2.181	0.023
rno-miR-532-5p	2.165	0.0004
rno-miR-29c-5p	2.149	0.014
rno-miR-26a-5p	2.132	0.048
rno-miR-741-3p	2.123	0.001
rno-miR-210-3p	2.122	0.004
rno-miR-188-5p	2.112	0.003
rno-miR-181a-2-3p	2.058	0.018
rno-miR-3068-3p	2.025	0.025
rno-let-7d-5p	2.003	0.002
Down-regulated miRNAs in ICP		
rno-miR-463-3p	0.175	0.048
rno-miR-3560	0.197	0.031
rno-miR-154-5p	0.208	0.001
rno-miR-344a-5p	0.312	0.035
rno-miR-3596d	0.393	0.023
rno-miR-1188-3p	0.402	0.009
rno-miR-295-5p	0.429	0.003
rno-miR-760-5p	0.454	0.026

Table 2. Cont.

Gene	Fold change	P value
rno-miR-539-3p	0.468	0.009
rno-miR-409b	0.468	0.011
rno-miR-299b-5p	0.472	0.016
rno-miR-183-3p	0.474	0.039
rno-miR-3593-3p	0.474	0.043
rno-miR-3591	0.477	0.001
rno-miR-878	0.479	0.025
rno-miR-200c-5p	0.494	0.016

analysis to spot the target gene, which was closely related to angiogenesis.

Reverse-transcription and real-time Polymerase Chain Reaction (PCR)

As is described in the previous part, two groups of cells were further divided according to the time of proliferation, migration and tube formation, the miRNA expression of Rps6kb1, HIF-1a, VEGF, MAPK, PI3K and Akt was detected by applying real-time PCR.

Western blot analysis

As is described in the previous part, two groups of cells were further divided according to the time of proliferation, migration and tube formation, the gene expression of Rps6kb1, HIF-1a, VEGF, MAPK, PI3K and Akt was detected by applying Western-blot [26]. Total protein extraction kit was used to extract the total protein of the samples. The density of the samples was measured according to the instruction of BCA protein fluorometric kit. The protein was ionophortically separated after the prepared sample and prestained protein marker were loaded respectively. The filter paper cellulose gel interlayer was assembled according to the instruction of Bio-Rad protein transferring device. Non specific binding on the closing membrane was incubated at room temperature in 5% skim milk powder solution. First antibody was added into sealed membrane to achieve the antigen antibody union. HRP labeled second antibody was added to unite first antibody. HRP labeled β-actin antibody was added to detect the content of β-actin simultaneously. The membrane was incubated with chemiluminescence substrate and developed after X film exposure. The pictures were scanned and GIS1000 Software was applied to digitalize the grey level of every specific band of the pictures. The grey level of the target protein was divided by that of β-actin to get alignment error, of which the outcome stood for the relative content of the target protein of the specific sample.

Statistical analysis

All data are expressed as mean±standard deviation (SD) from at least three separate experiments. The differences between groups were analyzed using Student's t test. Differences were of statistical significance when $P<0.05$.

Results

Rats myocardial infarction model building and cell culture

After the rat's left anterior descending coronary artery (LAD) was ligated, electrocardiograms indicated ST segment elevated significantly (Fig. 1A), which proved the model building was successful. There were two rats failed in respiration and circulation in 24 hours after mice model establishment, and breathing machine and intravenous injection of 0.1% adrenaline 1 mL were given, and finally these two rats died despite the rescuing efforts. Finally 38 of the myocardial infarction model rats were established and 36 were survived (success rate was 94.7%). Under reverted microscope, cells were observed to disassociate out of the tissue block and bespread the bottom of the culture flask, during which typical morphological and functional changes with typical CMECs characteristics (Fig. 1B) were found. Immunocytochemical stain revealed that VIII factor and CD31 expressed positively in cells (Fig. 1C), which proved that the cultured cells were CMECs.

Cell growth curve and proliferation

MTT colorimetry method was used to protract the cell growth curve, the normal CMECs grew slowly during the first 2 days, proliferated vigorously on the third day at a logarithmic growth, and then went into a cell growth plateau. Ischemic CMECs grew slowly during the first 5 days, and proliferated vigorously on the sixth day, during which there was no obvious plateau (Fig. 2A). The window phases of cell proliferation of both groups were found respectively from the dynamic observation (Table 1). The cell proliferation ratio of ischemic CMECs decreased significantly compared with that of the normal CMECs ($P<0.05$) (Fig. 2B).

Cell migration and tube formation

The number of cell migration of ischemic CMECS decreased significantly compared with that of the normal CMECs (Fig. 3A). The window phases of cell migration of both groups were found respectively from the dynamic observation (Table 1). The cell migration ratio of ischemic CMECs decreased significantly compared with that of the normal CMECs ($P<0.01$)(Fig. 3B). The number of tube formation of ischemic CMECS decreased significantly compared with that of the normal CMECs (Fig. 4A). The window phases of cell tube formation of both groups were found respectively from the dynamic observation (Table 1). The tube formation ratio of ischemic CMECs decreased compared with that of the normal CMECs, but that was of no statistical significance ($P>0.05$) (Fig. 4B).

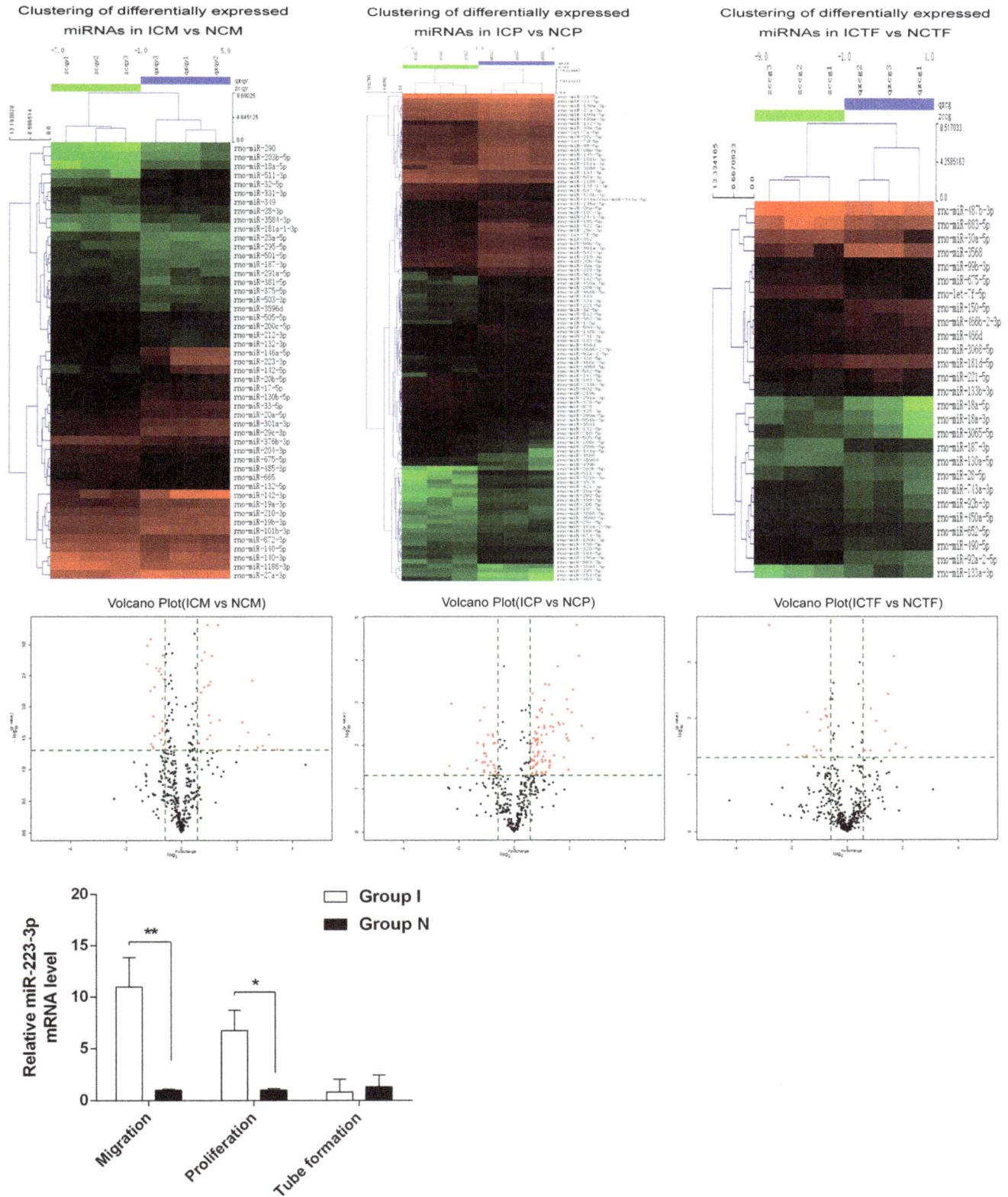

Figure 5. MicroRNA expression profiling in ischemic CMECs proliferation(ICP), ischemic CMECs tube formation (ICTF)and ischemic CMECs migration (ICM)compared with that of normal CMECs proliferation(NCP), normal CMECs tube formation (NCTF) and normal CMECs migration (NCM). A. Differentially expressed miRNAs in ICP(n = 3), ICTF(n = 3) and ICM(n = 3) compared with NCP(n = 3), NCTF(n = 3) and NCM(n = 3). The heat map diagram showed the result of the two-way hierarchical clustering of miRNAs and samples. Each row represented a miRNA and each column repressentsed a sample. The miRNA clustering tree was shown on the left, and the sample clustering tree appeared at the top. The

color scale shown at the top illustrated the relative expression level of a miRNA in the certain slide: red color represented a high relative expression level; green color represented a low relative expression levels. n = 3 in each group. B. Volcano Plots were useful tool for visualizing differential expression between two different conditions. They were constructed using fold-change values and p-values, and thus allowing visualizing the relationship between fold-change (magnitude of change) and statistical significance (which took both magnitude of change and variability into consideration). They also allowed subsets of genes to be isolated, based on those values. The vertical lines corresponded to 1.5-fold up and down, respectively, and the horizontal line represented a p-value of 0.05. So the red point in the plot represented the differentially expressed miRNAs with statistical significance. C. Confirmation of mir-223-3p in the same set of samples as used in microarray assay by means of real-time PCR. ΔCt values were normalized to U6 levels. Relative expression was calculated with respect to normal CMECs. The results were expressed as Log10 ($2^{-\Delta\Delta Ct}$). *P< 0.05, **P<0.01.

The differential expression of miRNAs during the angiogenesis of ischemic CMECs

At present, the expression and function of miRNAs in ischemic CMECs at different stages of angiogenesis is largely unknown. This study explored the expression profile of miRNAs during the different stages of angiogenesis of CMECs by applying miRNAs chip for the first time. Based on the "window" feature of normal/ischemic CMECs angiogenesis process, two groups of cells were further divided according to the time of proliferation, migration and tube formation. Compared with normal CMECs, ischemic CMECs had 40 up-regulated miRNAs and 16 down-regulated miRNAs during proliferation, normal CMECs proliferation (NCP), ischemic CMECs proliferation(ICP) (Table 2), ischemic CMECs had 7 up-regulated miRNAs and 7 down-regulated miRNAs during tube formation, normal CMECs tube formation (NCTF), ischemic CMECs tube formation (ICTF) (Table 3), and ischemic CMECs had 16 up-regulated miRNAs and 6 down-regulated miRNAs during migration, normal CMECs migration (NCM), ischemic CMECs migration (ICM) (Table 4). According to the significance of differential expression and its relationship with angiogenesis, mir-142-5p was confirmed as the key miRNA of the ischemic CMECs proliferation; mir-223-3p was confirmed as the key miRNA of the ischemic CMECs migration; mir-221-5p was confirmed as the key miRNA of the ischemic CMECs tube formation (Table 5). Mir-223-3p had the most significant up-regulation during angiogenesis of ischemic CMECs, in which it increased 3.679 times during proliferation and 11.022 times

during migration. These data indicated that up-regulated mir-223-3p played an important role in the angiogenesis of ischemia CMECs. Finally mir-223-3p was confirmed as the core miRNA of ischemic CMECs. Expression heat maps of the data were presented in Figure 5A. Volcano Plots were presented in Figure 5B.

The result of miRNAs chip analysis was tested and verified by applying real-time RT-PCR, the group division was made as previously described, the result of real-time RT-PCR detection was consistent with that of miRNAs chip analysis. Compared with normal CMECs, mir-223-3p up-regulated significantly during the ischemic CMECs proliferation ($P<0.05$) and migration ($P<0.01$) and down-regulated significantly during the tube formation ($P>0.05$) (Figure 5C).

Rps6kb1 was identified as the direct and functional target of mir-223-3p

MiRNAs functioned by regulating the expression of target genes [27], two-step sequential approach was used to analyze and confirm the direct and functional target of mir-223-3p: (I) three databases of the target gene of mir-223-3p –mirbase, miranda and mirdb were retrieved to predict the target genes possibly related to the angiogenesis. The genes predicted simultaneously in these three databases were chosen as potential target genes to decrease false positive rate (Fig. 6A), 8 genes were filtered: Acsl3, Alcam, Asz1, Cbfb, Cdk2, Ddit4, Rhoj and Rps6kb1. Next, these genes were analyzed by using pathway, during which Rps6kb1 was

Table 3. The differential expression of miRNAs in ICTF and in NCTF (n = 3 in each group).

Gene	Fold change	P value
Up-regulated miRNA in ICTF		
rno-miR-133a-3p	4.334	0.034
rno-miR-3568	3.401	0.029
rno-miR-150-5p	3.233	0.001
rno-miR-221-5p	2.919	0.037
rno-miR-187-3p	2.802	0.004
rno-miR-133b-3p	2.586	0.017
rno-miR-3068-5p	2.073	0.011
Down-regulated miRNAs in ICTF		
rno-miR-92a-2-5p	0.144	0.0002
rno-miR-18a-5p	0.230	0.029
rno-miR-3065-5p	0.329	0.047
rno-miR-18a-3p	0.362	0.046
rno-miR-743a-3p	0.369	0.007
rno-miR-490-5p	0.437	0.032
rno-miR-883-5p	0.467	0.037

Table 4. The differential expression of miRNAs in ICM and in NCM (n = 3 in each group).

Gene	Fold change	P value
Up-regulated miRNA in ICM		
rno-miR-223-3p	11.022	0.049
rno-miR-511-3p	8.907	0.028
rno-miR-142-3p	7.591	0.042
rno-miR-142-5p	6.739	0.045
rno-miR-18a-5p	5.868	0.003
rno-miR-146a-5p	5.326	0.026
rno-miR-32-5p	4.581	0.017
rno-miR-290	4.287	0.042
rno-miR-203b-5p	2.597	0.016
rno-miR-33-5p	2.503	0.0004
rno-miR-101b-3p	2.138	0.001
rno-miR-3584-3p	2.095	0.018
rno-miR-29c-3p	2.055	0.004
rno-miR-331-3p	2.054	0.028
rno-miR-349	2.010	0.004
rno-miR-20b-5p	2.008	0.013
Down-regulated miRNAs in ICM		
rno-miR-132-3p	0.428	0.002
rno-miR-23a-5p	0.428	0.001
rno-miR-375-5p	0.465	0.001
rno-miR-501-5p	0.468	0.005
rno-miR-381-5p	0.475	0.039
rno-miR-132-5p	0.495	0.043

found to regulate angiogenesis by participating in HIF-1signal pathway, therefore, it was predicted that Rps6kb1 (Gene ID: 83840) might be the target gene of mir-223-3p.(II) Western blot was applied to detect the protein expression of Rps6kb1, compared with normal CMECs, the protein expression of Rps6kb1 of ischemic CMECs decreased significantly ($P<0.01$) during proliferation and migration, and there was so significant change in tube formation. The mRNA expression of Rps6kb1 was detected by using real-time PCR in order to clarify the reasons of protein expression decreasing: compared with normal CMECs, the mRNA expression of Rps6kb1 of ischemic CMECs had no significant difference, which proved that down-regulation of Rps6kb1 of ischemic CMECs occurred posttransriptionally, the segregation phenomenon of the gene and protein expression of Rps6kb1 conformed to the regulating laws of miRNA, suggesting that Rps6kb1 might be the direct and functional target of mir-223-3p.

mir-223-3p   UGUCAGUUUGUCAAAUACCCC
Rps6kb1   241 C**AACTGAC**TG...... 301 GCCGTA**AACT-GAC**AGTATTA

Mir-223-3p inhibiting the angiogenesis of ischemic CMECs by affecting RPS6KB1/hif-1a signal pathway

More and more studies had found that many growth factors caused by ischemia and hypoxia functioned via Hif-1a signal pathway [28–29]. According to the results of miRNAs chip analysis, it was concluded that Rps6kb1 regulated the angiogenesis by taking part in hif-1a signal pathway. To study the mechanism of mir-223-3p's regulating the angiogenesis of ischemic CMECs; RPS6KB1/hif-1a signal pathway was used as a research target to analyze whether mir-223-3p regulated the angiogenesis via RPS6KB1/hif-1a signal pathway or not. The gene and protein expression of major molecules hif-1a, VEGF, MAPK, PI3K and Akt of RPS6KB1/hif-1a signal pathway were detected by applying

Table 5. Results of miRNA gene chip analysis.

Group	Gene name	Fold change	Regulation
ICM	mir-223-3p	11.02	up
ICP	mir-142-5p	5.02	up
ICTF	mir-221-5p	2.91	up

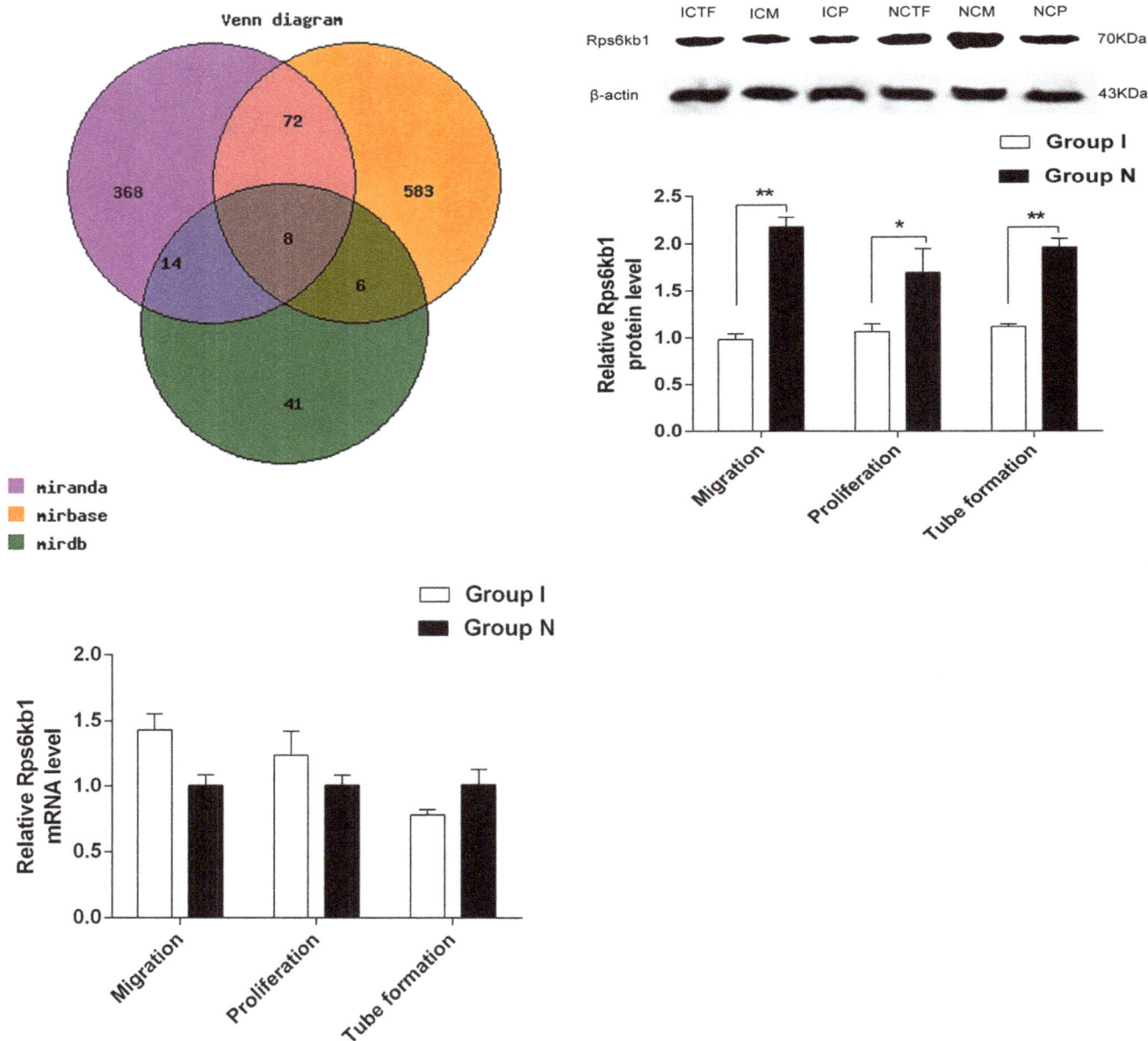

Figure 6. Rps6kb1 was determined as the direct and functional target of mir-223-3p. A. The Venn diagram displayed the overlap between three databases. B. Western blot analyzed the protein level of Rps6kb1 in ICM, ICP and ICTF when compared to that of NCM, NCP and NCTF. β-actin was used as internal controls. (C)Real-time PCR analysis showed no significant difference in RPS6KB1 mRNA expression in ICM, ICP and ICTF when compared to that of NCM, NCP and NCTF. *P<0.05, **P<0.01.

real-time PCR and Western bolt, compared with normal CMECs, the gene and protein expression of above mentioned molecules of ischemic CMECs decreased significantly (Figure 7) during proliferation and migration, and the difference in tube formation had no statistical significance, which proved that mir-223-3p decreased the expression of VEGF via RPS6KB1/hif-1a signal pathway, inhibited MAPK, PI3K and Akt in addition to affecting the proliferation and migration of cells, and finally decreased the angiogenesis.

Discussion

The angiogenic disorders such as decreased myocardial microvascular density and reduced collateral circulation formation etc. are the main pathological changes of ischemic heart diseases. The angiogenesis of microvascular matrix involved the degradation of extracellular matrix, the activation, proliferation, migration, and extension and cell reconstruction of vascular endothelial cells [30–31]. Vascular endothelial cells generally existed statistically and transformed into blood capillaries [32] only after the appropriate stimulation. When ischemic cardiovascular diseases

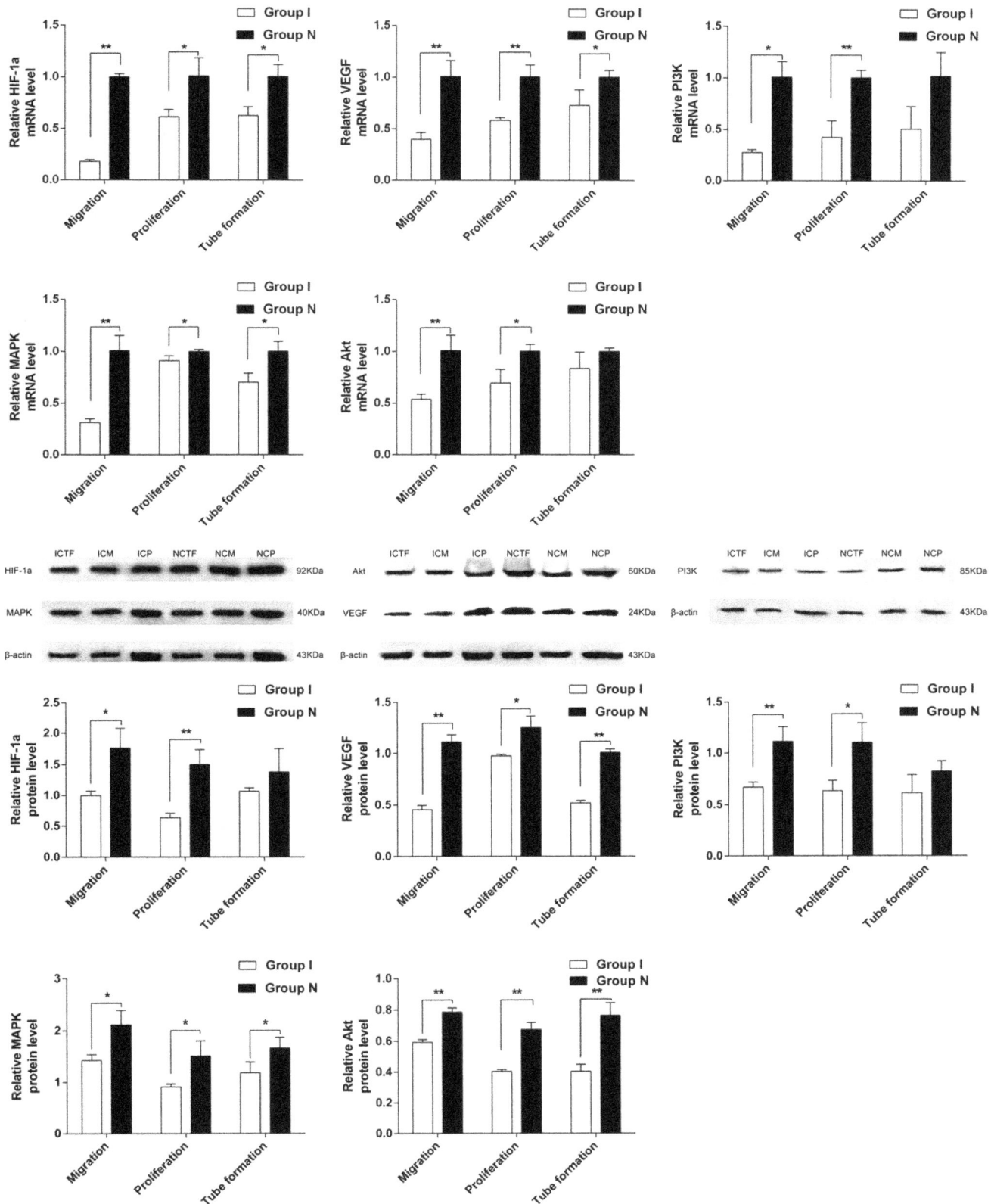

Figure 7. Mir-223-3p inhibited proliferation and migration via affecting RPS6KB1/hif-1a signal pathway. A. Real-time PCR analyzed the mRNA level of hif-1a, VEGF, MAPK, PI3K, Akt in ICM, ICP and ICTF when compared to that of NCM, NCP and NCTF. B. Western blot analyzes the protein level of hif-1a, VEGF, MAPK, PI3K, Akt in ICM, ICP and ICTF when compared to that of NCM, NCP and NCTF. β-actin was used as internal controls. *P< 0.05, **P<0.01.

attacked, the angiogenesis ability of vascular endothelial cells was limited; however, the characteristics of the angiogenesis of ischemic CMECs, the core miRNA of the angiogenesis of ischemic CMECs and its regulating laws were not clear up till now.

This study found the window phases of the angiogenesis of normal/ischemia CMECs in the process of proliferation, migration, and tube formation (Table 1) by establishing the dynamic model of angiogenesis. It was found that compared with normal CMECs, the proliferation period of ischemic CMECs was significantly delayed, the proliferation ratio and the migration ratio of the ischemic CMECs decreased significantly. In order to further explore the regulatory mechanism of the ischemic CMECs angiogenesis, this study divided them into groups according to the window phases of the proliferation, migration and tube formation in the progress in the normal/ischemic CMECs angiogenesis, miRNA chip hybridization was applied to analyze the expressional changes in the process of the ischemic CMECs angiogenesis and to filter the differentially expressed miRNAs, consequently, there were significant changes of the miRNA gene expression profiles at three different stages of angiogenesis: mir-142-5p up-regulated significantly in ischemic CMECs proliferation, mir-223-3p up-regulated significantly in ischemic CMECs migration and mir-221-5p up-regulated significantly in ischemic CMECs tube formation and, among which mir-223-3p up-regulated most significantly, increased 11.02 times in the migration, and increased 3.68 times in proliferation period, which indicated mir-223-3p played an important role in the process of ischemic CMECs angiogenesis. The mir-223-3p results which were verified via real-time PCR were consistent with those of the chip analysis. Bioinformatics predicted that Rps6kb1 was the potential target gene of mir-223-3p, interestingly, segregation phenomenon of Rps6kb1 mRNA and protein expression was found in the in mir-223-3p- increased-significantly group in the research focused on the expression of Rps6kb1, the segregation phenomenon was consistent with the expression of miRNA regulating gene, which indirect proved that Rps6kb1 probably was the functional target of mir-223-3p.

More and more studies had found that many growth factors caused by ischemia and hypoxia functioned via Hif-1a signal pathway. Pathway analysis indicated that Rps6kb1 regulated the angiogenesis by taking part in hif-1a signal pathway, this complex network contained lots of important molecules, among which mir-223-3p was a critical member. Further analysis revealed that the gene and protein expression of lots of important molecules such as VEGF, MAPK, PI3K and Akt of RPS6KB1/hif-1a signal pathway in the ischemic CMECs decreased significantly during the course of the proliferation and migration, and the difference in tube formation had no statistical significance, which suggested that mir-223-3p decreased the expression of VEGF via RPS6KB1/hif-1a signal pathway, inhibited MAPK, PI3K and Akt in addition to

affecting the proliferation and migration of cells ischemic CMECs, and finally decreased the angiogenesis.

Shi L [33] indicate that miR-223 is an antiangiogenic microRNA that prevents endothelial cell proliferation at least partly by targeting β1 integrin. The over-expression of precursor-miR-223 did not affect basal endothelial cell proliferation but abrogated vascular endothelial cell growth factor-induced and basic fibroblast growth factor-induced proliferation, as well as migration and sprouting. MiR-223 over-expression had no effect on the growth factor-induced activation of ERK1/2 but inhibited the vascular endothelial cell growth factor-induced and basic fibroblast growth factor-induced phosphorylation of their receptors and activation of Akt. β1 integrin was identified as a target of miR-223 and its down-regulation reproduced the defects in growth factor receptor phosphorylation and Akt signaling seen after miR-223 overexpression. Reintroduction of β1 integrin into miR-223-ovexpressing cells was sufficient to rescue growth factor signaling and angiogenesis.

Although we found Rps6kb1 could be taken as the potential functional target of mir-223-3p, Rps6kb1 was not the only target gene of mir-223-3p, the function of mir-223-3p came into true through regulating a set of target genes expression after transcription, so we should go on delving into other target genes of mir-223-3p in the future, and to get further comprehensive understanding of mir-223-3p in ischemic CMECs of the progress of angiogenesis. Otherwise, we selected many differentially expressed miRNAs by miRNA chip, mir-223-3p was the most significant of them, and there were other differentially expressed miRNA in ischemic CMECs which played a role in the progress of angiogenesis which needed further research. And then the present study just observed the expressed significantly difference of mir-223-3p in the angiogenesis of the ischemic CMECs, however, whether the intervention of mir-223-3p would improve ischemic CMECs angiogenesis or not remained to be confirmed by further experiments, and we would regulate the expression of mir-223-3p in the following experiments and observe the influence on the angiogenesis of the ischemic CMECs.

In conclusion, this study elucidated the miRNA regulating law in the angiogenesis of CMECs; mir-223-3p inhibited the process of migration and proliferation of ischemic CMECs via affecting RPS6KB1/hif-1a signal pathway, which in turn suppressed the angiogenesis. It is highly possible that mir-223-3p became a novel intervention core target in the treatment of angiogenesis of ischemic heart diseases.

Author Contributions

Conceived and designed the experiments: GHD. Performed the experiments: PZM XBS NL. Analyzed the data: TZ BW. Contributed reagents/materials/analysis tools: PZM XBS NL TZ BW. Wrote the paper: GHD PZM XBS NL.

References

1. Han YC, Park CY, Bhagat G, Zhang J, Wang Y, et al. (2010) MicroRNA-29a induces aberrant self-renewal capacity in hematopoietic progenitors, biased myeloid development, and acute myeloid leukemia. J Exp Med 207(3): 475–489.

2. Qin W, Shi Y, Zhao B, Yao C, Jin L, et al. (2010) MiR-24 regulates apoptosis by targeting the open reading frame (ORF) region of FAF1 in cancer cells. PLoS ONE 5(2): e9429.

3. Tie J, Pan Y, Zhao L, Wu K, Liu J, et al. (2010) MiR-218 inhibits invasion and metastasis of gastric cancer by targeting the Robo1 receptor. PLoS Genet 6(3): e1000879.

4. Filipowicz W, Bhattacharyya SN, Sonenberg N (2008) Mechanisms of post-transcriptional regulation by microRNAs: are the answers in sight. Nat Rev Genet 9(2):102–114.

5. Lewis BP, Burge CB, Bartel DP (2005) Conserved seed pairing, often flanked by adenosines, indicates that thousands of human genes are microRNA targets. Ceel 120(1):15–20.

6. Rajewsky N (2006) microRNA target predictions in animals. Nat Genet 38 Suppl: S8–S13.

7. Pasquinelli AE, Reinhart BJ, Slack F, Martindale MQ, Kuroda MI, et al. (2000) Conservation of the sequence and temporal expression of let-7 heterochronic regulatory RNA. Nature 408: 86–89.

8. Fish JE, Santoro MM, Morton SU, Yu S, Yeh RF, et al. (2008) MiR-126 regulates angiogenic signaling and vascular integrity. Dev Cell 15:272–284.

9. Poliseno L, Tuccoli A, Mariani L, Evangelista M, Citti L, et al. (2006) MicroRNAs modulate the angiogenic properties of HUVECs. Blood 108: 3068–3071.

10. Wang S, Aurora AB, Johnson BA, Qi X, McAnally J, et al. (2008) The Endothelial-specific microRNA miR-126 governs vascular integrity and angiogenesis. Dev Cell 15(2): 261–271.

11. Chen Y, Gorski DH (2008) Regulation of angiogenesis through a microRNA (miR-130a) that down-regulates antiangiogenic homeobox genes GAX and HOXA5Blood. 111(3): 1217–1226.

12. Lee DY, Deng Z, Wang CH, Yang BB (2007) MicroRNA-378 promotes cell survival, tumor growth, and angiogenesis by targeting SuFu and Fus-1 expression. Proc Natl Acad Sci USA 104(51):20350–20355.

13. Zhou Q, Gallagher R, Ufret-Vincenty R, Li X, Olson EN, et al. (2011) Regulation of angiogenesis and choroidal neovascularization by members of microRNA-23~27~24 clusters. Proc Natl Acad Sci U S A 108(20): 8287–8292.

14. Kim JH, Park SG, Song SY, Kim JK, Sung JH (2013) Reactive oxygen species-responsive miR-210 regulates proliferation and migration of adipose-derived stem cells via PTPN2. Cell Death Dis 4(4): e588.

15. Doebele C, Bonauer A, Fischer A, Scholz A, Reiss Y, et al. (2010) Members of the microRNA-17-92 cluster exhibit a cell-intrinsic antiangiogenic function in endothelial cells. Blood 115(23):4944–4950.

16. Mujahid S, Nielsen HC, Volpe MV (2013) MiR-221 and miR-130a regulate lung airway and vascular development. PLoS One 8(2):e55911.

17. Drexler H, Depenbusch JW, Truog AG, Zelis R, Flaim SF (1985) Effects of diltiazem on cardiac function and regional blood flow at rest and during exercise in a conscious rat preparation of chronic heart failure(myocardial infarction). Circulation 71(6):1260–1272.

18. Sadoshima J, Jahn L, Takahashi T, Kulik TJ, Izumo S (1992) Molecular characterization of the stretch-induced adaptation of cultured cardiac cells. J Biol Chem 267:10 551–10 560.

19. Manthey JA, Guthrie N (2002) Antiproliferative activities of citrus flavonoids against six human cancer cell lines. J Agric Food Chem 50:5837–5843.

20. Hwang YJ, Park SM, Yim CB, Im C (2013) Cytotoxic activity and quantitative structure activity relationships of arylpropyl sulfonamides. Korean J Physiol Pharmacol 17:237–243.

21. Lim JC, Park SY, Nam Y, Nguyen TT, Sohn UD (2012) The protective effect of eupatilin against hydrogen peroxide-induced injury involving 5-lipoxygenase in feline esophageal epithelial cells. Korean J Physiol Pharmacol 16:313–320.

22. Park SY, Sohn UD (2011) Inhibitory effect of rosiglitazone on the acid-induced intracellular generation of hydrogen peroxide in cultured feline esophageal epithelial cells. Naunyn Schmiedebergs Arch Pharmacol 383:191–201.

23. Cory G (2011) Scratch-wound assay. Methods Mol Biol 769: 25–30.

24. Yuan ZK, Mo L, Huang XP, Chen QH, Jian WX, et al. (2009) The impact of the effective components recipe of YangXinTongMai Formula on the angiogenesis of rat endothelium. Progress in Modern Biomedicine 9(8):1405–1408.

25. Kass RW, Kotler MN, Yazdanfar S (1992) Stimulation of coronary collateral growth: current developments in angiogenesis and future clinical applications. Am Heart J 123(2):486–96.

26. Chen C, Ridzon DA, Broomer AJ, Zhou Z, Lee DH, et al. (2005) Real-time quantification of microRNAs by stem-loop RT-PCR. Nucleic Acids Res 33:e179.

27. Bartel DP (2004) MicroRNAs: genomics, biogenesis, mechanism, and function. Cell 116: 281–297.

28. Koshiji M, Kageyama Y, Pete EA, Horikawa I, Barrett JC, et al. (2004) HIF-1alpha induces cell cycle arrest by functionally counteracting Myc [J].EMBO J 23(9):1949–1956.

29. Bardos JI, Chau NM, Ashcroft M (2004) Growth factor-mediated induction of HDM2 positively regulates hypoxia-inducible factor 1alpha expression [J]. Mol cell Biol 24(7):2905–2914.

30. Sellke FW, Simons M (1999) Angiogenesis in cardiovascular disease: current status and therapeutic potential. Drugs 58(3):391–396.

31. Pu LQ, Sniderman AD, Brassard R, Lachapelle KJ, Graham AM, et al. (1993) Enhanced revascularization of the ischemic limb by angiogenic therapy. Circulation 88(1):208–215.

32. Choi DW, Maulucci GM, Kriegstein AR (1987) Glutamate neurotoxicity in cortical cell cuhure. J Neurosci 7(2):357–368.

33. Shi L, Fisslthaler B, Zippel N, Frömel T, Hu J, et al. (2013) MicroRNA-223 antagonizes angiogenesis by targeting β1 integrin and preventing growth factor signaling in endothelial cells. Circ Res 113(12):1320–1330.

3

An *In Vitro* Cord Formation Assay Identifies Unique Vascular Phenotypes Associated with Angiogenic Growth Factors

Beverly L. Falcon[1◐], **Michelle Swearingen**[1], **Wendy H. Gough**[2], **Linda Lee**[1], **Robert Foreman**[3], **Mark Uhlik**[1], **Jeff C. Hanson**[4], **Jonathan A. Lee**[2], **Don B. McClure**[5], **Sudhakar Chintharlapalli**[1*◐]

1 Department of Cancer Angiogenesis, Eli Lilly and Company, Lilly Corporate Center, Indianapolis, Indiana, United States of America, 2 Department of Quantitative Biology, Eli Lilly and Company, Lilly Corporate Center, Indianapolis, Indiana, United States of America, 3 Department of In Vivo Pharmacology, Eli Lilly and Company, Lilly Corporate Center, Indianapolis, Indiana, United States of America, 4 Department of Informatics Capabilities, Eli Lilly and Company, Lilly Corporate Center, Indianapolis, Indiana, United States of America, 5 Department of BioTDR, Eli Lilly and Company, Lilly Corporate Center, Indianapolis, Indiana, United States of America

Abstract

Vascular endothelial growth factor (VEGF) plays a dominant role in angiogenesis. While inhibitors of the VEGF pathway are approved for the treatment of a number of tumor types, the effectiveness is limited and evasive resistance is common. One mechanism of evasive resistance to inhibition of the VEGF pathway is upregulation of other pro-angiogenic factors such as fibroblast growth factor (FGF) and epidermal growth factor (EGF). Numerous *in vitro* assays examine angiogenesis, but many of these assays are performed in media or matrix with multiple growth factors or are driven by VEGF. In order to study angiogenesis driven by other growth factors, we developed a basal medium to use on a co-culture cord formation system of adipose derived stem cells (ADSCs) and endothelial colony forming cells (ECFCs). We found that cord formation driven by different angiogenic factors led to unique phenotypes that could be differentiated and combination studies indicate dominant phenotypes elicited by some growth factors. VEGF-driven cords were highly covered by smooth muscle actin, and bFGF-driven cords had thicker nodes, while EGF-driven cords were highly branched. Multiparametric analysis indicated that when combined EGF has a dominant phenotype. In addition, because this assay system is run in minimal medium, potential proangiogenic molecules can be screened. Using this assay we identified an inhibitor that promoted cord formation, which was translated into *in vivo* tumor models. Together this study illustrates the unique roles of multiple anti-angiogenic agents, which may lead to improvements in therapeutic angiogenesis efforts and better rational for anti-angiogenic therapy.

Editor: Domenico Ribatti, University of Bari Medical School, Italy

Funding: All of the authors are employed with Eli Lilly and Company. The funder provided support in the form of salaries for all the authors, but did not have any additional role in the study design, data collection and analysis, decision to publish, or preparation of the manuscript. The specific roles of these authors are articulated in the "author contributions" section.

Competing Interests: The work is funded by Lilly Research Laboratories. All of the authors are employees of Eli Lilly and Company and received salary from them. There are no patents, products in development or marketed products to declare.

* Email: chintharlapalli_sudhakar@lilly.com

◐ These authors contributed equally to this work.

Introduction

Angiogenesis, the formation of new blood vessels from existing vessels, is a complex multistep process involving numerous growth factors. These steps include initiation, tip formation and sprouting, migration, proliferation, lumen formation, anastamosis, and maturation [1]. While numerous growth factors have been shown to play a role in the angiogenic process, vascular endothelial growth factor (VEGF) appears to have a dominant role [1].

Inhibitors targeting the VEGF pathway have had some success in the clinic; however, the effects of anti-angiogenic therapy tend to result in transitory improvements measured in months. These treatments result in tumor stasis and shrinkage with some resulting in increased survival. Inevitably, however, the tumors return to growth and progression in many patients. A number of possible evasive resistance pathways have been proposed [2]. One feasible evasive resistance mechanism of anti-angiogenic therapies is the induction of other pro-angiogenic factors to re-establish the tumor vasculature. In fact, profiling of gene expression changes associated with resistance to VEGF inhibitors in xenograft models, showed that EGFR and FGFR pathways were upregulated in the stroma [3]. bFGF has also been shown to drive revascularization in the RIP-Tag2 model after acquiring resistance to anti-VEGFR2 therapy [4]. Targeting VEGF and bFGF with a dual inhibitor, has subsequently been shown to inhibit tumor progression after resistance to VEGF inhibition [4,5].

Numerous in vitro and in vivo assays have been developed to examine the various steps in the angiogenic process including sprouting and tip formation, migration, differentiation, proliferation, lumen formation, and tube or cord formation [6]. Many of these assays are driven by VEGF or have multiple growth factors in the medium. Little is known about the distinct phenotypes and roles of other angiogenic factors in driving angiogenesis. We have developed a basal medium that allows the characterization of other angiogenic growth factors on cord formation. We found that growth factors such as HGF, EGF, and bFGF can induce cord formation in this system. Interestingly, each of the growth factors induces a unique phenotype that can be differentiated and growth factor combinations indicate dominant growth factor phenotypes. This co-culture system with minimal basal medium also allows for the identification of unique pro-angiogenic drugs or factors and translates into in vivo xenograft models.

Methods

ADSC and ECFC co-culture cord formation assay

Human adipose derived stem cells (ADSCs) and endothelial colony forming cells (ECFCs) purchased from Lonza (Allendale, NJ) were cultured as previously described [7]. ADSC and ECFC co-culture assays were performed in basal medium (MCDB-131 medium with 30 µg/mL L-ascorbic acid 2-phosphate, 1 µM dexamethasone, 50 µg/mL tobramycin, 10 µg/mL r-transferrin AF, and 10 µg/mL insulin). ADSCs were plated in 96 well plates at 40–50K cells per well and incubated overnight at 37°C, 5% CO_2. The next day, the media was removed and 4–5K ECFCs were plated on the ADSC monolayer, incubated at 37°C, 5% CO_2 for 3–6 hours to allow ECFC attachment before the addition of growth factors and/or inhibitors (2–5X) to achieve the indicated final concentrations. The differences in cell counts reflect differences observed with different cell counters. For validation experiments, a modified assay to increase pericyte association was used whereby 15K ADSCs and 3K ECFCs were plated in a 384-well plate. When indicated cell bound growth factors were removed from the ADSC monolayer by a 60 minute treatment with 500 µg/mL sodium heparin (Sigma) in basal medium prior to ECFC addition. Co-cultures were grown for 3 days, at which time they were fixed, stained, and imaged as described below.

Growth factors and inhibitors

Multiple doses of growth factors were used to determine the optimal dose to use for subsequent studies (data not shown). Vascular endothelial growth factor (VEGF; R&D Systems) was used at 10–20 ng/mL, hepatocyte growth factor (HGF; R&D Systems) at 100 ng/mL basic fibroblast growth factor (bFGF; Invitrogen) at 50 ng/mL, and epidermal growth factor (EGF; Invitrogen) at 20 ng/mL. To block VEGF and HGF signaling, antibodies to VEGF (Bevacizumab; 10 µg/mL) and HGF (R&D Systems; 10 µg/mL) were used. To examine whether additional growth factors were dependent on each other to induce cords, inhibitors to VEGFR2 (Ramucirumab), bFGF (bFGF antibody; Invitrogen), or EGFR (Gefitinib) were used in basal, VEGF, bFGF, and EGF driven cords. Finally, a TGF-β inhibitor (LY2157299), an inactive control (LY596144), and a multikinase inhibitor (SU11248, Sutent) were tested to examine increases in cord or tumor vessels.

Fixation, staining, imaging, and quantification of the cords

Following completion of the assay, the ADSC/ECFC co-culture was fixed and permeabilized with either 70% ice cold ethanol or 80% ethanol (which gives equivalent staining; data not shown) for 10–20 minutes. Cells were stained essentially as previously described [7]. Endothelial cells were detected with a sheep anti-CD31 (PECAM-1; Sigma; 1:200) antibody, smooth muscle actin (SMA) was detected with either a Cy3 conjugated mouse anti-smooth muscle actin (Sigma; 1:200) or a mouse anti-human SMA antibody (Sigma; 1:200), and nuclei was detected with Hoechst 33342 (Invitrogen; 1:1000). Secondary AlexaFluor 488 or 647 conjugated anti-sheep and anti-mouse antibodies were used for detection (Invitrogen; 1:400).

Cord formation images were capture with either a Cellomics Arrayscan VTI or an Acumen eX3 microplate cytometer. Images taken on the Arrayscan were read at a 5X magnification and the tube formation bio-application was used to detect CD31 staining. Total tube area was calculated from 9 fields for each well with 3–4 wells for each treatment. SMA index was calculated from the intensity of the SMA staining and related to the number of cords as previously described [7]. Tiff images of the entire well were collected with the Acumen eX3. The images were then analyzed with a customized Image Pro algorithm to assess the nuclear area, cord area, and SMA area. In addition, custom built Image J software analysis was used to measure over 100 different descriptors (**Table S1**) to differentiate and assess the different growth factor dependent morphologies. Clustering of the different descriptors were performed in an unsupervised manner as to not place particular meaning on each individual parameter, but rather to utilize these characteristics as unique phenotypes.

Analysis of growth factors secreted by the cord formation assay

Basal medium, media collected from ADSC monocultures, media collected from ADSC/ECFC co-cultures, and media collected from cocultures treated with VEGF were analyzed for growth factors using Luminex beads according to the manufacturers' protocol (R&D Systems and Millipore).

Effects of TGF-β inhibition in A549 in vivo study

A549 NSCLC tumor cells (5×10^6 cells) were mixed 1:1 with Matrigel (BD Biosciences) and injected subcutaneously into the flank of CD1 nu/nu male mice. Tumors were allowed to grow to ~150 mm³ (~7–10 days) prior to treatment. Animals were orally treated by oral gavage with twice a day (BID) dosing of vehicle, a TGF-β inhibitor (LY2157299; 75 mg/kg), an inactive control (LY596144; 100 mg/kg), or a multi-tyrosine kinase inhibitor targeting VEGF (Sutent, SU11248; 20 mg/kg) for 5 days prior to fixation and staining. Tumors were fixed in Zn Tris, processed, and embedded in paraffin. Four micron sections were cut and stained with a CD31 antibody (PECAM; Pharmingen 550274) and Alexa Fluor 488 conjugated secondary antibodies. Each tumor was imaged at 10× with an inverted fluorescence microscope looking at multiple fields residing completely within the tumor that were well-separated and non-overlapping. The number of fields imaged ranged between 2 to 11 fields and depended upon the size of tumor and amount of non-necrotic tissue present. The following total number of fields was imaged for each group: non-treated (43), LY2157299 (45), LY596144 (31), and Sutent (45). The field data for total area of blood vessels (using CD31) as a ratio of total tissue area (using Hoechst 33342) for individual tumors was averaged to derive the individual tumor vessel density values. The individual tumor values within a group were averaged to derive the group vessel density values expressed with standard errors and P-values. Four to eight animals were analyzed in each treatment group.

Statistical analysis

Results were expressed as means ±SEM. Statistical differences were analyzed by ANOVA with a Tukey or Dunnett's posthoc test using JMP software.

Results

Characterization of growth factors present in the ADSC/ECFC co-culture system

Studies indicate that co-cultures of ADSCs and ECFCs lead to robust cord formation with associated SMA positive pericyte-like structures in response to VEGF (**Figure 1A, Figure S1**) [7,8]. This assay can be run in 96 and 384 well format with qualitative analysis on either an ArrayScan or an Acumen ([7] and **Figure S2**). Quantitative validation was performed on a similar assay ran on the Acumen eX3 in a 384 well format (Z' score = 0.68 or 0.70 and MSR = 1.69 or 1.99 for tube area and SMA area analysis respectively; **Figure S2**).

To examine the ability of other angiogenic growth factors to induce cord formation we developed a basal cord formation media which lacks serum and other growth factors typically found in traditional assay systems [7,9,10]. To determine which factors were endogenously produced in the ADSC/ECFC co-culture system, Luminex profiling of multiple angiogenic growth factors was examined. Compared to basal medium alone, ADSCs secreted VEGF and HGF into the medium (**Figure 1B**). Co-culturing ADSCs with ECFCs without exogenous growth factors appeared to reduce the levels of VEGF secretion into the medium, but did not alter the secretion of HGF (**Figure 1B**). Interestingly, the addition of VEGF to ADSC monocultures did not change the secretion of any of the factors we examined, however VEGF treatment of the co-cultures increased accumulated secretion of TGF-β and Ang1 at 96hrs and Ang2 at 48 and 96 hours (**Figure 1B**). Additional angiogenic factors such as bFGF, PDGF, and EGF were not secreted above basal levels at any of the time points or culture conditions (data not shown).

To confirm the importance of HGF in basal cord formation, antibodies targeting VEGF or HGF were tested (**Figure 2**). Treatment of basal cords with an anti-VEGF antibody did not reduce the cord formation or the associated SMA. Basal cords were significantly reduced, however, when treated with an antibody targeting HGF. SMA was still associated with the few remaining cords causing the SMA index to increase (**Figure 2**).

Cord formation phenotypes driven by different angiogenic factors

Most in vitro angiogenesis assays are dependent on VEGF. However, multiple angiogenic factors have been described. Because bFGF and EGF upregulation has been demonstrated in resistance to inhibitors of the VEGF pathway [2–5] and are not endogenously present within our co-culture system, we chose to focus our studies on EGF and bFGF driven cords and how they may differ from VEGF and HGF driven cords (**Figure 3**). VEGF stimulation in the ADSC and ECFC co-culture system led to a robust increase in total tube area, a greater branching index, and increased length to width ratio which was inhibited by an anti-VEGF antibody (Bevacizumab; **Figure 3**). Exogenous addition of HGF, which was highly expressed in the basal system (**Figure 1**), did not increase cord formation. If, however, a heparin wash prior to plating ECFCs was performed, which may strip bound-HGF from the basal system, HGF driven cords were seen (**Figure S3**). Exogenous bFGF and EGF, two growth factors that had no detectable expression in the basal system, were able to induce cords in the ADSC/ECFC co-culture system (**Figure 3**). Both of these angiogenic factors increased total tube area, branching, and length to width ratio of the cords; but both had less SMA associated with the cords (**Figure 3**). Qualitatively, bFGF cords appeared to have thicker nodes and EGF thinner nodes compared to VEGF driven cords. Interestingly, while bFGF-driven cords

were not affected by Bevacizumab, EGF driven cords had small decreases in some of the readouts (**Figure 3**). Taken together these results indicate that the in vitro basal medium ECFC/ADSC cord formation assay responds to multiple pro-angiogenic factors as observed in tumor models in vivo [4].

To determine which phenotypes were dominant, growth factor combinations were used to induce cord formation (**Figure 4**). Combining VEGF with HGF led to a phenotype that was similar to the VEGF driven cords (**Figure 4**). Similarly, the combination of bFGF and HGF had cords that phenotypically look like bFGF cords (**Figures 3 and 4**). This was likely because (as shown with the single growth factors) the endogenous levels of HGF secreted by the system itself were already high. Interestingly, when VEGF and bFGF were combined the phenotype was almost a hybrid of each growth factor alone (**Figures 3 and 4**). These cords were highly branched and had some SMA coverage similar to the VEGF driven cords, but had large nodes indicative of bFGF-driven cords (**Figure 3**). When VEGF was inhibited with Bevacizumab, the phenotype looked more similar to bFGF driven cords (**Figures 3 and 4**). When bFGF was combined with EGF, the EGF phenotype appeared dominant as the large nodes and lack of SMA associated with bFGF driven cords was not seen. Instead the cords had some SMA and were long with very small nodes (**Figure 4**). Combining HGF with EGF and bFGF had a phenotype similar to EGF or the bFGF and EGF combo (**Figure 4**). To further understand these vascular phenotypes associated with the different growth factors driving cord formation, an Image J algorithm was developed to measure 101 different endothelial and pericyte descriptors (**Table S1**) from whole well images of the various growth factor driven cords (**Figure 5**). Basal, HGF, bFGF, EGF, and bFGF + HGF driven cord phenotypes were able to differentiate from one another and other treatments using three readouts: branch width, branch node quad connection, and tube area (**Figure 5**). The five remaining growth factor driven phenotypes could then be separated by four additional parameters. bFGF + EGF and HGF+EGF+bFGF were able to be differentiated from the rest based on the nuclear intensity in the segment area, SMA area and branch node quad connection (**Figure 5**). Finally, VEGF, VEGF+bFGF, and VEGF+HGF phenotypes were able to be separated by looking at SMA area, branch node SMA area, and standard deviation of the nuclear intensity in the nuclei area (**Figure 5**). These results also confirm the observations made with the ArrayScan that EGF is the dominant phenotype when combined with bFGF, as the combinations cluster more closely to EGF driven cords. This analysis also indicates that while the addition of HGF to VEGF or bFGF originally didn't show a difference compared to VEGF or bFGF alone, use of a multiparametric analysis can differentiate phenotypes and indicates that the addition of HGF has subtle effects on endothelial-pericyte network phenotypes.

To evaluate whether the phenotypes associated with different growth factor driven cord formation is a direct effect of the growth factors or some secondary signaling, we assessed the effects of inhibition on cord formation. Inhibition of VEGFR-2 with IMC-1121B (Ramucirumab; Ram) blocked basal (IC50 = 0.32 μg/ml), VEGF (IC50 = 0.96 μg/ml), and EGF (IC50 = 0.14 μg/ml) driven cords, but not bFGF driven cords (IC50>10 μg/ml) (**Figure 6**). In contrast, inhibition of cord formation with an anti-bFGF antibody uniquely affected FGF driven cords with (IC50 = 0.013 μg/ml) and a small molecule EGFR inhibitor (Gefitinib) specifically inhibited EGF driven cords (IC50 = 3.1 μM) unless given at high concentrations (**Figure 6**). The IC50 values for anti-bFGF antibody on VEGF and EGF driven cords were greater than 10 μg/ml.

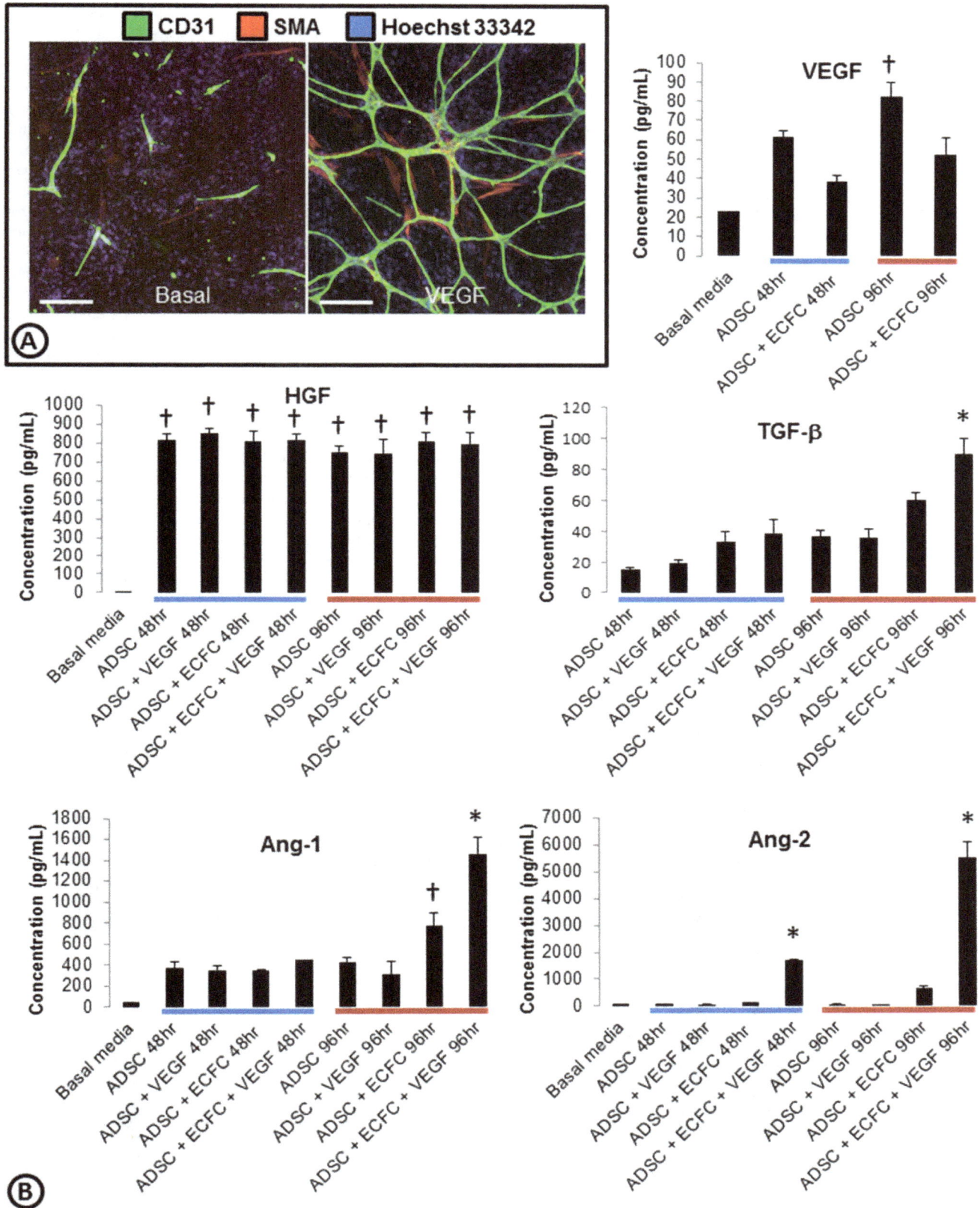

Figure 1. Characterization of growth factors present in the ADSC/ECFC co-culture system. (**A**) Basal or VEGF driven co-cultures of ADSCs and ECFCs were stained for cords (CD31; green), smooth muscle actin (SMA; red), and nuclei (Hoechst 33342; blue). (**B**) Media was collected from ADSCs alone or ADSC/ECFC co-cultures in basal or VEGF driven conditions at 48 (blue bar) and 96 hrs (red bar). Examination of angiogenic growth

factors present in the collected media was measured using Luminex. VEGF, HGF, TGF-β, Ang1, and Ang2 had detectable levels above basal media, while bFGF, EGF, and PDGF were not detected (data not shown). n = 3–4 per group with similar results found on two separate experiments. * = p< 0.05 vs. all other treatment groups. † = p<0.05 vs. basal media. Scale bars are 250 μm.

Pro-angiogenic activity of small molecules

Development of a medium for the ECFC/ADSC cord formation assay which lacks serum or growth factors allows testing of potential pro-angiogenic small molecules without interference from angiogenic growth factors. It is known that TGF-β inhibits endothelial cell proliferation [11–13]. Therefore a TGF-β type 1 receptor inhibitor (LY2157299) was tested in the cord formation assay. LY2157299 increased total tube area by 149% (**Figure 7**) when tested in basal medium but only increased VEGF driven cords by 37%. To assess whether these observations would be translated in vivo, we tested LY2157299 in a xenograft model and observed that the vessel area of A549 tumors significantly increased (**Figure 7C**). In contrast, a structural analog of LY215299 that served as an inactive control compound (LY596144) did not increase vessel area and Sutent (SU11248), a multi-targeted receptor tyrosine kinase targeting VEGFR, decreased the vessel area (**Figure 7C**). A significant increase in tumor vessel area with LY2157299 was also seen in the U87MG glioblastoma tumor xenograft model (data not shown). These results provide a qualitative correlation between these in vitro and in vivo models of angiogenesis, an important aspect if considering an in vitro system for phenotypic drug discovery [14].

Discussion

Neo-vascularization is a complex process with coordinated cellular signaling between precursor and mature forms of endothelial cells with stromal cells (fibroblasts, smooth muscle cells, and pericytes) coupled with morphological changes including endothelial tube formation, anastomosis, endothelial sprouting, and endothelial vessel stabilization by pericyte recruitment/ differentiation. While vascular endothelial growth factor, VEGF, is recognized as the dominant pro-angiogenic factor, other factors such as fibroblast growth factor, epidermal growth factor, hepatocyte growth factor, angiopoietins, thrombomodulin, notch ligands, and transforming growth factor- β are involved as well. Endothelial cord formation in co-cultures of mature endothelial and smooth muscle cells are dependent on addition of VEGF, bFGF, and EGF (16) but do not inform on pericyte differentiation. Development of a basal media co-culture system of progenitor endothelial and stromal cells provide an opportunity to study the roles of multiple angiogenic factors on endothelial cord formation and pericyte differentiation. We found that HGF, bFGF, EGF, and VEGF can all drive cord formation in this system, but each has a unique phenotype that can be differentiated using multiparametric analysis. In general, we find that VEGF has small nodes with many branched and connected tubes and is associated with high levels of SMA. In contrast, bFGF driven cords have thick nodes that are not associated with SMA and EGF has thin nodes with less branching and intermediate levels of SMA. When growth factors were combined, we found that EGF drives a dominate phenotype, while other growth factors have a mixed phenotype when combined (ie VEGF + bFGF). Together these results demonstrate the unique roles of different growth factors in inducing angiogenesis and while different growth factors can induce angiogenesis, the blood vessels that form may not be the

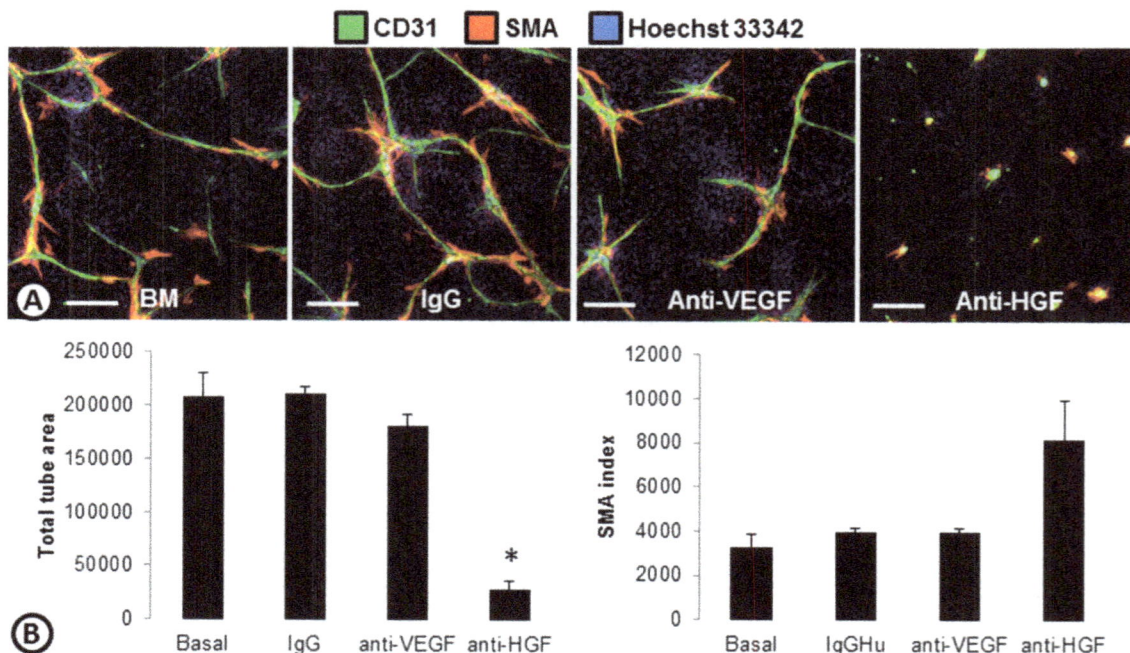

Figure 2. The role of endogenous growth factors in basal cord formation. (**A**) Basal cords made with ADSCs and ECFCs without the addition of growth factors were treated with IgG, or anti-VEGF or anti-HGF antibodies and stained for cords (CD31; green), smooth muscle actin (SMA; red), and nuclei (Hoechst 33342; blue). (**B**) Basal cords treated with IgG, anti-VEGF, or anti-HGF were quantified on the ArrayScan and the total tube area (left) and SMA index (right) are shown. * p<0.0001 vs basal. n = 3 per group. Scale bars are 250 μm.

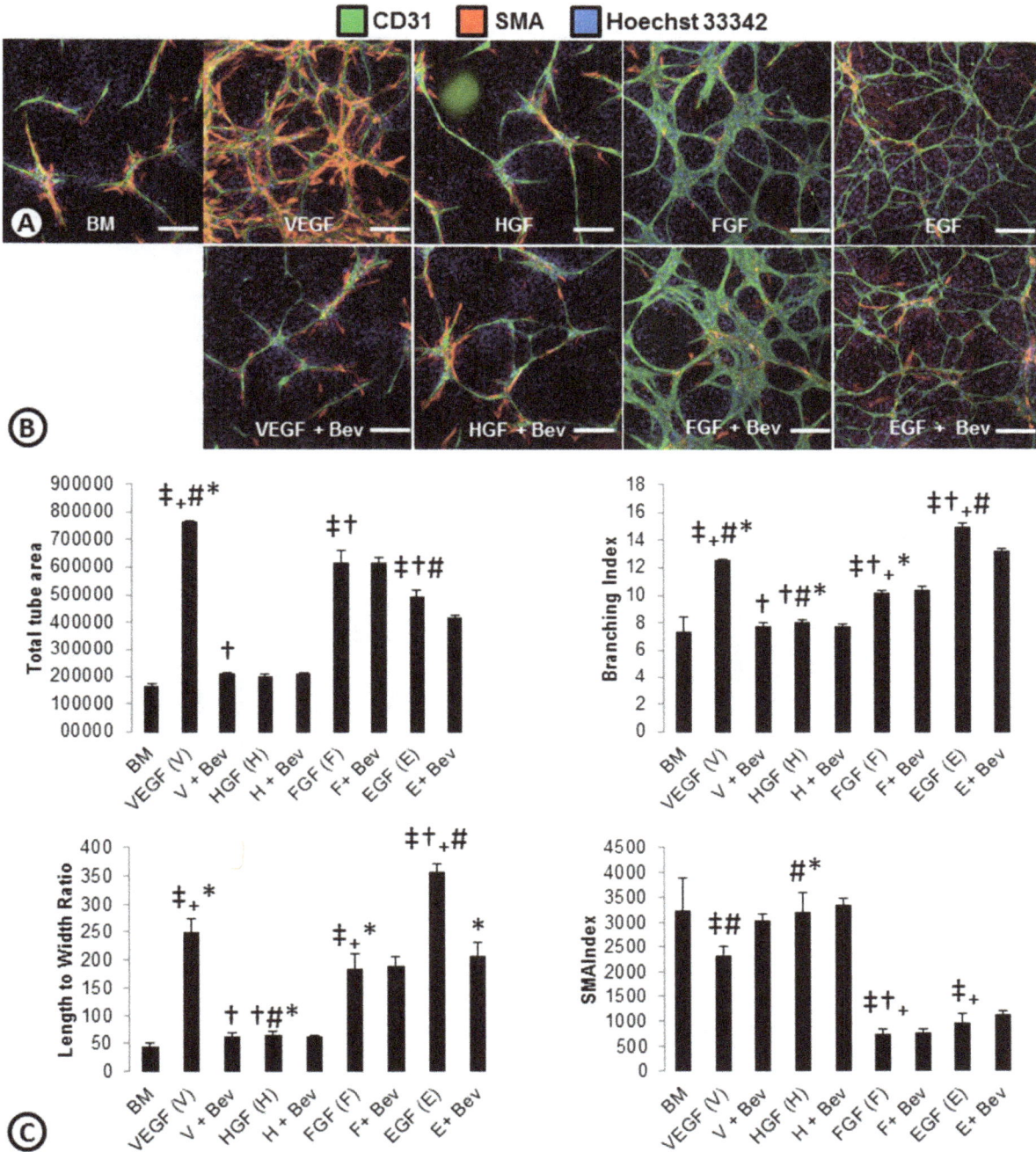

Figure 3. Cord phenotypes driven by angiogenic growth factors. (**A**) ADSC and ECFC co-cultures were stimulated with angiogenic growth factors; VEGF, HGF, bFGF, or EGF and stained for cords (CD31; green), smooth muscle actin (SMA; red), and nuclei (Hoechst 33342; blue). (**B**) To assess whether the cord induction was dependent on VEGF, cords were treated with the different angiogenic factors plus an anti-VEGF antibody (Bevacizumab; Bev). (**C**) ArrayScan quantification of total tube area, branching index, length to width ratio and SMA index are shown as an indication of phenotypes associated with the VEGF, HGF, bFGF, or EGF driven cords. n = 3 per group. ‡ = p<0.05 vs. BM. † = p<0.05 vs. VEGF. # = p<0.05 vs. bFGF. ₊ = p<0.05 vs. HGF. * = p<0.05 vs. EGF. Scale bars are 250 μm.

same. In addition, we show that use of a basal medium allows one to interrogate these individual roles of the growth factors and allows for the identification of other proangiogenic factors and drugs such as an inhibitor of TGF-β receptor.

Evaluation of growth factors in the ADSC and ECFC co-cultures revealed expression of VEGF, HGF, TGF-β and Ang1 by the feeder layer (ADSCs). Addition of ECFCs decreased the level

of VEGF in the medium. This may be a reflection of internalization and degradation of the ligand by endothelial cells [15]. High levels of HGF are secreted by ADSCs and are the main driver of basal cord formation in our system as inhibition of HGF by an antibody almost completely eliminates basal cord formation. Addition of HGF to the system doesn't induce more cord formation, but this is likely due to saturation of the system by

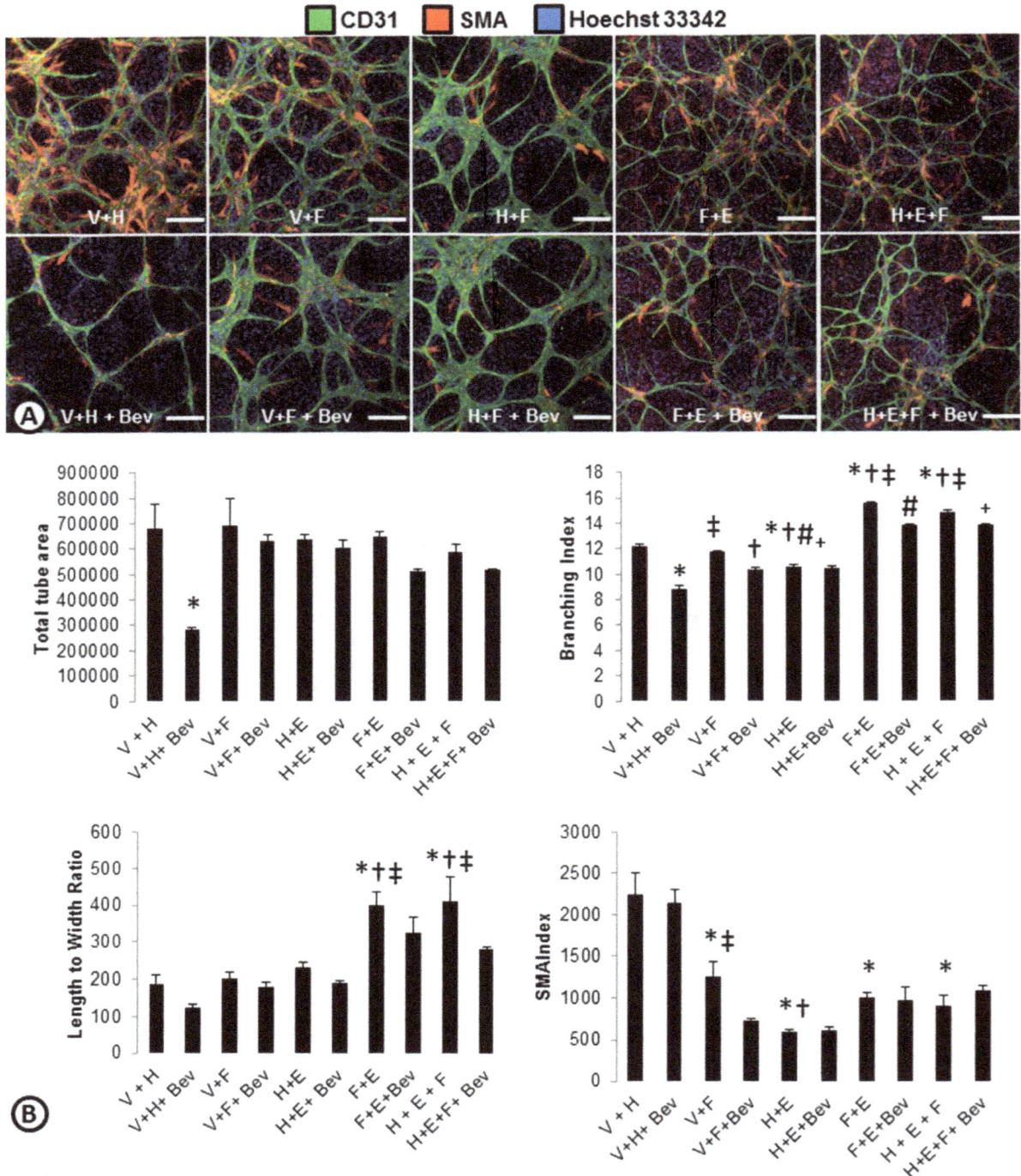

Figure 4. Phenotypes of angiogenic growth factor combinations. (A) ADSC and ECFC co-cultures were treated with combinations of angiogenic growth factors (V = VEGF, H = HGF, F = bFGF, E = EGF) with or without anti-VEGF (Bevacizumab; Bev) and stained for cords (CD31; green), smooth muscle actin (SMA; red), and nuclei (Hoechst 33342; blue). (B) ArrayScan quantifications of total tube area, branching index, length to width ratio, and SMA index of samples treated with combinations of growth factors with and without bevacizumab. n = 3 per group. * = p<0.05 vs. V+H. † = p<0.05 vs. V+F. ‡ = p<0.05 vs. H+E. # = p<0.05 vs. F+E. + = p<0.05 vs. H+E+F. Scale bars are 250 µm.

bound HGF, as a heparin wash removal of bound HGF prior to addition of HGF leads to significant cord formation. Interestingly, Ang1 is produced to some extent by ADSCs alone, but at the later timepoints there is more Ang1 in the medium when ADSCs and ECFCs are co-cultured. This increase in Ang1 is likely from pericytes associated with the endothelial cells. Ang1 is secreted by pericytes and previous studies have shown that pericyte association with cords began on day 3 and increased with time [7]. Therefore, there are likely only enough pericytes present at the 96 hr time point to effectively increase the Ang1 concentration. Furthermore,

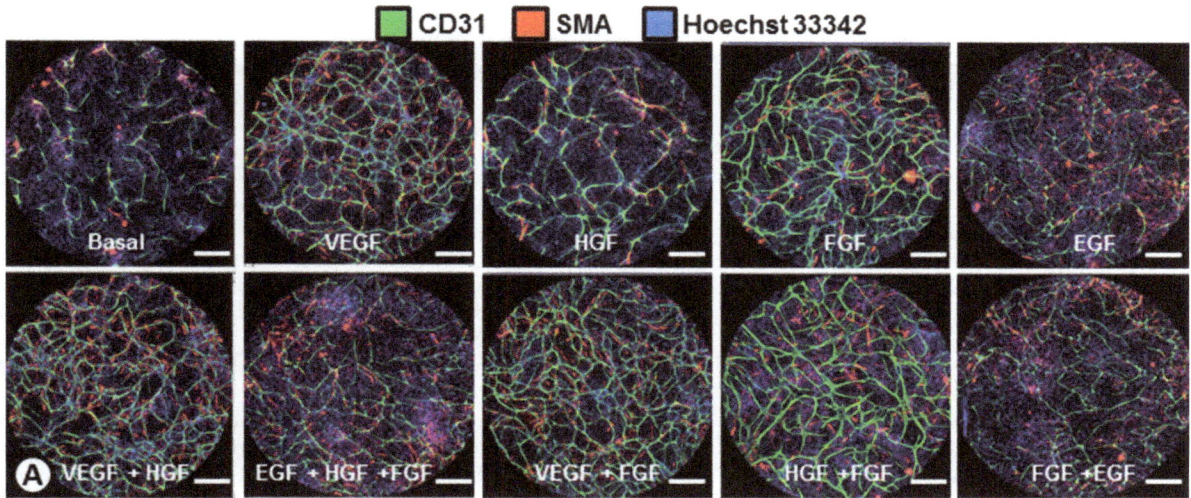

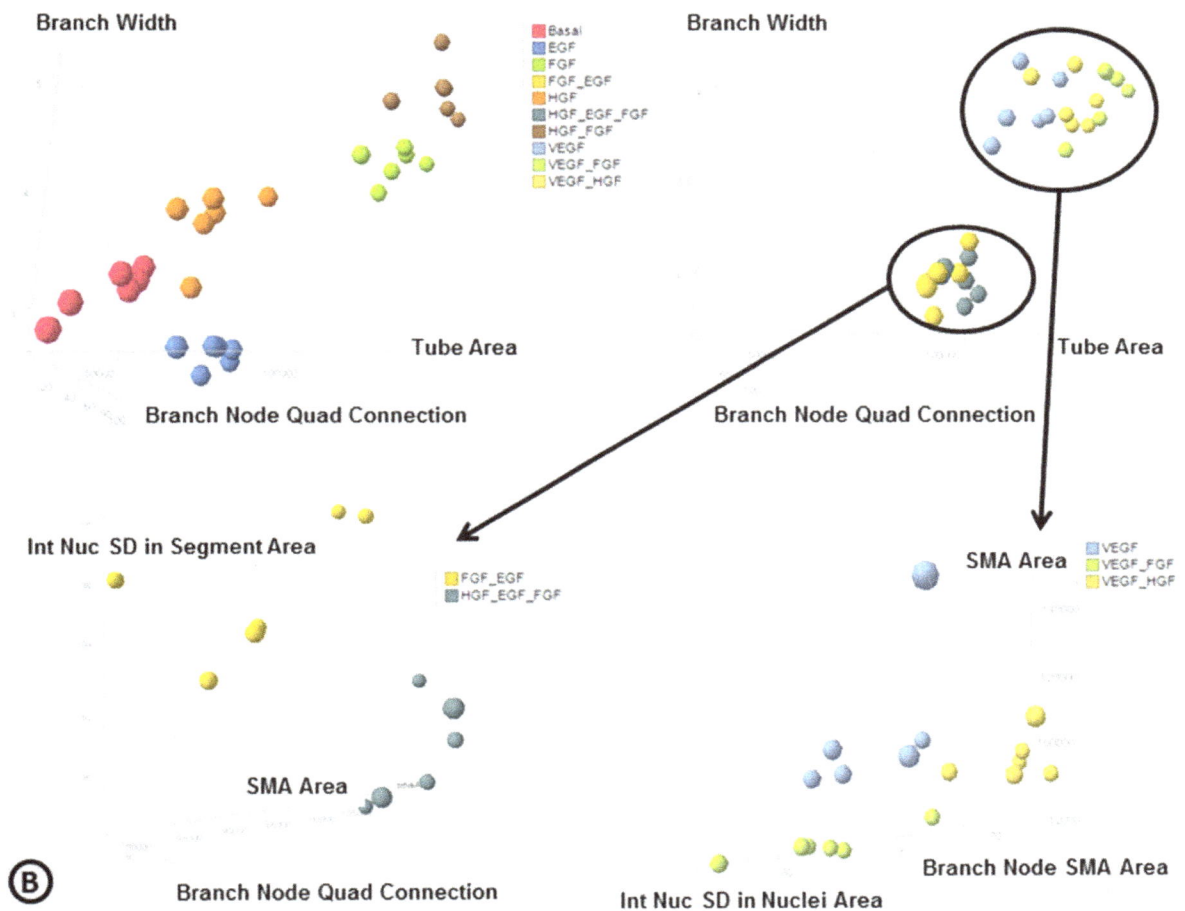

Figure 5. Cluster analysis of phenotypes associated with angiogenic growth factors. (**A**) Whole-well Acumen images of ADSC and ECFC co-cultures treated with angiogenic growth factors or combinations of growth factors following a heparin wash and stained for cords (endothelial cells; CD31; green), smooth muscle actin (SMA; red), and nuclei (Hoechst 33342; blue). (**B**) Cluster analysis based on the top phenotypes from the 101 ImageJ descriptors (Table S1) differentiate the phenotypes of cords driven by angiogenic growth factors or growth factor combinations. The output from statistics comparing the same populations in terms of all the dimensions is shown in Table S2. A p-value less than 0.05 indicate the means of the two groups were significantly different in at least one dimension. Scale bars are 1000 um.

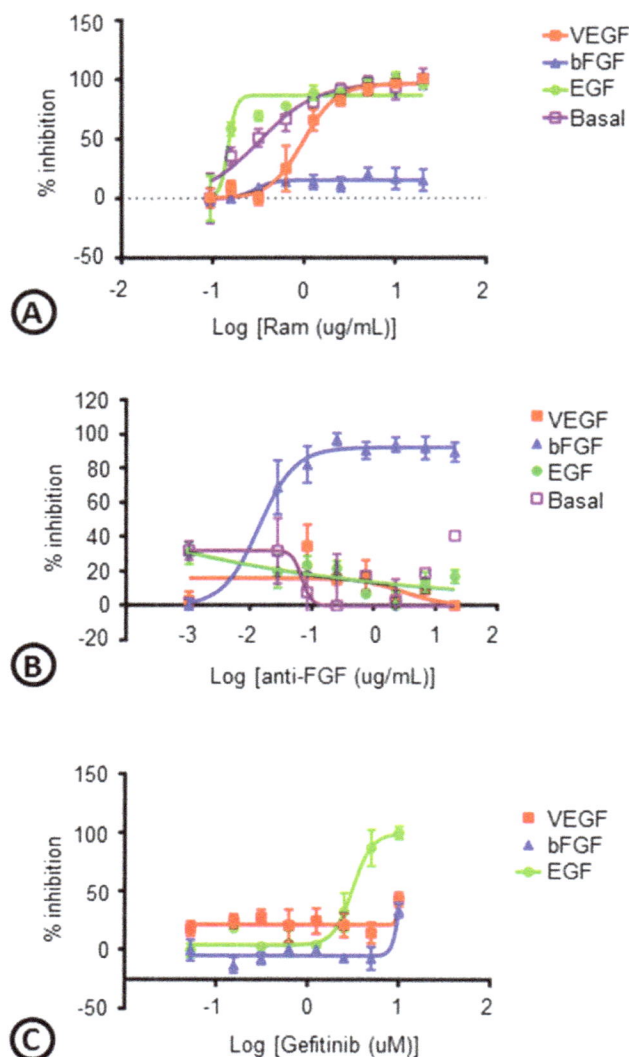

Figure 6. Cross-talk between angiogenic growth factors. Basal, VEGF-, bFGF-, or EGF-driven cords were treated with a VEGFR-2 antibody (IMC-1121B; Ramucirumab; Ram), a bFGF antibody (anti-bFGF), or an EGFR inhibitor (Gefitinib) and the percent inhibition of total tube area from the ArrayScan was graphed. n = 3 per group.

recent cell lots of ADSCs that do not produce as much SMA-associated cells do not see a spike even at these later time points (data not shown). Finally, the increase in Ang2 in co-cultures of ADSCs and ECFCs with VEGF stimulation is in alignment with the association between Ang2 and VEGF. Ang2 is secreted by endothelial cells and increases in response to VEGF to induce pericyte dissociation [16–18].

bFGF and EGF signaling have been shown to play a role in revascularization of tumors after development of resistance to anti-VEGF/VEGFR2 therapy [3–5]. Because these factors were not endogenously present within our co-culture system, we examined the effects of bFGF and EGF driven cord formation. We found that similar to VEGF, both bFGF and EGF can induce cords, but phenotypic differences were observed. These phenotypic differences could reflect differences in mitogenic, sprouting, and survival potencies of the different growth factors. bFGF driven cords were larger in caliber and lacked pericyte coverage. This is consistent

with a previous report examining the relationships between VEGF and bFGF in tumor models designed to overexpress both growth factors. Interestingly, pericyte association and maturation was decreased when only bFGF was expressed after inhibition of VEGF expression [19]. Previous reports have also shown that bFGF induced ERK signaling antagonizes TGF-β induced smooth muscle gene expression [20], which may explain the loss of SMA association in bFGF driven cords. EGF driven cords appeared thinner with increased length to width ratios. Based on multiple phenotypic parameters, we were able to differentiate cords driven by individual or multiple factors and were able to establish that cords driven by some growth factors have dominant phenotypes compared to others. This may illustrate an ability to define blood vessels into different classes. Quantitative correlation of the various endothelial-pericyte morphologies with the various growth factors and combinations may lead to predictive biomarkers for inhibiting blood vessels driven by VEGF, bFGF, or EGF.

In addition to bFGF and EGF driving different phenotypic cords, we were able to demonstrate that their ability to induce cord formation is independent of VEGF. Numerous growth factors have been shown to drive angiogenesis, but many of these induce angiogenesis through upregulation of VEGF rather than a direct effect. In our system, we stimulate cord formation with VEGF, bFGF, or EGF but only the VEGF driven cords are dramatically altered by inhibition of VEGF with bevacizumab (a VEGF antibody). Even with growth factor combinations, only the VEGF driven phenotypes appeared to be blocked by the addition of bevacizumab. Similarly, inhibition of bFGF with an antibody only blocked bFGF driven cords. Likewise, an EGFR inhibitor only blocked EGF driven cords. This indicates that these angiogenic growth factors act independent of one another, but can work together to elicit particular angiogenic phenotypes. This also highlights the redundancy in proangiogenic factors and the ability of multiple growth factors to drive angiogenesis. This is particularly important in response to inhibition of a particular pathway, as what has been seen with bFGF driving angiogenesis in response to inhibition of the VEGF pathway [4]. In contrast, we observed some reductions of EGF driven cords with inhibition of the ligand (bevacizumab) or the receptor (ramucirumab). Previous studies have shown that the oncogenic properties of EGFR may be mediated by up-regulation of VEGF, which may explain why we see these effects [21].

In addition to the examination of phenotypic differences between cords driven by various growth factors and the study of dominant growth factor phenotypes in combination treatments, this ADSC/ECFC co-culture system can be used to screen for pro-angiogenic factors or drugs. To address whether this assay system can be used to identify factors that can promote cord formation and potentially be pro-angiogenic, we used a TGF-β inhibitor (LY2157299) in the cord formation assay. TGF-β is known to inhibit endothelial cell proliferation [11–13], so one would expect to see increased cord formation with the addition of LY2147299. When LY2157299 was added to VEGF-driven cords or cords in optimized medium, an induction in cords was not apparent. However, when LY2157299 was added into basal medium a significant induction in cord formation was observed. This indicates that some agents that may promote cord formation may be masked in the presence of a milieu of growth factors. Thus, because we have developed a basal medium without exogenously added growth factors, this assay may aid in the identification of new angiogenic factors or drugs that may be useful for driving therapeutic angiogenesis. In addition, the basal medium allows for the identification of other factors that may be combined or inhibited with current anti-angiogenic therapies. This highlights

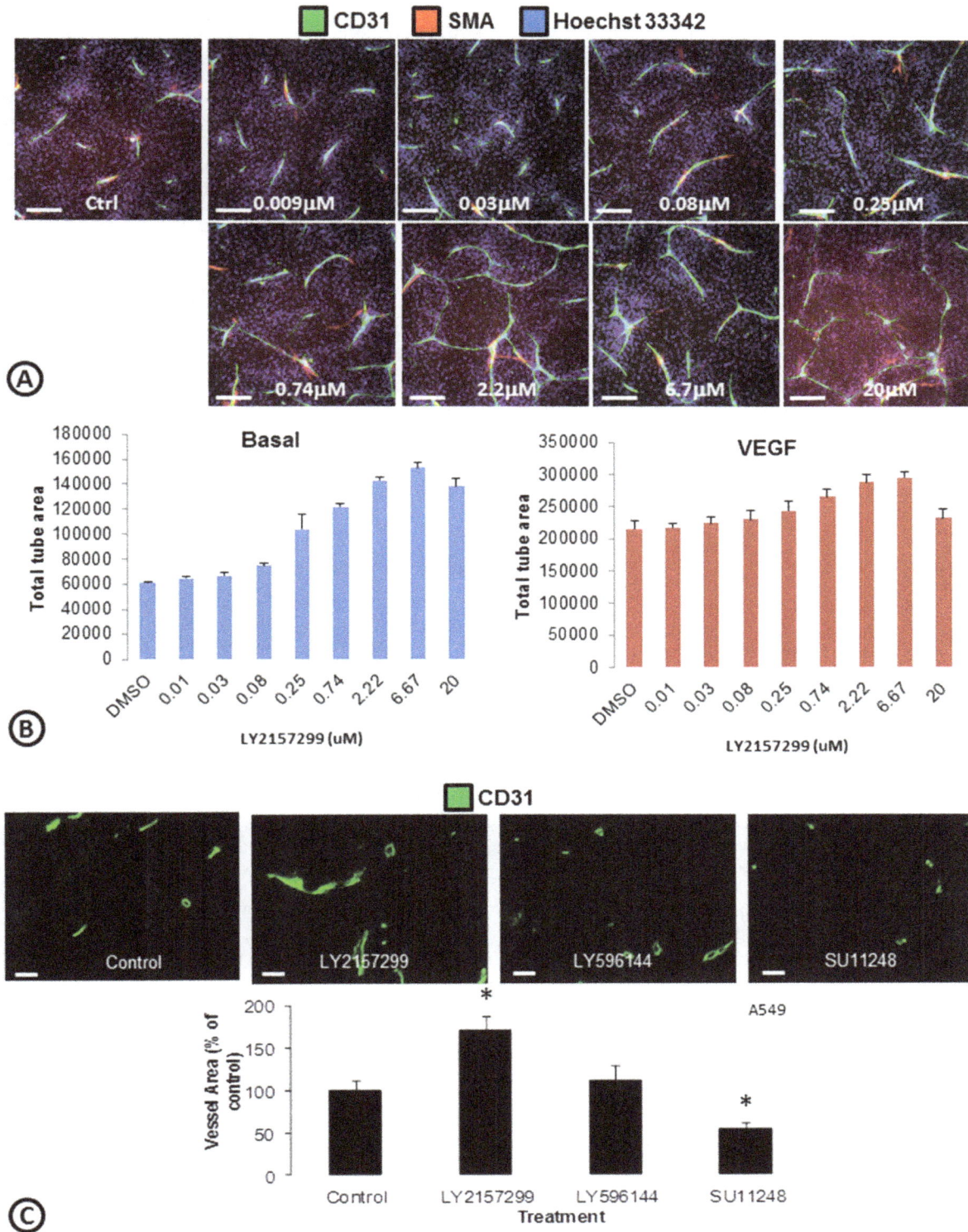

Figure 7. Induction of cord formation with a TGF-β inhibitor. (**A**) Co-cultures of ADSCs and ECFCs were treated with a TGF-β inhibitor (LY2157299) and stained for cords (CD31; green), smooth muscle actin (SMA; red), and nuclei (Hoechst 33342; blue). (**B**) ArrayScan quantifications of total tube area following treatment with LY2157299 in basal medium (left) versus VEGF driven cords (right). n = 6 per group. (**C**) Mice harboring A549 tumor xenografts were treated with a TGF-β inhibitor (LY2157299), an inactive control (LY596144), or sunitinib (Sutent; SU11248) for 5 days. Tumors were fixed, sectioned, stained for tumor vessels (CD31; green), and quantified using Image J. *=p<0.05 vs. control. n = 4–6 per treatment group. Scale bars in A are 250 μm. Scale bars in B are 50 μm.

the need to perform these sorts of assays in as minimal of medium as possible to support cord formation without the addition of exogenous angiogenic factors.

In normal epithelial and endothelial cells TGF-β is antiproliferative. However, in tumor cells, parts of the TGF-β signaling pathway are mutated and TGF-β no longer controls the cells. Both tumor and stromal cells have been shown to have increased TGF-β production which is associated with increased tumor invasiveness [11–13]. Thus, while in the normal setting TGF-β is antiproliferative, it has been shown to be an effective anti-tumor target. Despite the increases in tumor angiogenesis we observed with the TGF-β inhibitor, this drug has been shown to elicit antitumor effects (Yingling et al. manuscript in preparation). This may reflect differential effects of the inhibitor on endothelial cells versus tumor cells. In addition, previous studies have shown that the number of tumor blood vessels does not necessarily correlate with tumor growth [22–25]. Thus, an increase in tumor angiogenesis does not necessarily mean the tumors will grow faster. In fact, this is what we have observed with LY2147299 (Yingling et al. manuscript in preparation).

Despite the evidence that numerous growth factors drive angiogenesis, the majority of the in vitro studies examine a single factor or are performed in media or matrix with numerous growth factors. These studies limit one's ability to understand the different phenotypes driven by the growth factors and how combinations may lead to a particular phenotype versus another. In addition, without the use of a growth factor free medium, many proangiogenic factors may be missed. It would be interesting to relate these phenotypes with function in an in vivo setting to determine whether these phenotypes are also associated with other functional or physiological differences. This may lead to improvements in therapeutic angiogenesis efforts and or better rational for anti-angiogenic therapy in different pathological settings.

Supporting Information

Figure S1 Association of SMA-positive cells to endothelial cords. Co-cultures of ADSCs and ECFCs were stained for cords (CD31) and smooth muscle actin (SMA) and imaged with the ArrayScan. High magnification images show a close association of the SMA-positive pericyte-like structures with the endothelial cords. Scale bars are 250 μm.

Figure S2 High throughput quantitative validation of the assay. (**A**) Co-cultures of ADSCs and ECFCs were stained for nuclei (Hoechst), cords (CD31), and smooth muscle actin (SMA) and whole wells were imaged with the ArrayScan. Grayscale images show the image of each marker and the black and white image shows what was analyzed. (**B**) Quantitative validation of Acumen eX3 images was performed in a 384 well assay format. Maximum, minimum and concentration response curves for total tube area and SMA area were used to calculate the overall Z′ and minimum significant ratio (MSR) for each parameter. Scale bars are 250 μm.

Figure S3 Induction of cords with HGF following heparin wash. (**A**) To address whether HGF can induce cord formation in the ADSC/ECFC co-culture assay, a heparin wash was performed prior to addition of HGF. After 3 days, the cords were fixed and stained for cords (CD31; green), smooth muscle actin (SMA; red), and nuclei (Hoechst 33342; blue). (**B**) ArrayScan quantification of heparin washed HGF induced total tube area and inhibition with an anti-HGF antibody. * p<0.05 vs basal. n = 3 per group. Scalebars are 250 μm.

Acknowledgments

The authors would like to thank Jonathan Yingling and Kuldeep Neote for helpful scientific discussions, Xioling Xia for technical assistance, and Bronislaw Pytowski and Laura Benjamin for critical review of the manuscript.

Author Contributions

Conceived and designed the experiments: BLF MS WHG LL RF MU JAL DBM SC. Performed the experiments: BLF MS WHG LL RF JCH SC. Analyzed the data: BLF MS WHG LL MU JCH DBM SC. Contributed reagents/materials/analysis tools: BLF MS WHG LL MU JCH DBM SC. Contributed to the writing of the manuscript: BLF WHG MU JAL SC.

References

1. Bergers G, Benjamin LE (2003) Tumorigenesis and the angiogenic switch. Nat Rev Cancer 3: 401–410.
2. Bergers G, Hanahan D (2008) Modes of resistance to anti-angiogenic therapy. Nat Rev Cancer 8: 592–603.
3. Cascone T, Herynk MH, Xu L, Du Z, Kadara H, et al. (2011) Upregulated stromal EGFR and vascular remodeling in mouse xenograft models of angiogenesis inhibitor-resistant human lung adenocarcinoma. J Clin Invest 121: 1313–1328.
4. Casanovas O, Hicklin DJ, Bergers G, Hanahan D (2005) Drug resistance by evasion of antiangiogenic targeting of VEGF signaling in late-stage pancreatic islet tumors. Cancer Cell 8: 299–309.
5. Allen E, Walters IB, Hanahan D (2011) Brivanib, a dual FGF/VEGF inhibitor, is active both first and second line against mouse pancreatic neuroendocrine tumors developing adaptive/evasive resistance to VEGF inhibition. Clin Cancer Res 17: 5299–5310.
6. Staton CA, Reed MW, Brown NJ (2009) A critical analysis of current in vitro and in vivo angiogenesis assays. Int J Exp Pathol 90: 195–221.
7. Falcon BL, O'Clair B, McClure D, Evans GF, Stewart J, et al. (2013) Development and characterization of a high-throughput in vitro cord formation model insensitive to VEGF inhibition. J Hematol Oncol 6: 31.
8. Merfeld-Clauss S, Gollahalli N, March KL, Traktuev DO (2010) Adipose tissue progenitor cells directly interact with endothelial cells to induce vascular network formation. Tissue Eng Part A 16: 2953–2966.
9. Chen Y, Wei T, Yan L, Lawrence F, Qian HR, et al. (2008) Developing and applying a gene functional association network for anti-angiogenic kinase inhibitor activity assessment in an angiogenesis co-culture model. BMC Genomics 9: 264.
10. Lee S, Chen TT, Barber CL, Jordan MC, Murdock J, et al. (2007) Autocrine VEGF signaling is required for vascular homeostasis. Cell 130: 691–703.
11. Goumans MJ, Valdimarsdottir G, Itoh S, Rosendahl A, Sideras P, et al. (2002) Balancing the activation state of the endothelium via two distinct TGF-β type I receptors. EMBO J 21: 1743–1753.
12. Muller G, Behrens J, Nussbaumer U, Bohlen P, Birchmeier W (1987) Inhibitory action of transforming growth factor β on endothelial cells. Proc Natl Acad Sci U S A 84: 5600–5604.
13. Takehara K, LeRoy EC, Grotendorst GR (1987) TGF-β inhibition of endothelial cell proliferation: alteration of EGF binding and EGF-induced growth-regulatory (competence) gene expression. Cell 49: 415–422.
14. Lee JA, Berg EL (2013) Neoclassic Drug Discovery: The Case for Lead Generation Using Phenotypic and Functional Approaches. J Biomol Screen.
15. Gourlaouen M, Welti JC, Vasudev NS, Reynolds AR (2013) Essential role for endocytosis in the growth factor-stimulated activation of ERK1/2 in endothelial cells. J Biol Chem 288: 7467–7480.
16. Augustin HG, Koh GY, Thurston G, Alitalo K (2009) Control of vascular morphogenesis and homeostasis through the angiopoietin-Tie system. Nat Rev Mol Cell Biol 10: 165–177.
17. Daly C, Eichten A, Castanaro C, Pasnikowski E, Adler A, et al. (2013) Angiopoietin-2 functions as a Tie2 agonist in tumor models, where it limits the effects of VEGF inhibition. Cancer Res 73: 108–118.

18. Gerald D, Chintharlapalli S, Augustin HG, Benjamin LE (2013) Angiopoietin-2: an attractive target for improved antiangiogenic tumor therapy. Cancer Res 73: 1649–1657.

19. Giavazzi R, Sennino B, Coltrini D, Garofalo A, Dossi R, et al. (2003) Distinct role of fibroblast growth factor-2 and vascular endothelial growth factor on tumor growth and angiogenesis. Am J Pathol 162: 1913–1926.

20. Kawai-Kowase K, Sato H, Oyama Y, Kanai H, Sato M, et al. (2004) Basic fibroblast growth factor antagonizes transforming growth factor-β1-induced smooth muscle gene expression through extracellular signal-regulated kinase 1/2 signaling pathway activation. Arterioscler Thromb Vasc Biol 24: 1384–1390.

21. Petit AM, Rak J, Hung MC, Rockwell P, Goldstein N, et al. (1997) Neutralizing antibodies against epidermal growth factor and ErbB-2/neu receptor tyrosine kinases down-regulate vascular endothelial growth factor production by tumor cells in vitro and in vivo: angiogenic implications for signal transduction therapy of solid tumors. Am J Pathol 151: 1523–1530.

22. Falcon BL, Pietras K, Chou J, Chen D, Sennino B, et al. (2011) Increased vascular delivery and efficacy of chemotherapy after inhibition of platelet-derived growth factor-B. Am J Pathol 178: 2920–2930.

23. Noguera-Troise I, Daly C, Papadopoulos NJ, Coetzee S, Boland P, et al. (2006) Blockade of Dll4 inhibits tumour growth by promoting non-productive angiogenesis. Nature 444: 1032–1037.

24. Ridgway J, Zhang G, Wu Y, Stawicki S, Liang WC, et al. (2006) Inhibition of Dll4 signalling inhibits tumour growth by deregulating angiogenesis. Nature 444: 1083–1087.

25. Thurston G, Noguera-Troise I, Yancopoulos GD (2007) The Delta paradox: DLL4 blockade leads to more tumour vessels but less tumour growth. Nat Rev Cancer 7: 327–331.

4

A Differential Role for CD248 (Endosialin) in PDGF-Mediated Skeletal Muscle Angiogenesis

Amy J. Naylor[1¶], Helen M. McGettrick[1,2¶], William D. Maynard[1], Philippa May[1], Francesca Barone[1], Adam P. Croft[1], Stuart Egginton[3], Christopher D. Buckley[1,2*]

[1] Rheumatology Research Group, Centre for Translational Inflammation Research, University of Birmingham, Birmingham, West Midlands, United Kingdom, [2] Systems Science for Health, University of Birmingham, Birmingham, West Midlands, United Kingdom, [3] Faculty of Biological Sciences, University of Leeds, Leeds, West Yorkshire, United Kingdom

Abstract

CD248 (Endosialin) is a type 1 membrane protein involved in developmental and pathological angiogenesis through its expression on pericytes and regulation of PDGFRβ signalling. Here we explore the function of CD248 in skeletal muscle angiogenesis. Two distinct forms of capillary growth (splitting and sprouting) can be induced separately by increasing microcirculatory shear stress (chronic vasodilator treatment) or by inducing functional overload (extirpation of a synergistic muscle). We show that CD248 is present on pericytes in muscle and that CD248[-/-] mice have a specific defect in capillary sprouting. In contrast, splitting angiogenesis is independent of CD248 expression. Endothelial cells respond to pro-sprouting angiogenic stimulus by up-regulating gene expression for HIF1α, angiopoietin 2 and its receptor TEK, PDGF-B and its receptor PDGFRβ; this response did not occur following a pro-splitting angiogenic stimulus. In wildtype mice, defective sprouting angiogenesis could be mimicked by blocking PDGFRβ signalling using the tyrosine kinase inhibitor Imatinib mesylate. We conclude that CD248 is required for PDGFRβ-dependant capillary sprouting but not splitting angiogenesis, and identify a new role for CD248 expressed on pericytes in the early stages of physiological angiogenesis during muscle remodelling.

Editor: Atsushi Asakura, University of Minnesota Medical School, United States of America

Funding: AJN was supported by Arthritis Research UK Programme Grant (19791), HMM was supported by Arthritis Research UK Career Development Fellowship (19899) and the Systems Science for Health Initiative, University of Birmingham (5212). WDM and PM were supported by the Arthur Thomson Trust. SE was supported by a grant from the British Heart Foundation PG/08/018/24599. The funders had no role in study design, data collection and analysis, decision to publish, or preparation of the manuscript.

Competing Interests: The authors have declared that no competing interests exist.

* Email: c.d.buckley@bham.ac.uk

¶ These authors are joint first authors on this work.

Introduction

Angiogenesis is the physiological process through which new blood vessels are formed from cells of the existing vasculature. This can be achieved by one of two processes, splitting or sprouting, that require different levels of pericyte involvement (reviewed in [1–2]). Splitting angiogenesis depends on the reorganisation of existing cell populations, where opposing vascular endothelial cells extend lamellipodia into the lumen until they contact with the opposite side of the lumen, effectively splitting the vessel in two. In contrast, sprouting angiogenesis is characterised by the migration and proliferation of endothelial cells towards an angiogenic stimulus in the tissue.

Pericytes play an essential role in stabilising the developing vessel in sprouting angiogenesis [3]. Indeed, a loss or lack of pericytes results in weaknesses in the capillaries, and has been associated with micro-aneurysms and loss of sight [4–5]. Pericytes are a heterogeneous population of perivascular cells located in close proximity to endothelial cells beneath a common basement membrane [2,6–7]. To date, no specific pan-pericyte marker has been identified. Pericytes are defined as cells expressing either

platelet-derived growth factor receptor beta (PDGFRβ), neuron glial antigen 2 (NG2), alpha smooth muscle actin (αSMA) or CD248 (endosialin) in close proximity to CD31 positive endothelial cells (reviewed in [1,8]).

During physiological angiogenesis, platelet-derived growth factor-B (PDGF-B) secreted by endothelial cells dimerises and activates pericyte PDGFRβ, which ultimately induces their proliferation and migration towards the newly developing vessel [5]. Importantly, lack of PDGFRβ or PDGF-BB, and therefore lack of pericyte function, results in the formation of disorganised vessels leading to perinatally lethal haemorrhaging and oedema [9–11].

CD248 (endosialin; tumour endothelial marker 1) is a C-type lectin-like domain family member highly expressed during embryogenesis [12], and upregulated on pericytes in vascularised brain tumours and sarcomas [13–14]. Despite confusion in early literature on the subject (eg. [15]), CD248 expression is not seen on endothelial cells, but rather is a marker of neighbouring pericytes and stromal cells where it has the potential to influence the process of angiogenesis [16–17]. For example, tumour growth and large vessel formation *in vivo* are markedly reduced by genetic deletion of CD248 [18] or removal of its cytoplasmic tail [19]. Similarly, antibody blockade of CD248 interfered with pericyte migration and tube formation *in vitro* [12]. CD248 has also been shown to regulate the kinetics of vessel pruning during developmental vasculogenesis, ensuring only correctly organised and viable vessels survive [20].

Recent evidence suggests that CD248 may exert its effects through regulation of the PDGF pathway as PDGF-BB-induced phosphorylation of extracellular signal-regulated kinase (ERK), but not phosphorylation of PDGFRβ itself, was markedly diminished in CD248-deficient pericytes [21]. Thus, CD248 may function to enhance or modify PDGF-BB signalling acting downstream of PDGFRβ but upstream of ERK1/2 by an as yet unknown mechanism.

CD248 is required for pathological angiogenesis and developmental vasculogenesis [18–20]; however little is known about its function in physiological angiogenesis and whether this differs according to the form of capillary growth elicited (splitting *vs.* sprouting). Here we have examined the role of CD248 within skeletal muscle. Skeletal muscle displays a highly organised microvascular network with a consistent relationship between the number of capillaries and the number of muscle fibres; any increase in the capillary to fibre ratio (C:F) strongly indicates an angiogenic response [22–23]. We explored this relationship and demonstrated that CD248-deficient mice display a specific defect in sprouting, but not splitting, angiogenesis in skeletal muscle and demonstrate for the first time that CD248-positive pericytes are required during the early stages of physiological angiogenesis.

Methods

In vivo studies of angiogenesis

Male C57Bl/6 WT (Harlan, UK) and C57Bl/6 CD248$^{-/-}$ mice (bred as described in Nanda *et al.* [18] donated by D.L. Huso, Johns Hopkins Medical Institutions, Baltimore, MD, USA) were studied between 8–12 weeks of age. All experiments were carried out at the University of Birmingham, UK (project licence number 40/9475) following strict guidelines governed by the UK Animal (Scientific Procedures) Act 1986 and approved by the local ethics committee (BERSC: Birmingham Ethical Review Subcommittee). Mice were housed in individually ventilated cages in groups of 3–6 individuals on a 12 hour light-dark cycle with *ad libitum* access to standard laboratory mouse chow diet and water. 6 mice were used for each experiment.

Extirpation of the tibialis anterior (TA) muscle was performed under isoflurane general anaesthesia in aseptic conditions, to produce overload of the synergist extensor digitorum longus (EDL), as previously described [24]. Alternatively, prazosin hydrochloride (50 mg/l; Tocris Bioscience, UK) supplemented with 0.5 g/l granulated sucrose (Amresco, UK) was administered orally *ad libitum* in drinking water which was replaced every 3 days [25]. Imatinib mesylate (15 mg/ml in dH$_2$0; Santa Cruz Biotechnology, USA) was administered daily by gavage, equivalent to a therapeutic dose of 150 mg/kg/day [26].

Mice were carefully monitored throughout all treatment programs by the Named Animal Care and Welfare Officer. Opiate-based pain relief was administered for 24 hours following surgical intervention. No weight loss or other adverse effects were observed in response to any of the treatments given. All treatments lasted for 7 days, after which time mice were sacrificed by cervical dislocation. The EDL was dissected immediately and either snap frozen in (i) liquid nitrogen-cooled isopentane for tissue sectioning or (ii) liquid nitrogen for gene expression analysis. All samples were stored at -80°C until use.

Immunofluorescence

Transverse 8 μm cryosections of the EDL muscle were cut at −20°C, air dried for 1 hr, fixed in acetone at 4°C for 20 minutes and stored at −20°C until use. Sections were rehydrated and blocked at room temperature for 30 minutes in phosphate buffered saline (PBS) with 1% bovine serum albumin (PBSA; Sigma-Aldrich, UK) for capillary: fibre ratio studies, or for 15–20 minutes first in 0.05% Avidin, then 0.005% biotin and finally 10% horse serum diluted in PBS (all from Sigma) for pericyte imaging. Sections were incubated with the following primary antibodies for 1 hr at room temperature or overnight at 4°C: anti-CD31 (1:100: AbD Serotec, BioRad, USA; clone 2H8); anti-CD248 (1:400; clone p13, gift from Claire Isacke, The Institute of Cancer Research, London, UK); anti-NG2 (1:75; Upstate, Merck Millipore, USA; clone 132.38); anti-αSMA (1:100; Neomarkers, ThermoScientific, USA; clone 1A4); anti-PDGFRβ biotin (1:100; eBioscience, USA; clone APB5), anti-collagen IV (1:200; Abcam, Life Technologies, UK; polyclonal; ab19808), anti-phospho ERK (1:100; Cell Signaling Technologies, UK; Phospho-p44/42 MAPK (Erk1/2) (Thr202/Tyr204) Antibody #9101). Subsequently, slides were incubated with secondary and then tertiary antibodies and Hoechst 33342 (10 μg/ml; Invitrogen, UK) for 30–60 min each before mounting with either Prolong Gold Antifade (Molecular Probes, Life Technologies, UK) or Dabco (Sigma-Aldrich, UK).

In some cases (Figure 1A, B and C), in order to visualise all pericytes at once, tissues were incubated with a cocktail of primary antibodies to PDGFRβ, NG2 and αSMA which were detected with specific secondary antibodies that all shared the same fluorophore so that all pericytes, regardless of protein expression phenotype, were visible at once. Alternatively, the pericyte markers NG2, αSMA and CD248 were analysed on separate tissue sections, each of which was counterstained with CD31 and PDGFRβ (Figure 1D).

Fluorescence microscopy and image analysis

For quantification of capillarity, images were acquired using a Leica DM6000 fluorescence microscope controlled by Leica Advanced Fluorescence software. A fibre was defined as an isolated non-stained, convex area surrounded by collagen IV as previously described [22]. A capillary was defined as a CD31-positive structure that was <8 μm in diameter that appears either as a circle in cross section or elongated structures when sectioned obliquely. Individual branches were counted as single capillaries. Images were blinded prior to analysis. Figure S1 shows example images from each genotype for control, prazosin and extirpated mice. The differences in response to treatment become most apparent following analysis of exact capillary and fibre number, counted using ImageJ (NIH) and plotted as capillary to fibre ratio (C:F) as previously described [22].

To determine pericyte phenotype, confocal images were acquired for the entire muscle tissue section using a Zeiss LSM 510-UV confocal microscope, resolution (1024×768 pixels per image), magnification (x63) giving 120 μm by 120 μm for each co-localisation image. The average number of capillaries counted per field was 14 (range 3–28). Images were analysed using LSM Image Browser (Zeiss). Capillaries were defined as above, and pericytes defined as cells positive for ≥1 pericyte marker and located within 3 μm of a capillary. Pericyte coverage of capillaries was calculated as the percentage of capillaries surrounded by cell bodies or cell processes positive for ≥1 pericyte marker. For quantification of

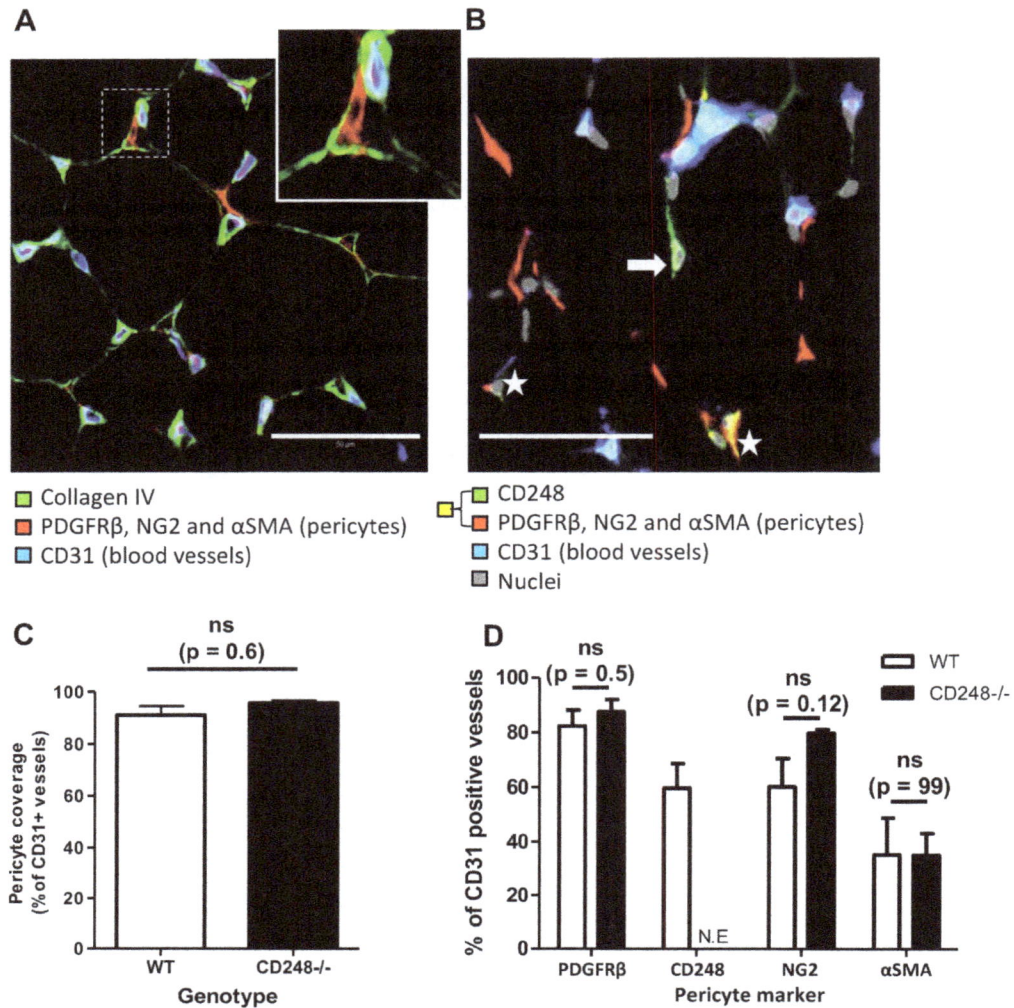

Figure 1. Phenotype of pericytes in wildtype and CD248 knockout skeletal muscle. Immunofluorescence and confocal microscopy of EDL muscle sections from wildtype mice stained with antibodies to either (**A**) Collagen IV (green), CD31 (blue) and pericyte markers αSMA, NG2 and PDGFRβ (all red) or (**B**) CD248 (green), CD31 (blue), pericyte markers αSMA, NG2 and PDGFRβ (all red) and nuclei (grey). CD248 was detected alone (green – marked with arrow) or co-localised with the other pericyte markers (yellow – marked with star). Enlarged region (dashed box) shows a pericyte (red) surrounded by the collagen IV basement membrane. (**C**) Pericyte coverage expressed as a percentage of CD31 positive vessels positive for ≥1 pericyte marker. (**D**) Expression of individual pericyte markers, expressed as percentage of CD31 positive vessels positive for either PDGFRβ, NG2 or αSMA. Empty bars are WT, filled bars are CD248$^{-/-}$. Data are mean ± SEM from 3 independent animals. N.E = not expressed. ns = no significant difference assessed by (C) t-test or (D) ANOVA with Bonferroni post-test. Scale bars are 50 microns.

expression levels (phospho-ERK only) pixel counting was performed using Zen pro 2012 imaging software (Carl Zeiss, UK). 2 images per section were taken from 3 separate mice. Results are the sum of pixels with an expression intensity >10 normalised to untreated control tissue.

Gene expression analysis by quantitative PCR

Messenger RNA (mRNA) was isolated from murine skeletal muscle tissue using the RNeasy Fibrous Mini Kit (following manufacturer's instructions, Qiagen, UK) and stored at -80°C until use. Isolated mRNA was converted to cDNA using High Capacity cDNA conversion kit (as per manufacturer's instructions; Applied Biosystems, UK) in a Techne TC-Plus thermal cycler (Techne, UK) and stored at −20°C until use. Gene expression was analysed by quantitative PCR (qPCR) on isolated cDNA with

TaqMan 2xPCR Master Mix (Applied Biosystems, Life Technologies, UK) and FAM-labelled primers (Assay on Demand kits from Applied Biosystems, Life Technologies, UK). Samples were amplified using the 7900HT Real-Time PCR machine and analysed using SDS 2.2 (Applied Biosystems, Life Technologies, UK). Data were expressed as relative expression units ($2^{-\Delta Ct}$) relative to 18S.

Western blotting

Transverse frozen sections of EDL muscle (100×20 μm sections) were pooled for protein isolation in 50 μl RIPA buffer (Sigma Aldrich, UK) containing a protease inhibitor cocktail (Roche, UK: cOmplete, mini) phosphatase inhibitors (Roche, UK: PhosSTOP phosphatase inhibitor tablets) as per manufacturer's instructions. Samples were incubated on ice for 30 minutes with periodic vortexing. Insoluble debris was removed using QiAShredder columns (Qiagen, UK) and samples were boiled in SDS page buffer for 5 minutes. Criterion TGX precast gels (Bio-Rad, UK) were used for electrophoresis and protein was transferred using the trans-blot turbo transfer system (Bio-Rad, UK). Membranes were blocked in 5% non-fat milk in TBS containing 0.1% Tween-20. Primary antibodies were incubated at a 1:1000 dilution performed overnight at 4°C in block. Primary antibodies were as follows: Total ERK (Cell Signaling Technologies, UK, p44/42 MAPK (Erk1/2) clone #9102), phospho-ERK (Cell Signaling Technologies, UK, Phospho-p44/42 MAPK (Erk1/2) (Thr202/Tyr204) clone #9101). Anti-rabbit HRP-linked secondary antibody (Cell Signaling Technologies, UK, #7074) was used at 1:1000 for 1 hour at room temperature. ECL Western blotting substrate (Pierce, UK) reagent was used to visualise the resulting bands.

Statistical analysis

Data are presented as mean ± SEM of n experiments. Variation between multiple treatments was evaluated using analysis of variance (ANOVA) followed by Bonferroni post-hoc test. Where appropriate, differences between individual treatments were evaluated by unpaired t-test unless stated otherwise in the figure legend. P values<0.05 were considered statistically significant.

Results

CD248 is expressed in skeletal muscle by a subset of pericytes

We initially characterised the phenotype of pericytes in resting skeletal muscle from wildtype (WT) and CD248$^{-/-}$ animals. Pericytes were identified histologically with a panel of antibodies against PDGFRβ, NG2 and αSMA and clearly visible under the collagen IV basement membrane in close association with CD31-positive capillaries (Figure 1A). In both WT and CD248$^{-/-}$ tissue almost all CD31 positive vessels within the skeletal muscle (>90%) were associated with pericyte cell bodies or processes (Figure 1C) expressing a heterogeneous mix of PDGFRβ, NG2 and αSMA (Figure 1D), thus confirming previous studies demonstrating that pericyte processes cover 99% of capillary length in normal skeletal muscle [6]. CD248 was visible on some of these pericytes (Figure 1B, examples marked with a star) and also occasionally on cells where none of the three other pericyte markers used were detectable (Figure 1B, example marked with an arrow). There were no significant differences in pericyte coverage (Figure 1C), or expression of the different pericyte markers in tissue from CD248$^{-/-}$ compared to WT mice (Figure 1D). The majority of pericytes were positive for PDGFRβ, with 60-80% expressing NG2 and/or CD248, and ~40% positive for αSMA (Figure 1D). Approximately 45% of CD248 positive pericytes also expressed PDGFRβ (data not shown). As expected, CD248 expression on pericytes was not expressed (NE) in CD248$^{-/-}$ muscle tissue (Figure 1D) but this did not affect the relative expression of other markers. Following extirpation of WT mice we also found no statistically significant differences in the expression of any of the four pericyte markers (Figure S2).

WT and CD248$^{-/-}$ muscle display the same characteristics before treatment

As pericytes are critical for the stabilisation of the capillary network, we sought to examine whether genetic deletion of CD248 could affect the normal architecture of the capillary network in skeletal muscle. We observed no difference in the capillary density (CD) or the capillary to fibre ratio (C:F) in WT and CD248$^{-/-}$ animals at baseline (Figure 2A and B respectively). Similarly, both WT and CD248$^{-/-}$ showed the same inverse, non-linear relationship between CD and fibre size as previously described [23], with CD progressively declining as the area of the fibre increased (Figure 2C). No overt phenotypic differences in the organisation of the capillary network were observed between WT and CD248$^{-/-}$ by confocal microscopy (Figure 2D).

Both WT and CD248$^{-/-}$ mice mount a splitting angiogenic response induced by prazosin treatment

We used prazosin to increase blood flow within skeletal muscle, thereby increasing shear stress and inducing a splitting angiogenic response [25]. As expected, we observed a significant increase in C:F ratio following treatment in WT animals and a similar increase was seen in the CD248$^{-/-}$ muscle (Figure 3A), thus suggesting CD248 is not required for splitting angiogenesis.

CD248$^{-/-}$ mice are unable to mount a sprouting angiogenic response to muscle overload

Sprouting angiogenesis requires extensive pericyte involvement to co-ordinate endothelial cell migration [2,27–28]. We examined the potential importance of CD248 in this process in vivo by using surgical extirpation of the tibialis anterior muscle. This procedure, causing overload in the EDL muscle, triggers a compensatory angiogenic response based only on sprouting that can be observed in the operated limb in rats [3,24] and in mice [29–30]. Induction of sprouting angiogenesis in WT animals was demonstrated by a significant increase in C:F when compared to untreated, control mice (Figure 3B), as previously described [24]. In contrast, this response was completely ablated in CD248$^{-/-}$ animals (Figure 3B), indicating that CD248 is required for sprouting angiogenesis in this model of muscle remodelling. Of note, we observed no gender-specific differences in these responses for either genotype (data not shown).

Recent evidence suggests that CD248 may function to enhance or modify PDGF-BB signalling by acting upstream of ERK1/2 phosphorylation in pericytes [21]. In skeletal muscle, we observed an up-regulation of ERK phosphorylation following extirpation in the WT but not in the CD248$^{-/-}$ muscle by Western blot (Figure 3E) and immunofluorescence (Figure 3F). Interestingly, extirpation-induced ERK phosphorylation was ablated with Imatinib treatment (Figure 3E–F). Collectively these data support the concept that CD248 modulation of PDGF-BB signalling occurs upstream of ERK phosphorylation.

We next aimed to evaluate the response of genes known to regulate the angiogenic response by using quantitative RT PCR (Figure 4). In both WT and CD248$^{-/-}$ mice, extirpation significantly increased the levels of PDGF-B and its receptor PDGF receptor β, angiopoietin 2 and HIF1α mRNA (Figure 4). A moderate but insignificant increase was also observed for the angiopoietin receptor homologue of Tie2, TEK (Figure 4B). Prazosin treatment did not induce the expression of these genes in either WT or CD248$^{-/-}$ animals. Tissue-wide expression of VEGF-A mRNA expression was not altered following either extirpation or prazosin treatment regardless of CD248 genotype (Figure 4E). The effects of these treatments on HIF1α, VEGF-A and Ang2 expression are broadly in agreement with previous findings [29]. To our knowledge the effect of extirpation or prazosin treatment on the expression of the other genes shown here has not been previously reported in the literature.

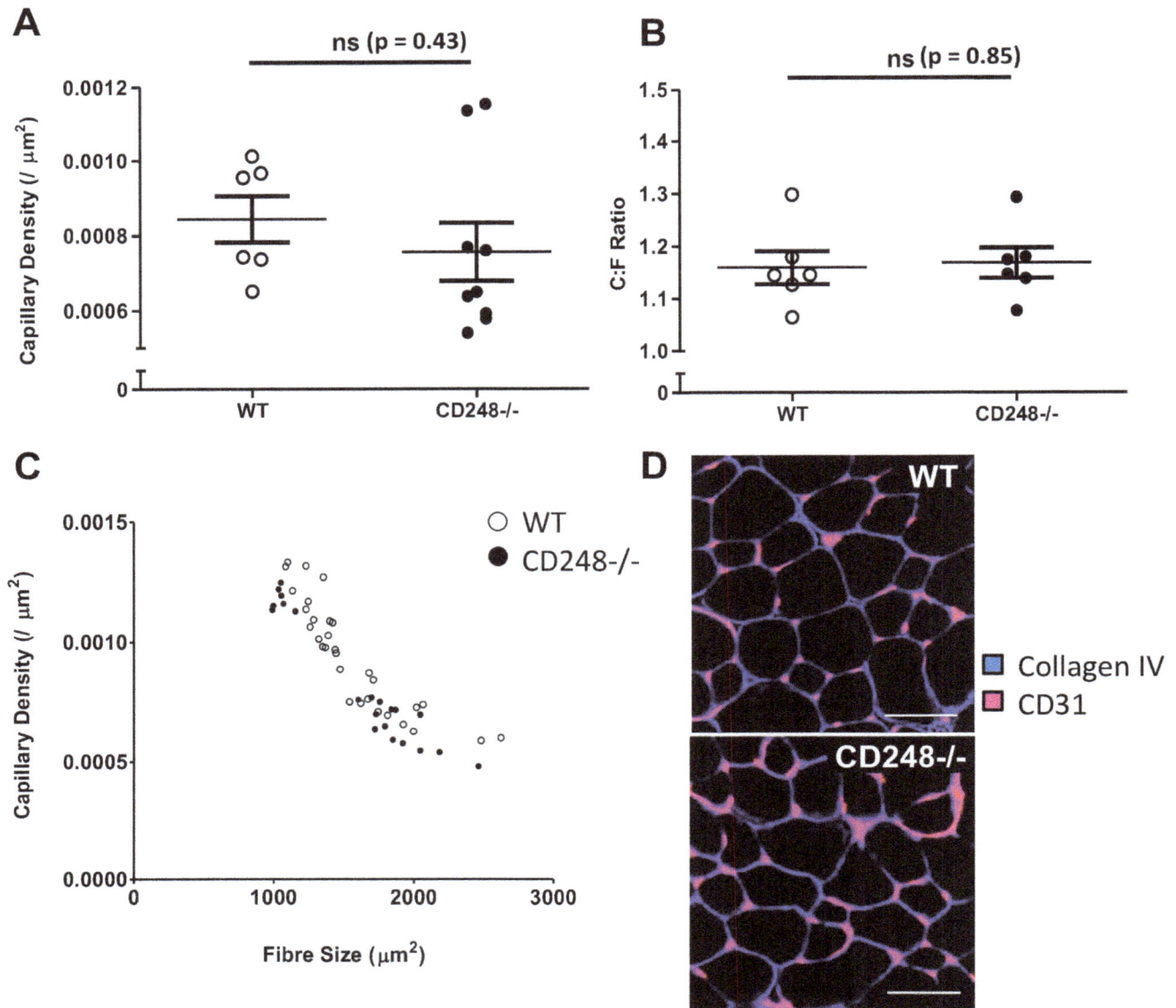

Figure 2. Effects of CD248$^{-/-}$ on the architecture of skeletal muscle in control animals. (**A**) Average capillary density (capillary/μm^2) and (**B**) capillary to fibre ratio were determined from tissue sections of untreated EDL muscle by immunofluorescence. In (**A**) and (**B**) each point represents the mean value obtained for 3–5 sections per animal. The mean for all animals is represented by the wide line and the error bars show the 95% confidence interval. (**C**) In both genotypes a non-linear relationship is seen between muscle fibre size and capillary density. Empty circles are WT, filled circles are CD248$^{-/-}$. Each circle represents the mean value for one animal, subjected to control, extirpation or prazosin treatment. (**D**) Immunofluorescence and confocal microscopy of EDL tissue sections from untreated 8-12 week old wildtype (top) or CD248$^{-/-}$ (bottom) mice. Sections were stained with antibodies to Collagen IV (blue) to mark the basement membrane and CD31 (red/magenta) to mark the blood vessels. Scale bars are 50 microns. ns = no significant difference by t-test.

Wildtype mice treated with Imatinib mesylate mirror the defect in sprouting angiogenesis observed in CD248$^{-/-}$ mice

CD248 is known to be required for effective PDGF signalling in pericytes [21] therefore we tested whether selective inhibition of PDGF signalling could replicate the CD248$^{-/-}$ phenotype that we observed in the sprouting angiogenic response to muscle overload. Imatinib mesylate is a tyrosine kinase inhibitor of Bcr Abl chimeric protein, c Kit and a competitive inhibitor of PDGF signalling, known to effectively block phosphorylation of the PDGF Receptor β thereby preventing downstream signalling [26]. Imatinib

treatment alone had no effect on C:F ratio in untreated WT or CD248$^{-/-}$ mice when compared to genotype-matched controls. Similarly, Imatinib treatment had no effect on the prazosin-induced increase in C:F in either WT or CD248$^{-/-}$ mice (Figure 3C), implying that PDGF signalling is not required for splitting angiogenesis. In contrast, Imatinib completely abolished extirpation-induced angiogenesis in WT mice (Figure 3D), mirroring the effect of CD248 knockout (Figure 3B).

Interestingly, Imatinib prevented the up-regulation of PDGF-B, PDGFRβ, angiopoietin 2, TEK and HIF1α mRNA in both WT and CD248$^{-/-}$ muscle (Figure 5), suggesting the dependency of all

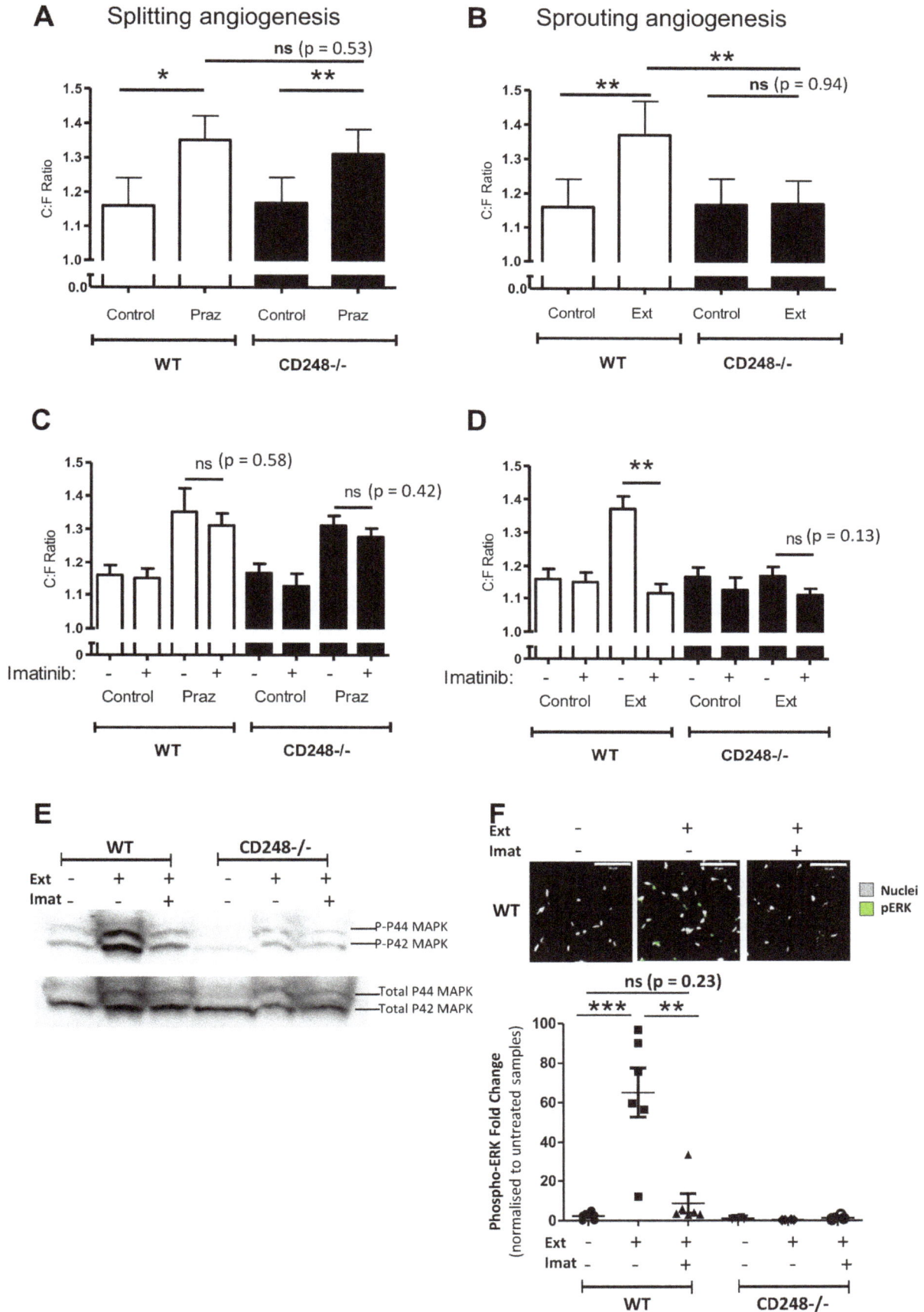

Figure 3. Effect of Prazosin and Extirpation treatment on muscle angiogenesis. Effects of (**A**) prazosin treatment (Pra) and (**B**) extirpation (Ext) on the capillary to fibre ratio (C:F) in wildtype and CD248$^{-/-}$mice. The capillary to fibre ratio (C:F) was calculated for each group. Alternatively mice underwent (**C**) prazosin treatment or (**D**) extirpation surgery either alone or in the presence (+) or absence (-) of the PDGF inhibitor Imatinib (150 mg/kg/day). In each case, control animals received no treatment. Empty bars are WT, filled bars are CD248$^{-/-}$. (**E**) Western blot of EDL muscle from WT and CD248$^{-/-}$ mice undergoing extirpation (Ext) surgery either alone or in the presence (+) or absence (-) of the PDGF inhibitor Imatinib (Imat) at 150 mg/kg/day. Upper blot shows levels of phospho-ERK expression whilst the lower blot is a loading control showing levels of total ERK. (**F**) Top: Representative images of phospho-ERK expression by confocal microscopy from control, extirpated (Ext) and extirpated plus Imatinib (Imat). Phospho-ERK (green) nuclei (grey). Scale bar is 50 microns. Below: Pixel counts (expressed as fold change from genotype-matched control) from confocal immunofluorescence images of phosphorylated ERK from muscle sections with (+) and without (-) extirpation (Ext) and/or Imatinib (Imat) treatment. Data are mean ± SEM from 6 animals (A-D) and 3 animals (E–F). (A–D) ANOVA with Bonferroni post-test shows a significant effect of treatment and genotype on the response to stimulus. (F) Students t-test was used to identify significance * = $P<0.05$, ** = $P<0.01$, *** = $P<0.001$, ns = non-significant.

these genes on the PDGF signalling pathway. Again, no change was seen in VEGF-A mRNA expression following Imatinib treatment, regardless of genotype (Figure 5E).

Discussion

Appropriate regulation of angiogenesis is crucial in allowing tissues to respond to changing physiological requirements and pericytes are known to play a crucial role in the control of these processes. In this manuscript we have shown that CD248 is expressed on some, but not all, pericytes surrounding the capillaries within resting muscle tissue and we have demonstrated a role for CD248 in sprouting angiogenesis. PDGFRβ and NG2 are widely used as pericyte markers, but are neither specific for pericytes nor expressed on all pericytes at all times [28]. While CD248 sometimes co-localised with PDGFRβ and NG2, CD31 positive capillaries were also seen closely surrounded by CD248 single-positive perivascular cells, in a location expected to be occupied by pericytes i.e. within the collagen IV basement membrane. This suggests that CD248 can be useful in identifying a pericyte subset that would otherwise be missed if only the traditional pericyte markers are used.

Angiogenesis can occur via a process of vessel splitting, where one vessel is reorganised longitudinally to become two, or by sprouting where an entirely new vessel is formed [1]. Prazosin causes an increase in microvascular flow through an α-adrenoreceptor antagonised arteriolar relaxation [31], elevating shear stress on the luminal capillary walls and triggering angiogenesis by longitudinal splitting. This is a mostly pericyte-independent process occurring through reorganisation of the endothelium with little requirement for basement membrane remodelling or an increase in pericyte number [3]. Our results demonstrate that muscle is able to effectively mount a microvascular response to increased shear stress in CD248$^{-/-}$ mice.

CD248$^{-/-}$ mice were unable to mount a sprouting angiogenic response to extirpation-induced overload of the EDL muscle. Extirpation causes increased stretch on myocytes, seen as an increase in sarcomere length that leads to hypertrophy and hyperplasia, releasing growth factors into the local environment, and increasing stretch on the abluminal surface of adjacent capillaries [31]. This physical stretch is the trigger for abluminal sprouting as the sole mechanism of capillary growth, a mechanotransduction process which requires pericyte migration and activation. The observation that CD248$^{-/-}$ mice are unable to respond to these stimuli strongly suggests that CD248 expression on pericytes is required in the cascade of events leading to capillary sprout formation. Additionally, we observed that members of the PDGF, angiopoietin and HIF1α signalling pathways were upregulated only by extirpation and not by prazosin treatment. This extends the differential gene expression profile previously described between splitting and sprouting angiogenesis [29]. By Western blotting and immunofluorescence analysis we were able

to show that phosphorylation of ERK occurs following extirpation in the WT but not the CD248$^{-/-}$ muscle and that this phosphorylation can be blocked with Imatinib treatment, further implicating CD248 and the PDGF signalling cascade in this process.

Combining evidence in the literature and this most recent study, we propose the following model (Figure 6): when endothelial cells are subjected to mechanical stretch, such as that seen following extirpation, the transcription factor HIF-1α is up-regulated [32] and can bind to the angiopoietin 2 HIF-binding site resulting in up-regulation of angiopoietin mRNA [33]. Ang2 is known to be strongly upregulated at sites of active vessel remodelling [34] where it binds the receptor TEK on endothelial cells, inducing its phosphorylation [35]. This results in the up-regulation of PDGF-B protein which dimerises and binds to its receptor PDGFRβ on pericytes. In the presence of CD248, PDGFRβ signalling occurs which stimulates the migration of pericytes towards the endothelium and subsequently stabilises the capillary. Successful sprouting angiogenesis reduces the stretch experienced in the capillary bed, restoring HIF1α and angiopoietin gene expression to baseline levels. In the CD248$^{-/-}$ mouse sprouting cannot occur due to defective PDGF signalling resulting in persistently high levels of stretch and expression of its inducible genes, HIF1α, Ang2, TEK, PDGF-B and PDGFRβ.

We have to assume that PDGF signalling can occur normally in the absence of CD248 in most situations, and in cells where CD248 is not expressed (such as endothelial cells [36]). This is evidenced by the fact that the CD248$^{-/-}$ mouse does not phenocopy the PDGF-B or PDGFRβ knockout mice, both of which are embryonically lethal due to widespread microvascular bleeding caused by a severe shortage of vascular smooth muscle cells and pericytes [9–11]. In contrast, the CD248$^{-/-}$ has no overt phenotype and no increased mortality (unpublished observations). Imatinib blocks PDGF signalling in all cell types and by measuring its effects on mRNA expression within whole muscle we were unable to distinguish CD248-mediated PDGF signalling from non-CD248-mediated. Interestingly, Imatinib blocked up-regulation of HIF1α, TEK2, Ang2, PDGF-B and PDGFRβ mRNA whilst their expression was not prevented in the CD248$^{-/-}$ mouse. This can be explained by the non-specific nature of the inhibitor used. Recently, Chislock *et al.* [37] reported that Abelson (Abl) kinases (a target for Imatinib in addition to PDGFRβ) positively regulated TEK expression, explaining the reduction in the mRNA levels of this receptor following Imatinib treatment. In addition, Imatinib has been reported to reduce HIF1α protein expression in a model of prostate cancer by a hypoxia-independent process [38]. Given these findings, it is clear that Imatinib treatment can result in the blockade of many aspects of the HIF1α/angiopoietin/PDGF signalling process making it difficult to draw firm conclusions as to the exact role of CD248 within the cascade. Unfortunately, no specific PDGF-pathway inhibitors are available

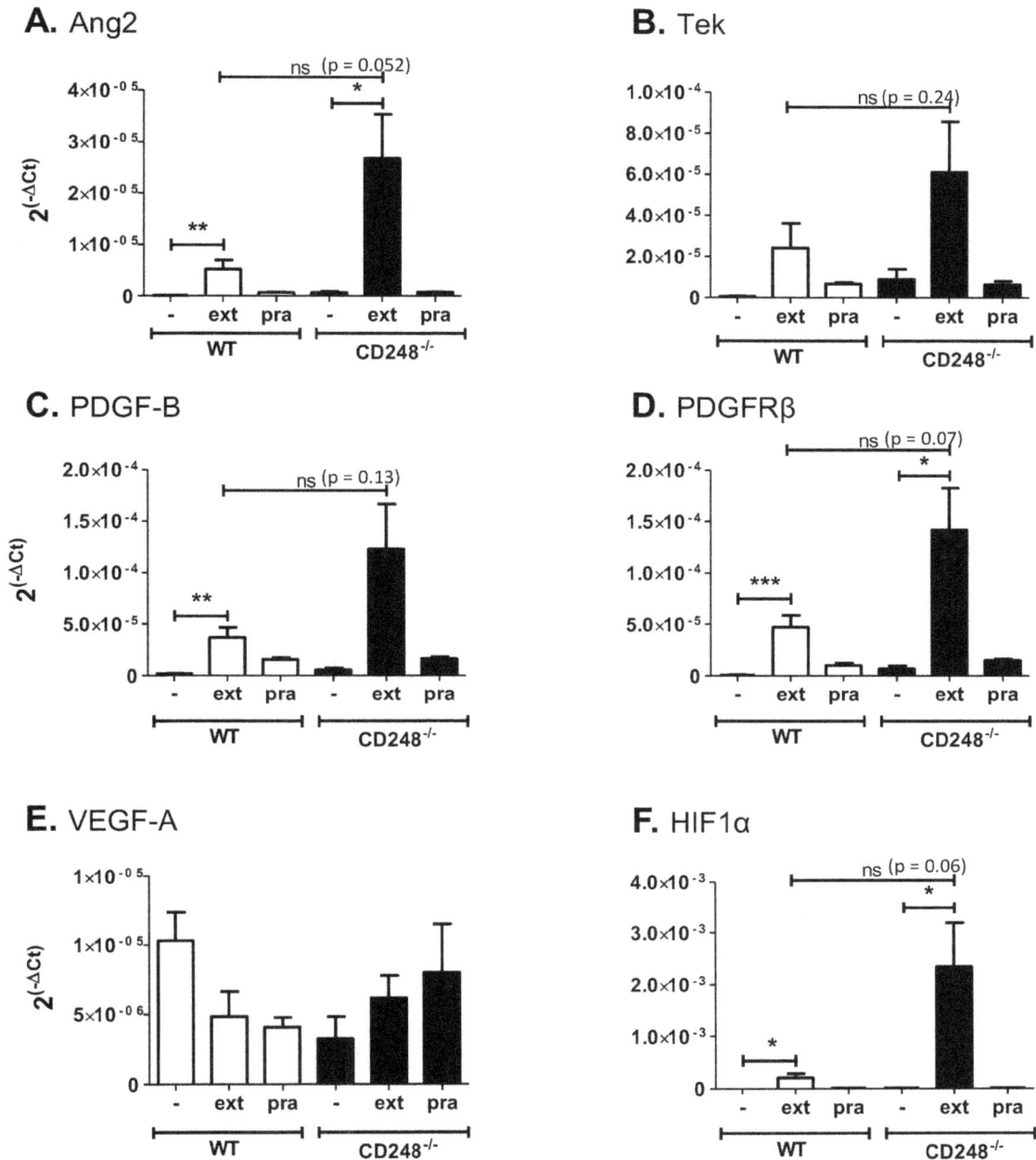

Figure 4. Effect of CD248 genotype on transcriptional response to Prazosin and Extirpation treatment. mRNA analysis of EDL muscle tissue by RT-PCR from WT and CD248$^{-/-}$ mice following either no treatment control (-), extirpation (ext) or prazosin (pra) treatment. Gene transcription data were acquired for angiopoietin2 (Ang2: **A**), endothelial tyrosine kinase (TEK: **B**), platelet-derived growth factor B (PDGF-B: **C**), platelet-derived growth factor receptor β (PDGFRβ: **D**), vascular endothelial growth factor A (VEGF-A: **E**) and hypoxia-inducible factor 1α (HIF1α: **F**). Data are shown as relative expression units (2−ΔCt) relative to 18S. Data are mean ± SEM from 6 animals. ANOVA with Bonferroni post-test shows a significant effect of treatment and genotype on the response to stimulus * = $P<0.05$; ** = $P<0.01$, *** = $P<0.001$, ns = non-significant.

to allow us to further dissect the role of PDGF signalling in this model of sprouting angiogenesis.

Whilst the nature of the interaction of Imatinib with the PDGF pathway is understood, its influence of CD248 on this pathway remains unclear. Tomkowicz *et al.* [21] reported that CD248 interacts downstream of the PDGF receptor and upstream of ERK by an unknown mechanism and with unknown intermediaries. Our results show that the induction of PDGF-B by endothelial cells and PDGFRβ by pericytes at the gene level does not require

CD248. However, downstream effects of CD248-mediated PDGF signalling that result in sprouting angiogenesis in this context seem to be dependent on CD248 expression. The intricacies of PDGF signalling have been exposed by the creation of an allelic series of PDGFRβ mice in which specific tyrosine residues were replaced with phenylalanine (reviewed in detail in [39–40]). All mouse strains generated were viable and fertile even when all 7 of the tyrosines that are known to be involved in PDGFRβ signalling were removed. This, compared to the PDGFRβ knockout, which

A. Imatinib Ang2

B. Imatinib Tek

C. Imatinib PDGF-B

D. Imatinib PDGFRβ

E. Imatinib VEGF-A

F. Imatinib HIF1α

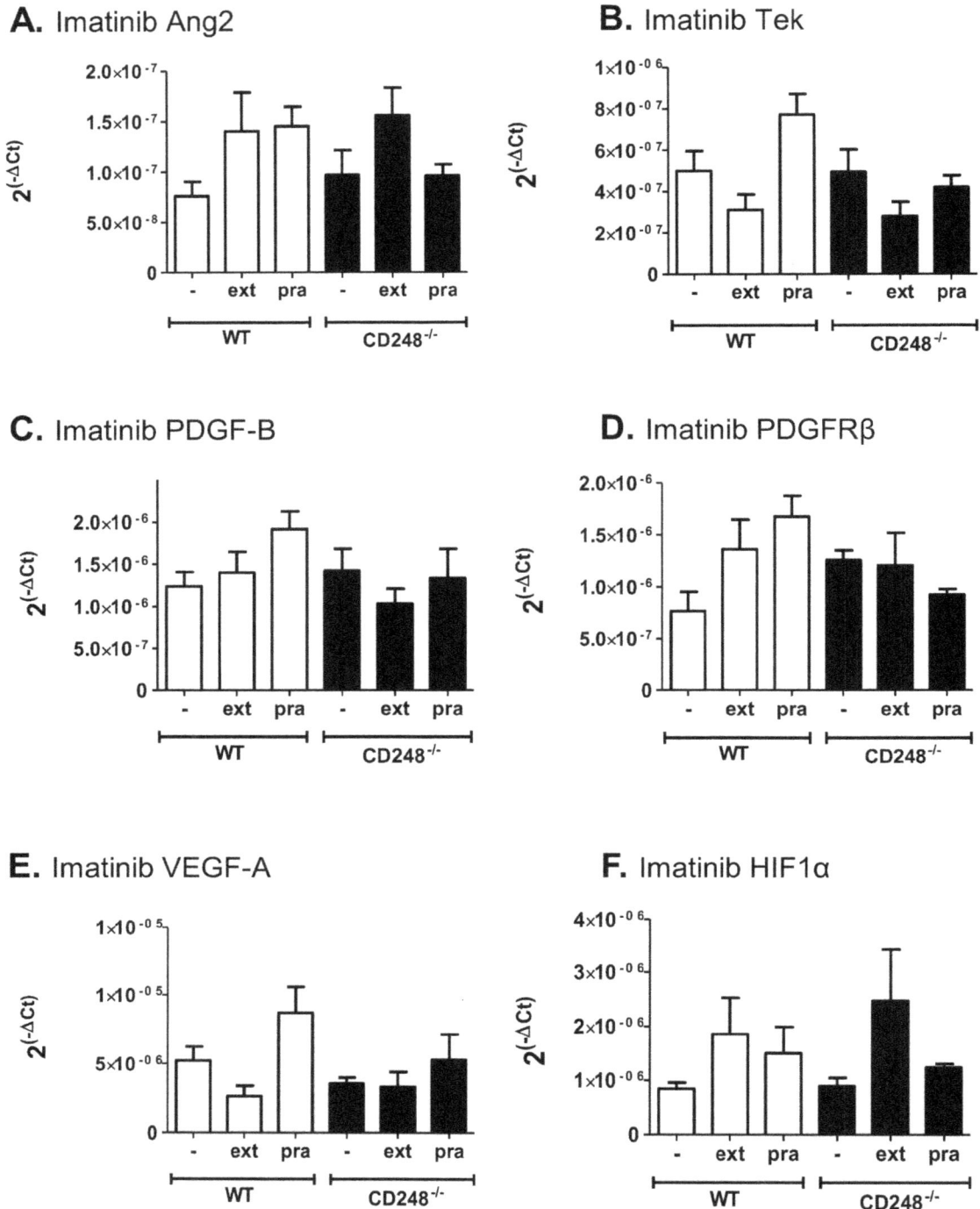

Figure 5. Effect of PDGF signalling inhibition by Imatinib on gene expression following Prazosin and Extirpation treatment. mRNA analysis of EDL muscle tissue by RT-PCR from WT and CD248$^{-/-}$ mice plus no treatment control (-), extirpation (ext) or prazosin (pra) treatment. In addition, all mice were treated with Imatinib throughout the experiment. Gene transcription data were acquired for angiopoietin2 (Ang2: **A**), endothelial tyrosine kinase (TEK: **B**), platelet-derived growth factor B (PDGF-B: **C**), platelet-derived growth factor receptor β (PDGFRβ: **D**), vascular endothelial growth factor A (VEGF-A: **E**) and hypoxia-inducible factor 1α (HIF1α: **F**). Data are shown as relative expression units (2−ΔCt) relative to 18S. Data are mean ± SEM from 6 animals. ANOVA with Bonferroni post-test was performed and no significant differences were observed between any treatments or genotypes.

is lethal at E18.5 [40] suggests that PDGFRβ has signalling capacity in the cytoplasmic tail beyond that of tyrosine phosphorylation. How CD248 interacts with the PDGF pathway has yet to be identified and is crucial in order to extend our understanding of this vital signalling pathway.

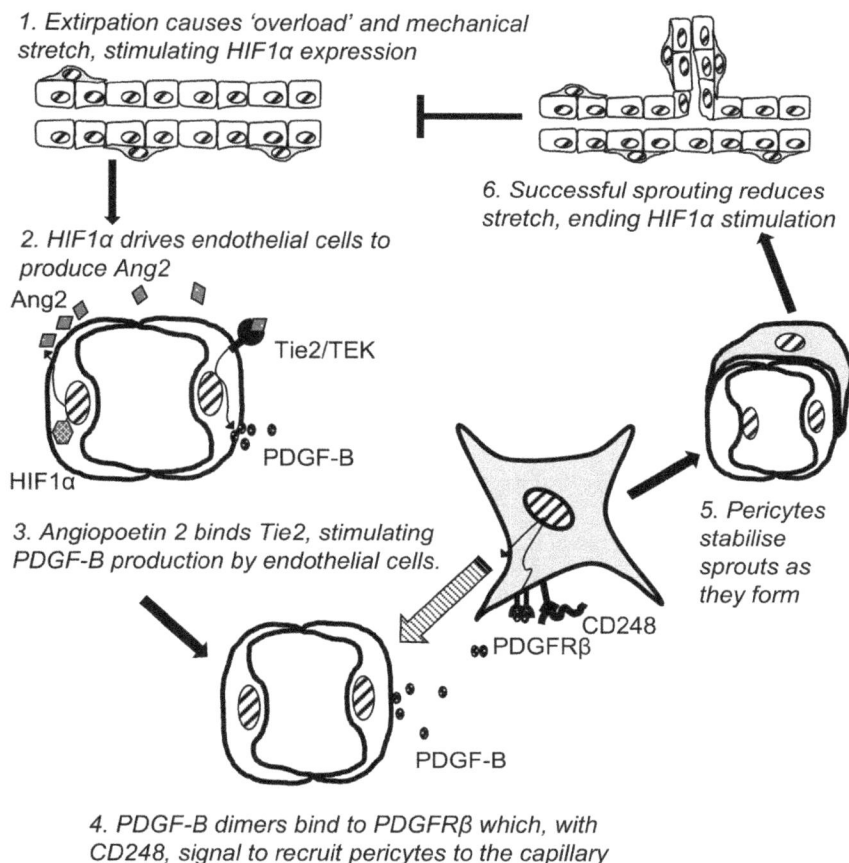

1. Extirpation causes 'overload' and mechanical stretch, stimulating HIF1α expression

2. HIF1α drives endothelial cells to produce Ang2

Ang2

Tie2/TEK

HIF1α

PDGF-B

3. Angiopoetin 2 binds Tie2, stimulating PDGF-B production by endothelial cells.

PDGF-B

4. PDGF-B dimers bind to PDGFRβ which, with CD248, signal to recruit pericytes to the capillary

CD248

PDGFRβ

5. Pericytes stabilise sprouts as they form

6. Successful sprouting reduces stretch, ending HIF1α stimulation

Figure 6. Model of the proposed role of CD248-mediated PDGF signalling in vessel sprouting. When endothelial cells are subjected to mechanical stretch, such as that seen following extirpation, the transcription factor HIF-1α is up-regulated and can bind to the HIF-binding site on the angiopoietin 2 gene. Angiopoietin 2 then binds to its receptor TEK on endothelial cells, inducing its phosphorylation. This results in upregulation of PDGF-B protein which dimerises and binds to its receptor PDGFRβ on pericytes. In the presence of CD248 this induces downstream signalling that stimulates migration of the pericyte to the endothelium and subsequent stabilisation of the capillary. When sprouting angiogenesis is successful the stretch on the capillary is reduced and HIF1α and angiopoietin gene expression can return to baseline.

Supporting Information

Figure S1 Confocal images used for capillary:fibre ratio analysis. Frozen sections from WT or CD248$^{-/-}$ mice either untreated, extirpated or prazosin treated. Sections were stained with antibodies to collagen IV (blue) to stain basement membrane and demarcate the fibre boundaries or CD31 (red/magenta) to mark capillaries. Images are representative of 3-6 animals per group. Scale bars are 50 microns.

Figure S2 Expression of individual pericyte markers following either sham operation or extirpation, ex- pressed as percentage of CD31 positive vessels positive for either PDGFRβ, NG2 or αSMA. Data are mean ± SEM from 3 independent WT animals. ns = no significant difference by ANOVA with Bonferroni post-test.

Author Contributions

Conceived and designed the experiments: AJN HMM FB APC SE CDB. Performed the experiments: AJN HMM WDM PM SE. Analyzed the data: AJN HMM WDM PM FB APC SE CDB. Contributed reagents/materials/analysis tools: SE. Contributed to the writing of the manuscript: AJN HMM FB APC SE CDB.

References

1. Bergers G, Song S (2005) The role of pericytes in blood-vessel formation and maintenance. J Neurooncol. 7: 452–64
2. Egginton S, Zhou AL, Brown MD, Hudlická O (2000) The role of pericytes in controlling physiological angiogenesis in vivo. In: Maragoudakis, M.E. (ed.) 'Angiogenesis: From the molecular to integrative pharmacology'. Kluwer Academic/Plenum Press, New York. Advances in Experimental Medicine and Biology. 476: 81–99
3. Egginton S, Zhou AL, Brown MD, Hudlická O (2001) Unorthodox angiogenesis in skeletal muscle. Cardiovasc Res. 49: 634–46
4. Wilkinson-Berka JL, Babic S, De Gooyer TE, Stitt AW, Jaworski K, et al. (2004) Inhibition of platelet derived growth factor promotes pericyte loss and angiogenesis in ischaemic retinopathy. Am J Path. 164: 1263–73
5. Hellstrom M, Kalén M, Lindahl P, Abramsson A, Betsholtz C (1999) Role of PDGF-B and PDGFRβ in recruitment of vascular smooth muscle cells and pericytes during embryonic blood vessel formation in the mouse. Development. 126: 3047–55
6. Egginton S, Hudlická O, Brown MD, Graciotti L, Granata AL (1996) In vivo pericyte-endothelial cell interaction during angiogenesis in adult cardiac and skeletal muscle. Microvasc Res. 51: 213–28
7. Ribatti D, Nico B, Crivellato E (2011) The Role of Pericytes in Angiogenesis. Int J Dev Biol. 55: 261–8
8. Tomkowicz B, Rybinski K, Foley B, Ebel W, Kline B, et al. (2007) Interaction of endosialin/Tem1 with extracellular Matrix Protein Mediates Cell adhesion and migration. Proc Natl Acad Sci USA. 104: 17965–70

9. Levéen P, Pekny M, Gebre-Medhin S, Swolin B, Larsson E, et al. (1994) Mice deficient for PDGF B show renal, cardiovascular, and hematological abnormalities. Genes Dev. 8: 1875–87

10. Soriano P (1994) Abnormal kidney development and hematological disorders in PDGF beta-receptor mutant mice. Gene Dev. 8: 1888–96

11. Lindahl P, Johansson BR, Levéen P, Betsholtz C (1997) Pericyte loss and microaneurysm formation in PDGF-B-deficient mice. Science. 277: 242–5

12. Bagley R, Honma N, Weber W, Boutin P, Rouleau C, et al. (2008) Endosialin/Tem1/CD248 is a Pericyte Marker of Embryonic and Tumor Neovascularization. Microvasc Research. 76: 180–8

13. Dolznig H, Schweifer N, Puri C, Kraut N, Rettig WJ, et al. (2005) Characterization of cancer stroma markers: in silico analysis of an mRNA expression database for fibroblast activation protein and endosialin. Cancer Immun. 5: 10

14. Carson-Walter E, Winans B, Whiteman M, Liu Y, Jarvela S, et al. (2009) Characterization of TEM1/endosialin in human and murine brain tumors. BMC Cancer. 9: 417

15. Rettig W, Garin-Chesa P, Healey JH, Su SL, Jaffe EA, et al. (1992) Identification of endosialin, a cell surface glycoprotein of vascular endothelial cells in human cancer. Proc Natl Acad Sci USA. 89: 10832–6

16. MacFadyen J, Haworth O, Robertson D, Hardie D, Webster MT, et al. (2005) Endosialin (TEM1,CD248) is a marker of stromal fibroblasts and is not selectively expressed on tumour endothelium. FEBS Lett. 579: 2569–75

17. Simonavicius N, Robertson D, Bax DA, Jones C, Huijbers IJ, et al. (2008) Endosialin (CD248) is a marker of tumor-associated pericytes in high-grade glioma. Modern Pathol. 21: 308–15

18. Nanda A, Karim B, Peng Z, Liu G, Qiu W, et al. (2006) Tumour Endothelial Marker 1 (Tem1) Functions in the Growth and Progression of Abdominal Tumours. Proc Natl Acad Sci USA. 103: 3351–6

19. Maia M, de Vriese A, Janssens T, Moons M, Lories RJ, et al. (2011) CD248 facilitates tumor growth via its cytoplasmic domain. BMC Cancer. 11: 162

20. Simonavicius N, Ashenden M, van Wevereijk A, Lax S, Huso DL, et al. (2012) Pericytes promote selective vessel regression to regulate vascular patterning. Blood. 120: 1516–27

21. Tomkowicz B, Rybinski K, Sebeck D, Sass P, Nicolaides NC, et al. (2010) Endosialin/TEM-1/CD248 regulates pericyte proliferation through PDGF receptor signaling. Cancer Biol Ther. 9: 908–15

22. Egginton S (1990) Morphometric analysis of tissue capillary supply. In Vertebrate Gas Exchange from Environment to Cell (ed. R. G. Boutilier). Advances in Comparative and Environmental Physiology. 6, 73–141. Berlin: Springer Verlag

23. Hudlická O, Brown MD, Egginton S (1992) Angiogenesis in skeletal and cardiac muscle. Physiol Rev 72: 369–417

24. Zhou AL, Egginton S, Brown MD, Hudlická O (1998) Capillary growth in overloaded, hypertrophic adult rat skeletal muscle: an ultrastructural study. Anat Rec. 252: 49–63

25. Zhou AL, Egginton S, Hudlická O, Brown MD (1998) Internal division of capillaries in rat skeletal muscle in response to chronic vasodilator treatment with alpha1-antagonist prazosin. Cell Tissue Res. 293: 293–303

26. Schultheis B, Nijmeijer B, Yin H, Gosden RG, Melo JV (2012) Imatinib mesylate at therapeutic doses has no impact on folliculogenesis or spermatogenesis in a leukaemic mouse model. Leukaemia Res. 36: 271–4

27. Gerhardt H, Betsholtz C (2003) Endothelial-pericyte interactions in angiogenesis. Cell Tissue Res. 314: 15–23

28. Armulik A, Genove G, Betscholtz C (2011) Pericytes: Developmental, Physiological and Pathological Perspectives, Problems, and Promises. Dev Cell. 21: 193–214

29. Williams JL, Weichert A, Zakrzewicz A, Da Siva-Azevedo L, Pries AR, et al. (2006) Differential gene and protein expression in abluminal sprouting and intraluminal splitting forms of angiogenesis. Clin Sci. 110: 587–95

30. Williams JL, Cartland D, Rudge JS, Egginton S (2006) VEGF trap abolishes shear stress- and overload-dependent angiogenesis in skeletal muscle. Microcirc. 13: 499–509

31. Hudlická O (1991) What Makes Blood Vessels Grow. J Physiol. 444: 1–24

32. Kim CH, Cho YS, Chun YS, Park JW, Kim MS (2002) Early expression of myocardial HIF-1α in response to mechanical stresses: regulation by stretch activated channels and the phosphatidylinositol 3-kinase signaling pathway. Circ Res. 90: E25–33

33. Simon MP, Tournaire R, Pouyssegur J (2008) The angiopoietin-2 gene of endothelial cells is up-regulated in hypoxia by a HIF binding site located in its first intron and by the central factors GATA-2 and Ets-1. J Cell Physiol. 217: 809–18.

34. Holash J, Maisonpierre PC, Compton D, Boland P, Alexander CR, et al. (1999) Vessel cooption, regression, and growth in tumors mediated by angiopoietins and VEGF. Science. 18: 1994–8

35. Thurston G (2003) Role of Angiopoietins and Tie receptor tyrosine kinases in angiogenesis and lymphangiogenesis. Cell Tissue Res. 314: 61–8

36. Beitz JG, Kim IS, Calabresi P, Frackelton AR Jr (1991) Human microvascular endothelial cells express receptors for platelet-derived growth factor. Proc Natl Acad Sci USA. 88: 2021–5

37. Chislock EM, Ring C, Perdergast AM (2013) Abl kinases are required for vascular function, Tie2 expression, and angiopoietin-1-mediated survival. Proc Natl Acad Sci USA. Early edition

38. Kimura Y, Inoue K, Abe M, Nearman J, Baranowska-Kortylewicz J (2007) PDGFRb and HIF-1a Inhibition with Imatinib and Radioimmunotherapy of Experimental Prostate Cancer. Cancer Biol Ther. 6: 1763–72

39. Betsholtz C (2004) Insight into the physiological functions of PDGF through genetic studies in mice. Cytokine and Growth Factor Rev. 14: 215–28

40. Tallquist MD, French WJ, Soriano P (2003) Additive effects of PDGF receptor beta signalling pathways in vascular smooth muscle cell development. PLoS Biol. 1:E52

5

Specific Matrix Metalloproteinases Play Different Roles in Intraplaque Angiogenesis and Plaque Instability in Rabbits

Xiao Qiong Liu[1,2], Yang Mao[1], Bo Wang[2], Xiao Ting Lu[1], Wen Wu Bai[1,2], Yuan Yuan Sun[1,2], Yan Liu[1], Hong Mei Liu[3], Lei Zhang[1]*, Yu Xia Zhao[2]*, Yun Zhang[1]

1 Key Laboratory of Cardiovascular Remodeling and Function Research, Shandong University Qilu Hospital, Jinan, Shandong, China, 2 Department of Traditional Chinese Medicine, Shandong University Qilu Hospital, Jinan, Shandong, China, 3 Department of Endodontics, Jinan Stomatologic Hospital, Jinan, Shandong, China

Abstract

Background: Ectopic angiogenesis within the intima and media is considered to be a hallmark of advanced vulnerable atherosclerotic lesions. Some studies have shown that specific matrix metalloproteinases (MMPs) might play different roles in angiogenesis. Therefore, we investigated the predominant effects of specific MMPs in intraplaque angiogenesis and plaque instability in a rabbit model of atherosclerosis.

Methods and Results: New Zealand rabbits underwent balloon injury of the abdominal artery and ingestion of a high-cholesterol (1%) diet to establish an atherosclerotic animal model. At weeks 4, 6, 8, 10, and 12 after balloon injury, five rabbits were euthanized and the abdominal aorta was harvested. Blood lipid analysis, intravascular ultrasound imaging, pathologic and immunohistochemical expression studies, and western blotting were performed. From weeks 4 to 12, the expression of MMP-1, -2, -3, and -9 and vascular endothelial growth factor A (VEGF-A) increased with atherosclerotic plaque development in the abdominal aorta, while the expression of MMP-14 substantially decreased. The vulnerability index (VI) gradually increased over time. Intraplaque neovessels appeared at week 8. The microvessel density (MVD) was greater at week 12 than at week 8. The VI, MVD, and VEGF-A level were positively correlated with the MMP-1, -2,-3, and -9 levels within plaques. Negative correlations were noted between the MMP-14 level and the VI, MVD, and VEGF-A level.

Conclusion: Upregulation of MMP-1, -2, -3, and -9 and downregulation of MMP-14 may contribute to intraplaque angiogenesis and plaque instability at the advanced stage of atherosclerosis in rabbits.

Editor: Christoph E. Hagemeyer, Baker IDI Heart and Diabetes Institute, Australia

Funding: This study was supported by the National 973 Basic Research Program of China (No. 2012CB518603), grants from National Natural Science Foundation of China (No. 81270351, 60971023, 81100103, 81302939), Natural Science Foundation of Shandong Province (ZR2011HQ020), and Doctoral Fund of Ministry of Education of China (20130131110045). The funders had no role in study design, data collection and analysis, decision to publish, or preparation of the manuscript.

Competing Interests: The authors have declared that no competing interests exist.

* Email: leilybao@163.com (LZ); yxzhao@sdu.edu.cn (YXZ)

Introduction

Atherosclerotic plaque rupture is a major cause of acute cardiovascular events. Thus, stabilization of vulnerable plaques is of great clinical importance [1]. Pathological studies have identified specific characteristics of atherosclerotic plaques that are associated with plaque instability and rupture, including the ongoing inflammatory response, matrix degradation, and cell death. These changes result in eventual thinning of the fibrous cap and an increase in the inflammatory and necrotic core content. Neovascularization is another crucial feature of atherosclerotic plaques. The number of neovessels increases with plaque progression, and such vessels are abundant in vulnerable plaques [2]. Neovessels within plaques are characterized by fragility and high perfusion, thus allowing for extravasation of lipoproteins and red blood cells that contribute to the formation of plaque lipids [3]. This process results in intraplaque hemorrhage, increases the permeability of inflammatory cells, and leads to plaque destabilization [4,5]. Ectopic angiogenesis within the intima and media is considered to be a hallmark of advanced vulnerable atherosclerotic lesions.

Angiogenesis is induced by various growth-inducing and -inhibiting factors. Multiple complex signal transduction pathways are involved in intraplaque angiogenesis. Proteinases are required for degradation of the extracellular matrix (ECM), creating an avenue for migrating endothelial cells during angiogenesis. The specific MMPs necessary for endothelial cell migration and tube formation [6] have attracted particular attention because they directly degrade ECM components. MMPs, also termed matrixins, are a family of more than 20 zinc-containing endopeptidases that degrade various components of the ECM [7]. MMPs are subdivided into at least five groups based on their structure and/or substrate specificities. MMP family members include collagenases (MMP-1, -8, -13, and -18), gelatinases (MMP-2 and -9), stromelysins (MMP-3, -10, and -11), matrilysins (MMP-7 and -26), and membrane-type MMPs (MMP-14 and -15).

It has become clear that MMPs contribute more to angiogenesis than just degrading ECM components. Various MMPs, including MMP-1, -2, -3, -9, and -14, have been shown to enhance angiogenesis [8–12]. Specific MMPs can also negatively contribute to angiogenesis [13–15]. However, the predominant effects of MMPs in intraplaque angiogenesis at the advanced stages of atherosclerosis remain inconclusive. In the present study, we investigated the roles of different MMPs in angiogenesis in patients with atherosclerosis.

Materials and Methods

Ethics statement

The experiment complied with the Animal Management Rule of the Ministry of Public Health, People's Republic of China (documentation 55, 2001), and the experimental protocol was approved by the Animal Care Committee of Shandong University. All surgical procedures were performed with the rabbits under general anesthesia, and all efforts were made to minimize suffering.

Animal protocol

Adult male New Zealand White rabbits (n = 52) weighing 1.7 to 2.1 kg were obtained from Jinan Xilingjiao Culture and Breeding Center (Jinan, Shandong Province, China). The animals were housed in individual cages at the Animal Care Center of Shandong University Qilu Hospital. All procedures were performed after general anesthesia had been induced. Maintenance of a slight corneal reflex was tested using saline drops.

A rabbit model of atherosclerosis was established as previously described [16–18] with modifications. All animals were fed an atherogenic diet (120–140 g/day of a 1% cholesterol and 99% standard rabbit diet) for 12 weeks. Twenty-seven rabbits underwent balloon-induced abdominal aortic endothelial injury under general anesthesia, while the other 25 rabbits underwent no injury (control group). Ten randomly chosen rabbits (aortic injury group, n = 5; control group, n = 5) were euthanized at the end of weeks 4, 6, 8, 10, and 12, and their abdominal aortas were harvested. Before euthanasia, the rabbits underwent intravascular ultrasound (IVUS) imaging to examine the morphological changes of the aortic plaques, and blood was drawn from the auricular artery after an overnight fast. The body weights of all rabbits were monitored throughout the experiment.

Blood lipid analysis

Blood samples were centrifuged at 3000 revolutions per minute for 10 min at 4°C. Serum samples were then collected and stored at −80°C. The serum levels of total cholesterol (TC), high-density lipoprotein cholesterol (HDL-C), low-density lipoprotein cholesterol (LDL-C), and triglycerides (TG) were measured by enzymatic assays using an automated biochemical analyzer (Roche Hitachi 917; Block Scientific, NY, USA).

IVUS assay

Each IVUS study was performed according to a standard procedure [19]. IVUS imaging was performed using a 3.2-F catheter containing a 40-MHz single-rotating-element transducer connected to an IVUS system (Galaxy; Boston Scientific, Fremont, CA, USA). The catheter was withdrawn to the abdominal aorta by a motorized pullback device at a constant speed of 0.5 mm/s. The lumen area (LA) and external elastic membrane area (EEMA) were measured on abdominal aortic cross-sectional images. The plaque area (PA) was calculated by EEMA − LA, and the plaque burden (PB, %) was calculated by PA/EEMA×100% [20].

Histopathology and immunohistochemistry

The abdominal aorta (2 cm long) was fixed in 4% formaldehyde for 24 h, and 5-μm-thick segments were then serially sectioned. Frozen sections were stained with Oil Red O (Santa Cruz Biotechnology, Santa Cruz, CA, USA) to determine the lipid content, and paraffin sections underwent Sirius red, hematoxylin and eosin, and immunohistochemical staining.

Immunohistochemical staining was performed using standard techniques as previously described [21]. Briefly, endogenous peroxidase activity was inhibited by incubation with 3% hydrogen peroxide. Sections were blocked with 5% goat serum in phosphate buffered saline and incubated overnight at 4°C with primary antibodies. After washing with phosphate buffered saline, the sections were incubated with secondary antibody at 37°C for 30 min. The immunohistochemical staining results were analyzed using a diaminobenzidine kit (Zhongshan Goldenbridge Biotechnology, Beijing, China). Hematoxylin was used to counterstain the nucleus. The primary antibodies were mouse anti-rabbit RAM-11 (1:200; Dako Glostrup, Denmark); α-smooth muscle cell (SMC) actin (1:200; Sigma Chemical, Santa Clara, CA, USA); CD31, MMP-1, -2, -9, and -14, vascular endothelial growth factor A (VEGF-A), and collagen I (1:20, 1:100, 1:100, 1:50, 1:100, 1:100, 1:100, respectively; Abcam, Cambridge, MA, USA); MMP-3 (1:100; Chemicon, Boston, MA, USA); and collagen III (1:200; Novus Biologicals, Littleton, CO, USA). The cross-reactivity between antibodies and rabbit antigens was tested in preliminary experiments and confirmed by negative-control experiments involving nonimmune IgG instead of primary antibodies.

Histopathological slides were analyzed using Image-Pro Plus 6.0 (Media Cybernetics, Cambridge, MA, USA). The intima–media thickness (IMT) of each aortic plaque was measured as follows. Eight randomly chosen fields in each cross section and five cross sections in each rabbit were selected for quantitative measurement, and the values were averaged [22]. The area of positive immunohistochemical staining was expressed as the proportion of the stained area divided by the total plaque area in at least 10 high-power fields (200×). The vulnerability index was calculated as follows: (macrophage staining % + lipid staining %)/(smooth muscle cell % + collagen fiber %) [21]. Ten random high-power fields (200×) were used for each sample to quantify the MVD in sections stained for CD31, and the microvessels were then quantified by the plaque area.

Western blot analysis

Protein was extracted and separated on 10% to 15% SDS-PAGE gel and transferred onto nitrocellulose membranes. After blocking with 5% nonfat milk for 2 h at room temperature, the membranes were incubated with the following primary antibodies overnight at 4°C: anti-MMP-1 (1:1000; Abcam, Cambridge, MA, USA), anti-MMP-2 (1:1000; Abcam, Cambridge, MA, USA), anti-MMP-3 (1:1000; Chemicon, Boston, MA, USA), anti-MMP-9 (1:1000; Abcam, Cambridge, MA, USA), and anti-MMP-14 (1:100; Abcam, Cambridge, MA, USA). After being washed in TBS-T, the membranes were incubated with horseradish peroxidase-conjugated secondary antibody for 2 h at room temperature. Signals were detected using an enhanced chemiluminescence kit (Millipore, Billerica, MA, USA). The protein levels were normalized to β-actin.

Statistical analysis

All data analyses were performed using Predictive Analysis Software 18.0 (SPSS Inc., Chicago, IL, USA). Intergroup comparisons involved one-way ANOVA followed by the least-squares difference test (with equal variances assumed) or Dunnett's T3 test (equal variances not assumed). Spearman's rank correlation coefficient was used for correlation analysis. All data are presented as mean ± standard error of the mean. A two-tailed P value of <0.05 was considered statistically significant.

Results

All rabbits showed full recovery without complications after balloon injury. Administration of the atherogenic diet was well tolerated by all rabbits, and no adverse effects were observed. Two rabbits that underwent balloon injury died of diarrhea at weeks 6 and 10.

In the control group, 12-week administration of the atherogenic diet resulted in fatty streak formation with lipid infiltration and only scarce plaques in the abdominal aorta (see supporting information for details; Figures S1–S4).

Serum lipid assay and body weight of balloon-injured rabbits

The serum levels of TC, HDL-C, LDL-C, and TG increased significantly after ingestion of the high-cholesterol diet (P<0.01) (Figure 1A–D). At the end of week 6, all four serum values were higher than at week 4 (P>0.05) (Figure 1A–D). At the end of weeks 8, 10, and 12, the serum levels of TC, HDL-C, and LDL-C were significantly higher than those at week 6 (P<0.05) (Figure 1A–C); however, the TG level showed no significant difference (P>0.05) (Figure 1D). The TG level was significantly higher at the end of week 12 than at week 6 (P<0.05) (Figure 1D). The body weights of the rabbits gradually increased over time (P<0.05) (Figure 1E).

IVUS measurements in the balloon-injured rabbits

The LA, EEMA, PA, and PB values increased throughout the duration of the experiment. The LA in the abdominal aorta did not differ among the 5 weeks (P>0.05) (Figure 2A, B). However, the EEMA, PA, and PB values were higher at weeks 10 and 12 than at week 4 (P<0.01), with no difference among weeks 4, 6, and 8 (P>0.05) (Figure 2A, C–E).

Histopathological examination of the balloon-injured rabbits

The IMT of the abdominal aortic plaques increased until week 12 and was higher at week 6 than at week 4 (P<0.01) (Figure 2F). The IMT was significantly thicker at weeks 8, 10, and 12 than at week 6 (P<0.01) (Figure 2F).

Immunohistochemical examination of the balloon-injured rabbits

The areas of α-actin-positive staining in the abdominal aortic SMCs gradually decreased over time (Figure 3A, B). The areas of α-actin-positive staining within the abdominal aorta significantly decreased at all weeks with the exception of week 4 (P<0.01) (Figure 3A, B). The SMC plaque content was significantly lower at week 8 than 6 and at week 12 than 10 (both P<0.01), with no difference between weeks 8 and 10 (P>0.05) (Figure 3A, B). RAM-11 staining showed that the relative content of macrophages within plaques increased from weeks 4 to 12, with differences among all weeks (all P<0.01) (Figure 3A, C). The lipid plaque content was higher at week 12 than at all other weeks (P<0.01) (Figure 3A, D) with increasing plaque area. The lipid content was significantly higher at week 10 than 4 (P<0.05), but no significant differences were observed among weeks 4, 6, and 8 (P>0.05) (Figure 3A, D). The positivity of Sirius red collagen staining did not differ among weeks 4, 6, and 8. Staining was more intense at weeks 10 and 12 than at any other weeks (P<0.05), but no significant difference was observed between weeks 10 and 12 (P>0.05) (Figure 3A, E). As a result, the VI gradually increased over time, with statistically significant differences among all weeks (Figure 3F).

The expression of MMP-1, -2, -3, and -9 significantly increased from weeks 4 to 12 (Figure 4A–E). The proportion of areas showing MMP-14-positive staining substantially decreased from weeks 4 to 12 (Figure 4A, F).

The collagen I level in plaques did not significantly differ among any weeks (P>0.05), but was slightly lower at week 12 than at

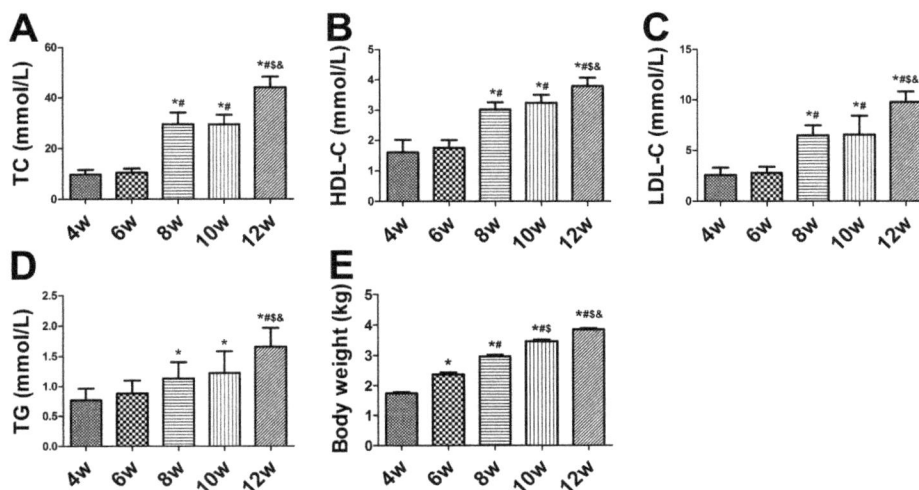

Figure 1. Biochemical measurements in balloon-injured rabbits. (A–D) Serum levels of total cholesterol (TC), high-density lipoprotein cholesterol (HDL-C), high-density lipoprotein cholesterol (LDL-C), and triglycerides (TG) in rabbits from weeks 4 to 12. (E) Body weights of rabbits in each group. *P<0.05 vs. week 4; #P<0.05 vs. week 6; $$P$<0.05 vs. week 8; &$P$<0.05 vs. week 10.

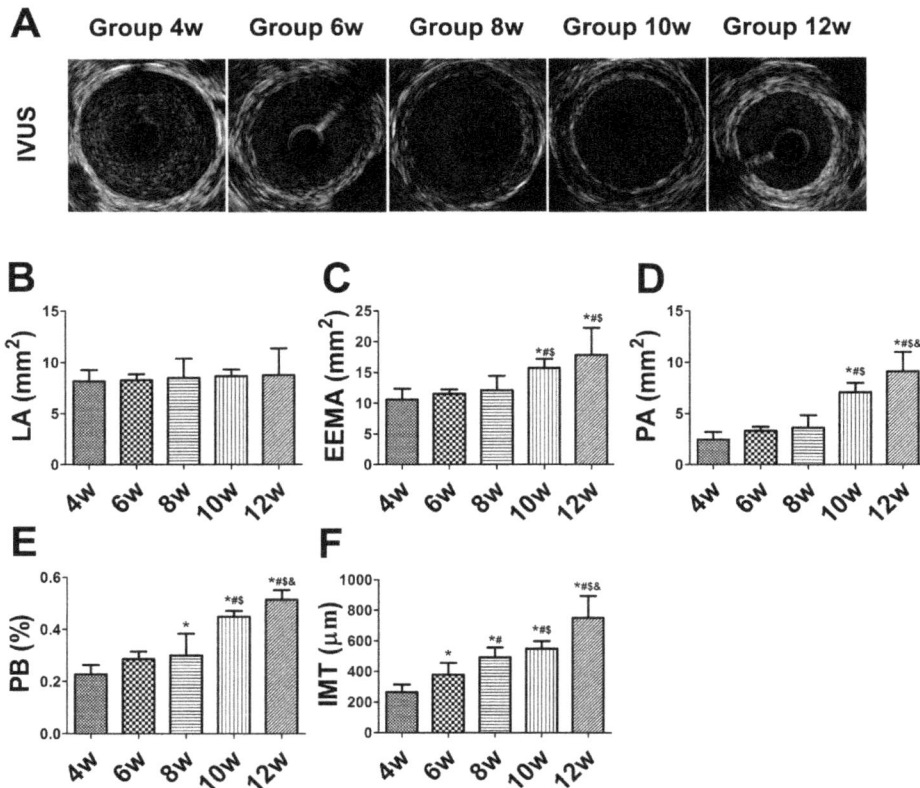

Figure 2. Intravascular ultrasound (IVUS) imaging and measurements in balloon-injured rabbits. (A) IVUS images. (B–F) Measurement of lumen area (LA), external elastic membrane area (EEMA), plaque area (PA), plaque burden (PB), and intima–media thickness (IMT). *$P<0.05$ vs. week 4; #$P<0.05$ vs. week 6; $$P<0.05$ vs. week 8; &$P<0.05$ vs. week 10.

week 4 ($P<0.05$) (Figure 5A, B). The relative content of collagen III in plaques increased from weeks 4 to 12, was higher at week 8 than at weeks 4 and 6 ($P<0.05$), and exhibited a significant change from weeks 8 to 12 ($P<0.05$) (Figure 5A, C). The expression of VEGF-A significantly increased from weeks 4 to 12 ($P<0.05$) (Figure 5A, D). Plaque neovessels appeared at week 8 (Figure 5A). The MVD was higher at week 12 than 8 ($P<0.05$), but no difference was observed between weeks 8 and 10 (both $P>0.05$) (Figure 5A, E).

Western blot analysis in the balloon-injured rabbits

The expression of MMP proteins exhibited the same trends as shown in the immunohistochemical results. The expression of MMP-1, -2, -3, and -9 significantly increased from weeks 4 to 12 (Figure 6A–E), while that of MMP-14 substantially decreased from weeks 4 to 12 (Figure 6A, F).

Correlation analysis in the balloon-injured rabbits

The correlation analysis results in the balloon-injured animals are shown in Table 1. All correlations between the VI and MMP-1, -2, -3, and -9 were positive (r = 0.767, 0.809, 0.890, and 0.887, respectively). The expression of MMP-1, -2, -3, and -9 was positively correlated with both the MVD in plaque (r = 0.762, 0.813, 0.884, and 0.769, respectively) and the VEGF-A in plaque (r = 0.760, 0.762, 0.858, and 0.789, respectively). The correlations between MMP-14 and the VI, MVD, and VEGF-A were all negative (r = –0.556, –0.424, and –0.525, respectively). The correlation between the VI and MVD was positive (r = 0.846).

Discussion

The most important finding in this study is that in this rabbit model of atherosclerosis, MMP-1, -2, -3, and -9 were positively correlated and MMP-14 was negatively correlated with intraplaque angiogenesis at the advanced stages of atherosclerosis.

Recent studies have found that MMPs participate and are indispensible in the process of angiogenesis. MMP-1 deficiency significantly decreases angiogenesis via the protease-activated receptor-1 pathway in lung tumors [8]. MMP-1 and -3 can degrade perlecan in basement membranes, releasing basic fibroblast growth factor (basic FGF) [9]. Likewise, MMP-2 and -3 degrade the ECM proteoglycan decorin, releasing latent tissue growth factor 1. MMP-2 and -9 can cleave latency-associated peptide to activate tissue growth factor β1, MMP-2 and MMP-9 have been shown to be critical for the "angiogenic switch in tumor angiogenesis [10,11]. However, different studies have shown different results. MMP-2 reportedly cleaves the ectodomain of FGF receptor 1, which retains FGF-binding activity, but is unable to signal and thus modulate the biological availability and mitogenic and angiogenic activities of FGFs [15]. In another study, reductions in MMP-9 levels by pharmacological methods in either wild-type or α1-knockout mice resulted in reduced angiostatin levels and increased tumor growth and vascularization [13]. Stable overexpression of MMP-9 in a mouse colon carcinoma cell line resulted in increased angiostatin levels and decreased tumor growth and angiogenesis *in vivo* [13]. The present study showed that MMP-1, -2, -3, and -9 are all strongly positive correlated with the MVD. Therefore upregulation of

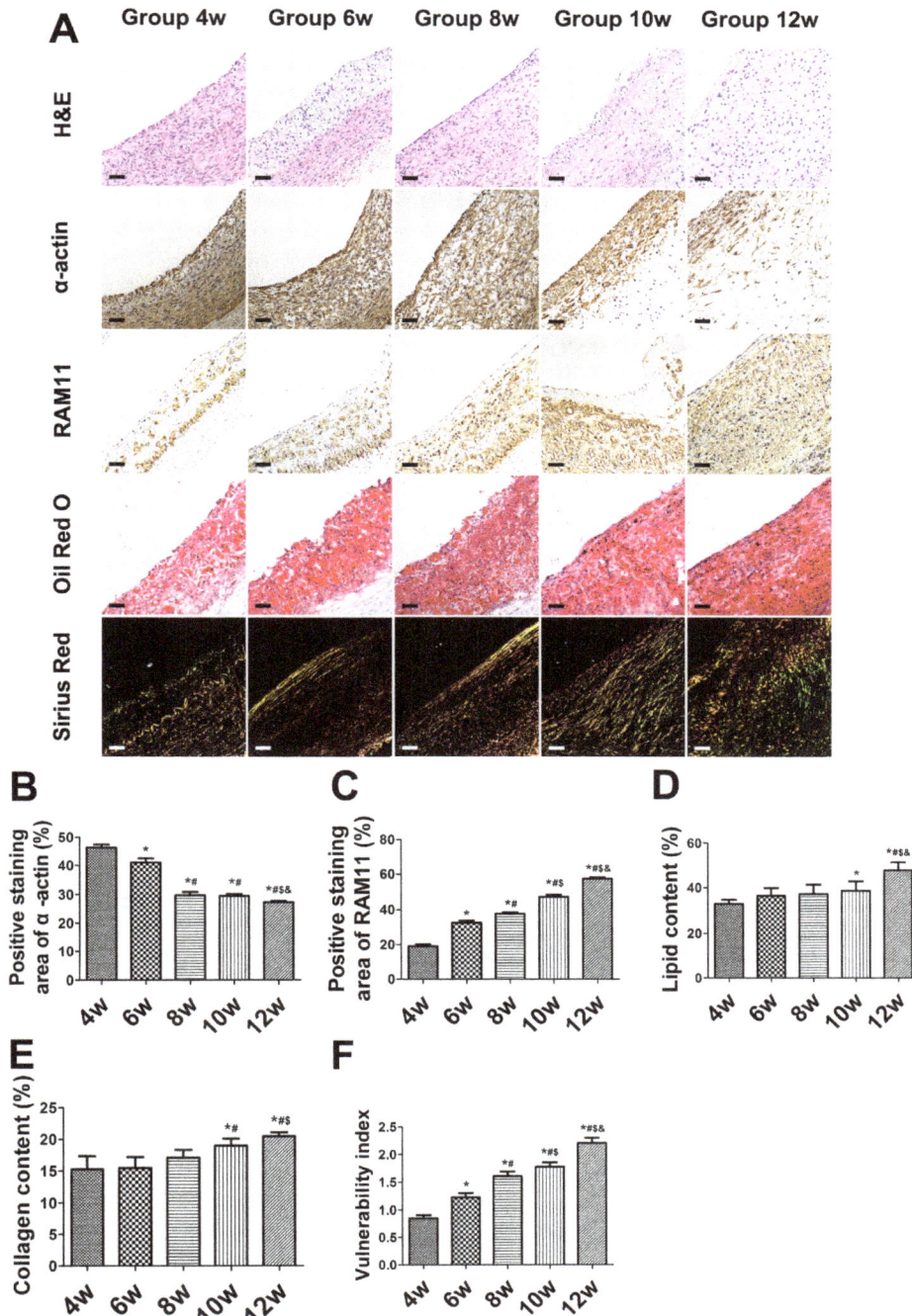

Figure 3. Immunohistochemical staining of plaque components in aortic plaques of balloon-injured rabbits. (A) Hematoxylin-and-eosin staining of abdominal aortic cross sections showing plaque area. α-actin staining for smooth muscle cells. RAM-11 staining for macrophages. Oil-red O staining for lipids. Sirius red staining for collagen. (B–E) Quantification of results in (A). (Bars = 20 μm). (F) Vulnerability index. *$P<0.05$ vs. week 4; #$P<0.05$ vs. week 6; $$P<0.05$ vs. week 8; &$P<0.05$ vs. week 10.

MMP-1, -2, -3, and -9 may enhance intraplaque angiogenesis at the advanced stage of atherosclerosis in rabbits.

A previous study showed that selective inhibition of MMP-14 blocks tumor angiogenesis [12]. Another showed that MMP-14 generates endogenous angiogenesis inhibitors by proteolytic cleavage of plasma proteins and ECM components. MMP-14 cleaves endoglin, a transforming growth factor-β coreceptor, at a site located close to the transmembrane domain. MMP-14 also upregulates the level of soluble endoglin, thus reducing the occurrence of spontaneous and VEGF-induced endothelial sprouting and inhibiting angiogenesis within tumors [14]. A placental study showed that MMP-14 acts as the cleavage protease for endoglin [23]. Cleavage of collagen XVIII by MMP-14 can generate endostatin, an angiogenesis inhibitor that blocks VEGF-induced endothelial cell migration [24]. In the present study, we found that MMP-14 is negatively correlated with angiogenesis at

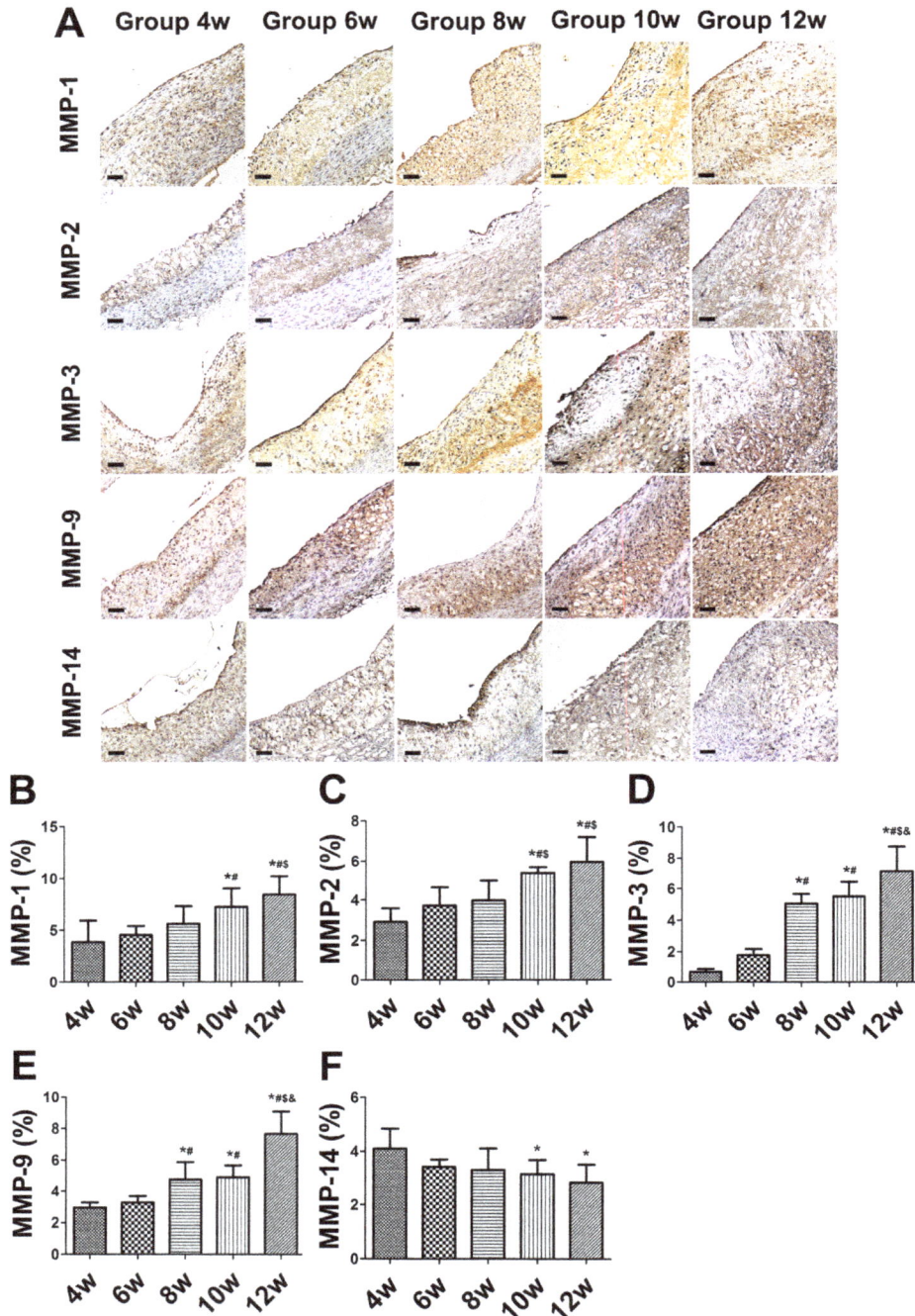

Figure 4. Immunohistochemical staining of matrix metalloproteinases (MMPs) and quantitative analysis in aortic plaques of balloon-injured rabbits. (A) Protein expression of MMP-1, -2,-3, -9, and -14. (B–F) Quantification. (Bars = 20 μm). *$P<0.05$ vs. week 4; #$P<0.05$ vs. week 6; $$P<0.05$ vs. week 8; &$P<0.05$ vs. week 10.

the advanced stages of atherosclerosis in rabbits. Therefore, downregulation of MMP-14 may participate in intraplaque angiogenesis at the advanced stages of atherosclerosis.

Angiogenesis is a critical factor in the development and progression of atherosclerosis. Pathological examination of unstable lesions has demonstrated that plaque rupture is associated with an increased density of microvessels. Angiogenesis of the intima is a consistent feature of plaque development in atherosclerosis [25]. Previous studies showed that the number of vasa vasorum was

two-fold higher in vulnerable plaques and up to four-fold higher in ruptured plaques than in stable plaques with severe luminal narrowing [26,27]. Mofidi *et al.* found strong associations between angiogenesis in atherosclerotic carotid plaques and plaque vulnerability [28]. The present study also showed that angiogenesis is correlated with plaque instability.

MMPs are correlated with changes associated with plaque vulnerability, such as macrophage ingress and apoptosis as well as loss of collagen and elastin [29,30]. MMP-3-knockout decreased

Specific Matrix Metalloproteinases Play Different Roles in Intraplaque Angiogenesis and Plaque Instability...

57

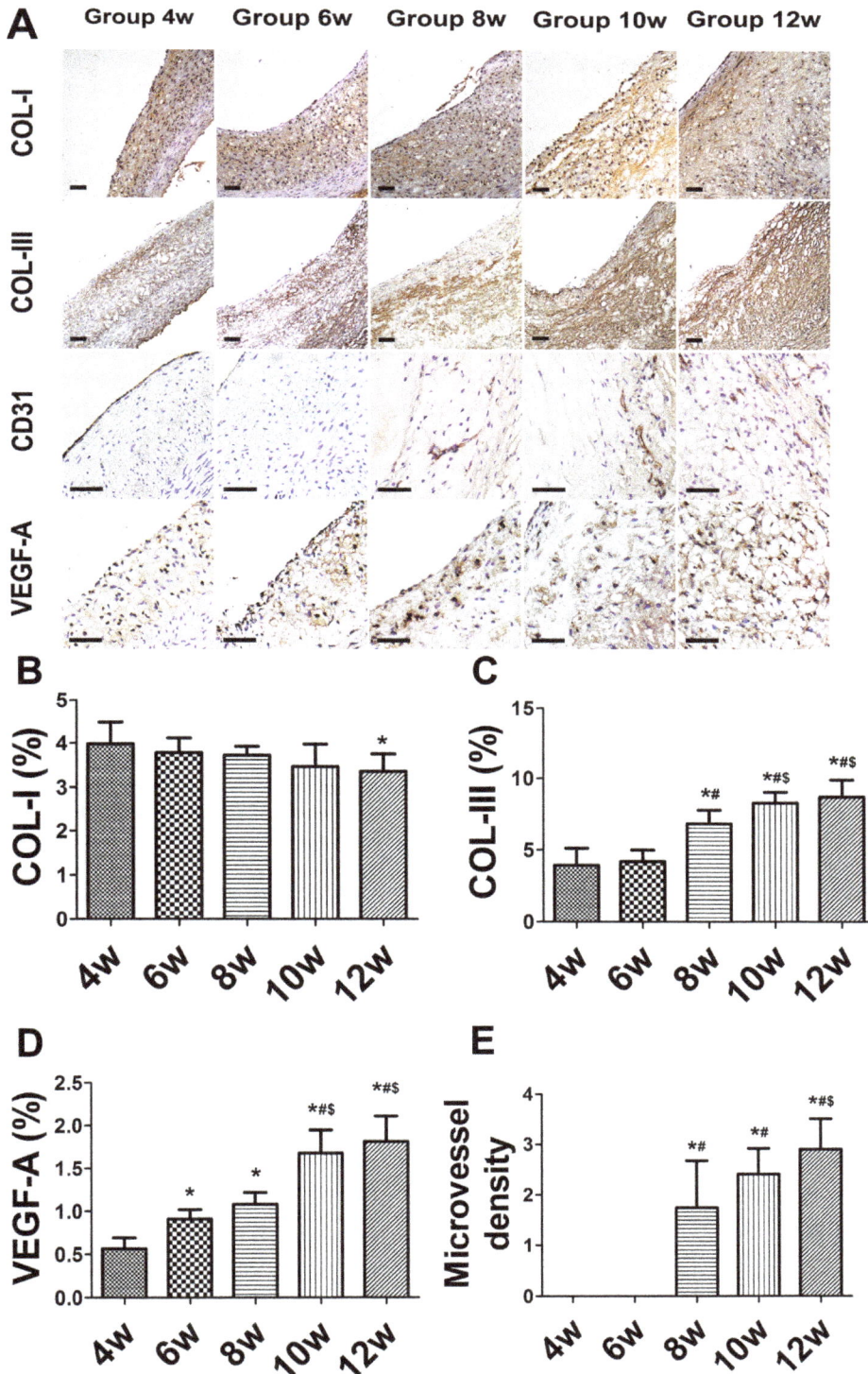

Figure 5. Immunohistochemical staining of collagen, CD31, and vascular endothelial growth factor A (VEGF-A) in aortic plaques of balloon-injured rabbits. (A) Protein expression of collagen I (COL-I), collagen III (COL-III), CD31, and VEGF-A. (B–E) Quantification. (Bars = 20 μm). *$P<0.05$ vs. week 4; #$P<0.05$ vs. week 6; $$P<0.05$ vs. week 8; &$P<0.05$ vs. week 10.

the incidence of elastin breaks [31], implying greater stability. Luttun et al. showed that MMP-9-knockout reduced plaque size, macrophage content, and elastin breaks, leading to plaque stability [32]. Overexpression of an autoactivated form of MMP-9 resulted in substantially greater plaque instability [33]. The correlation analysis in our study revealed that MMP-1, -2, -3, and -9 were positively correlated with the VI in plaques and that MMP-14 was significantly negatively correlated with the VI.

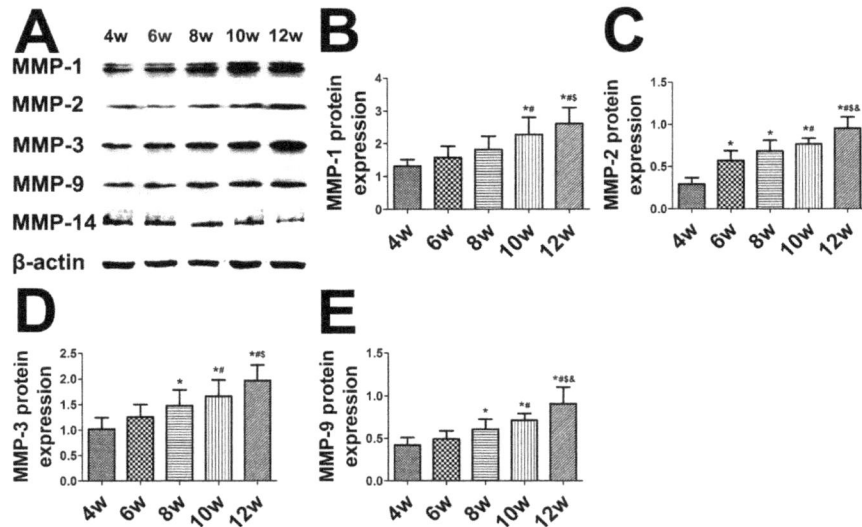

Figure 6. Western blot analysis and quantification of matrix metalloproteinase (MMP) protein expression in aortic plaques of balloon-injured rabbits. (A) Protein expression of MMP-1, -2, -3, -9, and -14. (B–F) Quantification. *$P<0.05$ vs. week 4; #$P<0.05$ vs. week 6; $P<0.05$ vs. week 8; &$P<0.05$ vs. week 10.

In the present study, the levels of MMP-1, -2, -3, and -9 were positively correlated with the expression of VEGF-A within plaques. MMPs are reportedly able to enhance the bioactivity of growth factors, and their expression is induced by angiogenic factors *in vitro*. Degradation of ECM releases membrane-sequestered VEGF [34]. MMP-1 promotes the expression of VEGF receptor 2 via stimulation of protease-activated receptor-1 and activation of NF-κB in endothelial cells [35]. VEGF-A-dependent phosphorylation of intracellular signaling molecules such as extracellular signal-regulated kinase and Akt has been observed within endothelial cells [35]. Connective tissue growth factor forms an inactive complex with VEGF-A, and cleavage of connective tissue growth factor by MMP-1 or -3 releases active VEGF-A within endothelial cells [36]. MMP-3 activates several MMPs, including proMMP-1, -7, and -9. Activated MMP-7 can in turn activate proMMP-1 and proMMP-9 [37,38]. Suppression of MMP-2 decreases integrin-αvβ3-mediated induction of PI3K/AKT, thus leading to decreased VEGF-A expression in lung cancer cells [39]. Recent studies have also demonstrated that adenovirus-mediated transfer of siRNA against MMP-2 results in impaired expression of VEGF and tumor-induced angiogenesis both *in vitro* and *in vivo* [40]. MMP-9 releases VEGF-A bound to proteoglycans within the ECM [41], thus enhancing the bioavailability of VEGF-A and potentially influencing plaque angiogenesis. Overexpression of MMP-9 in human breast cancer cells

increases VEGF–VEGF receptor 2 complex formation and tumor angiogenesis [42]. Thus, MMP-1, -2, -3, and -9 can promote the expression of VEGF-A either *in vitro* or within tumors. The processes triggered positive feedback cycles, enhancing the development of angiogenesis and finally leading to intraplaque hemorrhage and plaque rupture. These findings strongly support the influence of widespread MMP-1, -2, -3, and -9 expression within plaques on angiogenesis, in part by the role of these MMPs in activating VEGF-A.

Another important finding of the present study is that plaque neovessels first appeared at week 8. Angiogenesis is one of the key therapeutic factors in stabilization of atherosclerotic plaques; thus, inhibition of angiogenesis seems to be particularly important. Interest in intraplaque angiogenesis has been spurred by the potential to target plaque neovascularization with angiogenesis inhibitors [43]. Identification of the optimal time point at which to inhibit angiogenic growth within atherosclerotic lesions may lead to the development of therapies designed to stabilize plaques. Our findings may lead to the identification of this time point, thus assisting in the development of targeted drug or gene intervention therapy for intraplaque angiogenesis.

The present study contains several limitations. First, the sample size was relatively small. Further studies with larger samples are required to confirm our primary conclusions. Second, although the detailed molecular mechanisms of the influence of MMPs on

Table 1. Spearman correlations between matrix metalloproteinase (MMP) levels and the vulnerability index (VI), microvascular density (MVD), and vascular endothelial growth factor A (VEGF-A) level in balloon-injured rabbits.

	VI	MMP-1	MMP-2	MMP-3	MMP-9	MMP-14
VI	1.000	0.767**	0.809**	0.890**	0.887**	−0.556*
MVD	0.846**	0.762**	0.813**	0.884**	0.769**	−0.424*
VEGF-A	0.898**	0.760**	0.762**	0.858**	0.789**	−0.525**

*Statistically significant, $P<0.05$.
**Statistically significant, $P<0.01$.

plaque angiogenesis were investigated, further *in vitro* studies are required to fully elucidate the signal transduction pathways involved. Third, MMP gene interference is a preferred approach with which to determine the specific correlation between MMPs and intraplaque angiogenesis. Finally, the plaque formation in our animal model may not entirely simulate that in patients with acute coronary syndrome; the plaque-stabilizing effect of MMPs requires evaluation in clinical trials.

In conclusion, as shown in this rabbit model of atherosclerosis, upregulation of MMP-1, -2, -3, and -9 and downregulation of MMP-14 may participate in intraplaque angiogenesis at the advanced stages of atherosclerosis. Further investigation of MMPs may provide a novel approach for the prediction and treatment of vulnerable atherosclerotic plaques.

Supporting Information

Figure S1   Biochemical measurements of rabbits in the control group. The serum levels of total cholesterol (TC), high-density lipoprotein cholesterol (HDL-C), high-density lipoprotein cholesterol (LDL-C), and triglycerides (TG) significantly increased after ingestion of an atherogenic diet for 12 weeks ($P<0.05$). The body weights of the rabbits gradually increased over time ($P<0.05$).

Figure S2   Intravascular ultrasound (IVUS) imaging of rabbits in the control group. Only scarce plaque was present within the abdominal aorta after ingestion of an atherogenic diet for 12 weeks in the control group.

Figure S3   Hematoxylin-and-eosin (H&E) staining of abdominal aorta of rabbits in the control group. Only fatty streaks with lipid infiltration and no intimal injury were present in the abdominal aorta among rabbits without intimal injury after ingestion of an atherogenic diet for 12 weeks (bars = 20 µm).

Figure S4   Immunohistochemical staining of matrix metalloproteinases (MMPs) and CD31 in the abdominal aorta of rabbits in the control group. Rare MMPs are stained within smooth muscle cells in the control group. CD31 staining showed no angiogenesis after ingestion of an atherogenic diet for 12 weeks (bars = 20 µm).

Acknowledgments

We thank Drs. Shan Ying Huang and Xu Ping Wang for their technical assistance. We also thank Medjaden Bioscience Limited for linguistic advice.

Author Contributions

Conceived and designed the experiments: LZ YXZ YZ. Performed the experiments: XQL YM. Analyzed the data: XQL YM. Contributed reagents/materials/analysis tools: BW XTL WWB YYS YL HML. Contributed to the writing of the manuscript: XQL

References

1. Naghavi M, Libby P, Falk E, Casscells SW, Litovsky S, et al. (2003) From vulnerable plaque to vulnerable patient: a call for new definitions and risk assessment strategies: Part I. Circulation 108: 1664–1672.
2. Virmani R, Kolodgie FD, Burke AP, Finn AV, Gold HK, et al. (2005) Atherosclerotic plaque progression and vulnerability to rupture: angiogenesis as a source of intraplaque hemorrhage. Arterioscler Thromb Vasc Biol 25: 2054–2061.
3. Sluimer JC, Gasc JM, van Wanroij JL, Kisters N, Groeneweg M, et al. (2008) Hypoxia, hypoxia-inducible transcription factor, and macrophages in human atherosclerotic plaques are correlated with intraplaque angiogenesis. J Am Coll Cardiol 51: 1258–1265.
4. Lin HL, Zhang L, Liu CX, Xu XS, Tang MX, et al. (2010) Haemin-enhanced expression of haem oxygenase-1 stabilizes erythrocyte-induced vulnerable atherosclerotic plaques. British journal of pharmacology 160: 1484–1495.
5. Lin H-l, Xu X-s, Lu H-x, Zhang L, Li C-j, et al. (2007) Pathological mechanisms and dose dependency of erythrocyte-induced vulnerability of atherosclerotic plaques. Journal of molecular and cellular cardiology 43: 272–280.
6. Nguyen M, Arkell J, Jackson CJ (2001) Human endothelial gelatinases and angiogenesis. The international journal of biochemistry & cell biology 33: 960–970.
7. Nagase H, Woessner JF (1999) Matrix Metalloproteinases. Journal of Biological Chemistry 274: 21491–21494.
8. Foley C, Fanjul-Fernández M, Bohm A, Nguyen N, Agarwal A, et al. (2013) Matrix metalloprotease 1a deficiency suppresses tumor growth and angiogenesis. Oncogene.
9. Whitelock JM, Murdoch AD, Iozzo RV, Underwood PA (1996) The degradation of human endothelial cell-derived perlecan and release of bound basic fibroblast growth factor by stromelysin, collagenase, plasmin, and heparanases. Journal of Biological Chemistry 271: 10079–10086.
10. Imai K, Hiramatsu A, Fukushima D, Pierschbacher M, Okada Y (1997) Degradation of decorin by matrix metalloproteinases: identification of the cleavage sites, kinetic analyses and transforming growth factor-β1 release. Biochem J 322: 809–814.
11. Yu Q, Stamenkovic I (2000) Cell surface-localized matrix metalloproteinase-9 proteolytically activates TGF-β and promotes tumor invasion and angiogenesis. Genes & development 14: 163–176.
12. Devy L, Huang L, Naa L, Yanamandra N, Pieters H, et al. (2009) Selective inhibition of matrix metalloproteinase-14 blocks tumor growth, invasion, and angiogenesis. Cancer research 69: 1517–1526.
13. Pozzi A, LeVine WF, Gardner HA (2002) Low plasma levels of matrix metalloproteinase 9 permit increased tumor angiogenesis. Oncogene 21: 272–281.
14. Hawinkels IJ, Kuiper P, Wiercinska E, Verspaget HW, Liu Z, et al. (2010) Matrix metalloproteinase-14 (MT1-MMP)–mediated endoglin shedding inhibits tumor angiogenesis. Cancer research 70: 4141–4150.
15. Levi E, Fridman R, Miao H-Q, Ma Y-S, Yayon A, et al. (1996) Matrix metalloproteinase 2 releases active soluble ectodomain of fibroblast growth factor receptor 1. Proceedings of the National Academy of Sciences 93: 7069–7074.
16. Chen WQ, Zhang L, Liu YF, Chen L, Ji XP, et al. (2007) Prediction of atherosclerotic plaque ruptures with high-frequency ultrasound imaging and serum inflammatory markers. American Journal of Physiology-Heart and Circulatory Physiology 293: H2836–H2844.
17. Zhang L, Liu Y, Lu XT, Xu XS, Zhao YX, et al. (2009) Intraplaque injection of Ad5-CMV.p53 aggravates local inflammation and leads to plaque instability in rabbits. J Cell Mol Med 13: 2713–2723.
18. Zhang L, Liu Y, Zhang PF, Zhao YX, Ji XP, et al. (2010) Peak radial and circumferential strain measured by velocity vector imaging is a novel index for detecting vulnerable plaques in a rabbit model of atherosclerosis. Atherosclerosis 211: 146–152.
19. Mintz GS, Nissen SE, Anderson WD, Bailey SR, Erbel R, et al. (2001) American College of Cardiology clinical expert consensus document on standards for acquisition, measurement and reporting of intravascular ultrasound studies (ivus): A report of the american college of cardiology task force on clinical expert consensus documents developed in collaboration with the european society of cardiology endorsed by the society of cardiac angiography and interventions. Journal of the American College of Cardiology 37: 1478–1492.
20. Mintz GS, Nissen SE, Anderson WD, Bailey SR, Erbel R, et al. (2001) American College of Cardiology clinical expert consensus document on standards for acquisition, measurement and reporting of intravascular ultrasound studies (ivus) 33A report of the american college of cardiology task force on clinical expert consensus documents developed in collaboration with the european society of cardiology endorsed by the society of cardiac angiography and interventions. Journal of the American College of Cardiology 37: 1478–1492.
21. Torzewski M, Klouche M, Hock J, Mener M, Dorweiler B, et al. (1998) Immunohistochemical Demonstration of Enzymatically Modified Human LDL and Its Colocalization With the Terminal Complement Complex in the Early Atherosclerotic Lesion. Arteriosclerosis, Thrombosis, and Vascular Biology 18: 369–378.
22. Dong B, Zhang C, Feng JB, Zhao YX, Li SY, et al. (2008) Overexpression of ACE2 enhances plaque stability in a rabbit model of atherosclerosis. Arterioscler Thromb Vasc Biol 28: 1270–1276.

23. Kaitu'u-Lino TuJ, Palmer KR, Whitehead CL, Williams E, Lappas M, et al. (2012) MMP-14 is expressed in preeclamptic placentas and mediates release of soluble endoglin. The American journal of pathology 180: 888–894.

24. Chang J-H, Javier JA, Chang G-Y, Oliveira HB, Azar DT (2005) Functional characterization of neostatins, the MMP-derived, enzymatic cleavage products of type XVIII collagen. FEBS letters 579: 3601–3606.

25. Battegay E (1995) Angiogenesis: mechanistic insights, neovascular diseases, and therapeutic prospects. Journal of Molecular Medicine 73: 333–346.

26. Virmani R, Kolodgie FD, Burke AP, Farb A, Schwartz SM (2000) Lessons From Sudden Coronary Death: A Comprehensive Morphological Classification Scheme for Atherosclerotic Lesions. Arteriosclerosis, Thrombosis, and Vascular Biology 20: 1262–1275.

27. Kolodgie FD, Virmani R, Burke AP, Farb A, Weber DK, et al. (2004) Pathologic assessment of the vulnerable human coronary plaque. Heart 90: 1385–1391.

28. Mofidi R, Crotty T, McCarthy P, Sheehan S, Mehigan D, et al. (2001) Association between plaque instability, angiogenesis and symptomatic carotid occlusive disease. British journal of surgery 88: 945–950.

29. Sluijter JP, de Kleijn DP, Pasterkamp G (2006) Vascular remodeling and protease inhibition–bench to bedside. Cardiovascular research 69: 595–603.

30. Sluijter JP, Pulskens WP, Schoneveld AH, Velema E, Strijder CF, et al. (2006) Matrix metalloproteinase 2 is associated with stable and matrix metalloproteinases 8 and 9 with vulnerable carotid atherosclerotic lesions a study in human endarterectomy specimen pointing to a role for different extracellular matrix metalloproteinase inducer glycosylation forms. Stroke 37: 235–239.

31. Silence J, Lupu F, Collen D, Lijnen H (2001) Persistence of atherosclerotic plaque but reduced aneurysm formation in mice with stromelysin-1 (MMP-3) gene inactivation. Arteriosclerosis, thrombosis, and vascular biology 21: 1440–1445.

32. Luttun A, Lutgens E, Manderveld A, Maris K, Collen D, et al. (2004) Loss of matrix metalloproteinase-9 or matrix metalloproteinase-12 protects apolipoprotein E–deficient mice against atherosclerotic media destruction but differentially affects plaque growth. Circulation 109: 1408–1414.

33. Gough PJ, Gomez IG, Wille PT, Raines EW (2006) Macrophage expression of active MMP-9 induces acute plaque disruption in apoE-deficient mice. Journal of Clinical Investigation 116: 59–69.

34. Kalluri R (2003) Basement membranes: structure, assembly and role in tumour angiogenesis. Nature Reviews Cancer 3: 422–433.

35. Mazor R, Alsaigh T, Shaked H, Altshuler AE, Pocock ES, et al. (2013) Matrix metalloproteinase-1-mediated up-regulation of vascular endothelial growth factor-2 in endothelial cells. Journal of Biological Chemistry 288: 598–607.

36. Hashimoto G, Inoki I, Fujii Y, Aoki T, Ikeda E, et al. (2002) Matrix metalloproteinases cleave connective tissue growth factor and reactivate angiogenic activity of vascular endothelial growth factor 165. J Biol Chem 277: 36288–36295.

37. Ogata Y, Enghild J, Nagase H (1992) Matrix metalloproteinase 3 (stromelysin) activates the precursor for the human matrix metalloproteinase 9. Journal of Biological Chemistry 267: 3581–3584.

38. Fu X, Kassim SY, Parks WC, Heinecke JW (2001) Hypochlorous acid oxygenates the cysteine switch domain of pro-matrilysin (MMP-7) A mechanism for matrix metalloproteinase activation and atherosclerotic plaque rupture by myeloperoxidase. Journal of Biological Chemistry 276: 41279–41287.

39. Chetty C, Lakka SS, Bhoopathi P, Rao JS (2010) MMP-2 alters VEGF expression via αVβ3 integrin-mediated PI3K/AKT signaling in A549 lung cancer cells. International Journal of Cancer 127: 1081–1095.

40. Kargiotis O, Chetty C, Gondi CS, Tsung AJ, Dinh DH, et al. (2008) Adenovirus-mediated transfer of siRNA against MMP-2 mRNA results in impaired invasion and tumor-induced angiogenesis in vitro and inhibits tumor growth in vivo in glioblastoma. Oncogene 27: 4830–4840.

41. Bergers G, Brekken R, McMahon G, Vu TH, Itoh T, et al. (2000) Matrix metalloproteinase-9 triggers the angiogenic switch during carcinogenesis. Nature cell biology 2: 737–744.

42. Mira E, Lacalle RA, Buesa JM, de Buitrago GG, Jiménez-Baranda S, et al. (2004) Secreted MMP9 promotes angiogenesis more efficiently than constitutive active MMP9 bound to the tumor cell surface. Journal of cell science 117: 1847–1857.

43. Michel JB, Virmani R, Arbustini E, Pasterkamp G (2011) Intraplaque haemorrhages as the trigger of plaque vulnerability. Eur Heart J 32: 1977–1985, 1985a, 1985b, 1985c.

6

Retinoblastoma Binding Protein 2 (RBP2) Promotes HIF-1α–VEGF-Induced Angiogenesis of Non-Small Cell Lung Cancer via the Akt Pathway

Lei Qi[1], Feng Zhu[2], Shu-hai Li[1], Li-bo Si[1], Li-kuan Hu[1], Hui Tian[1]*

1 Department of Thoracic Surgery, Qi Lu Hospital, Shandong University, Jinan, Shandong Province, China, 2 Department of Thoracic Surgery, Shan dong Provincial Chest Hospital, Jinan, Shandong Province, China

Abstract

Background: Pathological angiogenesis plays an essential role in tumor aggressiveness and leads to unfavorable prognosis. The aim of this study is to detect the potential role of Retinoblastoma binding protein 2 (RBP2) in the tumor angiogenesis of non-small cell lung cancer (NSCLC).

Methods: Immunohistochemical staining was used to detect the expression of RBP2, hypoxia-inducible factor-1α (HIF-1α), vascular endothelial growth factor (VEGF) and CD34. Two pairs of siRNA sequences and pcDNA3-HA-RBP2 were used to down-regulate and up-regulate RBP2 expression in H1975 and SK-MES-1 cells. An endothelial cell tube formation assay, VEGF enzyme-linked immunosorbent assay, real-time PCR and western blotting were performed to detect the potential mechanisms mediated by RBP2 in tumor angiogenesis.

Results: Of the 102 stage I NSCLC specimens analyzed, high RBP2 protein expression is closely associated with tumor size ($P = 0.030$), high HIF-1α expression ($P = 0.028$), high VEGF expression ($P = 0.048$), increased tumor angiogenesis ($P = 0.033$) and poor prognosis ($P = 0.037$); high MVD was associated with high HIF-1α expression ($P = 0.034$), high VEGF expression ($P = 0.001$) and poor prognosis ($P = 0.040$). Multivariate analysis indicated that RBP2 had an independent influence on the survival of patients with stage I NSCLC ($P = 0.044$). By modulating the expression of RBP2, our findings suggested that RBP2 protein depletion decreased HUVECs tube formation by down-regulating VEGF in a conditioned medium. RBP2 stimulated the up-regulation of VEGF, which was dependent on HIF-1α, and activated the HIF-1α via phosphatidylinositol 3-kinase (PI3K)/Akt signaling pathway. Moreover, VEGF increased the activation of Akt regulated by RBP2.

Conclusions: The RBP2 protein may stimulate HIF-1α expression via the activation of the PI3K/Akt signaling pathway under normoxia and then stimulate VEGF expression. These findings indicate that RBP2 may play a critical role in tumor angiogenesis and serve as an attractive therapeutic target against tumor aggressiveness for early-stage NSCLC patients.

Editor: Vladimir V. Kalinichenko, Cincinnati Children's Hospital Medical Center, United States of America

Funding: The project was supported by the National Natural Science Foundation of China (No. 30571844), the Science and Technology Development Foundation of Shandong Province (No. 2009GG10002007), and the National Natural Science Foundation of Shandong Province (No. ZR2009CM090). The funders had no role in study design, data collection and analysis, decision to publish, or preparation of the manuscript.

Competing Interests: The authors have declared that no competing interests exist.

* Email: tianhuiy@sohu.com

Introduction

Non-small cell lung cancer (NSCLC) is among the most common malignancies leading to cancer-related death worldwide [1]. Despite numerous improvements in surgical techniques and adjuvant chemoradiotherapy for NSCLC over the last decades, the prognosis remains relatively poor [2]. A variety of new molecular markers and possible new targets have been found to treat the disease. However, tumor progression is a multistep process and the molecular mechanism underlying lung carcinogenesis is largely unclear.

Pathological angiogenesis is a relatively early event in carcinogenesis, and increased tumor angiogenesis is correlated with

invasive tumor growth and metastasis and a poor prognosis [3,4]. It has been proposed that vascular endothelial growth factor (VEGF) and hypoxia-inducible factor-1α (HIF-1α) play critical roles in tumor angiogenesis. VEGF, which is the most extensively characterized endothelial cell-specific angiogenic factor, leads to increased vascular permeability and plays a significant role in physiological and pathological angiogenesis [5,6]. Accumulating evidence has demonstrated that HIF-1α, a heterodimeric protein composed of HIF-1α and HIF-1β subunits, is associated with various aspects of cellular and physiologic process. Under normoxia, HIF-1α is prolyl-hydroxylated, ubiquitylated and degraded in proteasomes by binding to the von Hippel Lindau (VHL) complex. Following hypoxia stabilization, HIF-1α binds to

HIF-1β in the nucleus and initiates the transcription of target genes via the hypoxia-responsive element [7,8,9]. In recent years, many studies have suggested that HIF-1α also could lead to the elevated expression of various genes involved in diverse biological functions under normoxia, including cell proliferation, apoptosis, migration, invasion and angiogenesis [10,11].

Retinoblastoma binding protein 2 (RBP2), a member of the JARID family of proteins, is a nuclear phosphoprotein with demethylase activity for lysine 4 of histone H3 (H3-K4) [12,13,14]. It appeared that RBP2 exerts its function partly by repressing the transcription of target genes involved in differentiation and that binding to retinoblastoma protein (pRB) converts RBP2 from a transcriptional repressor to a transcriptional activator [15,16]. Recent research in lung cancer has established that RBP2 is correlated to tumor migration and invasion by directly binding to integrin β1 (ITGB1) promoters [17]. Another study demonstrated that RBP2 up-regulates the expression of N-cadherin and snail via the activation of Akt signaling [18]. Moreover, ITGB1 and Akt signaling are significantly correlated with tumor angiogenesis [19,20,21,22]. Taken together, these results suggest an oncogenic role for RBP2 in tumor angiogenesis and progression.

In this study, RBP2 expression was found to be increased in NSCLC cell lines as well as in the NSCLC tissues from patients. To further investigate the potential roles of RBP2 in tumor angiogenesis, we provide evidence showing that high RBP2 expression in NSCLC cell lines significantly promotes tumor angiogenesis and elucidate the mechanism involved in the activation of Akt signaling, induction of HIF-1α protein accumulation and VEGF expression under normoxia.

Materials and Methods

Ethics Statement

This study was approved by the Ethics Committee of Qilu Hospital. Written informed consent was obtained from each patient to publish the case details, and the acquisition of tissue specimens was carried out as prescribed by the institutional guidelines.

Patients

A total of 102 patients (71 men and 31 women, mean age 62±3.56 years) with stage I NSCLC who underwent complete tumor resection (lobectomy or pneumonectomy) with regional lymph node dissection between January 2006 and December 2008 at the department of Thoracic Surgery, Qilu Hospital, were included in the study. The histologic examination and grade of cancer cell differentiation were based on the classification system of the World Health Organization revised in 2004 and the TNM staging system of UICC 2009. In addition, 3 patients (2 cases with large cell cancer and 1 case with adenosquamous cancer) underwent complete tumor resection during this period were excluded owing to the too small sample size. The clinical characteristics of the 102 patients are presented in Table 1.

Immunohistochemistry

Immunohistochemical staining for RBP2, HIF-1α, VEGF and CD34 were carried out using the streptavidin-peroxidase method. In brief, 4-μm-thick sections were cut from paraffin-embedded blocks, and the slides were incubated with primary antibodies against RBP2 (Bethyl, Montgomery, TX, USA, dilution 1:100), HIF-1α (BD Biosciences, Pharmingen, Lexington, MA, USA, dilution 1:100), VEGF (A-20; Santa Cruz Biotechnologies, CA, USA, dilution 1:150) and CD34 (sc-19621; Santa Cruz Biotechnologies, CA, USA, dilution 1:100) overnight at 4°C. Subsequent-

ly, biotinylated secondary antibodies and peroxidase-conjugated streptavidin complex reagent were applied, followed by counterstaining with Mayer's hematoxylin. Positive and negative controls were included in each step. Expression of the RBP2 protein was evaluated by calculating a total immunostaining score as the product of both the intensity score (0, negative staining; 1, weak staining; 2, moderate staining; 3, strong staining) and proportion score (0, none; 1, <10%; 2, 10–50%; 3, 51–80%; 4, >80%). Thus, the total score ranged from 0 to 7. The immunostained slides were evaluated by two independent investigators in a blinded fashion and reevaluated by these investigators under a multihead microscope in discordant cases to reach a consensus. For evaluation of the positive staining of RBP2, at least 3 sections or areas from each sample were scored.

For tumor-associated angiogenesis quantification, microvessel density (MVD) was evaluated by counting CD34-positive immunostained endothelial cells. CD34-positive endothelial cells as well as clusters of endothelial cells that were clearly separate from adjacent microvessels were measured as countable microvessels [23,24,25]. To quantify the MVD, five highly vascular areas were scanned at low power to identify "hot spots" and counted microscopically in high-power (200× magnification) fields. The average count of ten vision fields was recorded as the final MVD (two observers and five vascular hot spots each).

The cutoff value for RBP2 and MVD expression was determined based on a heterogeneity value measured through a log-rank statistical analysis with respect to overall survival [26]. The final staining score of 4 was chosen as the cutoff point for the discrimination between high and low RBP2 expression. Therefore, tumors with a final staining score ≥4 were defined as overexpressing the RBP2 protein. Tumors with microvessels ≥ 57 were classified as high MVD; tumors with microvessels <57 were classified as low MVD. HIF-1α was regarded overexpressed when >1% of nuclei were positive as described before [27]. Tumors with a final staining score ≥3 were defined as overexpressing the VEGF protein [28].

Cell Lines, Culture Conditions, Transfection and Small Interfering RNA Treatment

The human lung adenocarcinoma cell lines A549, SPCA-1and H1975 were purchased from the National Cancer Institute (Bethesda, MD, USA). The human lung squamous cell line SK-MES-1 and the human bronchial epithelial cell line BEAS2B were obtained from American Type Culture Collection (Manassas, VA, USA). Human umbilical vein endothelial cells (HUVECs) were purchased from American Type Culture Collection (Manassas, VA, USA). The BEAS2B, A549, SPCA-1 and H1975 cells were cultured in Roswell's Park Memorial Institute (RPMI) 1640 medium (Hyclone, Logan, USA) supplemented with 10% fetal bovine serum (FBS; Gibco, Gaithersburg, USA). The SK-MES-1 cells were grown in MEM (Gibco, Carlsbad, CA, USA) supplemented with 20% FBS. HUVECs were cultured in endothelial cell growth medium M199 supplemented with 15% FBS, 1 mg/ml low serum growth supplements and 2 mM glutamine. All cells were incubated in 5% CO_2 at 37°C. RBP2 was overexpressed using pcDNA3-HA-RBP2, a generous gift from W.G Kaelin [12], and siRNA for RBP2 was purchased from Invitrogen (Carlsbad, CA, USA). The plasmid pcDNA3-HA-HIF-1α was purchased from Addgene (Plasmid 18949) [29], and siRNA for HIF-1α (ONTARGET plus SMART pool, L-004018) was purchased from Dharmacon RNA Technologies (Chicago, IL, USA). The plasmid pcDNA3 Myr HA Akt1 was purchased from Addgene (Plasmid 9008) [30]. For the small interfering RNA (siRNA) treatment, cells were incubated in 6-well plates (3.0×10^5/

Table 1. Correlation of clinicopathologic variables with RBP2 protein and MVD in NSCLC.

Category	No. of patients	RBP2			MVD		
		high	low	P^a	high	low	P^a
Age				0.570			0.405
<60 years	42	20	22		21	21	
≥60 years	60	32	28		25	35	
Sex				0.933			0.197
Male	71	36	35		35	36	
Female	31	16	15		11	20	
Smoking history				0.712			0.172
Smoker	59	31	28		30	29	
Non- smoker	43	21	22		16	27	
Histology				0.846			0.564
SCC	52	27	25		22	30	
Adeno	50	25	25		24	26	
Differentiation				0.247			0.500
Well	14	10	4		5	9	
Moderate	60	28	32		26	34	
Poor	28	14	14		15	13	
T stage				0.030			0.064
T1	48	19	29		17	31	
T2	54	33	21		29	25	
HIF-1α				0.028			0.034
high	64	38	26		34	30	
low	38	14	24		12	26	
VEGF				0.048			0.001
high	59	35	24		35	24	
low	43	17	26		11	32	

[a]Chi-square test.
SCC squamous cell cancer,
Adeno adenocarcinoma.

well) overnight and then transfection was performed using Lipofectamine 2000 (Invitrogen, Carlsbad, CA, USA). The following siRNA sequences were used in this study: RBP2 siRNA1 5′-UUGUGUACUCGUCAAACUCUACUCC-3′; RBP2 siRNA 2 5′-UUAACAUGCCGGUUAUCCAGGCUCU-3′; control siR NA 5′-UUCUCCGAAGGUGUCACGUTT -3′.

Preparation of Conditioned Medium

The RBP2-siRNA1 H1975 cells, RBP2-siRNA2 H1975 cells and control-siRNA H1975 cells were cultured under serum-free conditions in RPMI 1640 medium for 24 h, respectively. The supernatant was then collected, centrifuged, filtered through a 0.22-mm filter (Millipore, Billerica, USA) and stored at −20°C until used in the enzyme-linked immunosorbent assay (ELISA) and tube formation assay.

Endothelial Cell Tube Formation Assay

The tube formation assay was performed as described previously [31]. Briefly, HUVECs (1×10^4/well) were seeded in 96-well plates coated with Matrigel (50 μl) and then incubated at 37°C for 1 h to polymerize. HUVECs (1×10^4 cells) were seeded in wells with different conditioned media from RBP2-siRNA1 H1975 cells, RBP2-siRNA2 H1975 cells and control-siRNA H1975 cells. A VEGFR inhibitor (sunitinib malate, 2.5 μM) [32] was added to the conditioned medium of the control siRNA H1975 cells and recombinant human VEGF-165 (rhVEGF165, Millipore, Billerica, MA, USA, 2 ng/ml) was added to the conditioned medium of the RBP2-siRNA2 H1975 cells. The 96-well plates were incubated for 6 h, and tube formation was then photographed under an inverted microscope. The tube formation ability was quantified by counting the total number of complete tubes, and the average of three random ×200 fields per well was recorded as the value per well.

VEGF Enzyme-Linked Immunosorbent Assay (ELISA)

The VEGF levels in the different conditioned media were determined using an ELISA kit (R&D Systems, Minneapolis, MN, USA) according to the manufacturer's instructions and analyzed using a Labsystems Multiscan reader. The experiment was repeated twice with triplicate measurements in each experiment.

SDS-PAGE and Western Blotting

Proteins were extracted using RIPA lysis buffer. Equal amounts (20 μg) of protein were subjected to SDS–PAGE analysis, transferred onto nitrocellulose membranes and probed with primary antibodies against RBP2 (Cell Signaling Technologies, Danvers, MA, USA), HIF-1α (Cell Signaling Technologies, Danvers, MA, USA), VEGF (Santa Cruz Biotechnologies, Santa Cruz, CA, USA), Akt and phospho-Akt (Ser-473) (Cell Signaling Technologies, Danvers, MA, USA). LY294002 was purchased from Beyotime Institute of Biotechnology (Haimen, China). Protein bands were detected using the enhanced chemiluminescence method (Millipore, Billerica, MA, USA). The optical band density was quantified (Imager of Alpha Corporation, San Leandro).

RNA Extraction, Reverse-Transcription Polymerase Chain Reaction

Total cellular RNA in the cells from different treatments was extracted using Trizol (Invitrogen, Carlsbad, CA, USA). Complementary DNA (cDNA) was synthesized by SuperScript III First-Strand Synthesis System (Invitrogen, Carlsbad, CA, USA). Quantitative real-time PCR (QRT-PCR) was carried out using

SYBR Green Supermix (Bio-Rad) for HIF-1α and VEGF according to the manufacturer's instructions. The levels of HIF-1α and VEGF messenger RNA (mRNA) were normalized to the human β-actin expression level and calculated using the $2^{(-\Delta\Delta CT)}$ method [33]. The primers for HIF-1α were 5′-TTTTTCAAG-CAGTAGGAATTGGA-3′ (forward) and 5′-GTGATGTAG-TAGCTGCATGATCG-3′ (reverse). The primers for VEGF were 5′-ATCTTCAAGCCATCCTGTGTGTC- 3′ (forward) and 5′-CAAGGCCCACAGGGATTTTC-3′ (reverse). The primers for β-actin were 5′-GCATCCACGAAACTACCT-3′ (forward) and 5′-GAAAGGGTGTAACGCAAC-3′ (reverse). The cycling conditions were as follows: initial denaturation at 95°C for 30 s, followed by 40 cycles at 95°C for 5 s, 60°C for 30 s and 72°C for 15 s.

Follow-up

All patients discharged from the hospital were followed-up at the outpatient clinic every 3 to 6 months. The follow-up evaluation of patients consisted of physical examination, blood tests, computed tomography, ultrasound examination, chest X-ray and fiberoptic bronchoscopy if necessary. Follow-up was completed in all patients until December 2013, and the median follow-up period was 66 months (range: 16~96 months).

Statistical Analyses

All statistical analyses were examined using SPSS 17.0 statistical software. Quantitative data were expressed as the mean ± SD for each group, and comparisons were performed using Student's t-test. Chi-square tests were performed to examine the association between RBP2, MVD and various clinicopathologic factors. The correlation between intratumoral MVD and RBP2 protein levels was analyzed by a nonparametric test (Mann-Whitney U test). The follow-up time was censored if the patient was lost during follow-up. Survival curves were drawn using the Kaplan–Meier method and compared by the log-rank test. Multivariate Cox regression analysis was used to identify significant independent prognostic factors. P values were calculated from two-tailed statistical tests. A difference was considered statistically significant when $P<0.05$.

Results

1. Correlation of RBP2 protein and MVD with clinicopathologic factors

Immunohistochemistry with RBP2 (Fig. 1A and Fig. 1B) and HIF-1α (Fig. 1D and Fig. 1E) antibodies showed a positive reaction in the nucleus, and VEGF antibodies (Fig. 1F and Fig. 1G) showed a positive reaction in the cytoplasm of tumor cells. RBP2 was detected as being overexpressed in 52 (51%) of 102 NSCLC specimens according to the abovementioned criteria. Relationships between RBP2 protein expression and clinicopathologic factors were examined by the chi-square test and our data showed that RBP2 overexpression was associated with tumor size ($P = 0.030$), high HIF-1α expression ($P = 0.028$) and high VEGF expression ($P = 0.048$). However, there was no statistical significance in the relationships between RBP2 expression and other clinicopathologic variables ($P>0.05$, Table 1).

Intratumoral MVD was quantified by counting CD34-positive endothelial cells in the same series of lung cancer tissues (Fig. 1H and Fig. 1I), and the average number of microvessels in ten fields was counted as a measure of MVD for each sample. The average number of microvessels of MVD in each tumor sample ranged broadly, from 6.4 to 102. As described previously, tumors with microvessels ≥57 were classified as high MVD, and 46 cases (45.1%) showed high MVD. The chi-square test showed that high

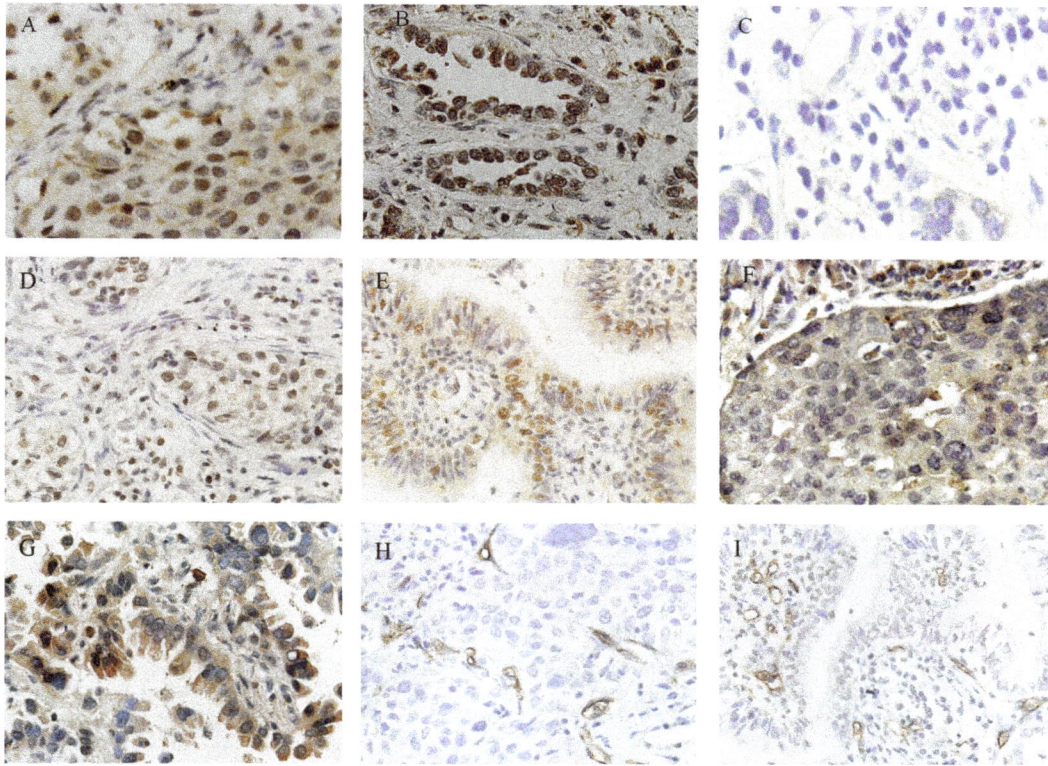

Figure 1. Immunohistochemical staining of the RBP2 protein and microvessels using the streptavidin–peroxidase method (magnification ×400). (A) High RBP2 protein expression in squamous cell cancer; (B) high RBP2 protein expression in adenocarcinoma; (C) negative RBP2 protein expression in NSCLC; (D) high HIF-1α expression in squamous cell cancer; (E) high HIF-1α protein expression in adenocarcinoma; (F) high VEGF expression in squamous cell cancer; (G) high VEGF in adenocarcinoma; (H) high CD34 expression in squamous cell cancer; (I) high CD34 expression in adenocarcinoma.

MVD was associated with high HIF-1α expression ($P = 0.034$) and high VEGF expression ($P = 0.001$), but no significant correlations were observed between MVD and other clinicopathologic factors ($P > 0.05$, Table 1).

Immunohistochemical staining of the serial sections of cancer tissues showed that the median MVD was 59.6 in the high RBP2 expression group (7.8 to 102) and 35.4 in the low RBP2 expression group (6.4 to 94). Furthermore, our statistical analysis demonstrated that high MVD was detected more frequently in tumors with RBP2 protein overexpression than in those without overexpression ($P = 0.033$, Mann-Whitney U test, Fig. 2A). These data suggest that RBP2 may promote pathological angiogenesis in NSCLC progression.

A Kaplan–Meier analysis of overall survival also demonstrated a poor 5-year overall survival rate in patients with RBP2 protein overexpression (53.8% versus 72.0%, $P = 0.037$; Fig. 2B) and high MVD (52.2% versus 71.4%, $P = 0.040$, Fig. 2C). All the statistically significant variables evaluated in the univariate analyses were included in a Cox proportional hazard regression model. The multivariate analysis indicated that only RBP2 had an independent influence on the survival of patients with stage I NSCLC ($P = 0.044$, Table 2).

2. RBP2 is overexpressed in human NSCLC cell lines

The protein level of RBP2 was up-regulated in lung cancer cell lines SK-MES-1, A549, SPCA-1 and H1975 compared to the human bronchial epithelial cell line BEAS2B (Fig. 3A). The expression level of RBP2 in H1975 cells was higher than that in BEAS2B, SK-MES-1, SPCA-1 and A549 cells.

Two pieces of siRNAs and pcDNA3-HA-RBP2 targeting RBP2 were employed for a functional analysis in H1975 and SK-MES-1 cells. As shown in Fig. 3B, the results demonstrated that RBP2-siRNA1 and RBP2-siRNA2 could significantly down-regulate the expression of the RBP2 protein in H1975 cells. In addition, the two siRNAs showed nearly the same RNAi effects, whereas the negative control siRNA did not significantly affect the expression of RBP2. Meanwhile, pcDNA3-HA-RBP2 significantly up-regulated the expression of RBP2 in SK-MES-1 cells, whereas pcDNA3-HA did not significantly affect RBP2 expression. Therefore, RBP2-siRNA1, RBP2-siRNA2 and pcDNA3-HA-RBP2 were selected to further study the functions of the RBP2 protein in vitro.

3. Depletion of the RBP2 protein decreases HUVEC tube formation induced by conditioned medium

To evaluate the functional significance of RBP2 in tumor angiogenesis, RBP2 was knocked down in H1975 cell lines. The results demonstrated that the number of complete tubes induced by the conditioned medium of RBP2-siRNA1 H1975 cells (12.33+ 3.06) and RBP2-siRNA2 H1975 cells (9.67+1.53) was significantly reduced compared to that of the control siRNA H1975 cells (38.67+2.52, Fig. 4 A–D, $P < 0.01$).

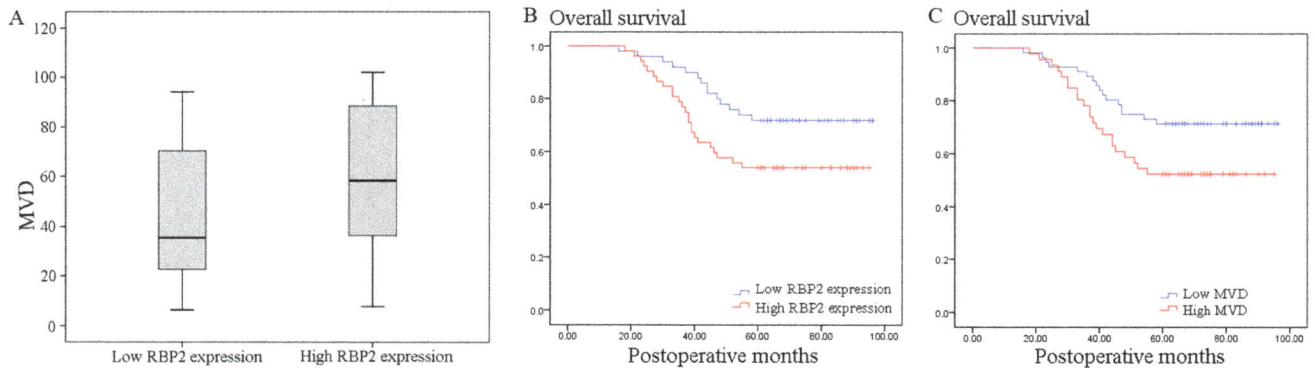

Figure 2. Correlation between RBP2 expression and MVD, and Kaplan–Meier curves of overall survival stratified according to RBP2 protein and MVD. (A) Correlation between RBP2 expression and MVD for stage I NSCLC. NSCLC with high RBP2 protein expression showed significantly higher intratumoral MVD than that with low RBP2 protein expression ($P = 0.033$, Mann-Whitney U test). (B) Kaplan–Meier curves of overall survival demonstrated a poor 5-year overall survival rate in patients with RBP2 protein overexpression (53.8% versus 72.0%, $P = 0.037$). (C) Kaplan–Meier curves of overall survival demonstrated a poor 5-year overall survival rate in patients with high MVD (52.2% versus 71.4%, $P = 0.040$).

4. Down-regulation of RBP2 protein decreases the expression levels of VEGF in conditioned medium

Given the fact that high MVD was associated with high VEGF expression (chi-square test, $P = 0.001$, Table 1), we next explored the association between RBP2 and VEGF protein levels in conditioned media using an ELISA assay. The results demonstrated that the VEGF protein levels in the conditioned media of RBP2-siRNA1 (0.99 ± 0.11 ng/ml) and RBP2-siRNA2 (0.94 ± 0.14 ng/ml) H1975 cells were significantly lower than in the control siRNA H1975 cells (1.87 ± 0.10 ng/ml), (Fig. 4E, $P < 0.01$). In addition, our results suggested that the tube formation induced by the conditioned medium of the control siRNA H1975 cells was blocked with the addition of a VEGFR inhibitor (sunitinib malate, 2.5 µM, 10.33+2.22, $P < 0.01$, Fig. 4F); the reduced tube formation induced by the conditioned medium of RBP2-siRNA2 H1975 cells was rescued by the addition of VEGF-165 (2 ng/ml, 41.03+3.25, $P < 0.01$, Fig. 4G).

5. RBP2 stimulates HIF-1α and VEGF mRNA and protein expression

HIF-1α is an important transcriptional factor and plays a crucial role in tumor angiogenesis. Moreover, the transcription factor HIF-1α regulates the expression level of various hypoxia-responsive genes, including VEGF [11]. We next investigated whether RBP2 could affect the expression of HIF-1α in ectopic RBP2-expressing SK-MES-1 cells. As shown in Fig. 5A, the enforced expression of RBP2 up-regulated the expression of the HIF-1α protein in a time-dependent manner under normoxic conditions, and the peak value of HIF-1α expression appeared at 36 hours after transfection was performed. However, HIF-1α was unstable and degraded by proteasomes under normoxia [9], and our results suggested that HIF-1α expression decreased after transfection was performed 48 hours. Therefore, to investigate the possible regulation of tumor angiogenesis by RBP2, we examined the expression of the transcription factors HIF-1α and VEGF in

Table 2. Univariate and multivariate analyses of prognostic variables.

Variable	Univariate analysis	Multivariate analysis		
	P	95% CI	RR	P
Sex	0.662	0.528–2.283	1098	0.802
Age	0.735	0.564–2.219	1.118	0.749
Histology	0.135	0.983–4.086	2.004	0.056
Differentiation	0.427	0.860–2.448	1.461	0.155
T stage	0.602	0.402–1.714	0.830	0.615
Smoking history	0.623	0.546–2.331	1.128	0.745
MVD	0.040	0.788–3.426	1.643	0.185
HIF-1α	0.306	0.236–1.606	0.616	0.322
VEGF	0.061	0.741–4.892	1.904	0.181
RBP2 protein	0.037	1.021–4.356	2.109	0.044

CI: confidence interval.

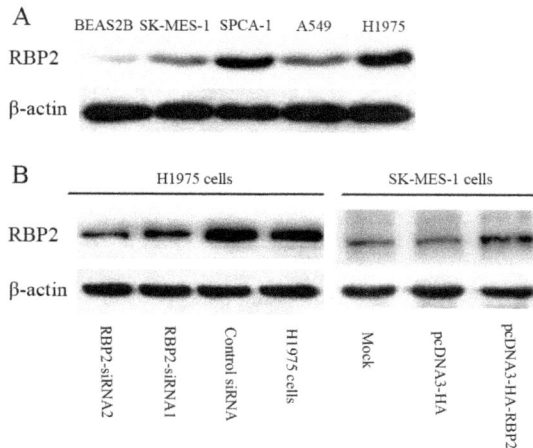

Figure 3. Expression of RBP2 in human NSCLC cell lines and the transfection efficiency of siRNA and pcDNA3-HA-RBP2. (A) RBP2 is overexpressed in human NSCLC cell lines SK-MES-1, A549, SPCA-1 and H1975 compared to the human bronchial epithelial cell line BEAS2B cells. (B) Effects of RBP2 siRNA1, RBP2 siRNA2 and pcDNA3-HA-RBP2 on the expression of the RBP2 protein.

RBP2-overexpressing and -depleted NSCLC cells under normoxia at 36 hours after transfection. As shown in Fig. 5B and Fig. 5C, the down-regulation of RBP2 in H1975 cells led to the decreased expression of HIF-1α and VEGF, whereas ectopic RBP2 expression in SK-MES-1 cells by pcDNA3-HA-RBP2 led to the up-regulation of HIF-1α and VEGF.

The mRNA expression levels of HIF-1α ($P^{\text{siRNA1}} = 0.006$, $P^{\text{siRNA2}} = 0.001$) and VEGF ($P^{\text{siRNA1}} = 0.000$, $P^{\text{siRNA2}} = 0.000$) were significantly decreased in RBP2-depleted H1975 cells. Moreover, HIF-1α ($P = 0.001$) and VEGF ($P = 0.000$) were increased in RBP2-overexpressing SK-MES-1 cells compared to the control cells (Fig. 5D and Fig. 5E). These findings suggested that RBP2 plays an important role in the process of tumor angiogenesis through the up-regulation of HIF-1α and VEGF.

6. RBP2 induction of VEGF is dependent on HIF-1α

To confirm the role of RBP2 in regulating HIF-1α in NSCLC cells, we modulated HIF-1α expression by transfecting cells with an siRNA specific against HIF-1α (si-HIF-1α) and a plasmid pcDNA3-HA-HIF-1α, and evaluated the expression of VEGF after 36 hours. As shown in Fig. 6A and Fig. 6B, knockdown of HIF-1α expression in ectopic RBP2-expressing SK-MES-1 cells led to the down-regulation of VEGF compared with the scramble non-specific control siRNA; up-regulation of HIF-1α expression in RBP2-depleted H1975 cells led to the up-regulation of VEGF. These results indicated that the RBP2-mediated tumor angiogenesis of NSCLC cells might partially be regulated through the activation of HIF-1α.

7. RBP2 activates HIF-1α via the PI3K/Akt signaling pathway

A recent study suggests that RBP2 regulates N-cadherin and snail through the activation of Akt signaling [18]. In addition, under normoxic conditions, the expression and activity of HIF-1α and the subsequent secreted angiogenic factors in cancer can be abnormally up-regulated by different signaling pathways [34,35,36] involving Akt and its downstream effectors [20,22]. Therefore, we hypothesized that RBP2 regulates HIF-1α through

the activation of Akt signaling, and we further sought to detect the signaling mechanisms involved in RBP2-mediated tumor angiogenesis. Our results revealed that silencing RBP2 expression with either RBP2-siRNA1 or RBP2-siRNA2 in H1975 cells significantly decreased the phosphorylation of Akt, whereas the forced expression of RBP2 with pcDNA3-HA-RBP2 in SK-MES-1 cells increased the activity of Akt (Fig. 7A). Moreover, when a constitutively active form of Akt in RBP2-siRNA2 H1975 cells was expressed, the expression of HIF-1α and VEGF were increased compared to the control; the PI3K/Akt inhibitor LY294002 significantly inhibited the expression of HIF-1α and VEGF in pcDNA3-HA-RBP2 SK-MES-1 cells (Fig. 7B). These data suggest that RBP2 promotes tumor angiogenesis through the activation of the PI3K/Akt signaling pathway in NSCLC cell lines.

VEGF has been shown to be a potent activator of Akt in some cases [37]. We next explored whether VEGF could activate Akt. As shown in Fig. 7C, treatment of RBP2-siRNA2 H1975 cells with recombinant human VEGF-165 (25 ng/mL) increased the activation of Akt within 15 to 30 minutes. Therefore, to investigate the possible regulation of Akt by VEGF, we examined the expression of p-Akt at 30 minutes after recombinant human VEGF-165 was added. As shown in Fig. 7D, in the presence of recombinant human VEGF-165 stimulation, the activation of Akt was increased in RBP2-depleted H1975 cells and RBP2-overexpressing SK-MES-1 cells (25 ng/mL, 30 minutes). Thus, our results suggested that VEGF indeed increases the activation of Akt, as regulated by RBP2.

Discussion

RBP2, a member of the JARID family, was originally identified as a tumor suppressor retinoblastoma protein (pRB) binding partner that possesses H3-K4 demethylase activity [12,13,14]. Previous studies demonstrated that the oncogenic protein RBP2 was overexpressed in gastric cancer and NSCLC, which correlated with tumor senescence, proliferation, migration and invasion [17,38]. However, the present study is the first study to investigate the role of the RBP2 protein in relation to angiogenesis of in NSCLC patients.

The data of our study showed that high RBP2 expression is common in stage I NSCLC tissues and is significantly associated with tumor size, high HIF-1α expression, high VEGF expression and a poor prognosis, suggesting that the RBP2 protein is involved in the aggressive progression of NSCLC. Pathological angiogenesis plays an essential role in tumor initiation, progression and metastasis and also has prognostic importance in various types of human solid tumors [39,40]. Tumor angiogenesis was evaluated by CD34-determined intratumoral MVD in the present study, and high MVD was also associated with high HIF-1α expression and high VEGF expression. Moreover, Mann-Whitney U test showed that high RBP2 expression was correlated with increased MVD in patients with stage I NSCLC, demonstrating a novel angiogenic role for RBP2 in NSCLC invasiveness and metastasis. Thus, the RBP2 protein may promote pathological angiogenesis through the up-regulation of HIF-1α and VEGF in NSCLC progression.

NSCLC is an angiogenesis-dependent tumor, and angiogenesis plays pivotal roles in progression and blood-borne metastases [41,42]. The pathological angiogenesis of tumors is a complex, multistep process involving various cytokines [43,44]. The possible angiogenic potential of the RBP2 protein in vitro was analyzed by the tube formation assay. Our results showed that down-regulation of the RBP2 protein could significantly decrease HUVEC tube formation induced by conditioned medium. VEGF is a key pro-

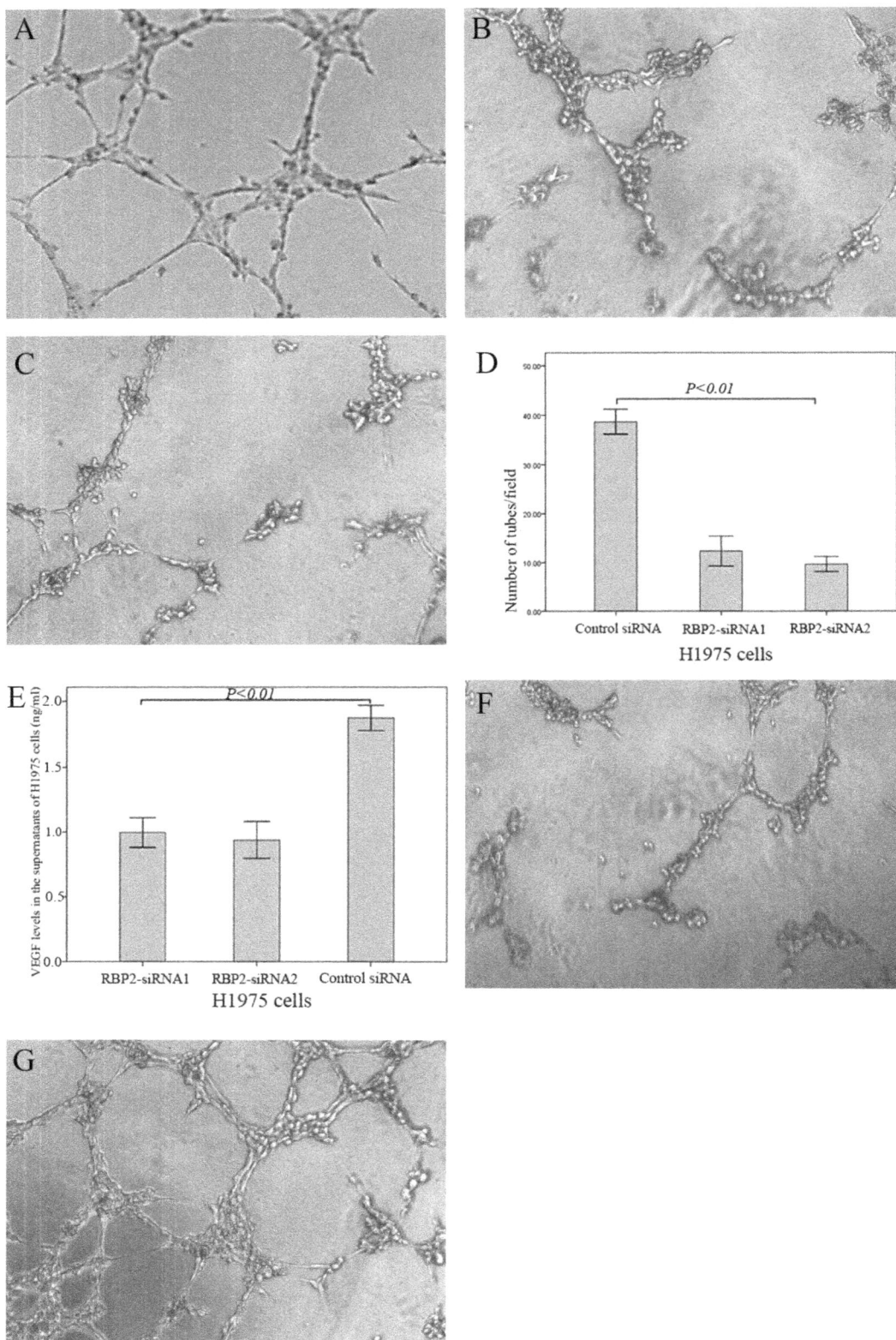

Figure 4. Down-regulation of the RBP2 protein decreased the tube formation by HUVECs induced by conditioned medium. Tube formation assay: (A) control-siRNA H1975 cells; (B) RBP2-siRNA1 H1975 cells; (C) RBP2-siRNA2 H1975 cells. (D) Quantitative analysis of the tube formation by HUVECs induced by conditioned medium; (E) Down-regulation of the RBP2 protein decreased the expression levels of VEGF in conditioned media. (F) The tube formation induced by the conditioned medium of control siRNA H1975 cells was blocked by the VEGFR inhibitor (sunitinib malate, 2.5 µM). (G) The reduced tube formation induced by the conditioned medium of RBP2-siRNA2 H1975 cells was rescued by adding VEGF-165 (2 ng/ml).

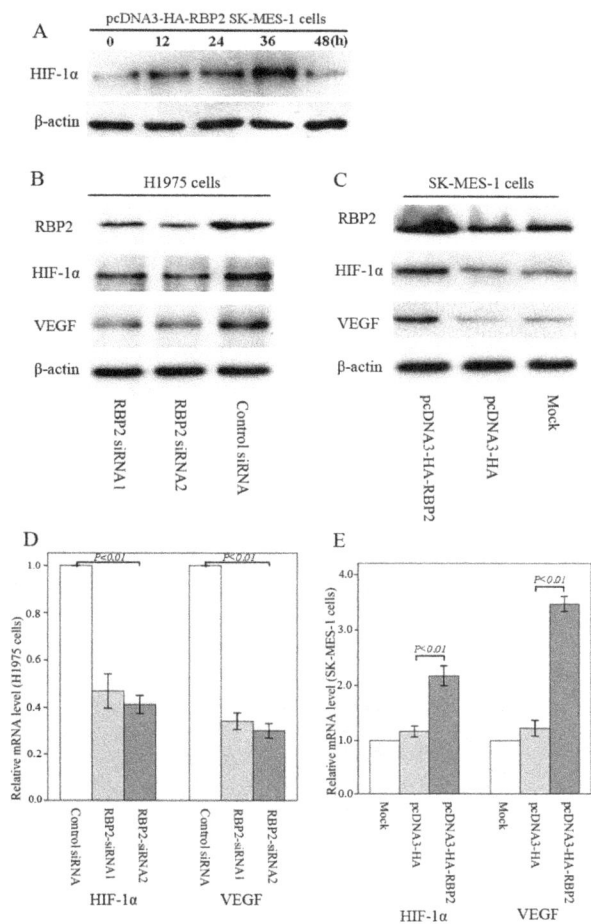

Figure 5. RBP2 stimulates the mRNA and protein expression of HIF-1α and VEGF. (A) RBP2 up-regulated the HIF-1α protein in a time-dependent manner under normoxic conditions. (B) Depletion of RBP2 decreased the expression of HIF-1α and VEGF in H1975 cells. (C) Up-regulation of RBP2 increased the expression of HIF-1α and VEGF in SK-MES-1 cells. (D) Real-time RT-PCR showed that the mRNA expression levels of HIF-1α and VEGF were significantly decreased in RBP2-depleted H1975 cells compared to control cells. (E) Real-time RT-PCR showed that the mRNA expression levels of HIF-1α and VEGF were significantly increased in RBP2-overexpressing SK-MES-1 cells.

angiogenic effector and plays a significant role in physiological and pathological angiogenesis [5,6], and we further detected the VEGF levels in different conditioned media. The results of our ELISA assay demonstrated that the VEGF protein levels in the conditioned medium of RBP2-siRNA H1975 cells were significantly lower than that of the control siRNA H1975 cells. In addition, the tube formation induced by the conditioned medium of control-siRNA H1975 cells was blocked by sunitinib malate which was a VEGFR inhibitor and the reduced tube formation induced by the conditioned medium of RBP2-siRNA2 H1975 cells was rescued by adding VEGF-165. These findings indicated that the tube formation induced by RBP2 might be VEGF dependent.

Transcription factor HIF-1α plays a crucial role in tumor angiogenesis and regulates the expression level of VEGF [11]. Many studies have suggested the importance of increased HIF-1α levels in the tumorigenesis and progression of various cancers by promoting tumor angiogenesis and the development of other hallmarks of cancer [45]. In addition, previous studies revealed that the expression of HIF-1α and VEGF is up-regulated in NSCLC and is related to a poor prognosis and worse overall survival [46,47,48]. We next explored the relationship between RBP2 and HIF-1α and VEGF protein expression in SK-MES-1 and H1975 cells. Our results suggested that the up-regulation of RBP2 leads to increased expression of HIF-1α and VEGF at both the mRNA and protein levels; in contrast, the depletion of RBP2 resulted in decreased expression levels of HIF-1α and VEGF. Interestingly, with RBP2 overexpression, the increased expression of VEGF induced by RBP2 was blocked by HIF-1α siRNA. Moreover, the enforced expression of HIF-1α in RBP2-depleted H1975 cells led to the up-regulation of VEGF. Therefore, our results confirmed that RBP2 is a non-hypoxic inducer of HIF-1α expression that modulates the process of tumor angiogenesis via HIF-1α-VEGF signaling. Targeting RBP2 signaling by novel approaches would be useful for reversing tumor angiogenesis.

The phosphatidylinositol 3-kinase (PI3K)/Akt signaling pathway plays a pivotal role in the core of the molecular signaling net work that governs proliferation, apoptosis, invasion and migration in many cell types [49,50]. Our observations showed that RBP2 increased the expression levels of HIF-1α and VEGF via the activation of PI3K/Akt signaling pathway. However, as VEGF has been shown to be a potent activator of Akt in some cases [37], we next explored the possible regulation of Akt by VEGF. Recombinant human VEGF-165 could stimulate the phosphorylation of Akt in RBP2-depleted H1975 cells and RBP2-overexpressing SK-MES-1 cells. As stated above, our results suggested that VEGF and Akt may be involved in a feedback loop.

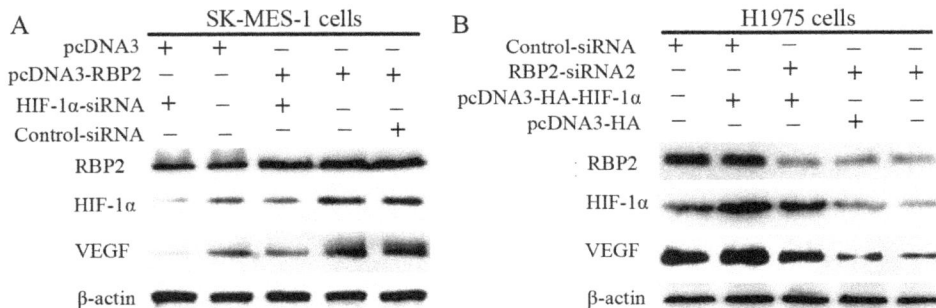

Figure 6. RBP2 induction of VEGF is dependent on HIF-1α. (A) Depletion of HIF-1α with an siRNA specific against HIF-1α in RBP2-overexpressing SK-MES-1 cells led to the down-regulation of VEGF compared with the scramble non-specific control siRNA. (B) Up-regulation of HIF-1α expression in RBP2-siRNA2 H1975 cells led to the up-regulation of VEGF.

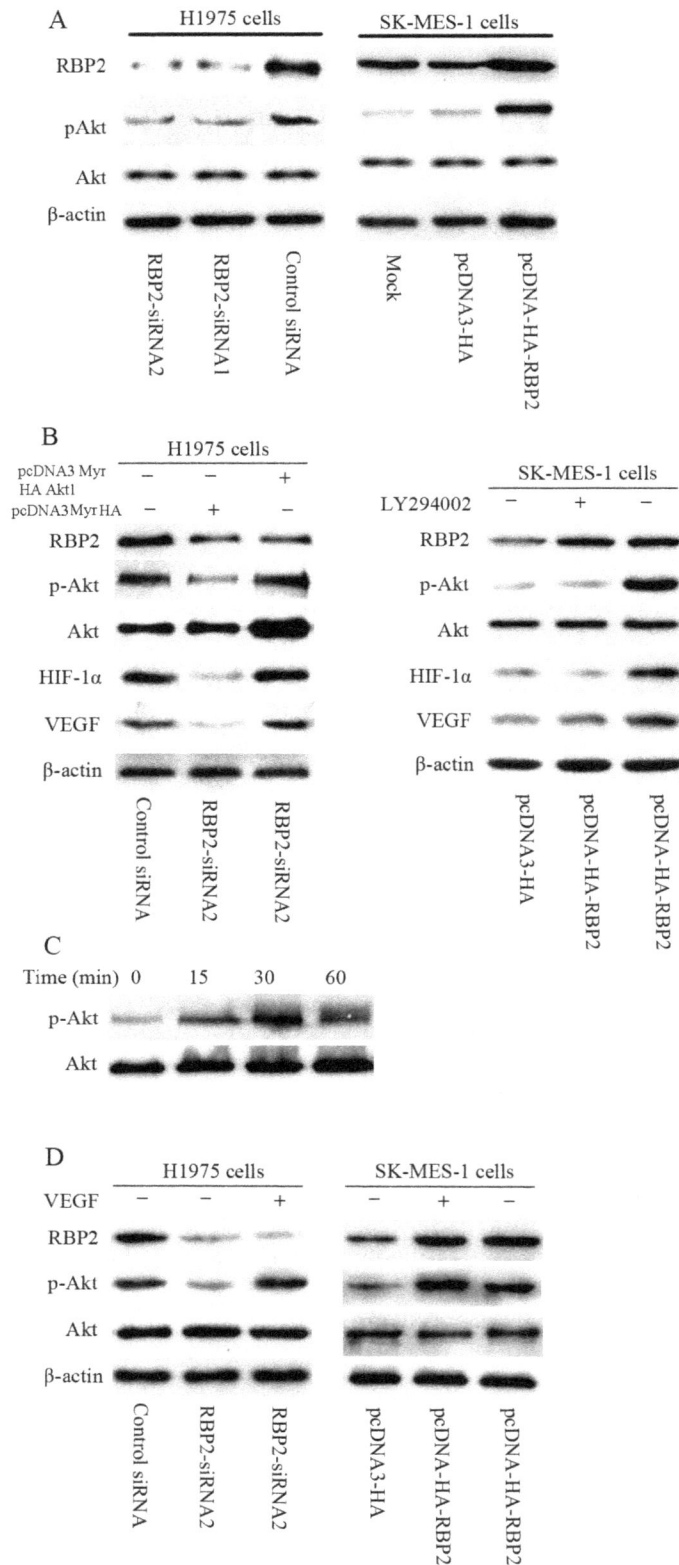

Figure 7. RBP2 activates HIF-1α via the PI3K/Akt signaling pathway. (A) Silencing RBP2 expression in H1975 cells significantly decreased the phosphorylation of Akt, and the forced expression of RBP2 in SK-MES-1 cells increased the activity of Akt. (B) When Akt was constitutively activated in RBP2-siRNA2 H1975, the expression of HIF-1α and VEGF were increased compared to the control. The PI3K/Akt inhibitor LY294002 significantly inhibited the expression of HIF-1α and VEGF in pcDNA3-HA-RBP2 SK-MES-1 cells. (C) Westernblots showing the time course of Akt phosphorylation in RBP2-siRNA2 H1975 cells due to VEGF-165 (25 ng/mL). (D) In the presence of recombinant human VEGF-165 stimulation, the activation of Akt was increased in RBP2-siRNA2 H1975 cells and RBP2-overexpressing SK-MES-1 cells (25 ng/mL, 30 minutes).

Integrins, a group of glycoprotein receptors, mediate cell adhesion and interaction with the extracellular matrix (ECM). In many cell types, integrins and other membrane receptors form macromolecular complexes, constituting signaling platforms at the adhesion sites. The Akt signaling pathway can be triggered by integrinβ1-mediated adhesion through Fak, which binds to the p85 subunit of PI3K, or via the Src–vinculin complex [51,52,53,54]. Interestingly, RBP2 was found to act as a transcription activator for integrinβ1 (ITGB1) by directly binding to its promoter, suggesting that ITGB1 is a direct and specific downstream target of RBP2 [17]. As stated above, the transcription of integrinβ1 activated by RBP2 may facilitate the activation of the Akt signaling pathway and play a critical role in RBP2-mediated tumor angiogenesis.

However, the activity, expression, synthesis and stability of HIF-1α are extremely complex, involving various factors such as MEK, PI3K, mTOR, eIF-4E, p70S6K, RACK1 and Hsp90 [55,56,57]. RBP2 plays a dual role by acting as a transcriptional repressor and transcriptional activator [15,16] and may have an affect on the activity, expression, synthesis and stability of HIF-1α. Therefore the precise mechanisms necessary for the RBP2 protein to induce HIF-1α still need to be further researched.

In conclusion, we provided evidence showing that high RBP2 expression and high MVD were common in stage I NSCLC tissues and closely associated with poor prognosis. In addition, high RBP2 expression was closely associated with tumor size, high HIF-1α expression, high VEGF expression and increased tumor angiogenesis. Multivariate analysis indicated that RBP2 had an independent influence on the survival of patients with stage I NSCLC. The RBP2 protein may play a critical role in NSCLC tumor angiogenesis by enhancing HIF-1α and VEGF expression under normoxia via the PI3K/Akt signaling pathway. Moreover, VEGF could increase the activation of Akt regulated by RBP2. These findings indicate that RBP2 could serve as an attractive therapeutic target against angiogenesis for early-stage NSCLC patients.

Acknowledgments

We would like to thank William G. Kaelin, Jr. (Howard Hughes Medical Institute, Dana-Farber Cancer Institute and Brigham and Women's Hospital, Harvard Medical School, USA) for the plasmids.

Author Contributions

Conceived and designed the experiments: HT. Performed the experiments: LQ FZ LBS. Analyzed the data: LQ FZ. Contributed reagents/materials/analysis tools: SHL LKH. Contributed to the writing of the manuscript: LQ HT.

References

1. Jemal A, Bray F, Center MM, Ferlay J, Ward E, et al. (2011) Global cancer statistics. CA Cancer J Clin 61: 69–90.
2. Pisters KM, Evans WK, Azzoli CG, Kris MG, Smith CA, et al. (2007) Cancer Care Ontario and American Society of Clinical Oncology adjuvant chemotherapy and adjuvant radiation therapy for stages I-IIIA resectable non small-cell lung cancer guideline. J Clin Oncol 25: 5506–5518.
3. Vamesu S (2008) Angiogenesis and tumor histologic type in primary breast cancer patients: an analysis of 155 needle core biopsies. Rom J Morphol Embryol 49: 181–188.
4. Vermeulen PB, van Golen KL, Dirix LY (2010) Angiogenesis, lymphangiogenesis, growth pattern, and tumor emboli in inflammatory breast cancer: a review of the current knowledge. Cancer 116: 2748–2754.
5. Tammela T, Enholm B, Alitalo K, Paavonen K (2005) The biology of vascular endothelial growth factors. Cardiovasc Res 65: 550–563.
6. Mac Gabhann F, Popel AS (2008) Systems biology of vascular endothelial growth factors. Microcirculation 15: 715–738.
7. Semenza GL (2003) Targeting HIF-1 for cancer therapy. Nat Rev Cancer 3: 721–732.
8. Semenza GL (2001) HIF-1, O(2), and the 3 PHDs: how animal cells signal hypoxia to the nucleus. Cell 107: 1–3.
9. Grimshaw MJ (2007) Endothelins and hypoxia-inducible factor in cancer. Endocr Relat Cancer 14: 233–244.
10. Cheng JC, Klausen C, Leung PC (2013) Hypoxia-inducible factor 1 alpha mediates epidermal growth factor-induced down-regulation of E-cadherin expression and cell invasion in human ovarian cancer cells. Cancer Lett 329: 197–206.
11. Crociani O, Zanieri F, Pillozzi S, Lastraioli E, Stefanini M, et al. (2013) hERG1 channels modulate integrin signaling to trigger angiogenesis and tumor progression in colorectal cancer. Sci Rep 3: 3308.
12. Christensen J, Agger K, Cloos PA, Pasini D, Rose S, et al. (2007) RBP2 belongs to a family of demethylases, specific for tri-and dimethylated lysine 4 on histone 3. Cell 128: 1063–1076.
13. Secombe J, Li L, Carlos L, Eisenman RN (2007) The Trithorax group protein Lid is a trimethyl histone H3K4 demethylase required for dMyc-induced cell growth. Genes Dev 21: 537–551.
14. Klose RJ, Yan Q, Tothova Z, Yamane K, Erdjument-Bromage H, et al. (2007) The retinoblastoma binding protein RBP2 is an H3K4 demethylase. Cell 128: 889–900.
15. Benevolenskaya EV, Murray HL, Branton P, Young RA, Kaelin WG Jr (2005) Binding of pRB to the PHD protein RBP2 promotes cellular differentiation. Mol Cell 18: 623–635.
16. Sims RJ 3rd, Reinberg D (2006) Histone H3 Lys 4 methylation: caught in a bind? Genes Dev 20: 2779–2786.
17. Teng YC, Lee CF, Li YS, Chen YR, Hsiao PW, et al. (2013) Histone demethylase RBP2 promotes lung tumorigenesis and cancer metastasis. Cancer Res 73: 4711–4721.
18. Wang S, Wang Y, Wu H, Hu L (2013) RBP2 induces epithelial-mesenchymal transition in non-small cell lung cancer. PLoS One 8: e84735.
19. Bolas G, de Rezende FF, Lorente C, Sanz L, Eble JA, et al. (2014) Inhibitory effects of recombinant RTS-jerdostatin on integrin alpha1beta1 function during adhesion, migration and proliferation of rat aortic smooth muscle cells and angiogenesis. Toxicon 79: 45–54.
20. Belaiba RS, Bonello S, Zahringer C, Schmidt S, Hess J, et al. (2007) Hypoxia up-regulates hypoxia-inducible factor-1alpha transcription by involving phosphatidylinositol 3-kinase and nuclear factor kappaB in pulmonary artery smooth muscle cells. Mol Biol Cell 18: 4691–4697.
21. Jahangiri A, Aghi MK, Carbonell WS (2014) beta1 integrin: Critical path to antiangiogenic therapy resistance and beyond. Cancer Res 74: 3–7.
22. Kim CH, Cho YS, Chun YS, Park JW, Kim MS (2002) Early expression of myocardial HIF-1alpha in response to mechanical stresses: regulation by stretch-activated channels and the phosphatidylinositol 3-kinase signaling pathway. Circ Res 90: E25–33.
23. Vermeulen PB, Gasparini G, Fox SB, Colpaert C, Marson LP, et al. (2002) Second international consensus on the methodology and criteria of evaluation of angiogenesis quantification in solid human tumours. Eur J Cancer 38: 1564–1579.
24. Igarashi M, Dhar DK, Kubota H, Yamamoto A, El-Assal O, et al. (1998) The prognostic significance of microvessel density and thymidine phosphorylase expression in squamous cell carcinoma of the esophagus. Cancer 82: 1225–1232.
25. Tanigawa N, Amaya H, Matsumura M, Shimomatsuya T, Horiuchi T, et al. (1996) Extent of tumor vascularization correlates with prognosis and hematogenous metastasis in gastric carcinomas. Cancer Res 56: 2671–2676.
26. Wolf D, Wolf AM, Rumpold H, Fiegl H, Zeimet AG, et al. (2005) The expression of the regulatory T cell-specific forkhead box transcription factor FoxP3 is associated with poor prognosis in ovarian cancer. Clin Cancer Res 11: 8326–8331.
27. Bos R, van Diest PJ, de Jong JS, van der Groep P, van der Valk P, et al. (2005) Hypoxia-inducible factor-1alpha is associated with angiogenesis, and expression of bFGF, PDGF-BB, and EGFR in invasive breast cancer. Histopathology 46: 31–36.
28. Saponaro C, Malfettone A, Ranieri G, Danza K, Simone G, et al. (2013) VEGF, HIF-1alpha expression and MVD as an angiogenic network in familial breast cancer. PLoS One 8: e53070.
29. Malhotra R, Tyson DW, Rosevear HM, Brosius FC 3rd (2008) Hypoxia-inducible factor-1alpha is a critical mediator of hypoxia induced apoptosis in cardiac H9c2 and kidney epithelial HK-2 cells. BMC Cardiovasc Disord 8: 9.
30. Kim SM, Park JH, Kim KD, Nam D, Shim BS, et al. (2014) Brassinin induces apoptosis in PC-3 human prostate cancer cells through the suppression of PI3K/Akt/mTOR/S6K1 signaling cascades. Phytother Res 28: 423–431.
31. Wang Z, Banerjee S, Kong D, Li Y, Sarkar FH (2007) Down-regulation of Forkhead Box M1 transcription factor leads to the inhibition of invasion and angiogenesis of pancreatic cancer cells. Cancer Res 67: 8293–8300.
32. Jamison J, Wang JH, Wells A (2014) PKCdelta regulates force signaling during VEGF/CXCL4 induced dissociation of endothelial tubes. PLoS One 9: e93968.
33. Livak KJ, Schmittgen TD (2001) Analysis of relative gene expression data using real-time quantitative PCR and the 2(−Delta Delta C(T)) Method. Methods 25: 402–408.

34. Keith B, Johnson RS, Simon MC (2012) HIF1alpha and HIF2alpha: sibling rivalry in hypoxic tumour growth and progression. Nat Rev Cancer 12: 9–22.
35. Dayan F, Mazure NM, Brahimi-Horn MC, Pouyssegur J (2008) A dialogue between the hypoxia-inducible factor and the tumor microenvironment. Cancer Microenviron 1: 53–68.
36. Pouyssegur J, Dayan F, Mazure NM (2006) Hypoxia signalling in cancer and approaches to enforce tumour regression. Nature 441: 437–443.
37. Takeshita K, Satoh M, Ii M, Silver M, Limbourg FP, et al. (2007) Critical role of endothelial Notch1 signaling in postnatal angiogenesis. Circ Res 100: 70–78.
38. Zeng J, Ge Z, Wang L, Li Q, Wang N, et al. (2010) The histone demethylase RBP2 Is overexpressed in gastric cancer and its inhibition triggers senescence of cancer cells. Gastroenterology 138: 981–992.
39. Folkman J (2007) Angiogenesis: an organizing principle for drug discovery? Nat Rev Drug Discov 6: 273–286.
40. Carmeliet P (2005) Angiogenesis in life, disease and medicine. Nature 438: 932–936.
41. Shijubo N, Kojima H, Nagata M, Ohchi T, Suzuki A, et al. (2003) Tumor angiogenesis of non-small cell lung cancer. Microsc Res Tech 60: 186–198.
42. D'Amico TA (2004) Angiogenesis in non-small cell lung cancer. Semin Thorac Cardiovasc Surg 16: 13–18.
43. Crabb SJ, Patsios D, Sauerbrei E, Ellis PM, Arnold A, et al. (2009) Tumor cavitation: impact on objective response evaluation in trials of angiogenesis inhibitors in non-small-cell lung cancer. J Clin Oncol 27: 404–410.
44. Maeda A, Nakata M, Yasuda K, Yukawa T, Saisho S, et al. (2013) Influence of vascular endothelial growth factor single nucleotide polymorphisms on non-small cell lung cancer tumor angiogenesis. Oncol Rep 29: 39–44.
45. Nakamura M, Bodily JM, Beglin M, Kyo S, Inoue M, et al. (2009) Hypoxia-specific stabilization of HIF-1alpha by human papillomaviruses. Virology 387: 442–448.
46. Rovina N, Hillas G, Dima E, Vlastos F, Loukides S, et al. (2011) VEGF and IL-18 in induced sputum of lung cancer patients. Cytokine 54: 277–281.
47. Charpidou A, Gkiozos I, Konstantinou M, Eleftheraki A, Demertzis P, et al. (2011) Bronchial washing levels of vascular endothelial growth factor receptor-2 (VEGFR2) correlate with overall survival in NSCLC patients. Cancer Lett 304: 144–153.
48. Park S, Ha SY, Cho HY, Chung DH, Kim NR, et al. (2011) Prognostic implications of hypoxia-inducible factor-1alpha in epidermal growth factor receptor-negative non-small cell lung cancer. Lung Cancer 72: 100–107.
49. Ha GH, Park JS, Breuer EK (2013) TACC3 promotes epithelial-mesenchymal transition (EMT) through the activation of PI3K/Akt and ERK signaling pathways. Cancer Lett 332: 63–73.
50. Lin JC, Wu YY, Wu JY, Lin TC, Wu CT, et al. (2012) TROP2 is epigenetically inactivated and modulates IGF-1R signalling in lung adenocarcinoma. EMBO Mol Med 4: 472–485.
51. Lee DY, Li YS, Chang SF, Zhou J, Ho HM, et al. (2010) Oscillatory flow-induced proliferation of osteoblast-like cells is mediated by alphavbeta3 and beta1 integrins through synergistic interactions of focal adhesion kinase and Shc with phosphatidylinositol 3-kinase and the Akt/mTOR/p70S6K pathway. J Biol Chem 285: 30–42.
52. Thamilselvan V, Craig DH, Basson MD (2007) FAK association with multiple signal proteins mediates pressure-induced colon cancer cell adhesion via a Src-dependent PI3K/Akt pathway. FASEB J 21: 1730–1741.
53. Moreno-Layseca P, Streuli CH (2014) Signalling pathways linking integrins with cell cycle progression. Matrix Biol 34: 144–153.
54. Poettler M, Unseld M, Braemswig K, Haitel A, Zielinski CC, et al. (2013) CD98hc (SLC3A2) drives integrin-dependent renal cancer cell behavior. Mol Cancer 12: 169.
55. Kalhori V, Kemppainen K, Asghar MY, Bergelin N, Jaakkola P, et al. (2013) Sphingosine-1-Phosphate as a Regulator of Hypoxia-Induced Factor-1alpha in Thyroid Follicular Carcinoma Cells. PLoS One 8: e66189.
56. Trisciuoglio D, Gabellini C, Desideri M, Ziparo E, Zupi G, et al. (2010) Bcl-2 regulates HIF-1alpha protein stabilization in hypoxic melanoma cells via the molecular chaperone HSP90. PLoS One 5: e11772.
57. Riddell JR, Maier P, Sass SN, Moser MT, Foster BA, et al. (2012) Peroxiredoxin 1 stimulates endothelial cell expression of VEGF via TLR4 dependent activation of HIF-1alpha. PLoS One 7: e50394.

7

Astaxanthin Inhibits JAK/STAT-3 Signaling to Abrogate Cell Proliferation, Invasion and Angiogenesis in a Hamster Model of Oral Cancer

J. Kowshik[1], **Abdul Basit Baba**[1], **Hemant Giri**[2], **G. Deepak Reddy**[3], **Madhulika Dixit**[2], **Siddavaram Nagini**[1]*

1 Department of Biochemistry and Biotechnology, Faculty of Science, Annamalai University, Annamalainagar, Tamil Nadu, India, 2 Laboratory of Vascular Biology, Department of Biotechnology, Indian Institute of Technology Madras, Chennai, Tami Nadu, India, 3 Medicinal Chemistry Research Division, Vishnu Institute of Pharmaceutical Education and Research, Narsapur, India

Abstract

Identifying agents that inhibit STAT-3, a cytosolic transcription factor involved in the activation of various genes implicated in tumour progression is a promising strategy for cancer chemoprevention. In the present study, we investigated the effect of dietary astaxanthin on JAK-2/STAT-3 signaling in the 7,12-dimethylbenz[a]anthracene (DMBA)-induced hamster buccal pouch (HBP) carcinogenesis model by examining the mRNA and protein expression of JAK/STAT-3 and its target genes. Quantitative RT-PCR, immunoblotting and immunohistochemical analyses revealed that astaxanthin supplementation inhibits key events in JAK/STAT signaling especially STAT-3 phosphorylation and subsequent nuclear translocation of STAT-3. Furthermore, astaxanthin downregulated the expression of STAT-3 target genes involved in cell proliferation, invasion and angiogenesis, and reduced microvascular density, thereby preventing tumour progression. Molecular docking analysis confirmed inhibitory effects of astaxanthin on STAT signaling and angiogenesis. Cell culture experiments with the endothelial cell line ECV304 substantiated the role of astaxanthin in suppressing angiogenesis. Taken together, our data provide substantial evidence that dietary astaxanthin prevents the development and progression of HBP carcinomas through the inhibition of JAK-2/STAT-3 signaling and its downstream events. Thus, astaxanthin that functions as a potent inhibitor of tumour development and progression by targeting JAK/STAT signaling may be an ideal candidate for cancer chemoprevention.

Editor: Shree Ram Singh, National Cancer Institute, United States of America

Funding: This work was supported by a grant from the Department of Biotechnology, New Delhi, India under the 7th FP of the Indo-EU Joint Collaborative Project on 'FUNCFOOD'. The funders had no role in study design, data collection and analysis, decision to publish, or preparation of the manuscript.

Competing Interests: The authors have declared that no competing interests exist.

* Email: s_nagini@yahoo.com

Introduction

Signal transducer and activator of transcription 3 (STAT3) protein is a latent cytoplasmic transcription factor that transmits signals from the cell surface to the nucleus when activated by cytokines and growth factors [1]. In particular, interleukin-6 (IL-6) or epidermal growth factor (EGF) stimulate the phosphorylation of STAT3 protein by Janus kinase and activated STAT3 forms a homodimer that translocates to the nucleus where it regulates the expression of genes critical for normal cellular processes such as cell development, differ-entiation, proliferation, survival, angio-genesis, and immune function [2–6].

Aberrant activation of JAK/STAT3 signaling has been documented in a wide variety of human tumors, including hematopoietic malignancies and solid tumors such as head and neck, breast, and prostate cancers [7,8]. Constitutive STAT3 activation contributes to proliferation and oncogenesis by modulating the expression of a variety of genes required for tumor cell survival, proliferation, and angiogenesis, as well as invasion and metastasis and commonly suggests poor prognosis [9–11]. Thus, JAK/STAT3 signaling plays a central role in tumorigenesis and is

considered an important therapeutic target for novel drug development.

Identification of agents that target STAT3 molecule is likely to be of significance in cancer chemoprevention. Several dietary antioxidants are recognized to block tumour development by targeting the STAT3 signaling network [12–15]. Astaxanthin, a non-provitamin A carotenoid predominantly found in microalgae, fungi, plants, sea foods and some birds such as flamingos and quail is a potent antioxidant [16]. Astaxanthin was found to exhibit the highest antioxidant activity among the carotenoids and is widely used in the prevention and treatment of various diseases [17]. AXT has also been demonstrated to exhibit anti-inflammatory and anticancer properties [18,19].

Recently, we demonstrated that dietary supplementation of AXT induces intrinsic apoptosis by inhibiting PI3/Akt, MAPK, NF-κB and Wnt/β-catenin signaling circuits in the 7,12-dimethylbenz[a]anthracene (DMBA)-induced hamster buccal pouch (HBP) carcinogenesis model [20]. These findings tempted us to hypothesize that AXT that induces apoptosis may block the opposing process of cell proliferation thereby preventing the sequential accumulation of mutations that eventually lead to tumour invasion and angiogenesis. Furthermore, AXT-induced inactivation of the transcription factors NF-κB and β-catenin, central hubs in oncogenic signaling could also impact the JAK/STAT3 pathway. In the present study we demonstrate that dietary AXT inhibits tumour progression based on abrogation of the JAK/STAT3 pathway and its downstream targets cyclin D1, MMP-2, -9, and VEGF in the HBP carcinogenesis model. Furthermore AXT decreased microvascular density, which plays an essential role in tumour development and progression. Cell culture experiments with the endothelial cell line ECV304 were also performed to substantiate the role of astaxanthin in suppressing hypoxia-induced angiogenesis.

Materials and Methods

Chemicals

Acrylamide, bovine serum albumin (BSA), bromophenol blue, 7,12-dimethylbenz[a]anthracene (DMBA), hydroxyurea, 2-mercaptoethanol, sodium dodecyl sulphate (SDS) N,N,N′,N′ - tetramethylene diamine (TEMED) and Trizol were purchased from Sigma Chemical Company, St. Louis, MO, USA. Astaxanthin was procured from Bio-Real, Sweden. DMEM-F12 medium, antibiotic solution consisting of penicillin and streptomycin and Alamar blue were from HiMedia Labs, Mumbai, India. Fetal bovine serum of South American origin was from GIBCO, Invitrogen, NY, USA. Power SYBR Green PCR master mix was obtained from Applied Biosystems, California, USA. Antibodies for IL-6, GAPDH, Cyclin D1, PCNA, p21, MMP-2, MMP-9, TIMP-2, RECK, VEGF, VEGFR2, HIF1α, were purchased from Santa Cruz Biotechnology, USA. pJAK-2$^{tyr1007/1008}$, JAK-2, pSTAT-3^{tyr705}, STAT-3 and histone (H2B) antibodies and BrdU, STAT-3^{tyr705}, total cyclin D1 and pVEGFR2^{tyr1175} ELISA kits were from Cell Signaling Technology, USA. CD-34 antibody was purchased from Novocastra, Germany. Matrigel was from BD Biosciences, USA. All other reagents used were of analytical grade.

Animals and ethics statement

Eight to ten weeks old male Syrian hamsters weighing between 100–110 g were used in this study. Animals were obtained from Central Animal House, Annamalai University, India. The animals were housed four to a cage and provided with standard pellet diet and water ad libitum. The animal health was monitored daily during the study. The protocols for the animal experiments were approved by the Institutional Animal Ethics Committee, Annamalai University and conducted according to the guidelines laid down by the Committee for the Purpose of Control and Supervision on Experiments on Animals (CPCSEA).

Treatment schedule

The animals were randomized into experimental and control groups and divided into 4 groups of 5 animals each. In group 1, the right buccal pouches of hamsters were painted with 0.5% DMBA in liquid paraffin three times a week for 14 weeks [21]. Group 2 animals received in addition to DMBA, a basal diet containing 15 mg/kg bw of astaxanthin [20,22]. Group 3 animals received astaxanthin (15 mg/kg bw) alone for 14 weeks. Group 4 animals received basal diet alone and served as an untreated control. The experiment was terminated at 14 weeks and all animals were sacrificed by cervical dislocation after an overnight fast. The buccal pouch tissues were immediately subdivided and processed for distribution to each experiment.

Cell culture

ECV 304 cell line was used and cultured in DMEM basal medium with 10% fetal bovine serum with antibiotics. ECV304 is an endothelial cell line derived from human umbilical vein endothelial cells (HUVECs) through spontaneous transformation [23]. Compared to primary HUVEC cultures, use of ECV304 cells has a practical advantage as these cells exhibit enhanced and reproducible capacity for in vitro angiogenesis are thus an ideal choice for cell culture based angiogenesis assays [24]. Confluent cultures of ECV304 cells were subcultured and maintained in CO_2 incubator at 37°C. For matrigel assay, cells were maintained in DMEM basal medium with 4% fetal bovine serum. For hypoxic condition, cells were incubated in hypoxia chamber with 1% O_2.

RNA extraction and quantitative real-time RT-PCR

Total RNA from the buccal pouch tissues was extracted using Trizol reagent as described previously [25]. The RNA concentration was determined from the optical density at a wavelength of 260 nm (using an OD260 unit equivalent to 40 μg/ml of RNA). 5 μg of isolated total RNA was reverse-transcribed to cDNA in a reaction mixture containing 4 μl of 5× reaction buffer, 2 μl of dNTP mixture (10 mM), 20 units of RNase inhibitor, 200 units of avian-myeloblastosis virus (AMV) reverse transcriptase and 0.5 μg of oligo(dT) primer (Promega, WI, USA) in a total volume of 20 μl. The reaction mixture was incubated at 42°C for 60 min and the reaction terminated by heating at 70°C for 10 min. The cDNA was stored at −80°C until further use.

Quantitative RT-PCR was performed using Power SYBR Green master mix according to the manufacturer's instructions using a StepOne Plus thermocycler (Applied Biosystems). To the 1×PCR master mix, 2.5 μl of each cDNA was added in a 20 μl final volume. The PCR conditions were as follows: 95°C for 5 min, 40 cycles of 30 s at 95°C, 30 s at 52 to 60°C (based on the target), and 60 s at 72°C. Relative quantitative fold change compared to control was calculated using the comparative Ct method, where Ct is the cycle number at which fluorescence first exceeds the threshold. The Ct values from each sample were obtained by subtracting the values for GAPDH Ct from the target gene Ct value. The specificity of resulting PCR products was confirmed by melting curves.

Western blotting

Proteins were extracted from tissue sample using lysis buffer containing 62.5 mM Tris (pH 6.8), 10% SDS, 5% 2-mercaptoethanol, 10% glycerol and bromophenol blue. Nuclear and cytoplasmic fractions were separated as described by Legrand-Poels et al. [26]. Equal amount of protein extracts were loaded onto SDS-PAGE and the resolved proteins were transferred to polyvinylidene difluoride membranes. The blots were then incubated for 2 h in 1X PBS containing 5% non-fat dry milk. The membranes were then probed with primary and secondary antibodies as per manufacturer's instructions. The proteins were visualized using enhanced chemiluminescence detection reagents (Sigma). Densitometry was performed on IISP flat bed scanner and quantitated with Total Lab 1.11 software.

ELISA

The levels of pSTAT^{tyr705}, total cyclin D1 and pVEGFR2^{tyr1175} were determined using sandwich ELISA kit (Cell Signaling Technology, USA) according to the manufacturer's instructions.

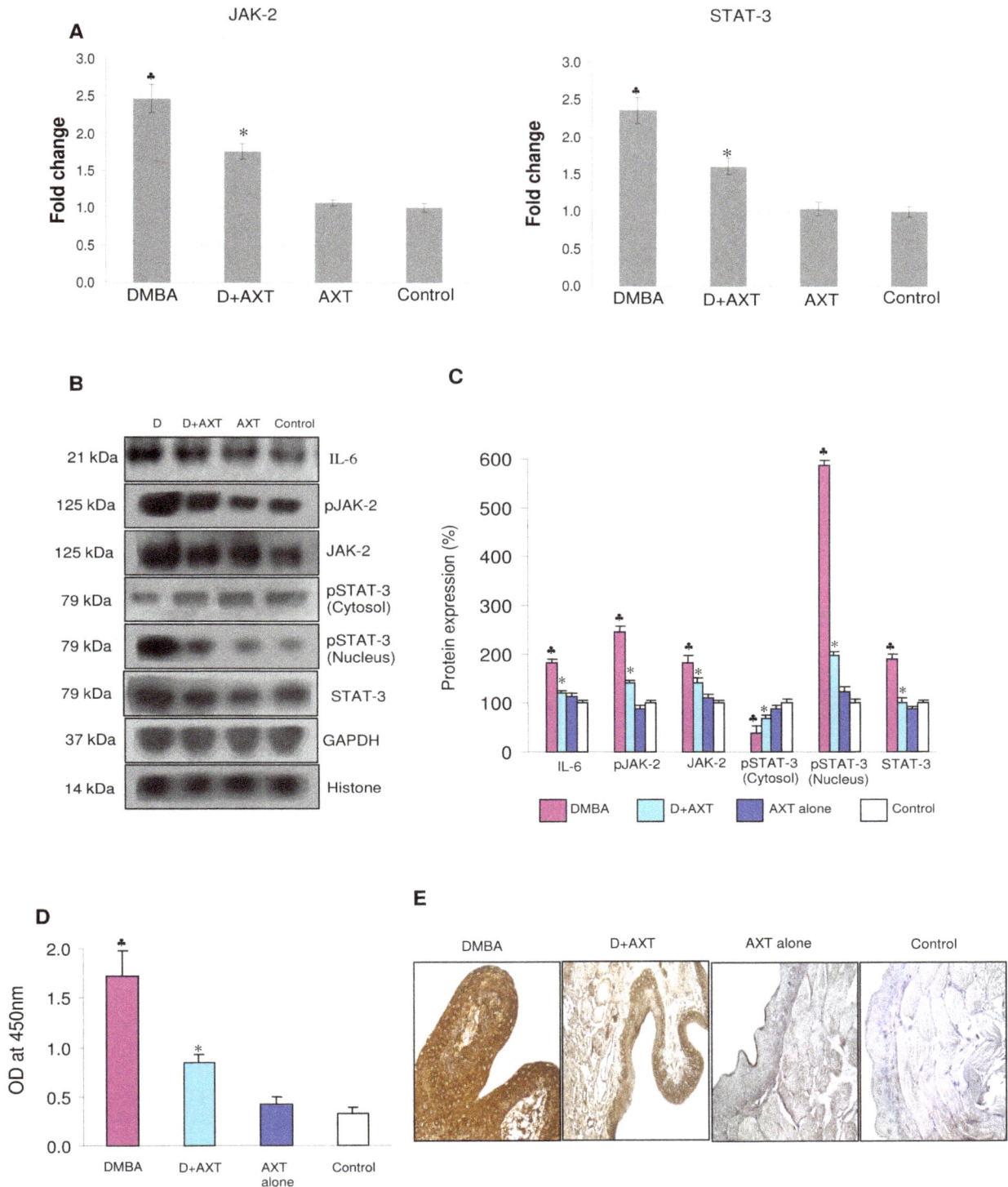

Figure 1. mRNA and protein expression of JAK-2 and STAT-3 in the buccal pouch tissues of experimental and control animals. (mean ± SD; n = 3). A. Transcript expression level of JAK-2 and STAT-3 in various experimental groups as determined by kinetic PCR. Data are the mean ± SD of three independent experiments. ♣p<0.05 versus control. *p<0.05 versus DMBA. B. Representative immunoblot analysis. Protein samples (100 μg/lane) resolved on SDS-PAGE were probed with corresponding antibodies. GAPDH was used as loading control for cytosol and whole tissue homogenates. Histone H2B was used as loading control for nuclear proteins. Phosphorylated proteins are normalized by their unphosphorylated form. C. Densitometric analysis. The protein expression from control lysates for three determinations was designated as 100% in the graph. Each bar represents the protein expression of three determinations. ♣p<0.05 versus control. *p<0.05 versus DMBA. D. Levels of pSTAT^{tyr705} (ELISA). E. Representative photomicrographs of immunohistochemical staining of pSTAT-3 in control and experimental animals (20X).

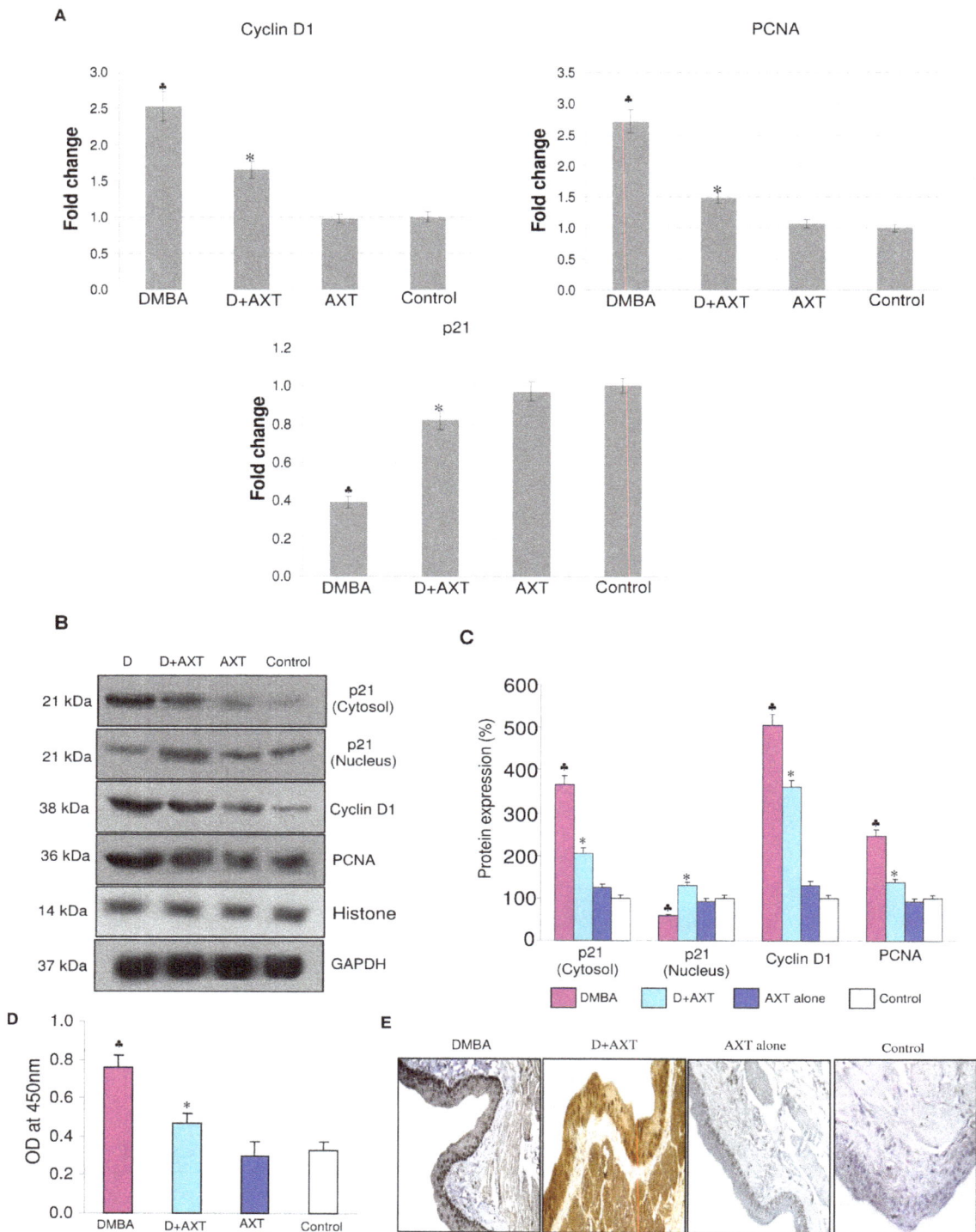

Figure 2. mRNA and protein expression of p21, Cyclin D1 and PCNA in the buccal pouch tissues of experimental and control animals. (mean $\pm$ SD; n = 3). A. Transcript expression level of p21, cyclin D1 and PCNA in various experimental groups as determined by kinetic PCR. Data are the mean $\pm$ SD of three independent experiments. ♣$p < 0.05$ versus control. *$p < 0.05$ versus DMBA. B. Representative immunoblot analysis. Protein samples (100 µg/lane) resolved on SDS-PAGE were probed with corresponding antibodies. GAPDH was used as loading control for cytosol and whole tissue homogenates. Histone H2B was used as loading control for nuclear proteins. C. Densitometric analysis. The protein expression from control lysates for three determinations was designated as 100% in the graph. Each bar represents the protein expression of three determinations. ♣$p < 0.05$ versus control. $p < 0.05$ versus DMBA. D. Levels of total cyclin D1 (ELISA). E. Representative photomicrographs of immunohistochemical staining of PCNA in control and experimental animals (20X).

A

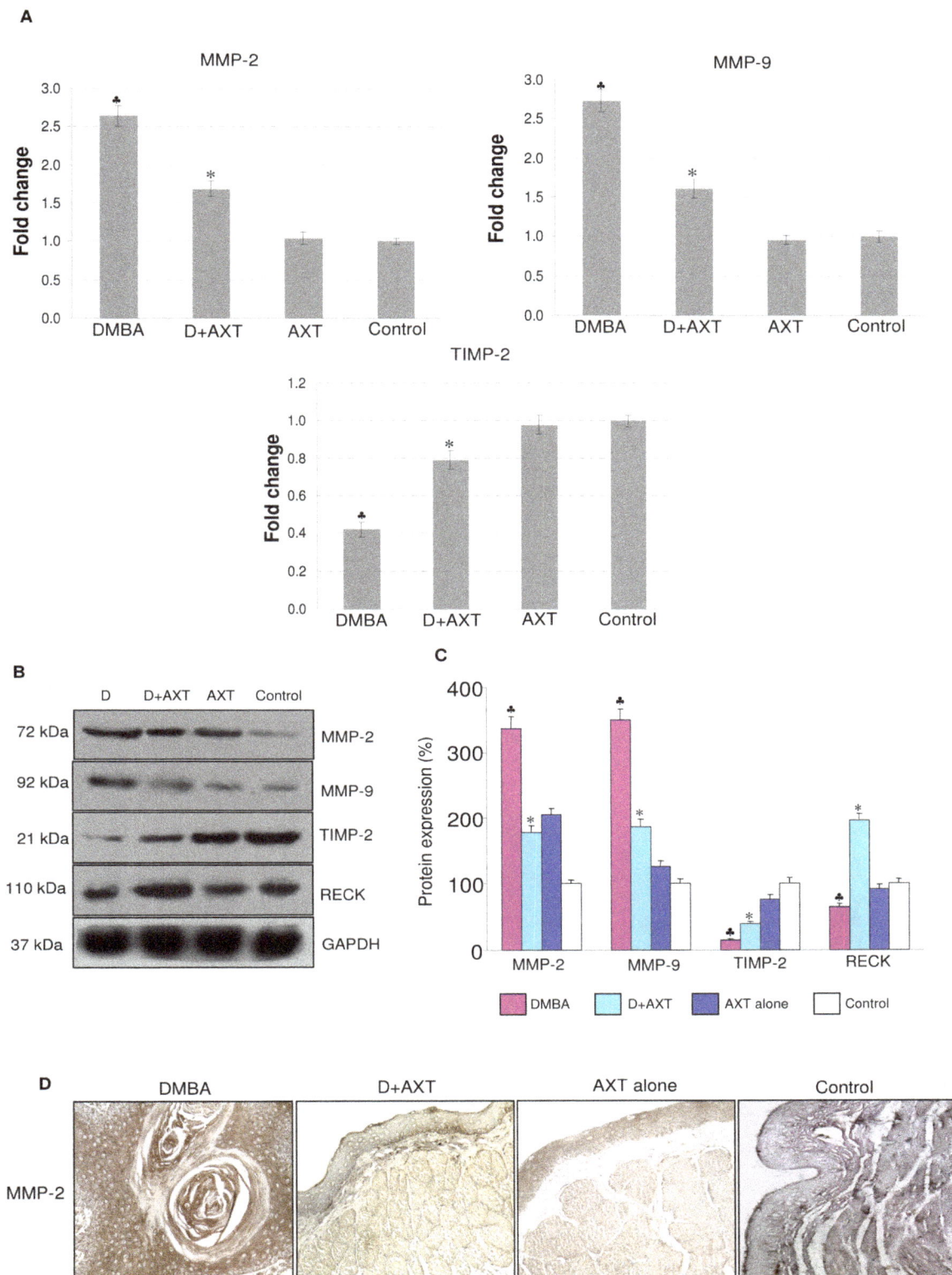

Figure 3. mRNA and protein expression of MMP-2, MMP-9, TIMP-2 and RECK in the buccal pouch tissues of experimental and control animals. (mean ± SD; n = 3). A. Transcript expression level of MMP-2, MMP-9 and TIMP-2 in various experimental groups as determined by kinetic PCR. Data are the mean ± SD of three independent experiments. ♣p<0.05 versus control. *p<0.05 versus DMBA. **B & C**. Representative immunoblots and bar graph representing the protein expression of MMP-2, MMP-9, TIMP-2 and RECK for minimum of three independent experiments. ♣p<0.05 versus control. *p<0.05 versus DMBA. D. Representative photomicrographs of immunohistochemical staining of MMP-2 in control and experimental animals (20X).

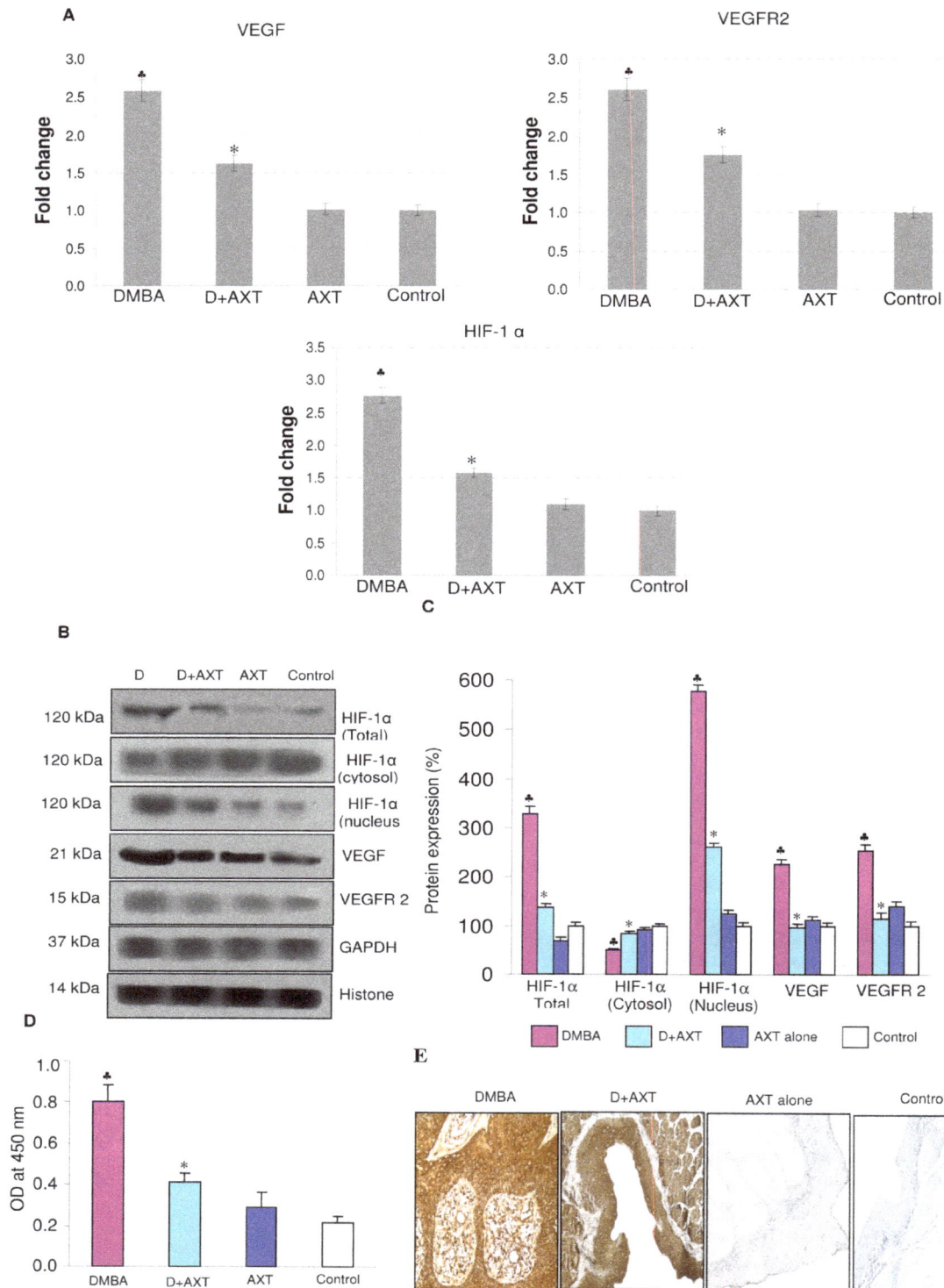

Figure 4. mRNA and protein expression of HIF-1α, VEGF and VEGFR2 in the buccal pouch tissues of experimental and control animals. (mean $\pm$ SD; n = 3). A. Transcript expression level of HIF-1α, VEGF and VEGFR2 in various experimental groups as determined by kinetic PCR. Data are the mean $\pm$ SD of three independent experiments. $^{\clubsuit}$p<0.05 versus control. *p<0.05 versus DMBA. B. Representative immunoblot analysis. Protein samples (100 µg/lane) resolved on SDS-PAGE were probed with corresponding antibodies. GAPDH was used as loading control for cytosol and whole tissue homogenates. Histone H2B was used as loading control for nuclear proteins. C. Densitometric analysis. The protein expression from control lysates for three determinations was designated as 100% in the graph. Each bar represents the protein expression of three determinations. $^{\clubsuit}$p<0.05 versus control. *p<0.05 versus DMBA. D. Levels of pVEGFR2^{tyr1175} (ELISA). E. Representative photomicrographs of immunohistochemical staining of VEGF in control and experimental animals (20X).

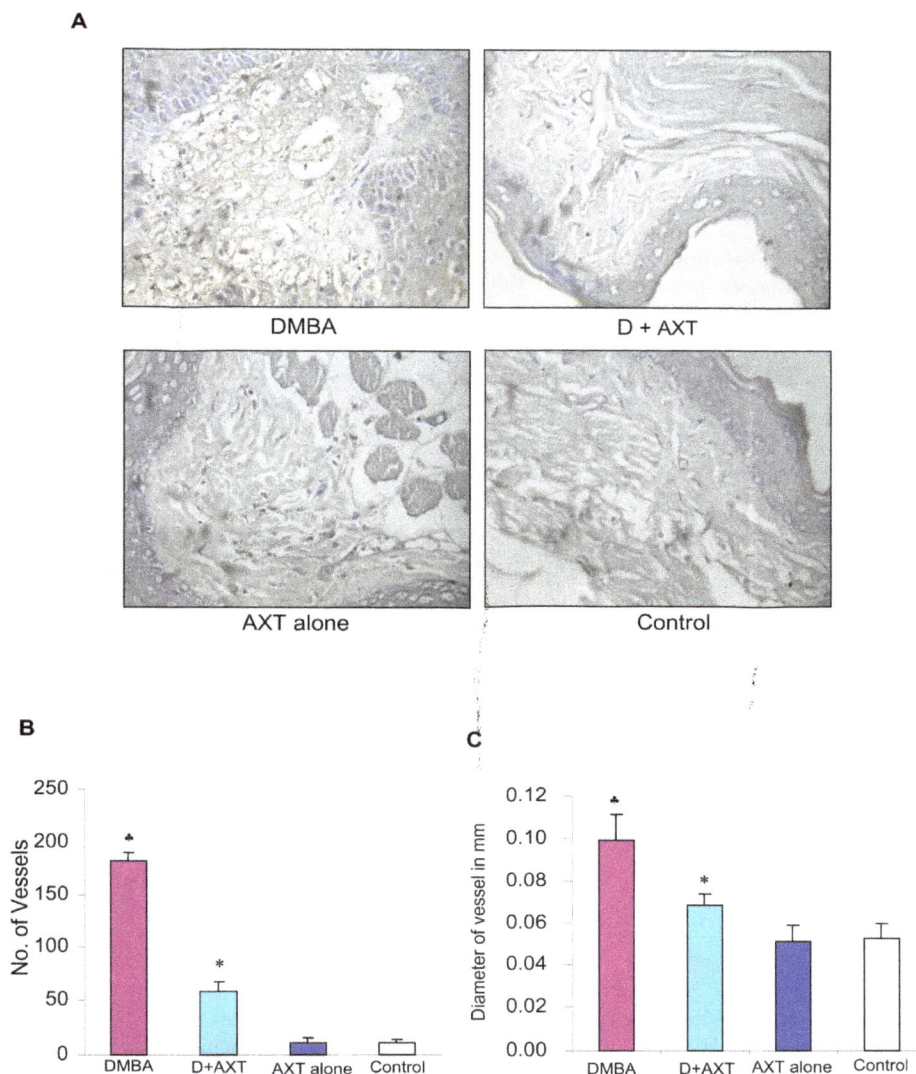

Figure 5. Effect of astaxanthin on microvascular density. A. Representative photomicrographs of microvascular density in control and experimental animals (40X). B. Bar graph representing number of vessels for minimum of three independent experiments. $^{\star}p < 0.05$ versus control. $^{*}p < 0.05$ versus DMBA. C. Bar graph representing vessel length for minimum of three independent experiments. $^{\star}p < 0.05$ versus control. $p < 0.05$ versus DMBA.

Immunohistochemistry

Paraffin embedded tissue sections were deparaffinised, rehydrated and subjected to antigen retrieval and endogenous peroxidase blocking. Then the sections were incubated with pSTAT-3 rabbit monoclonal, PCNA, MMP-2 and VEGF rabbit polyclonal antibodies at room temperature for 3 h. The slides were washed with TBS and then incubated with biotin-labeled secondary antibody followed by streptavidin–biotin–peroxidase (Dako, Carprinteria, CA, USA) for 30 min each at room temperature. The immunoprecipitate was visualized by treating with 3,3′-diaminobenzidine and counterstaining with hematoxylin. The tissues were then photographed using an Inverted Fluorescent Microscope (Leica Microsystem Vertrieb GmbH, Wetzler, Germany) attached with digital camera DFC295.

Microvascular density (MVD)

Microvascular density was assessed by immunohistochemical staining with anti-CD34 antibody. The areas of highest neovascularization were located and the images captured in a minimum of five different fields. Microvessels were counted by two independent investigators and the data represented as number of vessels/field of view.

Molecular docking

Molecular docking was done using Schrodinger suite 2013. Astaxanthin was retrieved from PubChem (www.ncbi.nlm.nih.gov/pccompound) and proteins STAT-3 and VEGF was retrieved from the protein databank with PDB ID: 3CWG and 3V2A respectively. Receptor grid generation and ligand docking were performed by employing Glide Xp docking algorithm.

A

B

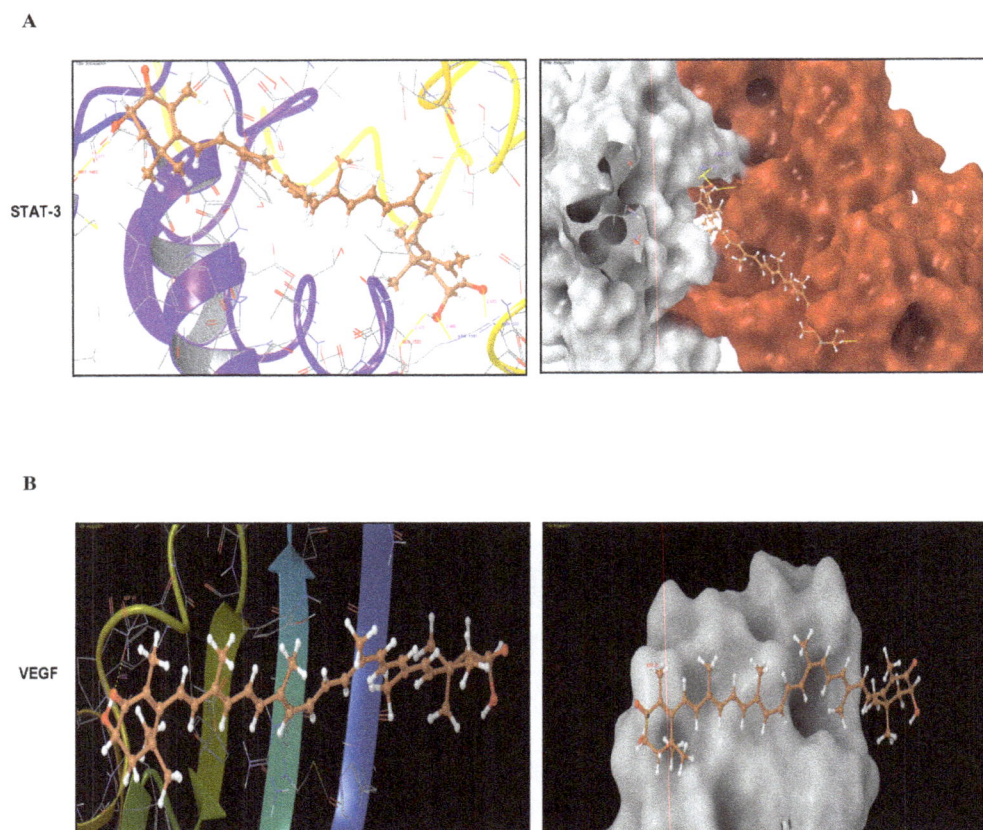

Figure 6. Molecular Docking. A. Represents AXT form hydrogen bond with Met 1428, Glu 1523, Arg 1593 and Asn 538 of STAT-3. B. Represents AXT form hydrogen bond with ASP 41 of VEGF.

Alamar blue assay

Cell viability was measured by Alamar Blue assay [27]. Briefly, Alamar blue (Resazurin sodium salt from Himedia) was dissolved in phosphate buffered saline pH 7.4 to make a stock of 5 mg/mL and a final working concentration of 0.1 mg/mL in cell culture medium. Resazurin is a redox indicator, which measures the reducing environment of the cell by reducing to a highly fluorescent resorufin. Astaxanthin at different concentrations (5, 10, 20, 50, 100, 200 and 400 µM) was added to the cells and after 24 h, Alamar blue dye was added and the plates were incubated at 37°C for 4 h. The color change was monitored colorimetrically at 595 nm and 570 nm to evaluate oxidized versus reduced forms respectively of the reagent by using multi-mode plate reader.

BrdU assay

Cell proliferation was analysed by measuring DNA synthesis with bromodeoxyuridine (BrdU) enzyme-linked immunosorbent assay (ELISA) kit (Cell Signaling Technology, USA), according to the manufacturer's instructions. Briefly, 1×10^4 cells were seeded into a 96-well microplate and cultured with or without astaxanthin (50 µM) for 24 h. The cells were then labelled with BrdU for 6 h. After fixation, the cells were incubated with 100 µl of anti-BrdU antibody for 60 min. After washing, 100 µl of secondary antibody was added and incubated for 30 min, then 100 µl of substrate (tetramethylbenzidine) was added to each well, and the plates were incubated at room temperature for 30 min. The absorbance at 450 nm was measured with an ELISA reader.

Migration assay

Confluent monolayers of ECV 304 cells in 24 well plates were scratched with a 200 µl pipette tip and incubated in normoxic and hypoxic condition with and without 50 µM astaxanthin. 5 mM hydroxyurea was also added to inhibit cell proliferation. Cells were photographed under a microscope at a magnification of 4x at 0 and 24 hours [28].

Matrigel tube formation assay

Pre-cooled 96 well plates were coated with 80 µl of matrigel (BD) and incubated at 37°C for half an hour. Equal number of cells (20,000/well) were added in each well with and without hypoxic condition and in presence and absence of astaxanthin (50 µM) and incubated in CO_2 incubator at 37°C for 14 hours. Images were captured in minimum five different fields and data represented finally as number of tubes/field of view [29].

Statistical analysis

Statistical analysis was carried out using a nonparametric Mann–Whitney test (Stats Direct, United Kingdom) for *in vivo* and Tukey posthoc test for *in vitro* experiments. A probability value of less than 0.05 was considered significant.

Results

Tumor incidence

The tumor incidence has been reported in an earlier study [20]. At the end of the experimental period the tumor incidence was

A

B

C

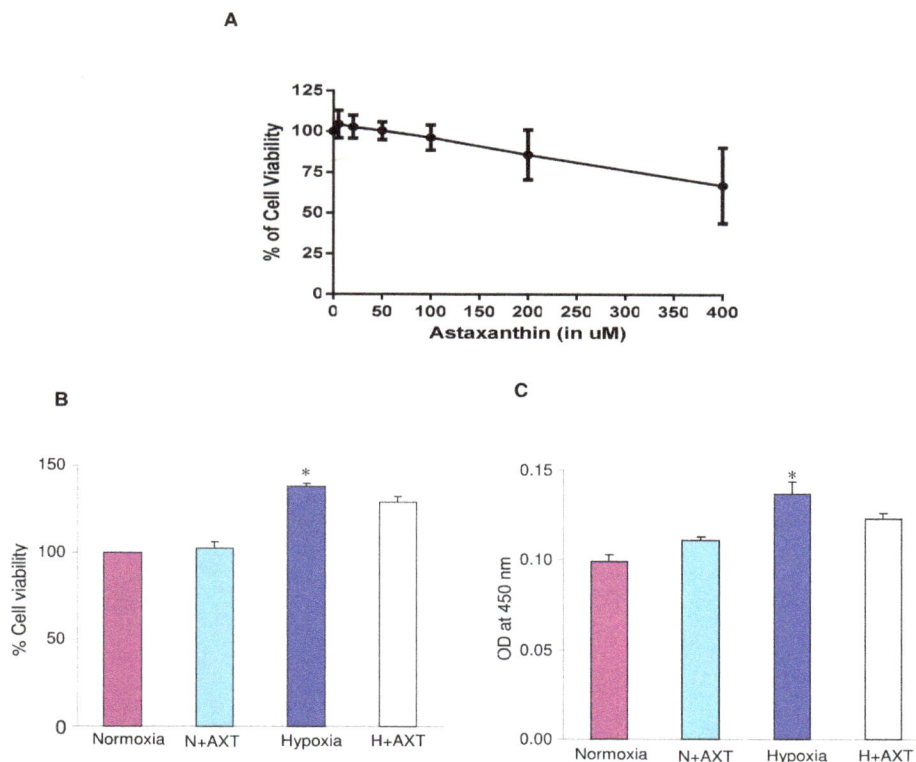

Figure 7. Effect of astaxanthin on cell viability and cell proliferation in ECV304 cells. A. IC_{50} value for astaxanthin on ECV304 cells (Alamar Blue assay). **B.** Effect of astaxanthin (50 μM) on hypoxia induced cell proliferation (Alamar blue assay). *$p < 0.05$ versus normoxia. **C.** Effect of astaxanthin (50 μM) on hypoxia induced cell proliferation (BrdU assay). *$p < 0.05$ versus normoxia.

100% with a mean tumor burden of 82.25 mm^3 in hamsters painted with DMBA (group 1). Dietary supplementation of astaxanthin (15 mg/kg bw) to DMBA painted hamsters did not induce any gross tumours in the buccal pouch and histological examination revealed only mild hyperplasia. In hamsters fed astaxanthin alone and in control groups, the epithelium was normal, intact, and continuous.

Astaxanthin inhibits JAK/STAT signaling by restraining the phosphorylation of STAT-3

As STAT 3 is constitutively activated in a wide range of malignancies, we first analyzed the mRNA expression of JAK-2 and STAT-3 by quantitative RT-PCR analysis. Our results revealed that dietary supplementation of astaxanthin significantly reduced the mRNA expression of key molecules involved In JAK/STAT signaling compared to DMBA-painted animals (Figure 1A). No significant differences were observed in animals treated with astaxanthin alone compared to control. Further to explore the mechanism by which astaxanthin regulates JAK/STAT signaling, we next determined the protein expression of IL-6, JAK-2, pJAK-2, STAT-3 and pSTAT-3 by western blotting. We found that topical application of DMBA significantly increased the expressions of these genes compared to control. Simultaneous dietary administration of astaxanthin inhibited JAK/STAT signaling by decreasing the levels of IL-6, JAK/STAT phosphorylated forms and subsequent translocation to the nucleus (Figure 1B & 1C). This was further confirmed by decreased level of pSTAT^{tyr705} (ELISA) in AXT treated group (Figure 1D). Immunohistochemical staining also confirmed that astaxanthin supplementation

resulted in significant decrease in the expression of pSTAT-3 compared to DMBA-painted animals (Figure 1E).

Astaxanthin impedes cell proliferation, invasion and angiogenesis via inhibiting JAK/STAT pathway

As STAT-3 activation regulates the transcription of genes involved in cell proliferation, invasion, and angiogenesis, we next investigated the effect of astaxanthin on markers of cell proliferation. Dietary supplementation of astaxanthin significantly reduced the mRNA and protein expression of cyclin D1 and PCNA. Furthermore, AXT increased nuclear p21 expression relative to the cytosolic fraction. In addition, AXT supplementation decreased total cyclin D1 level (ELISA) compared to DMBA group (figure 2). However, no statistically significant differences were noted between hamsters fed astaxanthin alone and the control group.

To determine whether inhibition of JAK/STAT pathway by astaxanthin impedes invasion, we next analyzed the expression of MMP-2, MMP-9 and their inhibitors. Dietary administration of astaxanthin significantly modulated the mRNA and protein expression of these molecules compared to group 1 animals. To further validate that astaxanthin regulates matrix metalloproteinases, we also examined protein expression of MMP-2 by immunohistochemical analysis. Our results revealed that astaxanthin administration markedly decreased the expression of MMP-2 compared to group 1 animals. On the other hand, no significant differences were observed in animals fed astaxanthin alone compared to control (figure 3).

As neovascularisation plays a major role in tumour growth and is one of the major downstream events triggered by the JAK/

A

Control   Control + AXT   Hypoxia   Hypoxia + AXT

B

C

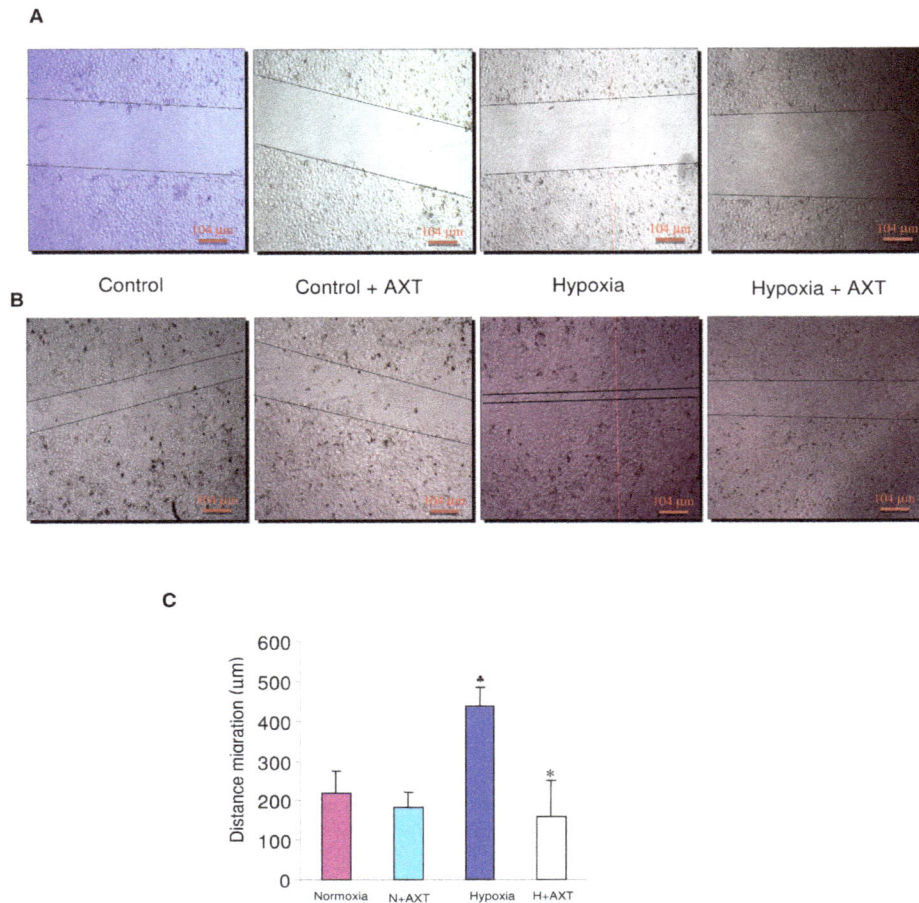

Figure 8. Effect of astaxanthin on the migration of ECV304 cells. A & B. Representative photomicrographs of migration assay in control and hypoxic ECV cells at 0 h and 24 h (4X). **C**. Bar graph representing distance migrated for minimum of three independent experiments. *p<0.05 versus normoxia. p<0.05 versus hypoxia.

STAT pathway, we investigated the effect of astaxanthin on angiogenesis. As shown in figure 4, dietary supplementation of astaxanthin significantly modulated the expression of VEGF, VEGFR2 and decreased HIF-1α nuclear translocation compared to DMBA-painted animals. Furthermore, AXT supplementation decreased the level of pVEGFR2 (ELISA). Immunohistochemical staining also confirmed decreased expression of VEGF in hamsters fed astaxanthin compared to DMBA-painted animals. No significant differences were observed in animals treated with astaxanthin alone compared to control.

As AXT decreased HIF-1α and VEGF expression, the key players involved in neovascularization, we next sought to determine whether inhibition of these molecules by AXT has any effect on vasculature by measuring the microvascular density. DMBA painted animals showed high vascularity with a mean MVD of 185 compared to control animals. Dietary supplementation of AXT significantly reduced the number of vessels compared to DMBA-painted animals, indicating the antiangiogenic potential of astaxanthin (figure 5).

To further confirm the inhibition of STAT-3 signaling and angiogenesis by astaxanthin, we performed molecular docking study for astaxanthin with STAT-3 and VEGF. AXT was found to bind with STAT-3 and VEGF with a docking score of −5.081 and −2.94 respectively. AXT interacts with the dimerization site of STAT-3 to form hydrogen bonds with Met 1482, Glu 1523, Arg

1593 and Asn 539 and interacts with VEGF through hydrogen bond with Asp 41 residue (Figure 6).

To test the antiangiogenic potential of astaxanthin *in vitro* we used ECV 304 cells. Angiogenesis is a complex process that involves cell proliferation, migration, and tube formation. First, we determined the concentration of astaxanthin at which it inhibits the viability of ECV cells by 50% (IC$_{50}$). We used varying concentrations of astaxanthin from 5 to 400 μM. We found that astaxanthin does not reduce the viability of ECV 304 cells to 50% at the concentrations tested. The viability of cells was 100% up to 50 μM of astaxanthin as shown in figure 7; therefore astaxanthin at 50 μM concentration was used for further experiments. To test whether astaxanthin inhibits proliferation of endothelial cells, we performed Alamar blue assay and BrdU assay. Hypoxia induced cell proliferation was not affected by astaxanthin as confirmed by both BrdU assay as well as Alamar blue assay (figure 7).

Migration of endothelial cells is one of the key steps in angiogenesis and metastasis; therefore we next determined the effect of astaxanthin on migration. Our results revealed that 50 μM astaxanthin significantly inhibited migration of endothelial cells. As shown in figure 8, hypoxic ECV cells migrated about 437 μm after 24 h; whereas AXT treated hypoxic cells migrated only about 192 μm, indicating the anti-migration potential of astaxanthin.

A

Control

Control + AXT

Hypoxia

Hypoxia + AXT

B

C

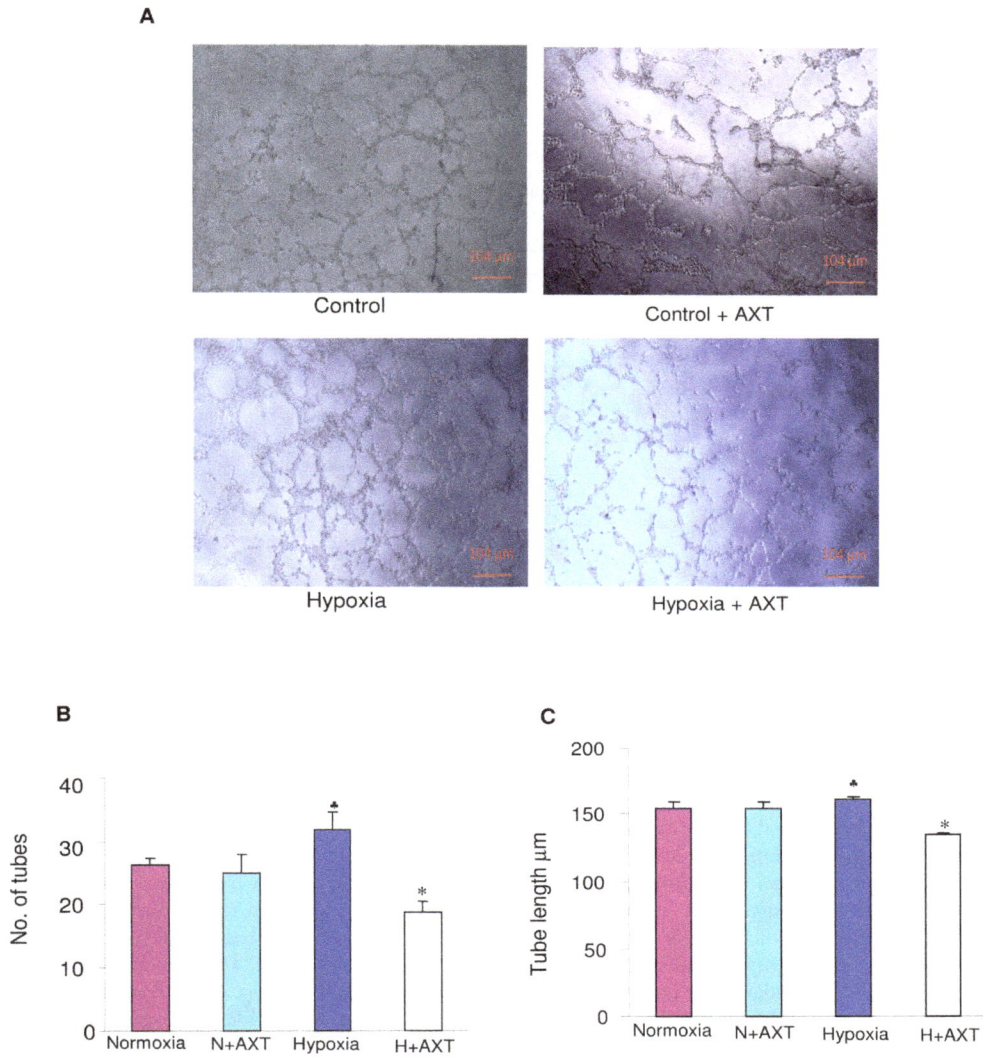

Figure 9. Effect of astaxanthin on tube formation in ECV304 cells. A. Representative photomicrographs of matrigel tube formation assay in control and hypoxic ECV cells (4X). B. Bar graph representing no. of tubes for minimum of three independent experiments. *p<0.05 versus normoxia. *p<0.05 versus hypoxia. C. Bar graph representing tube length for minimum of three independent experiments. *p<0.05 versus normoxia. *p<0.05 versus hypoxia.

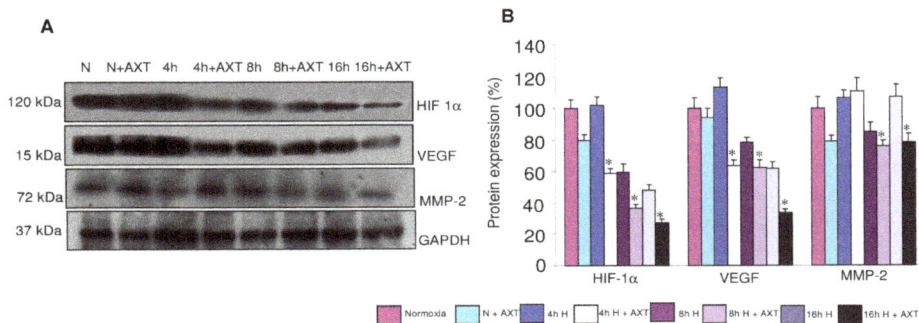

A

B

Figure 10. Effect of astaxanthin on the expression of HIF-1α, VEGF, and MMP-2 in normoxic and hypoxic ECV304 cells. A & B. Representative immunoblots and bar graph representing protein expression of HIF-1α, VEGF and MMP-2 for minimum of three independent experiments. *p<0.05 versus hypoxia.

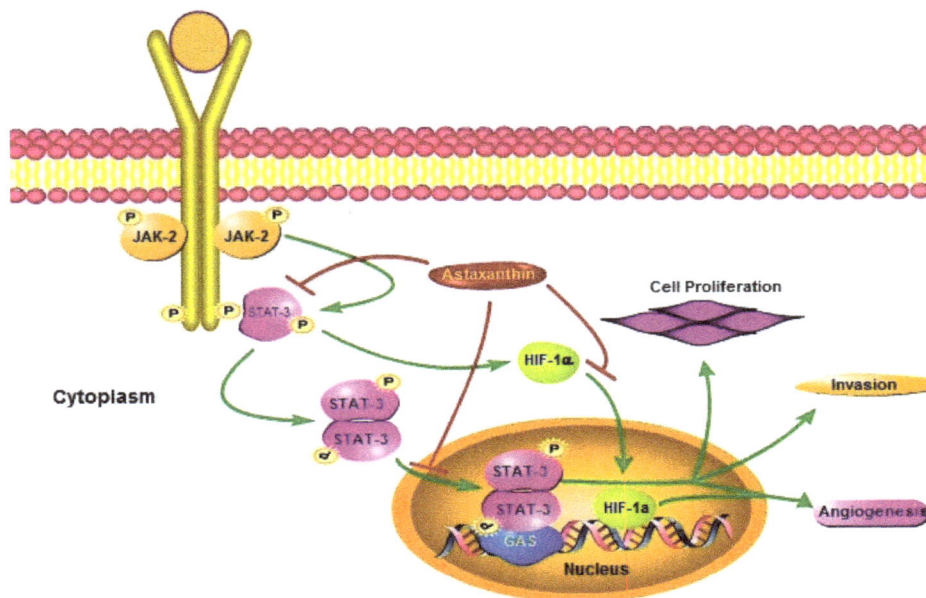

Figure 11. Schematic representation of the mechanism of action of astaxanthin in DMBA induced oral cancer. Dietary supplementation of astaxanthin abrogates DMBA induced oral cancer by targeting JAK/STAT-3 signaling. Astaxanthin prevents the phosphorylation and nuclear translocation of STAT-3 thereby prevents the transactivation of STAT-3 target genes which are involved in cell proliferation, invasion and angiogenesis. Furthermore astaxanthin also prevents nuclear translocation of HIF-1α, the master regulator of angiogenesis.

The principal step during angiogenesis is the formation and merging of tubes produced by endothelial cells forming a complex network of vessels, hence we next determined the effect of AXT on tube formation by performing matrigel tube formation assay. Under hypoxic condition, there was significant increase in the number of tubes formed as well as tube length compared to normoxic condition. Astaxanthin treatment significantly reduced the number of tubes and tube length under hypoxic condition. No significant differences were observed in cells treated with astaxanthin under normoxic condition (figure 9).

To know the mechanism by which AXT inhibits migration and tube formation of endothelial cells, we analyzed the expression of pro-angiogenic molecules in normoxic and 4 h, 8 h, and 16 h hypoxic ECV cells. Immunoblot analysis revealed an increase in HIF1α expression from 4 h that was sustained up to 8 h hypoxia. VEGF and MMP-2 expression increased from 8 h onwards and persisted till 16 h. Treatment with AXT reduced hypoxia-induced increase in the expression of these molecules (Figure 10).

Discussion

Several studies have documented that aberrant activation of the STAT-3 signaling pathway contributes to neoplastic transformation in various malignancies, and have validated STAT-3 as a promising target for cancer therapy [11,30,31]. The development of agents that target STAT-3 with adequate potency and tumour selectivity has proven to be a difficult task. Studies by others and us have indicated that phytochemicals are involved in cancer chemoprevention by modulating the signaling circuits aberrant in cancer [32–35]. In the present study, we demonstrate that astaxanthin inhibits the JAK/STAT-3 signaling pathway as well as its target genes in the HBP carcinoma model.

The functions of STAT-3 protein mainly depend on its phosphorylation and subcellular localization. In unstimulated cells, the STAT-3 proteins are present in the inactive form in the cytosol. Activation of STAT-3 occurs through phosphorylation of its tyrosine residue by cytokine or growth factor receptor signaling. Phosphorylated STAT-3 then dimerizes and translocates to the nucleus where it binds to IFN-gamma-activated site (GAS) in DNA and activates the transcription of target genes [12]. STAT-3 is found to be constitutively active in different carcinomas and inhibition of STAT-3 activation correlates with suppression of malignant cells both *in vitro* and *in vivo* [36,37]. The results of the present study provide evidence that astaxanthin supplementation abrogates constitutive activation of STAT-3 by preventing its phosphorylation and subsequent nuclear translocation. Furthermore, the interaction of AXT with the dimerization site of STAT-3 by molecular docking studies also validates the inhibition of STAT-3 by AXT. Astaxanthin was shown to inhibit rat hepatocellular carcinoma CBRH-7919 cells by modulating the JAK/STAT-3 signaling [38]. Taken together, these studies demonstrate that astaxanthin reduces the nuclear pool of STAT3, a key event in JAK/STAT-3 signaling.

Accumulating evidences have shown a positive correlation between the inhibition of STAT-3 signaling and suppression of tumor cell proliferation. Downregulation of the cell cycle regulatory proteins cyclin D1 and PCNA, biomarkers of the malignant phenotype and tumor progression with increased expression of p21 the most potent CDK inhibitor, underscore the antiproliferative effects of astaxanthin. These findings are substantiated by those of Zhang et al. [39] who demonstrated that astaxanthin inhibits cell proliferation in K562 cancer cells by modulating the expressions of cyclin D1 and p21. While targeting cyclin D1 can have far reaching implications in inhibiting cell proliferation, invasion, and angiogenesis, enforced nuclear localization of p21 seen in the present study can arrest the cell cycle by binding to PCNA [40,41].

Alterations in the levels and distribution of proteins involved in invasion have been documented in the HBP model [42]. Both STAT-3 and cyclin D1 are known to influence the expression of genes that promote migration and invasion [9,40]. Our results reveal that dietary astaxanthin significantly reduced the expression of matrix metalloproteinases (MMPs), MMP-2 and MMP-9, the crucial players involved in the degradation of the extracellular matrix and upregulated the expression of negative regulators of MMPs, TIMP-2 and RECK. In line with our findings, astaxanthin was shown to inhibit dimethylhydrazine induced rat colon carcinogenesis by modulating the expressions of MMPs, NF-κB and Erk [43].

Aberrant activation of STAT-3 signaling is also recognized to stimulate angiogenesis by activating VEGF, a pro-angiogenic molecule via direct binding with its promoter [44]. In the present study, abrogation of STAT-3 signaling by astaxanthin was found to be associated with downregulation of the key mediators of angiogenesis VEGF and VEGFR2. Interestingly, astaxanthin blocked nuclear translocation of HIF-1α, a master regulator of angiogenesis that transactivates several hypoxia responsive genes including VEGF and its receptors. The significant reduction in MVD in astaxanthin supplemented hamsters confirms its anti-angiogenic potential. Astaxanthin was also reported to inhibit the development of experimental choroidal neovascularization by modulating the expression of VEGF and VEGFR2 [45].

In tumours, hypoxia stimulates accumulation of HIF-1α by inhibiting proteasomal degradation which in turn stimulates angiogenesis by upregulating the expression of MMP-2 and VEGF [46,47]. Several phytochemicals have been reported to inhibit hypoxia induced angiogenesis by modulating the expression of pro-angiogenic molecules [48,49]. In the present study, astaxanthin inhibited hypoxia induced migration and tube formation of ECV 304 cells but did not significantly alter hypoxia induced cell proliferation. Immunoblotting analysis revealed that astaxanthin inhibited hypoxia induced angiogenesis by significantly decreasing the expression of HIF-1α, VEGF and MMP-2.

Inhibition of angiogenesis was further supported by molecular docking studies that showed interaction of AXT with VEGF.

Conclusion

In summary, the results of the present study provide substantial evidence that astaxanthin inhibits DMBA induced HBP carcinomas by attenuating JAK/STAT signaling (Figure 11). Astaxanthin appears to reduce the aberrant activation of STAT3 by various strategies including suppression of pSTAT3tyr705, blocking nuclear translocation of the active dimer and associated downstream signaling, and preventing transactivation of STAT3 target genes that play pivotal roles in cell proliferation, invasion, and angiogenesis. In addition, astaxanthin also inhibited endothelial cell migration and tube formation by modulating pro-angiogenic molecules. Our study supports the widely held tenet that inhibition of STAT-3 activation is an attractive strategy for modulating the expression of genes implicated in tumour development and progression. Dietary phytochemicals such as astaxanthin that function as potent inhibitors of JAK/STAT signaling are promising candidate agents for cancer chemoprevention and anticancer therapeutics.

Acknowledgments

The authors gratefully acknowledge the help of Dr. S. Mahalingam and K. Anbarasu, Indian Institute of Technology Madras, Chennai for help with the BrdU assay.

Author Contributions

Conceived and designed the experiments: SN MD JK ABB. Performed the experiments: JK ABB HG GDR. Analyzed the data: JK ABB HG GDR. Contributed reagents/materials/analysis tools: SN MD. Contributed to the writing of the manuscript: SN MD JK.

References

1. Yan S, Li Z, Thiele CJ (2013) Inhibition of STAT3 with orally active JAK inhibitor, AZD1480, decreases tumor growth in neuroblastoma and pediatric sarcomas In vitro and In vivo. Oncotarget 4: 433–445.

2. Matsui F, Meldrum KK (2012) The role of the Janus kinase family/signal transducer and activator of transcription signaling pathway in fibrotic renal disease. J Surg Res 178: 339–345.

3. Aparicio-Siegmund S, Sommer J, Monhasery N, Schwanbeck R, Keil E, et al. (2014) Inhibition of protein kinase II (CK2) prevents induced signal transducer and activator of transcription (STAT) 1/3 and constitutive STAT3 activation. Oncotarget 5: 2131–2148.

4. Bournazou E, Bromberg J (2013) Targeting the tumor microenvironment: JAK-STAT3 signaling. JAKSTAT 2: e23828.

5. Rajendran P, Li F, Shanmugam MK, Kannaiyan R, Goh JN, et al. (2012) Celastrol suppresses growth and induces apoptosis of human hepatocellular cancer through the modulation of STAT3/JAK2 signaling cascade in vitro and in vivo. Cancer Prev Res (Phila) 5: 631–643.

6. Silver-Morse L, Li WX (2013) JAK-STAT in heterochromatin and genome stability. JAKSTAT 2: e26090.

7. Samsonov A, Zenser N, Zhang F, Zhang H, Fetter J, et al. (2013) Tagging of genomic STAT3 and STAT1 with fluorescent proteins and insertion of a luciferase reporter in the cyclin D1 gene provides a modified A549 cell line to screen for selective STAT3 inhibitors. PLoS One 8: e68391.

8. Wang X, Crowe PJ, Goldstein D, Yang JL (2012) STAT3 inhibition, a novel approach to enhancing targeted therapy in human cancers (review). Int J Oncol 41: 1181–1191.

9. Subramaniam A, Shanmugam MK, Perumal E, Li F, Nachiappan A, et al. (2013) Potential role of signal transducer and activator of transcription (STAT) 3 signaling pathway in inflammation, survival, proliferation and invasion of hepatocellular carcinoma. Biochim Biophys Acta 1835: 46–60.

10. Gurbuz V, Konac E, Varol N, Yilmaz A, Gurocak S, et al. (2014) Effects of AG490 and S3I-201 on regulation of the JAK/STAT3 signaling pathway in relation to angiogenesis in TRAIL-resistant prostate cancer cells in vitro. Oncol Lett 7: 755–763.

11. Denley SM, Jamieson NB, McCall P, Oien KA, Morton JP, et al. (2013) Activation of the IL-6R/Jak/stat pathway is associated with a poor outcome in resected pancreatic ductal adenocarcinoma. J Gastrointest Surg 17: 887–898.

12. Trécul A, Morceau F, Dicato M (2012) Dietary compounds as potent inhibitors of the signal transducers and activators of transcription (STAT) 3 regulatory network. Genes Nutr 7: 111–125.

13. Zgheib A, Lamy S, Annabi B (2013) Epigallocatechin gallate targeting of membrane type 1 matrix metalloproteinase-mediated Src and Janus kinase/signal transducers and activators of transcription 3 signaling inhibits transcription of colony-stimulating factors 2 and 3 in mesenchymal stromal cells. J Biol Chem 288: 13378–13386.

14. Senggunprai z, Prawan A, Kukongviriyapan U (2014) Quercetin and EGCG Exhibit Chemopreventive effects in cholangiocarcinoma cells via suppression of JAK/STAT signaling pathway. Phytother Res 28: 841–848.

15. Yang CL, Liu YY, Ma YG, Xue YX, Liu DG, et al. (2012) Curcumin blocks small cell lung cancer cells migration, invasion, angiogenesis, cell cycle and neoplasia through Janus kinase-STAT3 signalling pathway. PLoS One 7: e37960.

16. Tanaka T, Shnimizu M, Moriwaki H (2012) Cancer chemoprevention by carotenoids. Molecules 17: 3202–3242.

17. Zhang J, Sun Z, Sun P, Chen T, Chen F (2014) Microalgal carotenoids: beneficial effects and potential in human health. Food Funct 5: 413–425.

18. Wang M, Zhang J, Song X, Liu W, Zhang L, et al. (2013) Astaxanthin ameliorates lung fibrosis in vivo and in vitro by preventing transdifferentiation, inhibiting proliferation, and promoting apoptosis of activated cells. Food Chem Toxicol 56: 450–458.

19. Maoka T, Tokuda H, Suzuki N, Kato H, Etoh H (2012) Anti-oxidative, anti-tumor-promoting, and anti-carcinogensis activities of nitroastaxanthin and nitrolutein, the reaction products of astaxanthin and lutein with peroxynitrite. Mar Drugs 10: 1391–1399.

20. Kavitha K, Kowshik J, Kishore TK, Baba AB, Nagini S (2013) Astaxanthin inhibits NF-κB and Wnt/β-catenin signaling pathways via inactivation of Erk/MAPK and PI3 K/Akt to induce intrinsic apoptosis in a hamster model of oral cancer. Biochim Biophys Acta 1830: 4433–4444.

21. Shklar G (1999) Development of experimental oral carcinogenesis and its impact on current oral cancer research. J Dent Res 78: 1768–1772.

22. Prabhu PN, Ashok Kumar P, Sudhandiran G (2009) Antioxidative and antiproliferative effects of astaxanthin during the initiation stages of 1,2-dimethyl hydrazine-induced experimental colon carcinogenesis. Fundam Clin Pharmacol 23: 225–234.

23. Takahashi K, Sawasaki Y, Hata J, Mukai K, Goto T (1990) Spontaneous transformation and immortalization of human endothelial cells. In Vitro Cell Dev Biol 26: 265–274.

24. Hughes SE (1996) Functional characterization of the spontaneously transformed human umbilical vein endothelial cell line ECV304: use in an in vitro model of angiogenesis. Exp Cell Res 225: 171–185.

25. Chomczynski P, Sacchi N (1987) Single-step method of RNA isolation by acid guanidinium thiocyanate-phenol-chloroform extraction. Anal Biochem 162: 156–159.

26. Legrand-Poels S, Schoonbrodt S, Piette J (2000) Regulation of interleukin-6 gene expression by pro-inflammatory cytokines in a colon cancer cell line. Biochem J 349: 765–773.

27. Ahmed SA, Gogal RM Jr, Walsh JE (1994) A new rapid and simple non-radioactive assay to monitor and determine the proliferation of lymphocytes: an alternative to [^{3}H]thymidine incorporation assay. J Immunol Methods 170: 211–224.

28. Liang CC, Park AY, Guan JL (2007) In vitro scratch assay: a convenient and inexpensive method for analysis of cell migration in vitro. Nat Protoc 2: 329–333.

29. Jeon KS, Na HJ, Kim YM, Kwon HJ (2005) Antiangiogenic activity of 4-O-methylgallic acid from Canavalia gladiata, a dietary legume. Biochem Biophys Res Commun 330: 1268–1274.

30. You Z, Xu D, Ji J, Guo W, Zhu W, et al. (2012) JAK/STAT signal pathway activation promotes progression and survival of human oesophageal squamous cell carcinoma. Clin Transl Oncol 14: 143–149.

31. Tu Y, Zhong Y, Fu J, Cao Y, Fu G, et al. (2011) Activation of JAK/STAT signal pathway predicts poor prognosis of patients with gliomas. Med Oncol 28: 15–23.

32. Bhatia D, Thoppil RJ, Mandal A, Samtani KA, Darvesh AS, et al. (2013) Pomegranate bioactive constituents suppress cell proliferation and induce apoptosis in an experimental model of hepatocellular carcinoma: Role of Wnt/β-catenin signaling pathway. Evid Based Complement Alternat Med 371813.

33. Wang D, Wise ML, Li F, Dey M (2012) Phytochemicals attenuating aberrant activation of β-catenin in cancer cells. PLos One 7: e50508.

34. Anitha P, Priyadarsini RV, Kavitha K, Thiyagarajan P, Nagini S (2013) Ellagic acid coordinately attenuates Wnt/β-catenin and NF-κB signaling pathways to induce intrinsic apoptosis in an animal model of oral oncogenesis. Eur J Nutr 52: 75–84.

35. Thiyagarajan P, Senthil Murugan R, Kavitha K, Anitha P, Prathiba D, et al. (2012) Dietary chlorophyllin inhibits the canonical NF-κB signaling pathway and induces intrinsic apoptosis in a hamster model of oral oncogenesis. Food Chem Toxicol 50: 867–876.

36. Darnell JE Jr (2002) Transcription factors as targets for cancer therapy. Nat Rev Cancer 2: 740–749.

37. Darnell JE (2005) Validating STAT3 in cancer therapy. Nat Med 11: 595–596.

38. Song XD, Zhang JJ, Wang MR, Liu WB, Lv CJ (2011) Astaxanthin induces mitochondria-mediated apoptosis in rat hepatocellular carcinoma CBRH-7919 cells. Biol Pharm Bull 34: 839–844.

39. Zhang X, Zhao WE, HU L, Zhao L, Huang J (2011) Carotenoids inhibit proliferation and regulate expression of peroxisome proliferation-activated receptor gamma (PPARγ) in K562 cancer cells. Arch Biochem Biophys 512: 96–106.

40. Elizabeth AM, Elizabeth C, Jane B, Andrew S, Robert LS (2011) Cyclin D as a therapeutic target in cancer. Nat Rev Cancer 11: 558–572.

41. Cmielova J, Rezacova M (2011) p21Cip1/Waf1 protein and its function based on a subcellular localization. J Cell Biochem 112: 3502–3506.

42. Harish Kumar G, Vidya Priyadarsini R, Vinothini G, Vidjaya Letchoumy P, Nagini S (2010) The neem limonoids azadirachtin and nimbolide inhibit cell proliferation and induce apoptosis in an animal model of oral oncogenesis. Invest New Drugs 28: 392–401.

43. Nagendraprabhu P, Sudhandiran G (2011) Astaxanthin inhibits tumor invasion by decreasing extracellular matrix production and induces apoptosis in experimental rat colon carcinogenesis by modulating the expressions of ERK-2, NFkB and COX-2. Invest New Drugs 29: 207–224.

44. Wei D, Le X, Zheng L, Wang L, Frey JA, et al. (2003) Stat3 activation regulates the expression of vascular endothelial growth factor and human pancreatic cancer angiogenesis and metastasis. Oncogene 22: 319–329.

45. Izumi-Nagai K, Nagai N, Ohgami K, Satofuka S, Ozawa Y, et al. (2008) Inhibition of choroidal neovascularization with an anti-inflammatory carotenoid astaxanthin. Invest Ophthalmol Vis Sci 49: 1679–1685.

46. Pugh CW, Ratcliffe PJ (2003) Regulation of angiogenesis by hypoxia: role of the HIF system. Nat Med 9: 677–684.

47. Ben-Yosef Y, Lahat N, Shapiro S, Bitterman H, Miller A (2002) Regulation of endothelial matrix metalloproteinase-2 by hypoxia/reoxygenation. Circ Res 90: 784–791.

48. Nagini S, Vidya Priyadarsini R, Veeravarmal V, Mishra R (2012) Chlorophyllin abrogates canonical Wnt/β-catenin signaling and angiogenesis to inhibit the development of DMBA-induced hamster cheek pouch carcinomas. Cell Oncol 35: 385–395.

49. Lamy S, Akla N, Ouanouki A, Lord-Dufour S, Béliveau R (2012) Diet-derived polyphenols inhibit angiogenesis by modulating the interleukin-6/STAT3 pathway. Exp Cell Res 318: 1586–1596.

8

In Vivo Evidence for Platelet-Induced Physiological Angiogenesis by a COX Driven Mechanism

Ian M. Packham[1], Steve P. Watson[1], Roy Bicknell[2], Stuart Egginton[1,3]*

1 Centre for Cardiovascular Sciences, School of Clinical and Experimental Medicine, College of Medical and Dental Sciences, University of Birmingham, Edgbaston, Birmingham, United Kingdom, 2 Centre for Cardiovascular Sciences, School of Immunity and Infection, College of Medical and Dental Sciences, University of Birmingham, Edgbaston, Birmingham, United Kingdom, 3 School of Biomedical Sciences, Faculty of Biological Sciences, University of Leeds, Leeds, United Kingdom

Abstract

We sought to determine a role for platelets in *in vivo* angiogenesis, quantified by changes in the capillary to fibre ratio (C:F) of mouse skeletal muscle, utilising two distinct forms of capillary growth to identify differential effects. Capillary sprouting was induced by muscle overload, and longitudinal splitting by chronic hyperaemia. Platelet depletion was achieved by anti-GPIbα antibody treatment. Sprouting induced a significant increase in C:F (1.42 ± 0.02 *vs.* contralateral 1.29 ± 0.02, $P<0.001$) that was abolished by platelet depletion, while the significant C:F increase caused by splitting (1.40 ± 0.03 *vs.* control 1.28 ± 0.03, $P<0.01$) was unaffected. Granulocyte/monocyte depletion showed this response was not immune-regulated. VEGF overexpression failed to rescue angiogenesis following platelet depletion, suggesting the mechanism is not simply reliant on growth factor release. Sprouting occurred normally following antibody-induced GPVI shedding, suggesting platelet activation *via* collagen is not involved. BrdU pulse-labelling showed no change in the proliferative potential of cells associated with capillaries after platelet depletion. Inhibition of platelet activation by acetylsalicylic acid abolished sprouting, but not splitting angiogenesis, paralleling the response to platelet depletion. We conclude that platelets differentially regulate mechanisms of angiogenesis *in vivo*, likely *via* COX signalling. Since endothelial proliferation is not impaired, we propose a link between COX1 and induction of endothelial migration.

Editor: Masuko Ushio-Fukai, University of Illinois at Chicago, United States of America

Funding: This work was funded by grant PG/08/018/24599 from the British Heart Foundation awarded to S.E., R.B., and S.W. The funders had no role in study design, data collection and analysis, decision to publish, or preparation of the manuscript.

Competing Interests: The authors have declared that no competing interests exist.

* Email: s.egginton@leeds.ac.uk

Introduction

At least two mechanisms of new vessel formation (angiogenesis) are now recognised, namely capillary sprouting and longitudinal splitting [1] (Figure 1A). Sprouting angiogenesis involves abluminal outgrowth, when mechanical deformation of capillaries stimulates endothelial cell (EC) activation and proliferation. Formation of filopodia and breakdown of the basement membrane results in expansion of the capillary bed under reduced fluid shear stress (FSS) [2]. Sprouting can be induced experimentally by extirpation of a skeletal muscle, leading to overload of the remaining synergists. In contrast, longitudinal splitting arises from sustained increases in blood flow, which stimulates formation of luminal lamellipodia that fuse, eventually dividing capillaries. Experimentally, splitting angiogenesis can be induced by administration of α_1-adrenoceptor antagonists, such as prazosin [3], causing vasodilatation to chronically elevate capillary FSS. Both forms of angiogenesis may be seen in various pathologies, apparently determined by the local shear environment [4], but possibly also by recruitment of endothelial mitosis that is markedly lower in neocapillary formation by splitting. There is no substantive difference between mouse and rat in the angiogenesis models utilised [4]. Although platelets are implicated as mediators of pathological angiogenesis, such as that driven by inflammation or tumour vascularisation [5], their contribution to non-repara-tive, physiological angiogenesis during tissue remodelling has not been studied.

Platelet involvement is thought to be due to: (i) release of growth factors or (ii) platelet-vessel interactions [5]. Platelets contain α-granules, dense granules, and lysosomes. The α-granule content includes both pro- and anti-angiogenic growth factors (including VEGF, FGF-2, PDGF, PF4, TSP-1 and endostatin) that are important regulators of some tumour growth [6,7]. Platelet releasate has been linked with *in* vitro and *in* vivo angiogenesis, involving neuropeptide Y and the angiopoietin pathway [8–10]. The mechanism of growth factor sequestration is unclear [11], but may involve endocytosis of circulating vascular endothelial growth factor (VEGF) or enhanced VEGF production by megakaryocytes (the platelet precursor cells). There has been an interest in non-haemostatic roles for platelets since the discovery that platelet depletion prevents growth of metastases [12]. Patients with cancers and inflammatory disorders that induce pathological angiogenesis demonstrate higher platelet levels of growth factors, including VEGF [13,14]. It is known that the higher VEGF levels parallels tumour progression, and platelets are activated in the circulation of such individuals [15]. Lyst^{bg} mice lacking dense granules and lysosomes demonstrate normal inflammatory angiogenesis [16], suggesting a role for α-granule release. Interestingly, pro-angiogenic and anti-angiogenic factors may be selectively released from platelets[17].

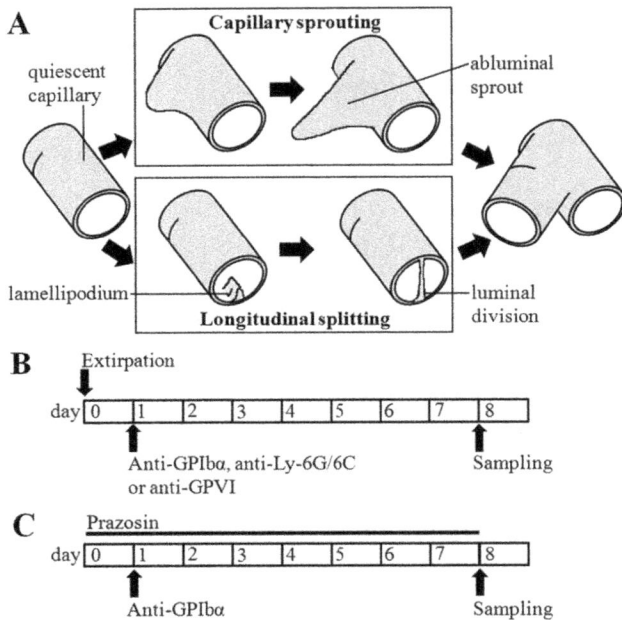

Figure 1. Different forms of angiogenesis and experimental protocols. A) Mechanisms of capillary sprouting and longitudinal splitting. B) Extirpation induced endothelial sprouting, with anti-GPIbα, anti-Ly6G/6C or anti-GPVI administration 24 h after surgery. C) Prazosin induced longitudinal splitting with anti-GPIbα. Sampling always occurred on the eighth day.

Evidence supporting the need for platelet adhesion includes unaffected *in vitro* endothelial tube formation in Matrigel by the addition of platelet secretate, which includes α-granule secretions, that is enhanced with the physical presence of platelets [18]. Also, platelet adhesion onto tumour endothelium is accompanied by VEGF release [19], and significantly more platelets have been observed adherent to angiogenic vessels compared to mature vasculature with intravital microscopy studies of dorsal skinfold chambers [20], supporting a role for platelet-vessel interactions. Whether platelets interact with endothelium or subendothelial structures remains unclear. While platelets bind subendothelial collagen after vessel injury during thrombosis, no evidence exists for a functional role of such interactions in physiological angiogenesis [21], nor for circulating platelet activation. Mice lacking GPVI, of central importance to direct platelet activation [22], demonstrate inflammatory angiogenesis in response to subcutaneous Matrigel implantation no differently from controls [16]. This suggests that intact collagen binding properties may not be required for angiogenesis to occur *in vivo*. Thus, platelet adhesion to endothelium may lead to angiogenesis as a result of releasate from activated platelets, but that secretion of pro-angiogenic factors may also occur without adhesion. For example, quiescent platelets may more effectively stimulate wound healing compared with activated platelets [23], possibly by enhancing fibroblast differentiation [24]. We therefore sought to identify a role for platelets using two *in vivo* models of physiological angiogenesis, sprouting and splitting forms of capillary growth [1] (Figure 1A), by examining the effect of platelet depletion by antibody treatment and pharmacological inhibition of platelet activation. We conclude that platelets differentially regulate mechanisms of angiogenesis *in vivo*.

Materials and Methods

In vivo experimentation

All procedures were performed in accordance with the UK Animals (Scientific Procedures) Act 1986, and approved by the University of Birmingham Biomedical Ethical Review Subcommittee. C57BL/6 (Charles River, Kent, UK), and MUC1-VEGF mice age and weight matched were used between 8–10 weeks of age (n = 4–9 per group). Weights did not differ between strains at 24.9 ± 0.3 and 23.0 ± 0.5 g respectively. Animals were housed at $21°C$ with 12:12 h light:dark cycle and *ad libitum* access to food and water. Longitudinal splitting angiogenesis was induced by 7 days oral *ad libitum* administration of 50 mg/L prazosin (Sigma, Poole, UK) a selective α_1-adrenoceptor antagonist, in drinking water [3]. Induction of endothelial sprouting was induced by muscle overload [2]. Unilateral extirpation of alternate *m. tibialis anterior* between animals causes hyperplasia and hypertrophy in the remaining *m. extensor digitorum longus* (EDL) since the muscles are synergistic. Sampling occurred on the eighth day after surgery. Surgery was performed by initially anaesthetising mice with 5% isoflurane (Novartis Animal Health UK Ltd., Hertfordshire, UK) in O_2 and sustaining anaesthesia with 2% isofluorane in O_2. Wounds of approximately 1.5 cm were sutured using 6-0 absorbable suture. Systemic analgesic (2.5 mL/kg buprenorphine, s.c.; Temgesic NVS, National Veterinary Services Ltd., Stoke-on-Trent, UK) and topical antibiotic (Duplocillin LA, NVS) were administered perioperatively. See Figure 1B-C for protocol, and [40] for representative data in mice.

Platelet depletion by antibody administration and pharmacological inhibition of platelet activation

Platelet depletion was achieved by single tail vein injection of 2 µg/g (4 µL/g) rat anti-mouse platelet glycoprotein Ibα (GPIbα) antibody (Emfret Analytics, Würzburg, Germany) or 4 µL/g 0.5% saline 24 h after overload or initiation of chronic vasodilatation [25], to permit coagulation of any bleeding during surgery. Antibody-induced platelet glycoprotein VI (GPVI) shedding was achieved by an identical regimen with rat anti-mouse GPVI antibody (Emfret) [26], dialysed to remove sodium azide preservative. Granulocytes/monocytes were depleted for 48 h with a single i.v. injection of 4 µg/g rat anti-mouse Ly6G/6C (Gr-1) antibody (BD Biosciences, Oxfordshire, UK) [27]. At 4, 24, and 48 h~10 µl of whole blood was collected in a container containing acid citrate dextrose anti-coagulant following tail-bleed. Whole blood smears were generated and stained with Diff-Quik solution (Dade Behring, Newark, USA). Smears were visualised for presence of cells with lobed nuclei (neutrophils). Untreated animals undergoing granulocyte/monocyte depletion underwent exsanguination to generate smears.

Pharmacological inhibition of platelets was initially achieved by 30 mg/kg clopidogrel hydrogensulfate plus 30 mg/kg acetylsalicylic acid (aspirin, ASA; both from Sigma) [28] or either compound alone were dissolved in drinking water and administered 24 h after overload/prazosin initiation for 72 h (Figure SI in File S1). A lower dose of 15 mg/kg ASA (LD-ASA) was administered similarly. Adequate inhibition of cyclooxygenase activity was demonstrated in dose-sighting experiments (Figure SII in File S1).

Tissue sampling for immunohistochemistry and VEGF protein quantification

Mice were killed by cervical dislocation. Muscles were immediately dissected and divided into two. One half was snap-frozen in liquid nitrogen for chemical analysis and the other in liquid nitrogen cooled isopentane (Sigma) mounted on 20 mm cork discs with OCT embedding matrix (both Raymond Lamb, Loughborough, UK) for sectioning. 10 μm sections for light microscopy were cut on a Bright Clinicut microtome at −20°C and mounted onto polysine™ slides (VWR International, Leuven, Belgium) and allowed to air dry. Samples were stored at −80°C and slides at −20°C.

For protein quantification, frozen tissue was powdered using a chilled pestle and mortar under liquid nitrogen, suspended in ice-cold lysis buffer (975 μl HEPES, 10 μl Protease Inhibitor Cocktail, 10 μl PMSF, 5 μl Na_3Va_4), and centrifuged at 5000 g for 20 min at 4°C. Samples were assayed in duplicate. Mouse and human VEGF protein (R&D Systems, Abingdon, UK), and PGF1α (Cambridge Biosciences, UK) was measured by enzyme linked immune sorbent assay (ELISA), according to manufacturer's instructions (5 animals/group). Total tissue protein concentration was determined by Bradford assay (using Bradford reagent, Sigma) performed in duplicate at the same time as the ELISA.

Immunohistochemistry

Slides were warmed to room temperature (RT) for 30 min and staining performed on EDL sections fixed with 4% w/v electron microscopy grade formaldehyde (TAAB, Berkshire, UK). Following 3×5 min PBS washes capillary/sarcolemma staining used 1:100 fluorescein *Griffonia simplicifolia* lectin-1 (Vector Laboratories Inc., Burlingame, CA): PBS for 1 h at RT in the dark was performed to permit quantification of capillary and fibre numbers (Figure 2C). Sections were washed in PBS and mounted on a coverslip with 1:10 Vectorshield plus DAPI: PBS (Vector Laboratories Inc.). Sections were examined at ×10 magnification. Four fields of view per section were analysed. *In vivo* platelet labelling with DyLight488-labelled GPIbβ (Emfret Analytics, Würzburg, Germany) was performed by i.v. injection of 0.1 μg/g body weight 10 min prior to tissue sampling (performed as described above). Sections were examined at ×40 magnification. Imaging was performed using a Zeiss Axioskop 2 plus fluorescent microscope and images captured using an Axiocam MRc digital camera and Axiovision software (Karl Zeiss, UK). Capillary and fibre numbers were determined by counts after data blinding.

BrdU pulse-labelling

The In Situ Cell Proliferation Kit, FLUOS (Roche, Mannheim, Germany) was used as per manufacturer's instructions. Briefly, animals were injected i.p. with bromo-deoxyuridine (BrdU) labelling reagent 16 h prior to tissue sampling. Immunostaining was also performed as instructed with the addition of 1:100 rhodamine *Griffonia simplicifolia* lectin-1 (Vector Laboratories Inc., Burlingame, CA) to allow co-localisation of BrdU-labelled cells with vascular structures. Slides were mounted using 1:10 Vectorshield plus DAPI: PBS to permit confirmation of nuclear localisation of BrdU-labelling.

Generation of platelet-rich plasma and platelet isolation

To generate washed platelets, whole blood was taken slowly into a syringe contained 100 μl anticoagulant acid citrate dextrose. Blood was transferred to 1.5 ml tubes containing 200 μl 30°C Tyrodes solution (130 mM NaCl, 0.34 mM Na_2HPO_4, 2.9 mM KCl, 12 mM $NaHCO_3$, 20 mM HEPES, 5 mM glucose, 1 mM $MgCl_2$) at pH7.3. The blood was mixed and microcentrifuged at 500 g for 5 min, producing platelet rich plasma (PRP). PRP and around one third erythrocytes was removed to a new 1.5 ml tube and centrifuged at 120 g for 6 min before removal of PRP to a third 1.5 ml tube. To prevent aggregation 1 μl 10 mg/ml prostacyclin was added to PRP before centrifugation at 1000 g

for 6 min. After supernatant removal, the platelet pellet was resuspended in 200 μl Tyrodes. Platelet numbers were determined with a Coulter counter (Beckman, High Wycombe, UK).

Flow cytometry

Whole blood was taken into a syringe containing acid citrate dextrose anticoagulant from the inferior vena cava under 2% isofluorane anaesthesia, which does not affect platelet function [29,30] to generate washed platelets before flow cytometry [31]. To determine GPVI expression following anti-GPVI administration 2 μl of FITC-conjugated antibody against GPVI (Emfret Analytics) was added to 100 μl of $1×10^6$ washed platelets resuspended in 30°C Tyrode's solution. Samples were rested for 30 min at RT in the dark. 200 μl PBS was added to stop the reaction, and samples analysed immediately.

Statistical Analysis

Data are presented as Mean±SEM. Statistical analysis used one-way ANOVA with Bonferroni post hoc analysis, * = $P<0.05$, ** = $P<0.01$, and *** = $P<0.001$ *vs.* untreated control or contralateral muscle as appropriate.

Results

Platelet depletion impairs angiogenesis by capillary sprouting but not longitudinal splitting

Administration of the anti-GPIbα antibody led to a rapid loss of circulating platelets in mice. At 24 h post injection, circulating platelet numbers dropped to <5% of normal values, as we and others have previously reported [25,31] (Table SI in File S1). Depletion was sustained for 48 h, with platelet numbers then rising to normal levels by 5 days post treatment (data not shown). Platelet depletion did not affect the capillary to fibre ratio (C:F) of untreated animals, a robust means of quantifying angiogenesis since capillary numbers increase while fibre numbers remain consistent within a given area [32] (Figure SIII in File S1).

The first form of angiogenesis we examined was capillary sprouting. Surgical ablation of *m. tibialis anterior* causes overload of the synergist *m. extensor digitorum longus* (EDL), stimulating endothelial filopodia formation by mechanotransduction of lateral strain [1]. This represents angiogenesis under reduced fluid shear stress (FSS) relative to prazosin-induced longitudinal splitting. The C:F increased by 11.7% at 7 days compared to contralateral muscles and muscles of untreated animals ($P<0.001$) (Figure 2A), consistent with our previous work [1]. Anti-GPIbα administration following induction of sprouting had no significant effect on the C:F of contralateral muscles, but prevented the increase in the C:F of ipsilateral muscles (n.s. *vs.* contralateral), indicating inhibition of sprouting angiogenesis.

Anti-GPIbα administration initiates an immune response by labelling platelets as foreign to the host, resulting in a rapid decrease in circulating leukocyte numbers during subsequent clearance of platelets, which had recovered by 24 h (Table SI in File S1). To confirm inhibition of sprouting angiogenesis resulted from *platelet* and not *leukocyte* depletion, we determined the effect of immune cell depletion alone. Administration of anti-Ly6G/6C causes depletion of granulocytes and monocytes lasting 48 h [27], but had no significant effect on platelet count (depleted $2.9×10^7$ *vs.* control $3.3×10^7$ platelets/ml total blood) or C:F (Figure 3) of otherwise untreated animals. Further, immune cell depletion did not alter sprouting angiogenesis, showing a similar rise in C:F as with untreated mice ($P<0.05$). These data indicate that the reduction in immune cell numbers resulting from platelet depletion did not contribute to the inhibition of angiogenesis.

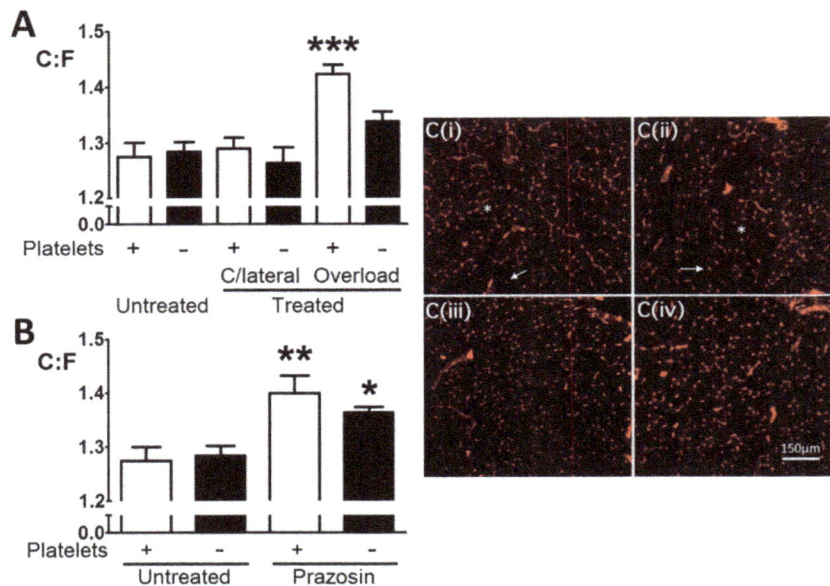

Figure 2. Platelet depletion differentially affects skeletal muscle angiogenesis. A) Capillary sprouting produced a significant capillary to fibre ratio (C:F) increase, abolished by platelet depletion following i.p. injection of anti-GPIbα(denoted by '-'). Depletion did not affect C:F of untreated or contralateral limbs. B) Longitudinal splitting caused a significant increase in C:F which was unaffected by platelet depletion. *$P<0.05$, **$P<0.01$, ***$P<0.001$ *vs.* untreated. C) Detail of representative images of lectin-stained mouse muscle cross-section showing fibres (asterisks) and capillaries (arrows) for extirpation with (i) or without (ii) platelets, and prazosin with (iii) or without (iv) platelets.

Angiogenesis induced by chronic vasodilatation leads to capillary growth through mechanotransduction of elevated FSS [3]. Induction of longitudinal splitting led to a 9.8% higher C:F in EDL after 7 days ($P<0.01$), in line with our previous work [1], with C:F also raised following platelet depletion ($P<0.05$; Figure 2B), suggesting the mechanism of longitudinal splitting angiogenesis is platelet-independent.

Activation of platelets *via* COX1 but not P2Y$_{12}$ is required to promote capillary sprouting angiogenesis

Having demonstrated that the induction of sprouting angiogenesis likely involves platelet mediation, we explored possible mechanisms by pharmacological inhibition of platelet activation. A combined regimen of clopidogrel hydrogensulfate with acetylsalicylic acid (ASA; aspirin) at varying concentrations is used clinically to inhibit platelet activation in order to limit thrombosis [33]. Clopidogrel antagonises the platelet specific P2Y$_{12}$ receptor. ASA irreversibly inhibits both cyclooxygenase (COX) 1 and 2, preventing thromboxane A2 (TXA$_2$) and prostacyclin (PGI$_2$) production, although platelets express COX1 alone. Dual clopidogrel/ASA treatment at doses of 30 mg/L for each drug blocked capillary sprouting angiogenesis (Figure 4A), supporting our findings with anti-GPIbα administration.

To clarify the underlying mechanism we induced sprouting angiogenesis with either clopidogrel or 30 mg/L ASA treatment alone. Clopidogrel treatment led to capillary sprouting (19.8% increase in C:F, $P<0.01$) similar to animals subjected to muscle overload without drug administration, suggests P2Y$_{12}$ signalling is not involved in sprouting angiogenesis. However, ASA markedly suppressed the angiogenic response to overload (Figure 4A), suggesting inhibition of TXA$_2$ or PGI$_2$ was responsible for the dual regimen inhibition of capillary sprouting.

A lower ASA dose (LD-ASA) was also investigated, as this is likely to generate a more platelet-specific response, which showed

similar results to the higher dose ASA (Figure 4A). LD-ASA inhibited sprouting angiogenesis ($P<0.05$), with no significant difference in the C:F observed ($P<0.05$). Quantification of the PGI$_2$ breakdown product PGF1α in plasma demonstrated a significant decrease in levels at day 7 ($P<0.05$) following LD-ASA treatment with overload (Figure 4C). We are therefore unable to distinguish between possible mediation of sprouting angiogenesis by TXA$_2$ or PGI$_2$, even at lower concentrations of ASA. In contrast to the anti-angiogenic effects, inhibition of platelet activation with ASA is dose-dependent (Figure SII in File S1).

We also inhibited COX-mediated platelet activation by ASA and LD-ASA from 24–96 h after initiation of longitudinal splitting, which demonstrated no effect with platelet depletion. ASA and LD-ASA treatment had no effect on the normal difference seen in the C:F ratio (both $P<0.05$; Figure 4B), paralleling the anti-GPIbα finding and adding further support to the hypothesis that platelets do not mediate longitudinal splitting. Induction of longitudinal splitting had no effect on plasma levels of PGF1α (Figure 4D), suggesting the chronic increase in FSS sustained PGI$_2$ levels but did not enhance them.

Increased muscle VEGF does not compensate for platelet depletion in sprouting angiogenesis

Previous reports suggest release of growth factors from secreted α-granules mediate pathological forms of sprouting angiogenesis [34]. VEGF is considered a key mediator of both pathological and physiological angiogenesis, and is contained within platelet α-granules [15]. Thus, inhibition of capillary sprouting by platelet depletion or inhibition could result from the absence or impairment of local VEGF delivery. To test this hypothesis, we determined whether tissue overexpression of VEGF compensated for loss of platelet VEGF after platelet depletion. We used a transgenic mouse line, MUC1-VEGF, expressing human VEGF$_{121}$ in addition to murine VEGF isoforms, resulting in

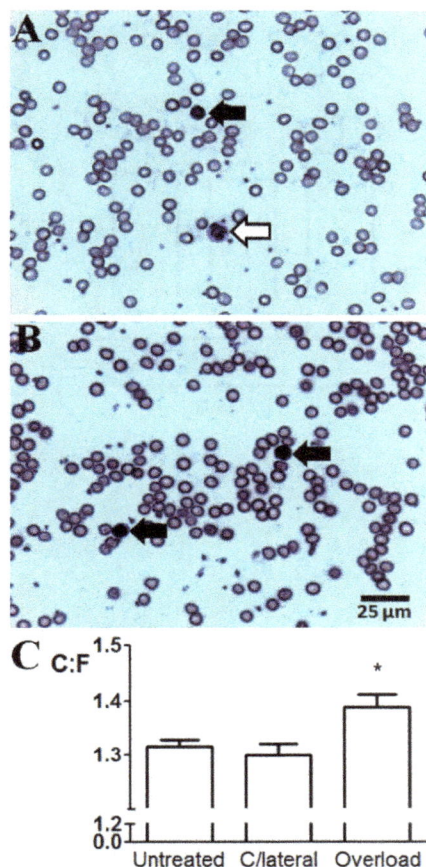

Figure 3. Granulocytes/monocytes do not mediate endothelial sprouting. A) Representative whole blood smears showing lymphocytes (black arrows) and granulocytes/monocytes (white arrow) were visualised in control animals. B) Following i.p. administration of anti-Ly6G/6C antibody only lymphocytes were readily visualised at 4, 24, and 48 h. C, Granulocyte/monocyte depletion did not alter the endothelial sprouting response normally observed ($P<0.01$).

significantly higher VEGF levels in all tissues examined [35]. Although contribution to tissue levels of VEGF by resident platelets is likely extremely low in the absence of adhesion, we determined platelet [VEGF]. Levels of the murine isoform were similar among strains, while human isoform expression was below ELISA detection limits (Table SII in File S1).

Compared to wildtype, MUC1-VEGF EDL muscles demonstrated ~50% higher overall (mouse + human) VEGF expression (Figure 5A). Untreated MUC1-VEGF mice had a higher C:F than wildtype animals ($P<0.05$), presumably resulting from chronic exposure to elevated VEGF. Following induction of sprouting angiogenesis, MUC1-VEGF mice increased the C:F ratio ($P<0.05$) compared to contralateral muscles to similar levels observed in wildtype animals (11.8% vs. 11.7% in wildtype mice). Further, platelet depletion by anti-GPIbα administration led to an inhibition of capillary sprouting comparable to that occurring in wildtype animals (Figure 5B). VEGF$_{121}$ overexpression is therefore unable to rescue sprouting angiogenesis following platelet depletion, indicating a more substantive role for platelets than α-granule secretion and local VEGF delivery.

Platelet mediation of capillary sprouting is independent of collagen-induced platelet activation

Since compensation for loss of platelet VEGF did not rescue sprouting angiogenesis we investigated whether platelet mediation required platelet-collagen interactions, as would occur during thrombosis, although no evidence has yet been found for collagen exposure during capillary sprouting [21]. *In vivo* platelet labelling at early (2 day) and later (7 day) stages of capillary growth confirmed that platelets can be observed within the vasculature (Figure 6), but were not localised to any specific element of the neovasculature. Indeed, we could identify no difference in platelet content of angiogenic loci between untreated and treated animals (data not shown). However, to exclude the requirement for activation following platelet-collagen interactions we induced sprouting angiogenesis followed by administration of an anti-GPVI antibody. The antibody caused shedding of about 70% GPVI as assessed by flow cytometry analysis at 7 days (Figure 7A). GPVI is of central importance to direct platelet activation by collagen, irrespective of FSS level [22], but shedding did not alter the extent of sprouting angiogenesis (C:F $P<0.05$ vs. contralateral control, Figure 7B). That loss of GPVI had no effect on capillary sprouting is consistent with the lack of an effect on pathological angiogenesis in GPVI knockout mice [16].

Platelet depletion has no effect on proliferation of capillary-associated cells in capillary sprouting

The total number of BrdU positive cells showed little increase following induction of muscle overload, although this reached statistical significance when induction of capillary sprouting followed platelet depletion ($P<0.05$) this still represented only ~3% of the total nuclei content (Figure 8A). We divided total BrdU counts into capillary-associated (endothelium, mural cells; Figure 8B), interstitial cells (e.g. fibroblasts; Figure 8C), or myocytes (Figure 8D) by co-localisation with rhodamine-linked isolectin B4. The increase in BrdU labelling after capillary sprouting resulted primarily from increased proliferation of interstitial cells at 7 days (Figure 8E). Numbers of proliferative capillary-associated cells were similar in sprouting angiogenesis with or without platelet depletion (Figure 8B). These data demonstrate that platelet depletion is not anti-angiogenic due to impaired EC proliferation, suggesting platelets may promote capillary sprouting *via* inhibition of another component of angiogenesis such as matrix proteolysis or EC migration.

Discussion

Platelets are normally regarded as effectors of haemostasis, but proteomic analyses suggest they may play a wider role in wound healing, tumour growth, inflammation and regeneration [36]. Our data show a differential role for platelets in mediating two distinct mechanisms of *in vivo* angiogenesis, namely capillary sprouting and longitudinal splitting. A failure to rescue platelet depletion by VEGF overexpression suggests the mechanism is more complex than α-granule secretion alone. It is difficult to directly assess platelet granule release *in vivo*, and monocyte-derived VEGF may play a role in some forms of angiogenesis [37], but these data are consistent with VEGF levels *per se* (irrespective of the source) not being responsible for angiogenesis ablation following platelet depletion. Maintenance of angiogenesis following loss of GPVI expression, although partial, indicates collagen-induced platelet activation is not the primary stimulus, while BrdU pulse-labelling suggests platelets do not affect endothelial cell (EC) proliferation.

Sprouting angiogenesis induced by muscle overload [2] causing elevated mechanical deformation of vessels and a resulting

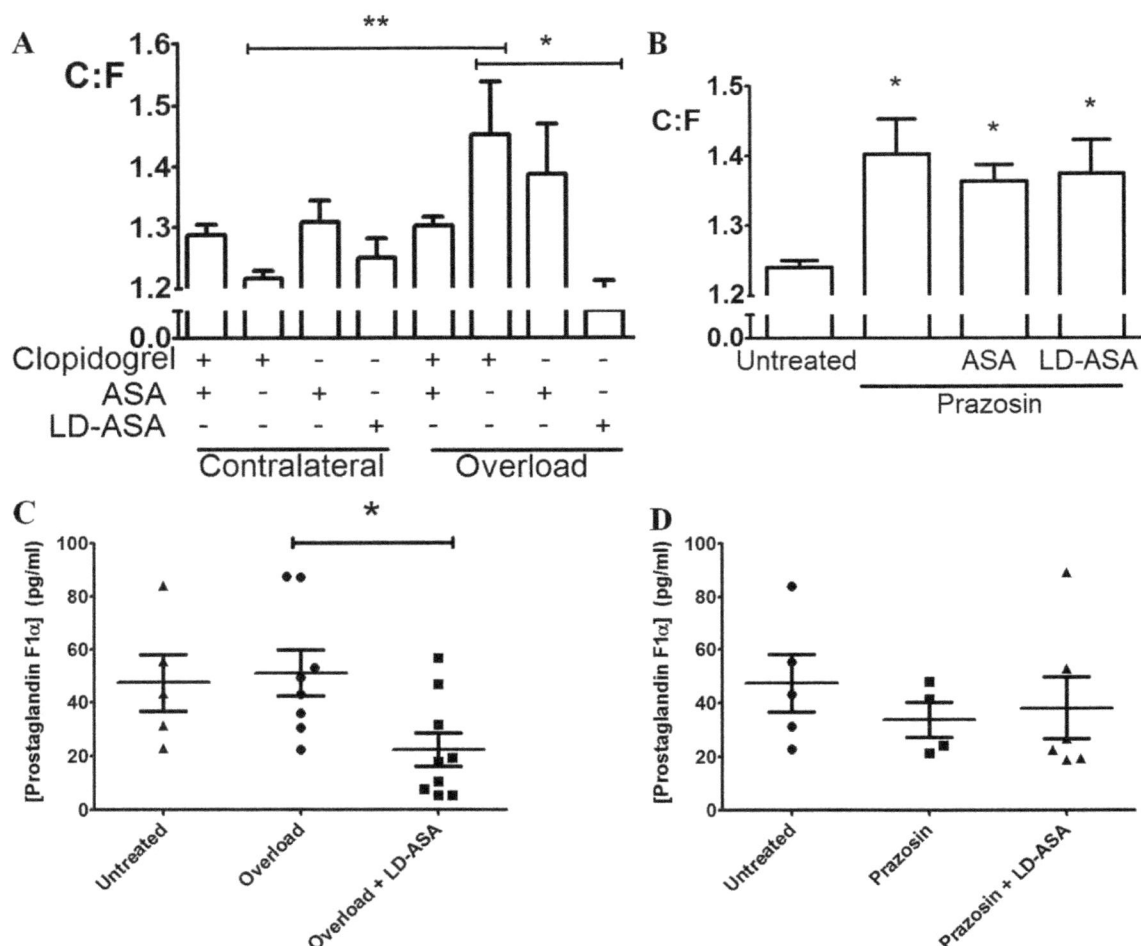

Figure 4. Platelets differentially affect angiogenesis *via* COX signalling. A) Dual clopidogrel/ASA regimen inhibited sprouting angiogenesis. Single regimens identified ASA as the active agent, with clopidogrel unable to alter the angiogenic response. B) Longitudinal splitting was unaffected by ASA or lower dose (LD)-ASA. C) PGF1α dropped significantly with overload + LD-ASA. D) Induction of longitudinal splitting did not alter PGF1α levels. *$P<0.05$, **$P<0.01$ between columns (A), or *vs.* untreated controls (B).

reduction in capillary FSS [1], was abolished by platelet depletion. In contrast, splitting angiogenesis is induced by elevated capillary FSS [3], and was unaffected by platelet depletion. Together, these data may suggest a shear-related response to platelet mediation of physiological angiogenesis. It is well known that higher FSS levels induce upregulation of vasoprotective genes in EC [38]. Indeed, while we observed significantly decreased levels of PGF1α with capillary sprouting there was no alteration in levels with longitudinal splitting. An alternative hypothesis is a difference in signalling between the angiogenic forms. For example, sprouting is dependent on matrix metalloprotease activity [39] while both forms require VEGF [40]. VEGF is found in both platelets and granulocytes, particularly neutrophils [41]. However, capillary sprouting was normal following granulocyte/monocyte depletion, demonstrating that despite the initial fall in immune cell numbers during platelet clearance after anti-GPIbα administration, it was depletion of platelets rather than immune cells that mediated angiogenesis.

Inhibition of capillary sprouting following treatment with a dual regimen of clopidogrel/ASA confirmed the platelet depletion result. ASA was identified as the active agent at both high and low dose regimens. The data are consistent with overload-induced

angiogenesis acting through COX signalling, and implicate COX inhibition of TXA$_2$ or PGI$_2$ synthesis as the anti-angiogenic target. Although ASA is not platelet specific, treatment may have a greater effect on platelets than EC depending on dose treatment regimen, since anucleate platelets are unable to initiate COX gene transcription. In addition, EC are primarily responsible for production of PGI$_2$, and platelets TXA$_2$, so that while PGI$_2$ levels are able to recover in this model, inhibition of TXA$_2$ is irreversible [42], suggesting that TXA$_2$ may be the target molecule. Our data suggests a graded response to different ASA doses with LD-ASA resulting in C:F similar to untreated animals, while ASA doses showed an increase. Further studies are required to fully define the *in* vivo mechanisms involved. Splitting angiogenesis was unaffected by ASA and LD-ASA treatment, confirming this form of angiogenesis does not require platelet mediation.

Having identified a role for platelets in physiologically-induced sprouting angiogenesis we sought to identify whether mediation required α-granule secretion alone or platelet-collagen interactions as with thrombosis. Animals lacking either platelet dense granules or lysosomes undergo angiogenesis in a manner unchanged from controls [16], suggesting α-granules are required for mediation of capillary sprouting. Studies into platelet mediation of pathological

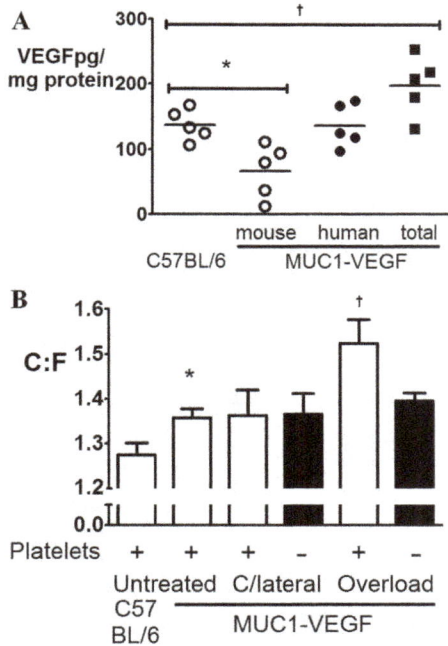

Figure 5. VEGF overexpression cannot rescue angiogenic deficit. A) Extensor digitorum longus muscle VEGF expression in wildtype and MUC1-VEGF mice. MUC1-VEGF human VEGF (●) plus mouse VEGF (○) resulted in a 45% increase in total content (■) vs. wildtype. B) MUC1-VEGF mice had higher initial C:F than wildtype. Capillary sprouting with or without platelets was no different from wildtype. *$P<0.05$ vs. C57 BL/6 controls, +$P<0.05$ vs. contralateral.

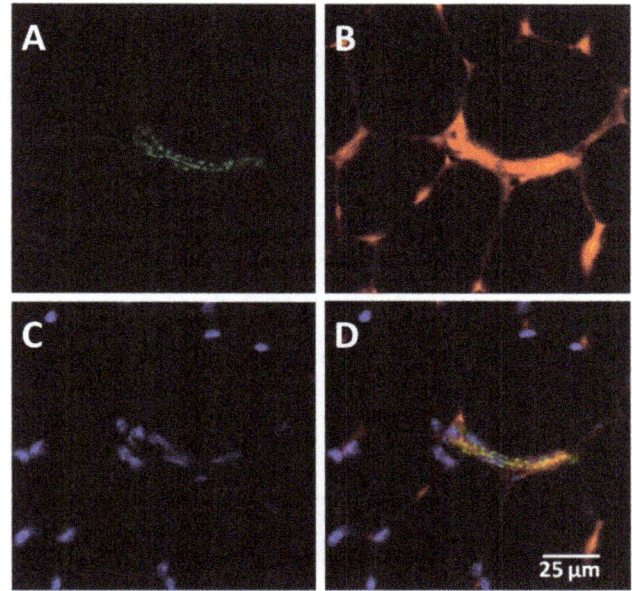

Figure 6. Platelets are observable in skeletal muscle vasculature. Platelets were labelled in vivo prior to muscle sampling. A) Imaging of muscle sections for the presence of platelets occurred under fluorescent microscopy in conjunction with B) rhodamine Griffonia simplicifolia lectin-1 staining for visualisation of vasculature, and C) DAPI for localisation of nuclei. D) A merged image of the three other panels depicts platelets within a venule, a potential locus for angiogenesis.

angiogenesis has concentrated on the role of VEGF, contained within α-granules [15] and widely seen as the most important growth factor to capillary growth. Indeed, endothelial sprouting is abolished without VEGF [40].

We reasoned that if α-granule content was responsible for mediation of capillary sprouting, compensating for the loss of platelet-derived VEGF after depletion may rescue the angiogenic response. We therefore induced sprouting angiogenesis in MUC1-VEGF transgenic mice, which have tissue VEGF levels 45% greater than wildtype mice due to expression of human $VEGF_{121}$ in addition to normal mouse isoforms. Although this overexpression was not detectable in platelets, levels of murine VEGF were similar to wildtype and hence we could detect any influence of altered tissue concentrations. In contrast to studies showing reliance of angiogenesis in VEGF, compensation of VEGF levels by overexpression did not rescue capillary sprouting, which was abolished in both wildtype and MUC1-VEGF mice with platelet depletion. Subsequent to submission of the original manuscript, intriguing in vitro data has suggested that platelet mediated angiogenesis is inhibited by ASA and may be independent of VEGF [43].

Capillary sprouting is therefore unlikely to be driven by release of VEGF from platelet α-granules, and so we tested the hypothesis that platelet-vessel interactions are responsible. During thrombosis, platelets become activated by exposed subendothelial collagen through GPVI. Mice with approximately 70% of GPVI shed demonstrated capillary sprouting in a similar manner to wildtype mice, suggesting collagen binding is not a significant mechanistic pathway during this form of angiogenesis. Indeed, we have previously identified no subendothelial exposure by electron micrograph analysis [21]. Our GPVI data is consistent with data

from GPVI knockout mice implanted with subcutaneous Matrigel to model inflammatory angiogenesis, [16], where no change was observed.

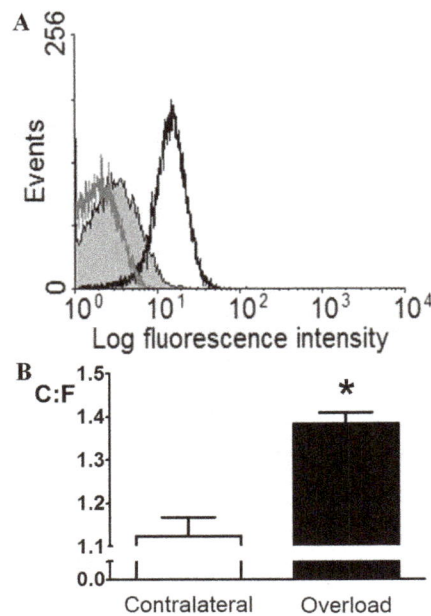

Figure 7. Angiogenesis is independent of collagen-induced platelet activation. A) Anti-GPVI resulted in ~70% GPVI shedding. Shaded grey peak, GPVI shed; clear black peak, control; clear grey peak, GPVI shed IgG expression. B) GPVI shedding did not alter capillary sprouting, with significantly increased C:F. *$P<0.05$ vs. contralateral.

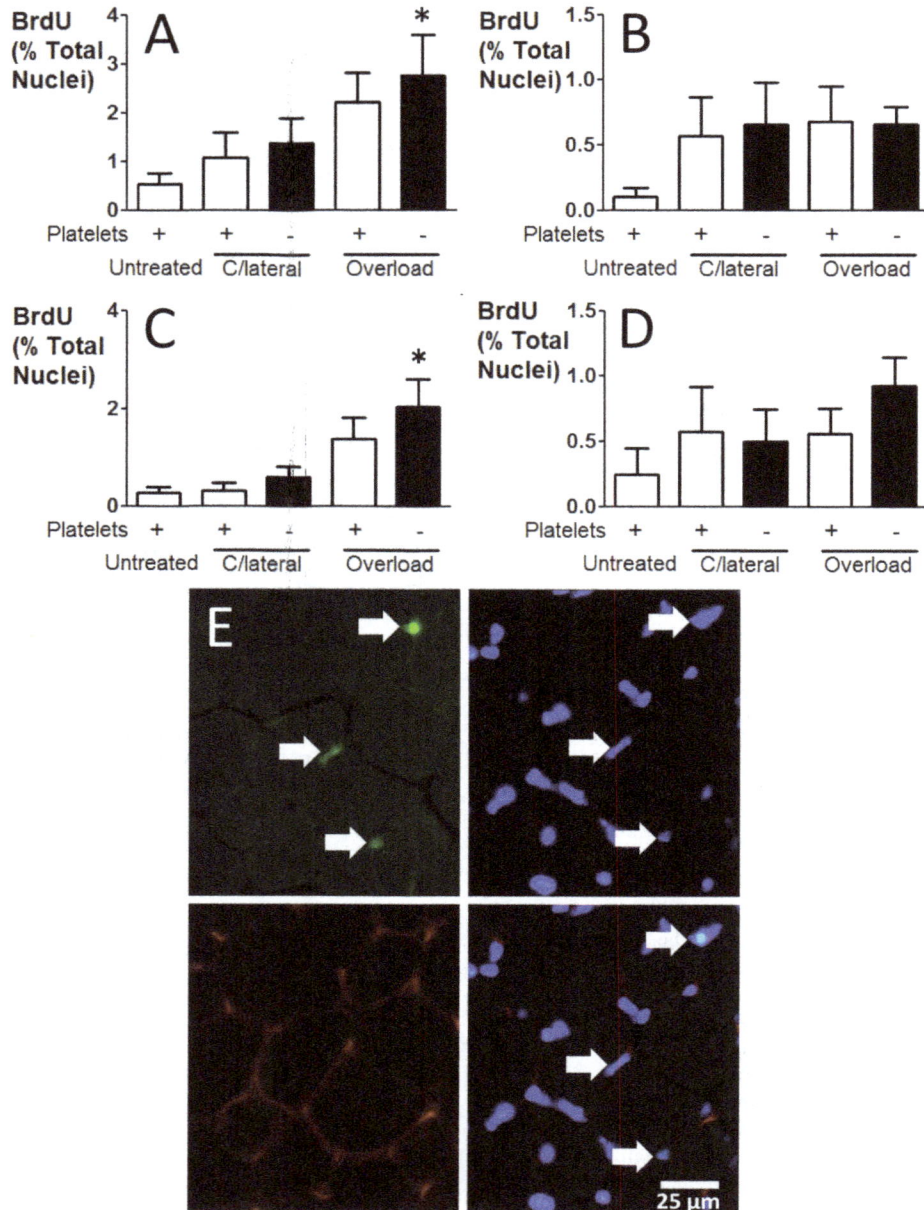

Figure 8. Platelet depletion did not affect proliferation of capillary-associated cells or myocytes. A) The total number of proliferating cells increased slightly in tissue after induction of capillary sprouting, but was not affected by platelet depletion. B) Capillary-associated cell proliferation was unaffected by platelet depletion. C) The increase in proliferating cell number with sprouting results from increased interstitial cell proliferation. D) The absence of platelets did not impair the proliferation of myocytes following muscle overload. E) BrdU labelling was performed in conjunction with rhodamine *Griffonia simplicifolia* lectin-1 staining (bottom left panel) for visualisation of vasculature, and DAPI (top right panel) to ensure BrdU staining observed was localised to nuclei. A merge (bottom right panel) of the three other panels with three BrdU-labelled interstitial cells (white arrows) is shown. Imaging was performed with fluorescent light microscopy as described in the methods at ×40 magnification. *$P < 0.05$ *vs.* contralateral.

Our data suggests a requirement for platelets at the initiation phase of the angiogenic response, since platelet depletion early on inhibits angiogenesis even 5 days after platelet numbers have normalised [25,31]. The increase in number of proliferating cells following induction of capillary sprouting remained after platelet depletion. Co-localisation analysis demonstrated that the labelling index of capillary-associated cells and myocytes remained unchanged after capillary sprouting with or without platelet depletion. The increase in BrdU-labelling was therefore a result of

increased proliferation of interstitial cells, and indicates that platelet depletion is not anti-angiogenic due to inhibition of EC proliferation. It is presumed, therefore, that platelets promote capillary sprouting *via* activation of another component of angiogenesis, such as endothelial migration and/or proteolytic modification of the extracellular matrix. In fact, inhibition of matrix metalloproteases required for extracellular matrix breakdown abolishes sprouting angiogenesis [39]. Additionally, it is conceivable that sphingosine-1-phosphate is required, since TXA_2

synthesis and thromboxane receptor activation mediate its release, while ASA inhibits its release [44].

In conclusion, using two distinct forms of capillary growth *in vivo* we have identified differential platelet mediation of physiological angiogenesis. Angiogenesis in high FSS environments is platelet independent, whereas angiogenesis under lower FSS is platelet mediated. Endothelial sprouting requires the presence of platelets, but not in delivery of pro-angiogenic growth factors released from α-granules alone, or platelet interactions with collagen. Platelet mediation did not result from alterations in proliferative potential of endothelium or perivascular cells, but platelet activation *via* COX is fundamental to sprouting angiogenesis.

Supporting Information

File S1 Table SI, Differential white cell count 24 h following platelet depletion ($\times 10^3.mm^{-3}$). Table SII, Platelets VEGF content is not altered by treatment (pg VEGF.10^{-6} platelets; mean±SEM). Figure SI, Experimental protocol for inhibition of platelet activation with clopidogrel and/or acetylsalicylic acid (ASA; aspirin). A) Endothelial sprouting was induced by extirpation of *m. tibialis anterior* causing overload of *m. extensor digitorum longus*. 24 h after surgery oral 30 mg/kg clopidogrel/ASA as dual or single regimens was administered for 72 h. B) ASA administration was begun 24 h after initiation of prazosin treatment, lasting 72 h. Prazosin induces longitudinal splitting. In both A and B, sampling occurred on the eighth day. **Figure SII, Inhibition of platelet activation with acetylsalicylic acid (ASA; aspirin) is dose-dependent.** Mice were administered aspirin *via* drinking water for 7 days. Experimental groups were 3 control mice, 3 low dose aspirin mice (30 mg/litre) and 3 high dose aspirin mice (300 mg/litre). Following 7 days aspirin treatment, blood was collected into sodium citrate and platelet-rich plasma (PRP) was prepared by centrifugation. Platelet aggregation was monitored by light transmission aggregometry in a Born lumi-aggregometer. Following stimulation with 0.5 mM arachidonic acid, platelets from the low dose aspirin treated mice aggregated normally (A) whereas platelets from the high dose aspirin treated mice showed only a minimal shape change response (B). Platelets from all mice aggregated normally to 500 mM PAR-4 peptide (C). **Figure SIII, Influence of scaling on muscle capillary supply.** In response to reviewer comments we offer an explanation for the choice of capillary to fibre ratio (C:F) as the most robust index of angiogenesis. It has been repeatedly been shown that other methods of quantifying angiogenesis (such as capillary density; Hudlická O, Brown MD, Egginton S. 1992. Angiogenesis in skeletal and cardiac muscle. Physiological Reviews 72: 369–417) have a bias due to alterations in fibre size often observed among experimental groups, that mask the changes in capillary number, whereas C:F is much less sensitive to these scaling effects (Egginton S. 1990. Morphometric analysis of tissue capillary supply. In: Boutilier RG (ed) Vertebrate Gas Exchange from Environment to Cell. Advances in Comparative and Environmental Physiology. 6: 73–141; Hudlická O, Brown MD, Egginton S. 1998. Angiogenesis: basic concepts and methodology. Chapt. 1, pp 3–19. In: Halliday A, Hunt BJ, Poston L, Schachter M (eds) An Introduction to Vascular Biology. CUP). The current experiment is no different: (1) contralateral muscle ± platelet depletion show minor, but reciprocal differences in CD and a(f). (2) extirpation without platelet depletion has a similar CD to contralateral muscle despite muscle hypertrophy that would be expected to reduce CD if angiogenesis had not occurred (C:F is significantly higher); in contrast extirpation with platelet depletion had both a similar CD and a(f) as contralateral muscles reflecting an absence of angiogenesis (C:F similar). (3) in the same way, relatively small differences in fibre size explain the modest difference in CD among prazosin groups, while the C:F is very similar (see Fig. 2 in the main text). Abbreviations: CD, capillary density; a(f), fibre cross-sectional area; C-, contralateral without platelet depletion; C+, contralateral with platelet depletion; E, extirpation; P, prazosin.

Acknowledgments

The authors wish to thank Alexandra Mazharian for assisting with the blood counts, as well as Marie Lordkipanidze and Craig Hughes for dose-sighting aspirin effects on platelet activity. This work was supported by the British Heart Foundation (BHF PG/08/018/24599).

Author Contributions

Conceived and designed the experiments: SE SW RB. Performed the experiments: IP SE. Analyzed the data: IP SE. Contributed reagents/materials/analysis tools: SW RB SE. Wrote the paper: IP SE SW RB.

References

1. Egginton S, Zhou AL, Brown MD, Hudlická O (2001) Unorthodox angiogenesis in skeletal muscle. Cardiovasc Res 49: 34–46.
2. Zhou AL, Egginton S, Brown MD, Hudlická O (1998) Capillary growth in overloaded, hypertrophic adult rat skeletal muscle: an ultrastructural study. Anat Rec 252: 49–63.
3. Zhou AL, Egginton S, Hudlická O Brown MD (1998) Internal division of capillaries in rat skeletal muscle in response to, chronic vasodilator treatment with alpha1-antagonist prazosin. Cell Tissue Res 293: 293–303.
4. Wragg JW, Durant S, McGettrick HM, Sample KM, Egginton S, et al. (2014) Shear stress regulated gene expression and angiogenesis in vascular endothelium. Microcirculation 21: 290–300.
5. Pinedo HM, Verheul HM, D'Amato RJ, Folkman J (1998) Involvement of platelets in tumour angiogenesis? Lancet 352: 1775–1777.
6. Wencel-Drake JD, Painter RG, Zimmerman TS, Ginsberg MH (1995) Ultrastructural localization of human platelet thrombospondin, fibrinogen, fibronectin, and von Willebrand factor in frozen thin section. Blood 65: 929–938.
7. Peterson JE, Zurakowski D, Italiano JE Jr, Michel LV, Connors S, et al. (2012) VEGF, PF4 and PDGF are elevated in platelets of colorectal cancer patients. Angiogenesis 15: 265–273.
8. Kakudo N, Morimoto N, Kushida S, Ogawa T, Kusumoto K (2014) Platelet-rich plasma releasate promotes angiogenesis in vitro and in vivo. Med Mol Morphol DOI: 10.1007/s00795-014-0083-y4

9. Tilan JU, Everhart LM, Abe K, Kuo-Bonde L, Chalothorn D, et al. (2013) Platelet neuropeptide Y is critical for ischemic revascularization in mice. FASEB J 27: 2244–2255.
10. Mammoto T, Jiang A, Jiang E, Mammoto A (2013) Platelet rich plasma extract promotes angiogenesis through the angiopoietin1-Tie2 pathway. Microvasc Res 89: 15–24.
11. Klement GL, Yip TT, Cassiola F, Kikuchi L, Cervi D, et al. (2009) Platelets actively sequester angiogenesis regulators. Blood 113: 2835–2842.
12. Gasic GJ, Gasic TB, Stewart CC (1968) Antimetastatic effects associated with platelet reduction. Proc Natl Acad Sci U S A 61: 46–52.
13. Adams J, Carder PJ, Downey S, Forbes MA, MacLennan K, et al. (2000) Vascular endothelial growth factor (VEGF) in breast cancer: comparison of plasma, serum, and tissue VEGF and microvessel density and effects of tamoxifen. Cancer Res 60: 2898–2905.
14. Solanilla A, Villeneuve J, Auguste P, Hugues M, Alioum A, et al. (2009) The transport of high amounts of vascular endothelial growth factor by blood platelets underlines their potential contribution in systemic sclerosis angiogenesis. Rheumatology (Oxford) 48: 1036–1044.
15. Salgado R, Benoy I, Bogers J, Weytjens R, Vermeulen P, et al. (2001) Platelets and vascular endothelial growth factor (VEGF): a morphological and functional study. Angiogenesis 4: 37–43.
16. Kisucka J, Butterfield CE, Duda DG, Eichenberger SC, Saffaripour S, et al. (2006) Platelets and platelet adhesion support angiogenesis while preventing excessive hemorrhage. Proc Natl Acad Sci U S A 103: 855–860.

17. Italiano JE Jr, Richardson JL, Patel-Hett S, Battinelli E, Zaslavsky A, et al. (2008) Angiogenesis is regulated by a novel mechanism: pro- and antiangiogenic proteins are organized into separate platelet alpha granules and differentially released. Blood 111: 1227–1233.

18. Pipili-Synetos E, Papadimitriou E, Maragoudakis ME (1998) Evidence that platelets promote tube formation by endothelial cells on matrigel. Br J Pharmacol 125: 1252–1257.

19. Salgado R, Vermeulen PB, Van Marck E, Benoy I, Dirix L (2001) Correspondence re: George ML, Eccles SA, Tutton MG, Abulafi AM, Swift RI (2000) Correlation of plasma and serum vascular endothelial growth factor levels with platelet count in colorectal cancer: clinical evidence of platelet scavenging? Clin. Cancer Res 6: 3147–3152. Clin Cancer Res 7: 1481–1483.

20. Manegold PC, Hutter J, Pahernik SA, Messmer K, Dellian M (2003) Platelet-endothelial interaction in tumor angiogenesis and microcirculation. Blood 101: 1970–1976.

21. Hansen-Smith FM, Hudlicka O, Egginton S (1996) In vivo angiogenesis in adult rat skeletal muscle: early changes in capillary network architecture and ultrastructure. Cell Tissue Res 286: 123–136.

22. Nieswandt B, Watson SP (2003) Platelet-collagen interaction: is GPVI the central receptor? Blood 102: 449–461.

23. Pietramaggiori G, Scherer SS, Mathews JC, Gennaoui T, Lancerotto L, et al. (2010) Quiescent platelets stimulate angiogenesis and diabetic wound repair. J Surg Res 160: 169–177.

24. Scherer SS, Tobalem M, Vigato E, Heit Y, Modarressi A (2012) Nonactivated versus thrombin-activated platelets on wound healing and fibroblast-to-myofibroblast differentiation in vivo and in vitro. Plast Reconstr Surg 129: p. 46e–54e.

25. Bergmeier W, Rackebrandt K, Schröder W, Zirngibl H, Nieswandt B (2000) Structural and functional characterization of the mouse von Willebrand factor receptor GPIb-IX with novel monoclonal antibodies. Blood 95: 886–893.

26. Massberg S, Gawaz M, Grüner S, Schulte V, Konrad I, et al. (2003) A crucial role of glycoprotein VI for platelet recruitment to the injured arterial wall in vivo. J Exp Med 197: 41–49.

27. Daley JM, Thomay AA, Connolly MD, Reichner JS, Albina JE (2008) Use of Ly6G-specific monoclonal antibody to deplete neutrophils in mice. J Leukoc Biol 83: 64–70.

28. Lorrain J, Lechaire I, Gauffeny C, Masson R, Roome N, et al. (2004) Effects of SanOrg123781A, a synthetic hexadecasaccharide, in a mouse model of electrically induced carotid artery injury: synergism with the antiplatelet agent clopidogrel. J Pharmacol Exp Ther 309: 235–240.

29. Hirakata H, Nakamura K, Sai S, Okuda H, Hatano Y, et al. (1997) Platelet aggregation is impaired during anaesthesia with sevoflurane but not with isoflurane. Can J Anaesth 44: 1157–1161.

30. Doğan IV, Ovali E, Eti Z, Yayci A, Göğüş FY (1999) The in vitro effects of isoflurane, sevoflurane, and propofol on platelet aggregation. Anesth Analg 88: 432–436.

31. Dhanjal TS, Pendaries C, Ross EA, Larson MK, Protty MB, et al. (2007) A novel role for PECAM-1 in megakaryocytokinesis and recovery of platelet counts in thrombocytopenic mice. Blood 109(10): 4237–4424.

32. Egginton S (1990) Numerical and areal density estimates of fibre type composition in a skeletal muscle (rat extensor digitorum longus). J Anat 168: 73–80.

33. Chen ZM, Jiang LX, Chen YP, Xie JX, Pan HC, et al. (2005) Addition of clopidogrel to aspirin in 45,852 patients with acute myocardial infarction: randomised placebo-controlled trial. Lancet 366(9497): 1607–1621.

34. Brill A, Elinav H, Varon D (2004) Differential role of platelet granular mediators in angiogenesis. Cardiovasc Res 63(2): 226–235.

35. Lui S (2004) Generation and characterisation of transgenic thymidine phosphorylase and vascular endothelial growth factor mice. DPhil, University of Oxford. pp. 408.

36. Gnatenko DV, Perrotta PL, Bahou WF (2006) Proteomic approaches to dissect platelet function: Half the story. Blood 108(13): 3983–3991.

37. Lopez-Holgado N, Alberca M, Sanchez-Guijo FM, Villaron EM, Rivas JV, et al. (2009) Prospective comparative analysis of the angiogenic capacity of monocytes and CD133+ cells in a murine model of hind limb ischemia. Cytotherapy 11(8): 1041–1051.

38. Chiu JJ, Chien S (2011) Effects of disturbed flow on vascular endothelium: pathophysiological basis and clinical perspectives. Physiol Rev 91(1): 327–387.

39. Haas TL, Milkiewicz M, Davis SJ, Zhou AL, Egginton S, et al. (2000) Matrix metalloproteinase activity is required for activity-induced angiogenesis in rat skeletal muscle. Am J Physiol Heart Circ Physiol 279(4): H1540–1547.

40. Williams JL, Cartland D, Rudge JS, Egginton S (2006) VEGF trap abolishes shear stress- and overload-dependent angiogenesis in skeletal muscle. Microcirculation 13(6): 499–509.

41. Kusumanto YH, Dam WA, Hospers GA, Meijer C, Mulder NH (2003) Platelets and granulocytes, in particular the neutrophils, form important compartments for circulating vascular endothelial growth factor. Angiogenesis 6(4): 283–287.

42. Masotti G, Galanti G, Poggesi L, Abbate R, Neri Serneri GG (1979) Differential inhibition of prostacyclin production and platelet aggregation by aspirin. Lancet 2(8154): 1213–1217.

43. Etulain J, Fondevila C, Negrotto S, Schattner M (2013) Platelet-mediated angiogenesis is independent of VEGF and fully inhibited by aspirin. Br J Pharmacol 170(2): 255–265.

44. Ulrych T, Böhm A, Polzin A, Daum G, Nüsing RM, et al. (2011) Release of sphingosine-1-phosphate from human platelets is dependent on thromboxane formation. J Thromb Haemost 9(4): 790–8.

9

Neem Leaf Glycoprotein Prophylaxis Transduces Immune Dependent Stop Signal for Tumor Angiogenic Switch within Tumor Microenvironment

Saptak Banerjee, Tithi Ghosh, Subhasis Barik, Arnab Das, Sarbari Ghosh, Avishek Bhuniya, Anamika Bose◕, Rathindranath Baral*◕

Department of Immunoregulation and Immunodiagnostics, Chittaranjan National Cancer Institute (CNCI), Kolkata, India

Abstract

We have reported that prophylactic as well as therapeutic administration of neem leaf glycoprotein (NLGP) induces significant restriction of solid tumor growth in mice. Here, we investigate whether the effect of such pretreatment (25µg/ mice; weekly, 4 times) benefits regulation of tumor angiogenesis, an obligate factor for tumor progression. We show that NLGP pretreatment results in vascular normalization in melanoma and carcinoma bearing mice along with downregulation of CD31, VEGF and VEGFR2. NLGP pretreatment facilitates profound infiltration of CD8[+] T cells within tumor parenchyma, which subsequently regulates VEGF-VEGFR2 signaling in CD31[+] vascular endothelial cells to prevent aberrant neovascularization. Pericyte stabilization, VEGF dependent inhibition of VEC proliferation and subsequent vascular normalization are also experienced. Studies in immune compromised mice confirmed that these vascular and intratumoral changes in angiogenic profile are dependent upon active adoptive immunity particularly those mediated by CD8[+] T cells. Accumulated evidences suggest that NLGP regulated immunomodulation is active in tumor growth restriction and normalization of tumor angiogenesis as well, thereby, signifying its clinical translation.

Editor: Rupesh Chaturvedi, Jawaharlal Nehru University, India

Funding: The work was partially supported by Council of Scientific and Industrial Research, New Delhi (grant no. 09/030(0050)/2008-EMR-I to S. Banerjee, grant no. 09/030(0063)/2011-EMRI to S. Barik and grant SRA, Scientists' Pool Scheme No: 8463A to A. Bose). The funders had no role in study design, data collection and analysis, decision to publish, or preparation of the manuscript.

Competing Interests: The authors have declared that no competing interests exist.

* Email: baralrathin@hotmail.com

◕ These authors contributed equally to this work.

Introduction

In 2000, Hanahan and Weinberg described angiogenesis as one of the most important hallmark criterion for cancer [1]. In spite of fundamental role of angiogenesis in fetal development and in many physiological conditions like wound healing [2,3] tumors exploit it to promote blood vessel growth and fuel a tumor's transition from benign to a malignant state [4,5]. Likewise, these malignant transformations need evasion from immune destruction, which has been included recently, in 2011, as another important hallmark of cancer growth [6]. Angiogenesis and immune evasion, these two apparently parallel cancer-intrinsic phenomenon actually possess bidirectional link and convergely promote malignant growth, metastasis and ultimately regulate therapeutic outcome [7]. In cancer, immune system can regulate angiogenesis with both pro- and anti-angiogenic activities [8,9]. Angiogenic molecules by differentially regulating immune system help in the development of sustained immunosuppressive mechanisms within tumor microenvironment (TME) [10,11]. This immunosuppressive mechanism may promote angiogenesis and tumor growth and inhibits infiltration and homing of activated immune cells within TME. Promoted angiogenesis then deregulates the proliferation and migration of vascular endothelial cells (VECs), thereby, causing neovascularization. These results in aberrant tumor vasculature associated with distorted and enlarged vessels, increased permeability, irregular blood flow and micro-hemorrhages [10,12,13]. Therefore, in recent years different works have shown that, for optimum immune-mediated tumor destruction, normalization of tumor vasculature is preferred over complete blockade of tumor angiogenesis [14].

Neem leaf glycoprotein (NLGP), a nontoxic immunomodulator reported previously have significant murine tumor growth restricting potential in prophylactic [15,16] as well as therapeutic [17,18] settings. NLGP facilitates anti-tumor activity by modulating both systemic and local immunity including: i) suppression of regulatory T cells [19], ii) activation of effector NK, NKT and T cells [20,21], iii) modulation of antigen presenting cells by maturating dendritic cells (DCs) towards DC1 phenotype [22,23] and macrophages [24], iv) regulation of cytokine-chemokine balance [25,26] and v) preventing anergy and exhaustion of effector T cells [17,18]. Recently in two consecutive studies, we have reported that therapeutic effectiveness of NLGP is associated with profound tumor infiltration of CD8[+] T cells [27] and normalization of tumor-immune-microenvironment [27,28].

Therefore, in the present study, we prophylactically applied NLGP in murine carcinoma and melanoma bearing mice to boost antitumor immune responses and subsequently analyzed the mode of NLGP counteraction on the tumor angiogenesis. We report that NLGP pretreatment associated immune-stimulation, particularly CD8[+] T cell activation, regulates the balance between pro- and anti-angiogenic molecules to induce vascular normalization without affecting normal physiological angiogenesis.

Results

NLGP prophylaxis prevents tumor angiogenesis and normalizes tumor vasculature

'Dormant' tumor requires both angiogenic switch and immune escape to proceed towards malignancy [7,9]. As prophylaxis with neem leaf preparation, precursor of NLGP, previously reported to be associated with significant immune-mediated tumor growth restriction [16,29], here, we intended to study how NLGP prophylaxis regulates pathological tumor angiogenesis. Consistent with our previous results prophylactic NLGP administration (4×) significantly restricts Ehrlich's carcinoma and B16 melanoma tumor growth (Figure 1a). Repeated investigations confirmed 4 immunizations with NLGP are required for optimum immune activation [15–18,27–29]. Angiogenic profiles were studied in mice after establishment of tumor (in between day 21 to 32) (Figure 1A.1 and A.2) and visual observations suggested a significant decrease in heavy, very thick, thick blood vessels, while thin blood vessels were retained substantially in NLGP pretreated carcinoma and melanoma tumor bearing mice group compared to PBS controls (Figure 1A.3). Additionally, histological analysis of tumor sections demonstrated less number of blood vessels with more regularized pattern in NLGP pretreated tumors than PBS mice. This regularized pattern of blood vessels is further evidenced by downregulation of CD31, a marker of VECs (Figure 1B). Correlating angiogenic profile with tumor volume revealed that normalized angiogenesis associated with NLGP prophylaxis represents restricted tumor growth, whereas, chaotic angiogenesis is correlated well with bigger tumor volume (Table 1; Figure 1C). Therefore, these data furnish evidences that NLGP can normalize tumor vasculature by decreasing only the thick and 'tortured' blood vessels while retaining the more compact thin blood vessels within tumor to maintain the optimum interstitial pressure and vaccine mediated immune benefits.

NLGP mediated vascular normalization is associated with down regulation of CD31, VEGF and VEGFR2

As VEGF-VEGFR2 signaling axis represents the key event in promoting tumor angiogenesis [30–32], expression of these molecules along with other pro-angiogenic molecules were next analyzed in NLGP pretreated carcinoma and melanoma bearing mice. Evidences obtained from RT-PCR (Figure 2A.1 and A.2)and Western Blot analyses demonstrated downregulation of VEGF, VEGFR2, CD31 in tumor from NLGP pretreated mice (Figure 2B.1 and B.2), in comparison to tumor obtained from PBS treated mice. Consistently, immunohistochemical analysis also revealed the significant decrease in expression level of VEGF and its receptor, VEGFR2, along with endothelial cell associated protein CD31 in harvested tumors with NLGP pre-therapy (Figure 2C.1). However, minimal decrease in VEGFR1 and NG2 level (Figure 2C.1 and C.2) was observed with similar treatment. Dual immunofluorescence staining of CD31 with NG2 (Figure 2C.3) indicated optimum and close pericyte coverage over VECs that may help in stabilization of blood vessels in NLGP treated mice group while, in PBS treated mice NG2[+] pericytes

were found detached from endothelial cells (Figure 2C.2), rendering the blood vessels thick, dilated and leaky. Therefore, obtained results clearly suggest that NLGP mediated alteration of pericytes' nature and/or that attachment along the vessel wall is intimately associated with observed vascular normalization within tumor.

NLGP mediated vascular normalization requires host's intact immune-system

Several recent studies have demonstrated that angiogenesis and suppressed cell-mediated immunity interdependently play central role in the pathogenesis of malignant disease facilitating tumor growth [33,34]. As NLGP prophylaxis reciprocally regulate tumor immune surveillance and angiogenesis to restrict murine tumor growth, next, we used two types of mice models (drug-induced immunosuppressive mice and immunocompromised athymic nude mice) to assess the immune involvement in NLGP mediated angiogenic modulation. As shown in (Figure 3A.1, A.2), mice were divided into three groups and two groups were injected with NLGP prophylactically, while one group was retained as control. Between these two NLGP pretreated mice groups, one group received immunosuppressant cyclosporine before EC tumor challenge as mentioned in 'Materials and Methods'. Analysis of their angiogenic profile revealed that NLGP pretreatment caused significant normalization of tumor vasculature than control group, as demonstrated in Figure 3A.1 However, in cyclosporine group, NLGP pretreatment failed to normalize angiogenesis, and so they showed prominent with prominent dilated and fragile blood vessels (Figure 3A.1, A.2-D.1, D.2). Observed results clearly indicated that NLGP modulates angiogenesis or vascular normal-ization by activating immune system.

Corroborately, in a separate set of experiments, tumor growth and associated angiogenesis were studied in three groups of NLGP-cyclosporin treated EC bearing mice. Two such groups of mice adoptively received non-adherent immune cells from either NLGP or PBS immunized normal mice (Figure 3A.3). Mice from all the 3 groups were sacrificed after tumor reached a considerable volume (1500 mm^3 to 2000 mm^3 approximately) and their angiogenic profiles were analyzed (Figure 3B.3–D.3). Enhanced angiogenesis related to the cyclosporine mediated immunosup-pression in NLGP pretreated mice was observed to be almost normalized due to adoptive transfer of splenic immune cells from NLGP treated mice (Figure 3B.3–D.3). These findings might further conclude that NLGP mediated normalization of angio-genesis is immune dependent.

To further validate the influence of NLGP-conditioned immune system to restrain tumor angiogenesis, immune-compromised athymic nude mice were pretreated with NLGP before tumor (EC) inoculation. However, NLGP pretreated nude mice failed to normalize tumor angiogenesis (Figure 3A.4–D.4) and adoptive transfer of syngenic non-adherent immune cells or isolated T cells of NLGP immunized normal mice showed tumor growth restriction and vascular normalization or inhibition in angiogenesis in comparison to PBS treated or only NLGP treated group (data not shown).

Tumors harvested from mice with different compromised immune systems with either pretreatment with NLGP or adoptive transfer of immune cells were analyzed for the expression status of VEGF, VEGFR2 and CD31, as we earlier found that NLGP downregulates the elevated expression levels of these molecules during tumor growth. Immunosuppression, either by means of cyclosporine treatment or in nude mice, abrogated the NLGP mediated downregulation of VEGF, VEGFR2 and CD31

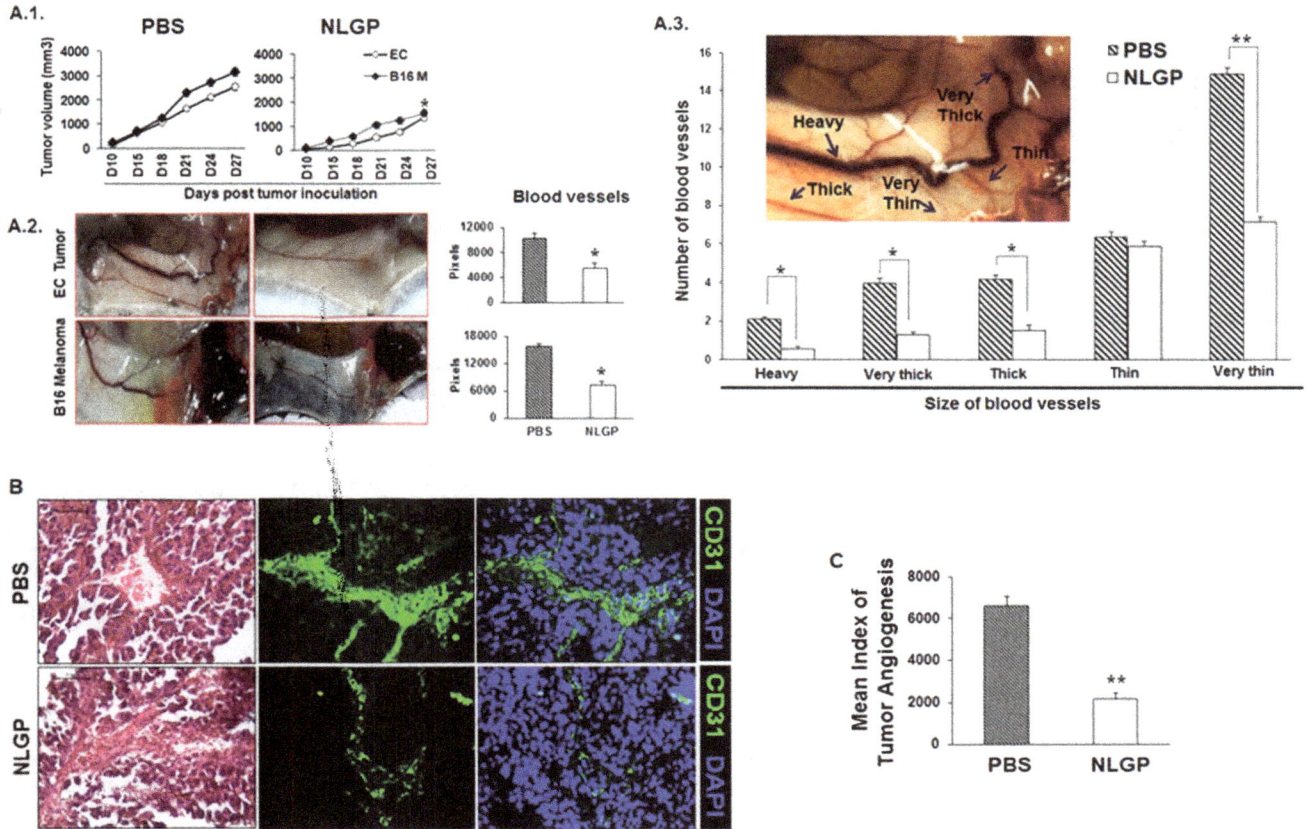

Figure 1. NLGP normalizes tumor vasculature. Swiss and C57BL/6 mice were pretreated with NLGP (25µg) once a week for four weeks in total followed by inoculation of EC (1×10^6 cells/mice) and B16 melanoma cells (2×10^5 cells/mice) subcutaneously. **A.1.** Tumor growth curve till day 27 is presented. *$p<0.01$. **A.2.** Mice were sacrificed and their angiogenic profile was studied and presented in photographs and bar diagrams (Mean±SD of pixel values). *$p<0.01$. **A.3.** Differentially dilated angiogenic vessels as shown in a representative figure (inset) were counted from NLGP and PBS treated mice and presented in bar diagram. *$p<0.05$; **$p<0.001$. **B.** Angiogenic blood vessels within tumors were studied by routine histology after H&E staining and CD31+ VECs were studied by immunofluorescence staining. Representative figures in each case are presented. **C.** Mean index of tumor angiogenesis is presented in bar diagram. **$p<0.001$.

Table 1. MITA* relating tumor volume and angiogenesis in NLGP pretreated mice.

PBS			NLGP		
Tumor Volume (in mm³)	Angiogenesis (in raw score)	Index for Tumor Angiogenesis	Tumor Volume (in mm³)	Angiogenesis (in raw score)	Index for Tumor Angiogenesis
220	+ (1)	220	126	+ (1)	126
600	++ (2)	1200	245	+ (1)	245
907	++ (2)	1814	665	++ (2)	1330
2025	++++ (4)	8100	1267	+++ (3)	3801
1152	+++ (3)	3456	445	+ (1)	445
3240	++++ (4)	12960	1568	++ (2)	3136
5292	++++ (4)	21168	1436	+++ (3)	4308
1352	+++ (3)	4056	1008	++ (2)	2016
Mean		**6622**			**1926**

*Mean index of tumor angiogenesis. Mean is presented in Figure 1C

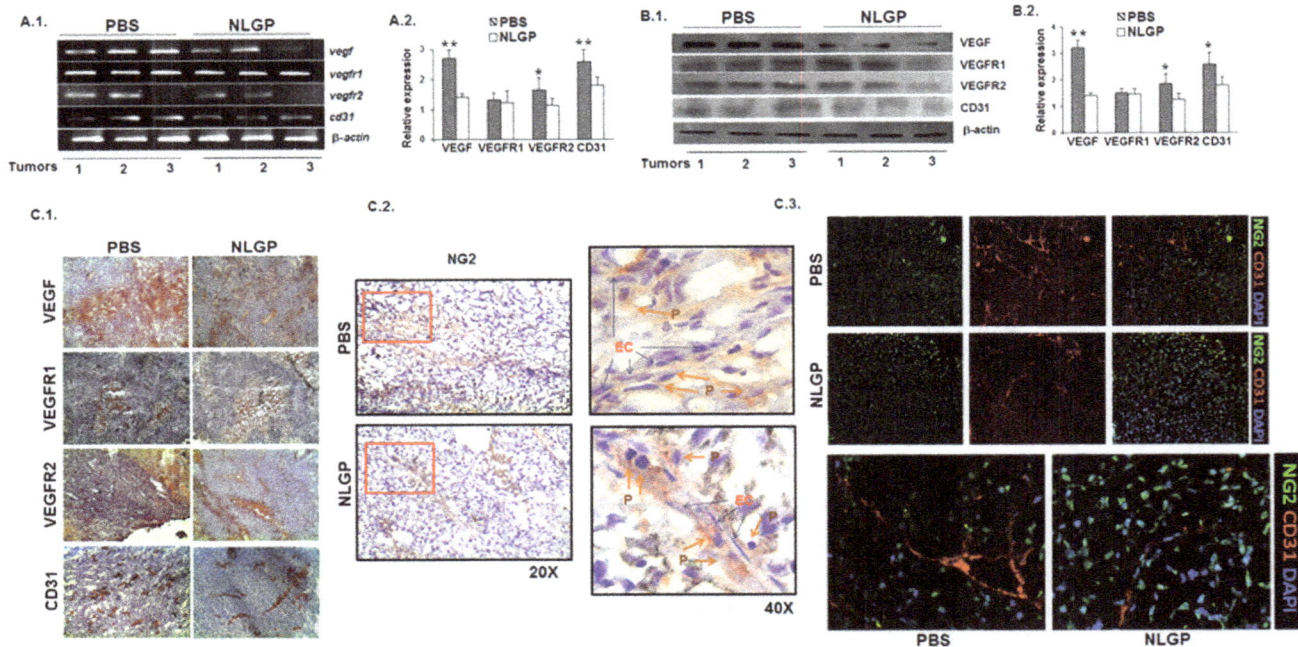

Figure 2. NLGP normalizes tumor microenvironment by downregulating expression of VEGF, VEGFR2 and CD31. B16 melanoma tumors (100 mm^3) harvested from either PBS or NLGP pretreated C57BL/6 mice representing tumor microenvironment were used for different analysis. **A.1.** Representative presentation of mRNA expression levels of *vegf, vegfr1, vegfr2, cd31* by RT-PCR analysis (n = 3). **A.2.** Densitometric analysis of three individual observations is presented with Mean ± SD. *$p < 0.05$; **$p < 0.01$. **B.1.** Another portion (100 mg) of tumors was lysed by freeze-thaw cycles in PBS used for Western Blotting to check the expression of various angiogenic proteins. Representative presentation of expression levels of different molecules as mentioned by Western blot analysis (n = 3) is shown. **B.2.** Densitometric analysis of three individual observations and Mean ± SD are presented. *$p < 0.05$; **$p < 0.01$. **C.1.** Immunohistochemistry with monoclonal antibodies, specific for VEGF, VEGFR1, VEGFR2 and CD31 and **C.2.** NG2 were detected on tumor sections. Arrows showed the pericyte coverage on endothelial cell lining on blood vessels. **D.** Fluorescence tagged monoclonal antibodies, specific for NG2$^+$ (green) and CD31$^+$ (Red) cells were used to study tumor vasculature. Nuclear staining was performed by DAPI.

(Figure 3E). Thus, NLGP may normalize angiogenesis by restricting availability of pro-angiogenic molecules.

CD8$^+$ T cells play vital role in NLGP mediated immune dependent vascular normalization

Since, above experiments clearly indicate that immune system has a regulatory role in NLGP driven normalization of tumor angiogenesis, next, we studied the histological sections from carcinoma and melanoma tumors of NLGP and PBS pretreated mice. Prominent infiltration of immune cells was noticed in tumors from NLGP pretreated mice (Figure 4A.1). Flow cytometric analysis of cells from PBMC of either PBS or NLGP treated tumor bearing mice revealed increased CD8$^+$ T cells in NLGP treated mice group (Figure 4A.2 and A.3). To validate the role of CD8$^+$ T cells (if any), such cells were depleted using specific antibody, as work plan is schematically presented in Figure 4B.1. CD8$^+$ T cell depletion was confirmed flow cytometrically (Figure 4B.2).

As we observed significant enhancement of CD8$^+$ T cells within tumors from NLGP pretreated mice, we wanted to decipher the contributing role of these effector cells in NLGP mediated normalization of angiogenesis by *in vivo* depletion of CD8$^+$ T cells as described in Materials and Methods and Fig. 4B.1. When mice were sacrificed on day 28 post B16F10 tumor inoculation, analysis of angiogenesis at that time point clearly suggested a predominant role for CD8$^+$ T cells in NLGP driven immune-mediated vascular normalization, since CD8$^+$ T cell depletion completely abolished anti-angiogenic potential of NLGP pretreatment (Figure 4C). NLGP mediated downregulation of VEGF,

VEGFR2 and CD31 was again upregulated in mice group with CD8$^+$ T cell depletion, as indicated by RT-PCR (Figure 4D.1, D.2) and immunohistochemical (Figure 4D.3) analysis.

NLGP mediated vascular normalization is not due to the T cell mediated apoptosis of CD31$^+$ cells rather due to unavailability of VEGF

Since CD8$^+$ T cells are found to be responsible for anti-angiogenic effect of NLGP-conditioned immune system (preferentially achieved by downregulation of VEGR2$^+$CD31$^+$ endothelial cells), initially we analyzed direct cytolytic effect of CD8$^+$ T cells on CD31$^+$ VECs. CD31$^+$ cells were flow sorted from solid B16F10 tumors (Figure S1) and exposed to CD8$^+$ T cells from NLGP pretreated tumor bearing mice. Co-incubation study suggested that CD8$^+$ T cells are unable to exert any direct cytolytic effect *in vitro* against tumor derived CD31$^+$ endothelial cells (Figure 5A). Furthermore, analysis of pro-apoptotic and apoptotic/necrotic VECs using Annexin V and PI respectively within tumor revealed that NLGP pretreatment has no effect on early apoptosis or late apoptosis/necrosis of CD31$^+$ cells (Figure 5B.1, B.2).

Analysing these two above mentioned results and considering the importance of VEGF as rate limiting factor for uncontrolled VEC proliferation and survival (necessary for neovascularization) next we assessed *in situ* VEGF concentration and its influence in NLGP mediated vascular normalization. Evidences obtained from ELISA clearly suggested that availability of VEGF is low in tumor

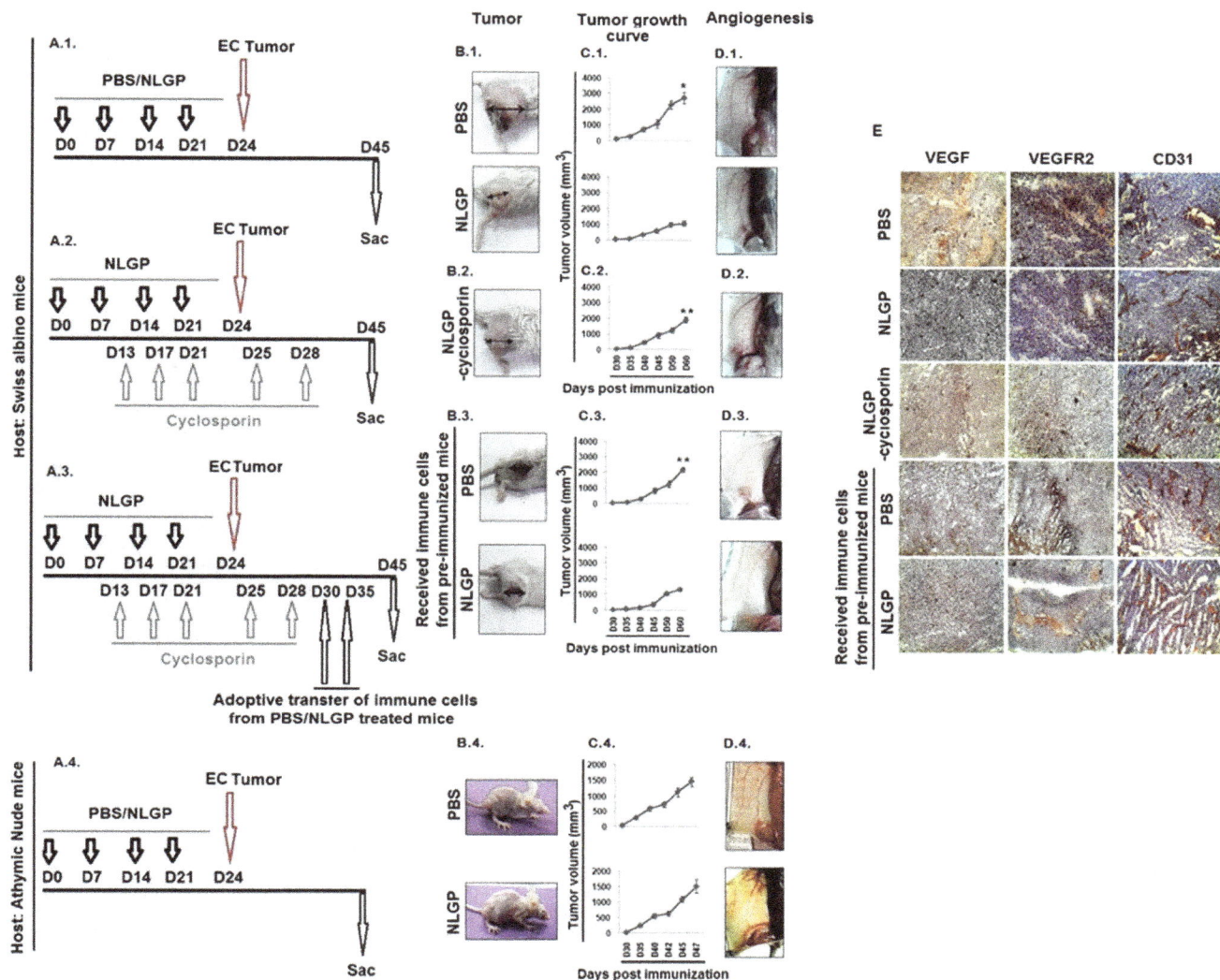

Figure 3. NLGP mediated normalization of angiogenesis is absent in immunocompromised mice. Schematic presentation of NLGP prophylaxis in **A.1.** normal mice, **A.2.** and **A.3.** cyclosporine treated/immunocompromised and **A.4.** athymic nude mice. **B.1.-B.4.** Representative photographs of murine tumors with **B.1.** PBS, NLGP, **B.2.** NLGP-Cyclosporin pretreatment, **B.3.** NLGP pretreatment with adoptive transfer of immune cells and **B.4.** NLGP and PBS pretreatment (athymic nude mice). **C.1.-C.4.** Tumor growth curve presenting Mean ± SD. *$p<0.001$, **$p<0.01$, in comparison to NLGP group with other above mentioned group and **D.1.-D.4.** Angiogenic profile of mice with **D.1.** PBS, NLGP, **D.2.** NLGP-Cyclosporin pretreatment, **D.3.** NLGP pretreatment with adoptive transfer of immune cells and **D.4.** NLGP and PBS pretreatment (athymic nude mice). **E.** Immunohistochemical detection of VEGF, VEGFR2 and CD31 in tumor sections as mentioned in **A.1–A.3.**

in situ from NLGP pretreated mice (Figure 5C), which might regulate CD31$^+$ endothelial cell proliferation. To further verify this possibility, CD31$^+$Ki67$^+$ proliferating cells were analyzed in B16F10 tumor from NLGP pretreated mice by flow cytometric (Figure 5D.1) and immunofluorescence analysis (Figure 5D.2). Consistently, *in vivo* BrdU labeling and analysis of CD31$^+$BrdU$^+$ proliferating cells within harvested cells from tumors indicated significant lowering of proliferating cells in tumor bearing mice pretreated with NLGP (Figure 5D.3). The obtained results clearly suggested that the presence of proliferating endothelial cells is significantly less in NLGP pretreated mice than control mice. Again, peripheral blood mononuclear cells (PBMC) from EC bearing PBS and NLGP treated mice were co-cultured with tumor (EC) cells and culture supernatant was analyzed for VEGF and IFNγ content. Analysis of such supernatants revealed low content of VEGF and high IFNγ (in NLGP-PBMC-EC cell co-culture), in comparison to those where PBS-PBMC was used (Figure 5E.1, E.2). Furthermore, flow-sorted CD31$^+$ cells were *in vitro* exposed to supernatants from NLGP-PBMC-EC cell co-culture and proliferation (monitored by Ki67 staining) of CD31$^+$ endothelial cells was monitored, where significantly less proliferation was noted due to supplementation of supernatant from NLGP-PBMC-EC cell co-culture (Figure 5E.3). Therefore, these results clearly pointed out the prominent role of VEGF downregulation caused after NLGP-instructed CD8$^+$ T cell infiltration in the reciprocal regulation of VEC proliferation and vascular normalization.

NLGP mediated vascular normalization has no adverse effect on normal wound healing process in mice

Given the potential safety concerns of systemic toxicity for strategies targeting tumor angiogenesis, we also intended to

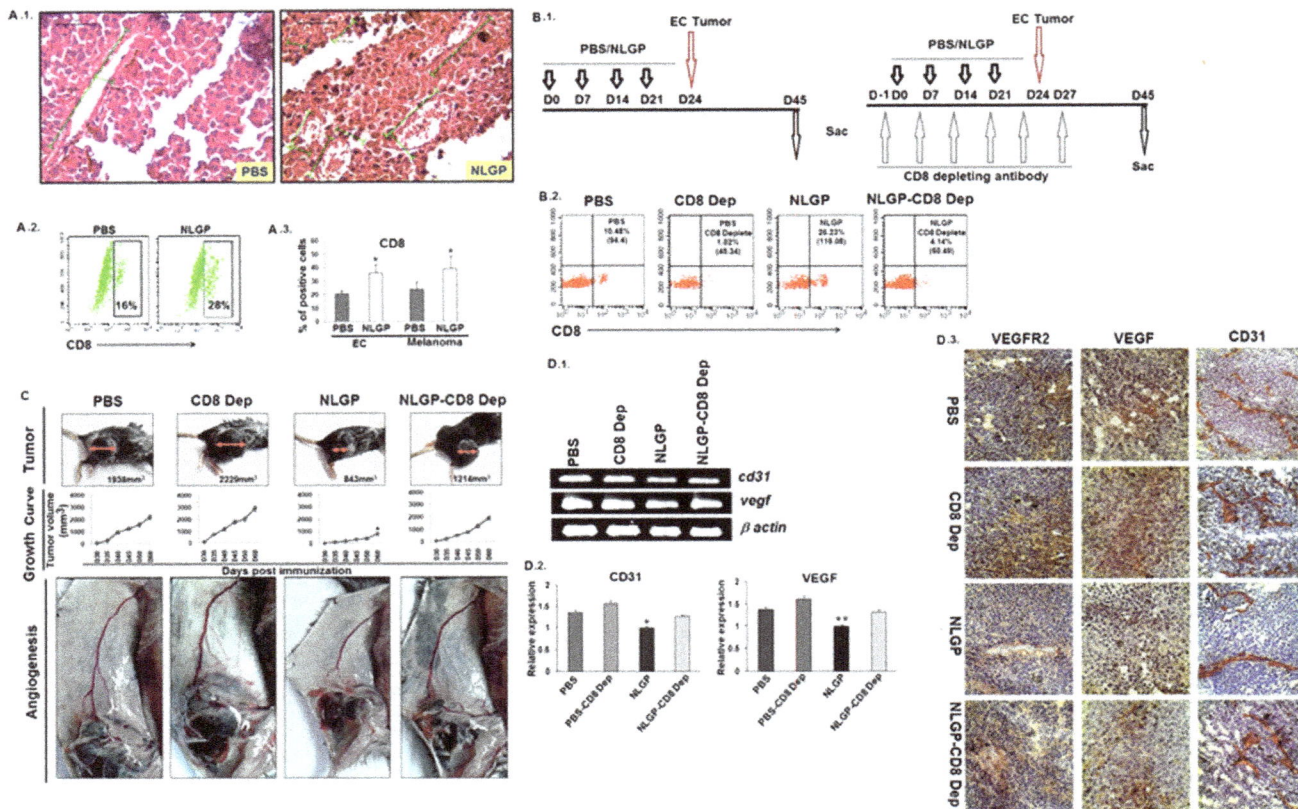

Figure 4. NLGP mediated normalization of tumor vasculature is dependent on CD8[+] T cells. B16 melanoma tumors were harvested from both PBS and NLGP pretreated C57BL/6 mice. **A.1.** Immune infiltration within tumors from PBS and NLGP treated mice were assessed histologically (H&E). **A.2.** Status of CD8[+] T cells in blood was assessed by flow cytometry. **A.3.** Bar diagram shows the status of CD8[+] T cells within carcinoma and melanoma tumors. *$p<0.01$. **B.1.** Schematic presentation of control and CD8[+] T cell depletion in either PBS or NLGP pretreated mice. **B.2.** Status of CD8[+] T cells in all four mice groups (PBS, NLGP, PBS-CD8 dep and NLGP CD8 dep) were presented with representative figures. **C.** Representative picture of tumors, tumor growth curve and angiogenesis of PBS and NLGP pretreated mice with or without CD8[+] T cell depletion. $p<0.001$. **D.1.** Total RNA was isolated from tumors of PBS, NLGP, PBS-CD8 depleted group (PBS-CD8 dep) and NLGP-CD8 depleted mice (NLGP-CD8-Dep) group (n = 3 in each case) to analyze genes, like, *cd31 and vegf* at transcriptional level by RT-PCR and **D.2.** densitometric analysis of band intensities from 3 individual observations (Mean ± SD) is presented. *$p<0.001$, **$p<0.01$. **D.3.** Immunohistochemical analysis of tumors obtained from PBS and NLGP pretreated mice with or without CD8 depletion were performed using monoclonal antibodies, specific for CD31, VEGF and VEGFR2.

evaluate the impact of NLGP on cutaneous wound healing process (model of physiological angiogenesis). Mice were treated with NLGP or PBS as described earlier and 4 mm^2 wounds were made in the skin of upper back. As shown in (Figure 6A) extent of wound closure in early days (between 4–7) was slightly higher in NLGP treated group, but in later stages (on day 9–14) healing was faster in PBS group and finally all wounds healed fully within a 2-week period. Furthermore, histological analysis revealed no observable differences in skin from both group of mice showing signature of wound healing (rapid epithelialization along with adipose layer were observed and hair follicles were formed) (Figure 6B). Immunofluorescence analysis on CD31[+] and NG2[+] cells on skin clearly showed no significant changes in wound healed skin from NLGP and PBS pretreated mice (Figure 6C). Therefore, our results clearly suggest that modulatory effect of NLGP on tumor angiogenesis does not hamper the normal physiological angiogenic process.

Discussion

We have reported significant restriction of murine sarcoma, carcinoma and melanoma growth due to administration of NLP/

NLGP in prophylactic [15,16,29] and therapeutic [17,18] settings. This tumor growth restriction is strictly dependent upon modulation of host-tumor immune interaction [20,25], since NLGP is unable to induce direct tumor cell apoptosis [19,35]. Apart from the already discussed immunomodulation by NLGP in cancer [18,20,22], angiogenic normalization property of this molecule is described here for the first time.

As results suggest, prophylactic administration of NLGP (with an interval of 7 days for 4 times) is inhibitory towards neovascularization initiated after tumor challenge and the antiangiogenic effect is indeed associated with the decrease in heavily dilated (thick)/fragile as well as very thin blood vessels. However, the thin and compact vessels were observed to be retained, probably to facilitate the trafficking of immune effector cells. Based on the available data, we reasoned that NLGP pretreatment causes significant reduction in proliferating Ki67[+]CD31[+] VECs within tumor and thereby reduces the tumor micro vessel density (an indicator of tumor angiogenesis). Since proliferation of CD31[+] cells corroborates neovascularization [36,37], such reduction plays a great role in angiogenic normalization. Unlike VECs, NLGP do not decrease the number of NG2[+] pericytes, but effectively preserve their maturity and coverage of these cells on blood

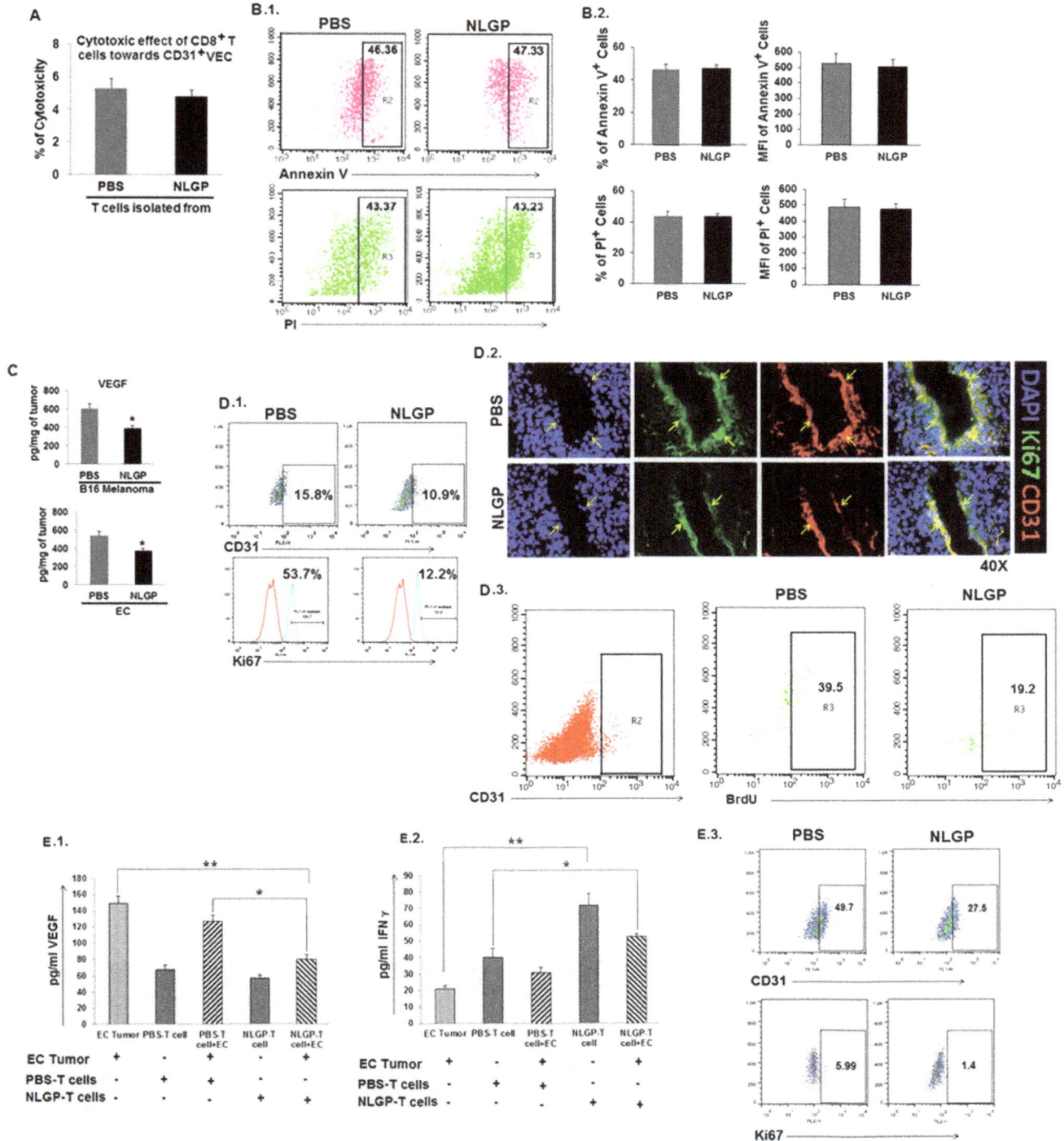

Figure 5. NLGP mediated vascular normalization is not due to CD8[+] T cell mediated apoptosis of CD31[+] cells. Mice were inoculated with B16 melanoma cells (2×10^5 cells/mice) to grow tumor. After reaching the tumor volume to a considerable size (1372 mm[3] approximately), tumor was harvested and CD31[+] VECs were isolated by flow sorting. CD8[+] T lymphocytes were isolated from NLGP or PBS pretreated ($4\times$) mice by MACS purification and CD8[+] T cells were co-cultured with the CD31[+] VECs. **A.** Cytotoxicity was measured by LDH release assay. NLGP pretreated C57BL/6 mice were inoculated with B16 melanoma cells as mentioned earlier. **B.1.** As tumor reached a considerable volume (1372 mm[3] approximately), tumors were harvested, single cells prepared and stained with anti-CD31 antibody along with either Annexin V or Propidium Iodide (PI). Representative figures of Annexin-V and PI[+] cells from CD31 gated population. **B.2.** Bar diagram showing % positive cells and MFI. **C.** Cell lysates prepared from carcinoma and melanoma tumors of PBS and NLGP pretreated mice were used to quantitate the level of VEGF by ELISA. Cytokines were measured as pg/mg of tissue ± SE and Mean ± SD of 3 individual observations are presented in bar diagram. *$p<0.01$. **D.1.** Obtained cells as mentioned in **B.1**, were stained for CD31, along with Ki67. Gated CD31[+] population was assessed for Ki67 staining using Flowjo software and presented in histogram. **D.2.** Cryo-sections obtained from tumors of NLGP and PBS pretreated mice were stained with fluorescence labeled anti-CD31 (red) and anti-Ki67 (green) antibodies, along with DAPI (blue). Representative figures from 3 separate sets of experiments are presented. **D.3.**

PBS and NLGP pretreated tumor bearing mice were injected with BrdU within tumor and sacrificed after 48 hours. Single cells were prepared to check BrdU staining after gating the CD31 population, as shown in a representative figure. **E.1, E.2.** PBMC were isolated from both PBS and NLGP treated tumor bearing mice and cultured with EC cells (2×10^5 cells) for 24 hours and cell free supernatant were measured in pg/ml for VEGF (E.1) and IFNγ (E.2) by ELISA. Cytokines were quantitated as pg/ml $\pm$ SE. *$p<0.001$, **$p<0.01$. **E.3.** Flow sorted CD31$^+$ ECs isolated from tumor microenvironment were cultured with the above mentioned supernatants (NLGP-PBMC+EC vs PBS-PBMC+EC) for 48 hours and assessed for the EC proliferation flow cytometrically after Ki67 labeling.

vessels. Under NLGP influence, their tight association with VECs restore the vessel integrity and prevents leakiness. Therefore, by differentially regulating the two important stromal cell features, NLGP controls aberrant tumor vasculature. In context to host-antitumor benefits such results are encouraging as recent preclinical and clinical findings suggest that vascular normalization, rather than restriction of blood flow, is necessary to maintain the surge of effector immune cells and chemical regimens for cancer therapy [38].

Evidences are accumulated from present study suggesting the interference of NLGP in balancing tumor growth-supportive pro- and anti-angiogenic molecules. Several previous studies show that the VEGF family proteins, which signals through VEGFRs [39–41] are major factors involved in tumor-induced angiogenesis. Tumor and residing stromal cells secrete several growth factors particularly VEGF [42,43] to stimulate VEGFR$^+$ endothelial cell proliferation and in turn these cells provide the lining of newly formed blood vessels to supply nutrient to growing tumor [39]. Among all VEGFRs, VEGFR2 is mainly found on newly proliferating endothelial cells and targeting of VEGFR2 has been shown in some tumor models to reverse neo-vascularization [44].

Accordingly, NLGP selectively targets the VEGF-VEGFR2 signaling in proliferating endothelial cells to create a 'vascular normalization window' that might facilitate a decrease in interstitial pressure, enhanced tumor oxygenation and ultimately leads to a better therapeutic response [39,40] in terms of restricted tumor growth [27].

In view of our consistent observation on central involvement of immune system in NLGP-mediated eradication or prevention of murine tumor growth [17–20], the present study additionally evaluated the involvement of NLGP-instructed immune-modulation in controlling tumor-angiogenesis. Interestingly, we observed a significant abolition of NLGP mediated both anti-angiogenic and anti-tumor effect in cyclosporine [45,46] treated mice having prominent immunosuppression. However, adoptive transfer of immune cells from mice with NLGP therapy again restores both anti-angiogenic and tumor growth restricting effects of NLGP. Analysing these data, we speculated that NLGP-driven immune activation might be involved in anti-angiogenic process. To further validate our hypothesis, we used immunocompromised athymic nude mice and here also NLGP prophylaxis was unable to prevent neovascularization as well as tumor growth. Next, we directly

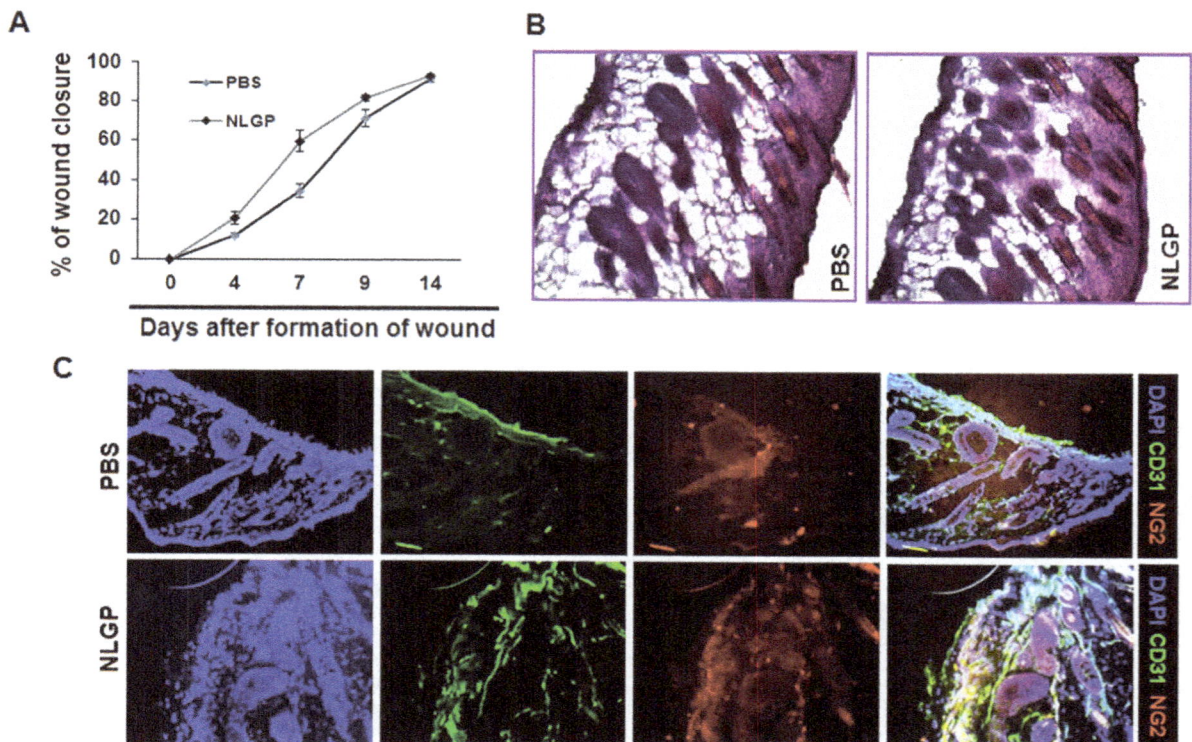

Figure 6. NLGP mediated vascular normalization has no adverse effect on normal wound healing process. Swiss mice were pretreated with NLGP (25µg) and PBS once in a week for four weeks and 4 mm^3 wound was made on the back of both groups of mice. **A.** Diameter of wounds was measured every two days and percentages of wound closure were calculated and data presented as Mean $\pm$ SD of 6 individual observations. **B.** Histological sections of wound beds were stained with H&E and assessed microscopically. Representative figures are presented. **C.** Cryo-sections of wound beds were stained with fluorescence labeled anti-CD31 (red) and anti-NG2 (green) antibodies along with DAPI.

focussed on the contribution of CD8$^+$ effector T cells, since NLGP selectively increases the trafficking of these effector cells into tumor parenchyma and therapeutic NLGP mediated tumor growth restriction is abrogated completely in CD8$^+$ T cell depleted mice [17,18]. However, infiltrating CD8$^+$ T cells often unable to show cytotoxic effect because, several tumor microenvironmental factors upregulate expression of inhibitory molecules like PD1 and CTLA4 on T cells to attenuate its effector functions and effector cytokine production [47]. In this context, modulatory effect of NLGP on TME is already reported [18,27,28]. More importantly, NLGP minimizes TME-induced anergy and exhaustion of CD8$^+$ T cells, as observed by downregulation of anergy related molecules DGKa, Grail, EGRs etc. [18] and exhaustion related molecules TIM3, LAG3, PD1 and CTLA4 [17,19] to preserve the optimum functional efficacy of infiltrated CD8$^+$ T cells. Likewise, in present study, NLGP administration followed by CD8$^+$ T cell depletion was unable to produce anti-angiogenic effect, as dilated tortuous (thick) blood vessels are seen in these groups of animals. Moreover, NLGP mediated reduction of proliferating CD31$^+$ endothelial cells or VEGF-VEGFR2 expression within tumor is abrogated in CD8$^+$ T cell depleted tumor bearing mice.

Considering this important contribution of CD8$^+$ T cells in NLGP mediated anti-angiogenesis, initially we assumed that CD8$^+$ T cells might be directly involved in killing of CD31$^+$ VECs. In several previous studies, it was demonstrated that VEGFR2-specific CTL can be directly involved in the killing of proliferating VECs [48]. Contrary to these reports in our system we do not observe any cytolytic activity of CD8$^+$ T cells isolated from NLGP treated mice towards flow sorted CD31$^+$ VECs. To solve this puzzle, we checked involvement of VEGF, for which sorted CD31$^+$ VECs were incubated with supernatants from co-culture of PBMC from NLGP/PBS EC bearing mice and EC cells. Interestingly, CD31$^+$ VECs proliferated less with NLGP-PBMC+EC cells culture supernatant (having comparatively high level of VEGF), which was again compensated with addition of recombinant VEGF. In vivo BrdU labeling study also suggests less number of CD31$^+$BrdU$^+$ proliferating cells within tumors from NLGP pretreated mice, where VEGF content is significantly less. Therefore, finally, we concluded that unavailability of VEGF might be the predominant rate limiting factor of reduced VEC growth and vascular normalization. Considering the infiltration and essential role of CD8$^+$ T cells, we further assumed that, NLGP treatment may enhance DC migration to lymph node to prime CD8$^+$ T cells, which eventually infiltrates tumor parenchyma to kill tumor cells (that serves as one of the prime source for VEGF). It could also be possible that infiltrated CD8$^+$ T cells produce IFNγ and/or infiltrated DC produce IL-12 and either of these immunomodulatory cytokines possess anti-angiogenic effects by altering pro-angiogenic mediators [29,49]. Interestingly, our previous studies suggested the effectiveness of NLGP to influence CD8$^+$ T cells and DC to produce IFNγ and IL-12 respectively [20–22]. On the other-hand, in a separate in vitro study, we observed that NLGP can directly modulate B16 melanoma tumor cells by reducing HIF1α and VEGF in normoxic as well in hypoxic condition (unpublished observation).

In summary, our results suggest that NLGP prophylaxis educate whole immune system in such a way that after tumor challenge antigen presenting cells efficiently prime effector CD8$^+$ T cells, which in due course kill tumor cells to reduce tumor promoting growth factor burden within TME. These reduced availability of growth factor especially VEGF subsequently impede the growth of endothelial cells without affecting the vessel integrity to maintain the proper trafficking of immune effector cells within TME. More importantly this strategy does not affect the normal wound healing

process, since immune-elimination is not obligate here. However, whether these infiltrated CD8$^+$ T cells affect other VEGF producing cells or any other parallel cascade operational in this NLGP-instructed immune system-mediated anti-angiogenic process needs further evaluation. Considering the limitation of anti-angiogenic immunotherapy [50,51] combination therapy integrating anti-angiogenic therapy along with immunotherapy or other conventional therapy was proposed by several groups [52,53]. In this context, NLGP treatment would be more promising in the field of cancer management because of its multidirectional fine tuning ability of tumor vasculature as well as of systemic/local immunity without any adverse physiological consequence.

Methods

Ethics statement on mice experiments

For maintenance and experimentation on mice, the relevant guidelines were followed and the Chittaranjan National Cancer Institute animal ethical committee approved the study.

Mice and tumors

Female C57BL/6 and Swiss mice (Age: 4–6 weeks; Body weight: 24–27 g) were obtained from the National Centre for Laboratory Animal Sciences (NCLAS), Hyderabad and Institutional Animal Care and Maintenance Department, Chittaranjan National Cancer Institute (CNCI), Kolkata, India respectively and maintained under standard laboratory conditions. Immunocompromised athymic nude mice (4–6 weeks old) were purchased from NCLAS, Hyderabad and maintained in a specific pathogen free facility. Autoclaved dry pellet diet (Epic Laboratory Animal Feed, West Bengal Govt, Kalyani, India) and water were supplied ad libitum. Ehrlich Carcinoma (EC) was maintained by regular in vivo intraperitoneal passage in Swiss mice. B16F10 melanoma cell line was cultured in vitro in DMEM supplemented with 10% (v/v) FBS, 2 mM L-glutamine and penicillin-streptomycin (100μg/ml) at 37°C humidified conditions. To develop solid tumors in vivo, C57BL/6 and Swiss mice were inoculated subcutaneously (s.c.) in right hind leg quarters with B16F10 melanoma cells (2×10^5) and EC cells (1×10^6) respectively.

Antibodies and reagents

RPMI 1640, DMEM, and FBS were purchased from Invitrogen (NY, USA). Lymphocyte separation media (LSM) was procured from MP Biomedicals, Irvine, CA, USA and HiMedia, Mumbai, India. Fluorescence conjugated different anti-mouse antibodies (CD4, CD8, Ki67) and purified CD31 were procured from either BD-Pharmingen or Biolegends (both in, San Diego, CA, USA). Fluorescence- or peroxidase-labeled secondary antibodies were procured from e-Biosciences (San Diego, CA, USA). Purified anti-mouse Foxp3, VEGF, VEGFR1, VEGFR2, were procured from Santa Cruz Biotech (California, USA). IFNγ/IL-10 estimation kits (OptEIA, BD Biosciences, San Jose, CA, USA) 3,3',5,5'-tetramethylbenzidine (TMB) substrate solutions (for ELISA), CytoFix/CytoPerm kit (for intracellular staining), AnnexinV-Propidium iodide apoptosis detection kit were obtained from BD Pharmingen, San Dieago, CA, USA. LDH release assay kit for cytotoxicity and BrdU kit for proliferation were obtained from Roche Diagnostics, Mannheim, Germany. Western lightning chemiluminescence and immunoperoxidase color detection kit were purchased from Pierce (Rockford, IL, USA) and Vector laboratories Inc (Burlingame, CA, USA) respectively. Optimal cutting temperature (OCT) compound was purchased from Sakura Finetek, Torrance, CA, USA. RT-PCR primers were procured from MWG-Biotech AG (Bangalore, India). DAPI was purchased from Sigma, St. Louis, MO, USA.

Neem leaf glycoprotein

Mature neem *(Azadirachta indica)* leaves of identical size and color (indicative of similar age), taken from a standard source were shed-dried and pulverized. Leaf powder was soaked overnight in phosphate buffered saline (PBS), pH 7.4 and supernatant was collected by centrifugation at 1500 rpm, termed neem leaf preparation (NLP) [16,54]. NLP was then extensively dialyzed against PBS and concentrated by Centricon Membrane Filter (Millipore Corporation, Bedford, MA, USA) with 10 KDa molecular weight cut off. Active component of this preparation is a glycoprotein, as characterized earlier [55] and designated as Neem leaf glycoprotein (NLGP). Protein concentration of NLGP solution was measured by Lowry's method [56] using Folin's Phenol reagent. Purity of the NLGP was confirmed by HPLC [22] before use.

NLGP injection and tumor growth restriction assay

Two groups (n = 8, in each group) of either C57BL/6 or Swiss mice were immunized once weekly (25μg/100μl PBS/mice s.c.) for 4 weeks in total at left hind leg quarter with NLGP, keeping other group as PBS control. Immunized mice were inoculated with B16F10 and EC tumors respectively as mentioned above to develop solid tumors. Growth of solid tumor (in mm^3) was monitored biweekly by caliper measurement using the formula: (width^2×length)/2. Survival of mice was noted regularly, till tumor size reached to 25 mm in either direction.

Angiogenesis study with blood vessels

To study the role of NLGP on tumor angiogenesis, both groups of NLGP and PBS pre-treated tumor bearing mice were sacrificed and skin were removed carefully from peritoneal region without disturbing the angiogenic vessels adjacent to tumors. These blood vessels were counted macroscopically using convex lens depending on the thickness of the blood vessels and categorized as heavy, very thick, thick, thin and very thin. Area of blood vessels was calculated using Photoshop software (Adobe Systems Incorporated, San Jose, California, USA) and presented in Pixels. Extent of angiogenesis was categorized as 4 (++++), 3 (+++), 2 (++) and 1 (+). Tumor volume (in mm^3) and extent of angiogenesis (in raw score) was multiplied to obtain an index for tumor angiogenesis. Mean of score from all mice was presented as Mean Index for Tumor and Angiogenesis (MITA).

Angiogenesis in immunocompromised mice

To study the role of immune system in tumor angiogenesis, Swiss mice were divided into three groups (n = 3) and two groups received NLGP immunization as said before, keeping other group as PBS control. One of these NLGP treated mice group was immune suppressed by three consecutive peritoneal cyclosporine injections (15 mg/Kg) on day 13, 17 and 21. Mice of all groups were inoculated s.c. with EC (1×10^6 cells) on day 24. Again, cyclosporine was injected on day 25 and 28. Similar study was conducted on immune compromised athymic nude mice, where one group received NLGP with another PBS control group. Following completion of immunization all mice received EC (1×10^5 cells) s.c. and tumor growth and survivability were monitored biweekly. Pattern of angiogenesis was noted after sacrificing the mice.

To reconfirm the same, NLGP immunized Swiss mice were similarly divided in three groups (n = 3, in each group) and

immunologically suppressed with consecutive peritoneal injection of cyclosporine as mentioned above. Then all three groups of mice were injected with 1×10^6 viable EC cells. Following establishment of tumor (64 mm^3 in average), first group was kept as control, second group received splenic immune cells (1×10^7) i.v. through tail vein from PBS treated mice and third group of mice received same number of immune cells from 4× NLGP (25μg/100μl/mice) immunized mice. When tumor reached a considerable volume (25 mm) in mice from PBS pretreated group, mice from both groups were sacrificed (on day 45) for comparative monitoring of angiogenesis, as described above. Identical experiment was performed in athymic nude mice with similar cell transfer from either PBS or NLGP injected mice.

Angiogenesis in CD8$^+$ T cell depleted mice

Within several immune cells, to study the specific role of CD8$^+$ T cells in the process of angiogenesis, C57BL/6 mice were divided in four groups (n = 4 in each group). Two groups of mice were immunized with NLGP as said before while other two groups of mice were injected with PBS. One NLGP and one PBS treated mice group were peritoneally injected with CD8 depleting antibody (100μg/50μl) on day -1, 6, 13, 20 and 27 as shown in Fig. 4BI. CD8$^+$ T cell depletion status was monitored regularly by analyzing peripheral blood using flow cytometry. On day 24, B16F10 tumors (2×10^5 cells/mice) were inoculated s.c. to the left flank of hind leg. Tumor volumes were monitored biweekly and on reaching a considerable size (25 mm) in mice from PBS pretreated group, mice from both groups (PBS and NLGP) were sacrificed for comparative monitoring in angiogenesis, as described above.

Tumor infiltrated immune cells

After attaining considerable size, tumors of either type were harvested from sacrificed mice. Portions of tumors were separately preserved for histology, immunohistochemistry, immunofluorescence studies, western blot, flow cytometry and RT-PCR analysis.

A piece of tumor was cleaned with PBS and chopped into small pieces and treated with mixture of collagenase (2μg/ml) and hyaluronidase (2μg/ml) and passed through the nylon mesh to prepare single cell suspensions. Tumor infiltrating lymphocytes (TILs) were then separated from tumor cells by differential gradient centrifugation at 2000 rpm for 30 minutes to analyze their proportions.

Histology, immunohistochemistry and immunofluorescence studies

Tumors were fixed in 10% formalin for standard histological preparations and embedded in paraffin. Sections (4–5 μm) were prepared and stained with hematoxylin-eosin (H&E) according to standard protocol. Representative tumors were selected for immunohistochemical analysis. Fresh tumor tissues were also frozen for cryo-sectioning. Sections were immunostained for CD31, NG2, VEGF, VEGFR1 and VEGFR2 by the method described [27]. In some cases, tumor or skin sections were snap-frozen in OCT compound. Sections (5 μm) were prepared using cryostat (Leica, Germany), air-dried and fixed in ice-cold methanol for 20-30 min. The sections were blocked with 5% BSA solution and stained with different anti-mouse antibodies (CD31-PE, NG2-FITC, Ki67-FITC) by the method described earlier [27].

Western blot analysis

Tumor lysate or cellular lysate (50 μg) were separated on 6–20% SDS–polyacrylamide gel and transferred onto a PVDF membrane for Western Blotting. Incubation was performed for different primary antibodies, e.g., CD31, NG2, VEGF, VEGFR1 and VEGFR2, and the procedure followed the method as published [18].

RT-PCR analysis

Total RNA was isolated from solid tumors (from PBS and NLGP treated mice) using the TRIZOL Reagent (Ambion, Austin, Texas, USA). The cDNA synthesis was carried out using RevertAid First Strand cDNA Synthesis Kit (Fermentas, K1622) following the manufacturer's protocol and RT-PCR was carried out using gene-specific primers. The primer sequences of mouse CD31, VEGF, VEGFR1, VEGFR2, NG2 and β-Actin are described in the Table 2. PCR products were identified by image analysis software for gel documentation (Gel Doc XR+ system, BioRad) following electrophoresis on 1.5%–2% agarose gels and staining with ethidium bromide [18,27].

Flow cytometric staining

Single cell preparation from harvested tumors were labeled with 0.5µl (for 1×10^6 cells) FITC or PE conjugated antibodies, specific for mouse CD8, CD31, Ki67 markers, and surface or intracellular flow cytometry was performed by the method described [17].

Annexin V-PI staining for apoptosis

Harvested tumors from PBS and NLGP treated mice were minced to make single cell suspension as mentioned before. Freshly collected single cells were mixed with $1 \times$ binding buffer (100 µl) and kept for 2 min at room temp. Then 5µl of each Annexin-V and PI were added and incubated for 15 mins and then finally analyzed by flow cytometry.

Flow sorting of CD31+ cells

Single cell suspension obtained from harvested tumors was washed with PBS (containing 1% FBS) and passed through cell strainer. This cell pellet was stained with primary anti-mouse-CD31 antibody (30 minutes) and further tagged with appropriate FITC labeled secondary antibody and CD31+ cells were purified by Flow sorting with BD FACS Aria, San Jose, CA.

Mechanistic studies on downregulation of CD31+ endothelial cells

CD8+ T cells were purified by MACS from the spleen of both PBS and NLGP treated tumor bearing mice by the method

described [17,18]. Flow sorted CD31+ endothelial cells were co-cultured with CD8+ T cells in 1:10 dilution in serum free media and checked for cytotoxicity by LDH release assay. Cell-free supernatants were used to measure the level of released LDH using the formula: % Cytotoxicity = (Lysis from Effector-Target Mixture − Lysis from Effector only) − Spontaneous Lysis/ (Maximum Lysis − Spontaneous Lysis) ×100.

In a separate experiment, splenic cells were purified from EC bearing PBS and NLGP treated mice and co-cultured with EC cells (10:1 ratio) for 24 hrs. Cell free culture supernatants were collected and assessed for VEGF and IFNγ content by ELISA. Purified CD31+ endothelial cells were also incubated with such culture supernatants for 48 hrs and their proliferation was assessed by Ki67 staining by the method described [15]. In a parallel experiment NLGP (4×) pretreated mice were injected with anti-mouse BrdU antibody injected in tumor as per manufacturer's manual. After 48 hours of injection both groups of mice were sacrificed to harvest tumors and single cells were prepared as described before. Single cells were stained with anti-CD31 antibody and assessed flow cytometrically as per standard protocol.

Wound healing assay

Mice were pretreated with PBS and NLGP as described earlier. Mice were then anesthetized with peritoneal injection of 0.3 ml of 2-2-2-tribromoethanol (Avertin, Sigma, St. Louis, MO) and back portion was properly shaved to remove all fur and cleaned with 70% alcohol. Subsequently using dual puncher 4 mm² wound was created on both side of their back and kept in sterile environment. After every 3 days interval wound closure was measured henceforth by a vernier caliper and the wound healing was analyzed. Finally on day 15 mice of both groups were sacrificed and their skins were fixed and sectioned using cryostat. Routine histology and immunofluorescence study was performed in skins.

Statistical analysis

All results represent the average of separate *in vivo* and *in vitro* experiments. Number of experiments is mentioned in result section and legends to figures. In each experiment a value represents the mean of three individual observations and presented as mean ± standard deviation (SD). Statistical significance was established by Student's t-test using INSTAT 3 Software (GraphPad Software, Inc.), with differences between groups attaining a p value <0.05 considered as significant.

Table 2. Primer sequences of various cytokine genes studied.

Name	Primer sequences (5′–3′)	Product size
β-Actin-forward	CAACCGTGAAAAGATGACCC	228 bp.
β-Actin-reverse	ATGAGGTAGTCTGTCAGGTC	
VEGFR2-forward	ACAGACAGTGGGGATGGTCC	271 bp
VEGFR2-reverse	AAACAGGAGGTGAGCGCAG	
VEGFR1-forward	CCAACTACCTCAAGAGCAAAC	315 bp
VEGFR1-reverse	CCAGGTCCCGATGAATGCAC	
CD31-forward	AGCCCACCAGAGACATGGAA	337 bp
CD31-reverse	CTGGCTCTGTTGGAGGCTGT	
VEGF-forward	GGACCCTGGCTTTACTGCTG	201 bp
VEGF-reverse	CACAGGACGGCTTGAAGATG	

Supporting Information

Figure S1   Purification of CD31⁺ cells by flow sorting.
Solid B16 melanoma tumors were harvested from PBS treated C57BL/6 mice and single cell preparation was made. Cells were labeled with anti-CD31 antibody and positive cells were sorted in flow cytometer (BD FACS Aria). A. FSC/SSC plot of single cell population under study. B. Unstained cell population in FL1 (CD31)/FSC plot. C. CD31⁺ cells in FL1 (CD31)/FSC plot. D. Purified CD31⁺ vascular endothelial cells after flow sorting.

Acknowledgments

We acknowledge Director, CNCI, Kolkata, India, for providing necessary facilities. Thanks to Dr. Subrata Laskar, Burdwan University, India, for his help in characterization of NLGP. Thanks to Dr. Abhijit Rakshit for providing experimental animals. We also extend our thanks to Dr. P. S. Dasgupta for his help and suggestions in angiogenic study.

Author Contributions

Conceived and designed the experiments: A. Bose S. Banerjee RB. Performed the experiments: S. Banerjee S. Barik TG SG AD A. Bhuniya. Analyzed the data: S. Banerjee A. Bose TG S. Barik RB. Contributed reagents/materials/analysis tools: RB. Wrote the paper: A. Bose S. Banerjee RB.

References

1. Hanahan D, Weinberg RA (2000) The hallmarks of cancer. Cell 7:57–70.
2. Breier G (2000) Angiogenesis in embryonic development- A review. Placenta 21:S11–15.
3. Tonnesen MG, Feng X, Clark RA (2000) Angiogenesis in wound healing. J Invest Dermatol Symp Proc 5:40–46.
4. Sihvo EI, Ruohtula T, Auvinen MI, Koivistoinen A, Harjula AL, et al. (2003) Simultaneous progression of oxidative stress and angiogenesis in malignant transformation of Barrett esophagus. J Thorac Cardiovasc Surg 126:1952–1957.
5. Khan M, Nayyar AS, Gayitri HC, Bafna UD, Siddique A (2012) Tumor angiogenesis: A potential marker of the ongoing process of malignant transformation in leukoplakia patients, removing the veil. Clin Cancer Invest J 1:127–134.
6. Sonnenschein C, Soto AM (2013) The aging of the 2000 and 2011 Hallmarks of Cancer reviews: A critique. J Biosci 38:651–663.
7. Hanahan D, Folkman J (1996) Patterns and emerging mechanisms of the angiogenic switch during tumorigenesis. Cell 86:353–364.
8. Zou W (2006) Regulatory T cells, tumour immunity and immunotherapy. Nat Rev Immunol 6: 295–307.
9. Ribatti D, Crivellato E (2009) Immune cells and angiogenesis. J Cell Mol Med 13:2822–2833.
10. Terme M, Colussi O, Marcheteau E, Tanchot C, Tartour E, et al. (2012) Modulation of Immunity. Antiangiogenic Molecules in Cancer. Clin Dev Immunol 2012:1–8.
11. Tartour E, Pere H, Maillere B, Terme M, Merillon N, et al. (2011) Angiogenesis and immunity: a bidirectional link potentially relevant for the monitoring of antiangiogenic therapy and the development of novel therapeutic combination with immunotherapy. Cancer Metastasis Rev 30:83–95.
12. Shiao SL, Ganesan AP, Rugo HS, Coussens LM (2011) Immune microenvironments in solid tumors: new targets for therapy. Genes Dev 25:2559–2572.
13. Munn LL (2003) Aberrant vascular architecture in tumors and its importance in drug-based therapies. Drug Discov Today 8:396–403.
14. Jain RK (2005) Normalization of tumor vasculature: an emerging concept in antiangiogenic therapy. Science 307:58–62.
15. Haque E, Mandal I, Pal S, Baral R (2006) Prophylactic dose of neem (Azadirachta indica) leaf preparation restricting murine tumor growth is nontoxic, hematostimulatory and immunostimulatory. Immunopharmacol Immunotoxicol 28:33–50.
16. Baral R, Chattopadhyay U (2004) Neem (Azadirachta indica) leaf mediated immune activation causes prophylactic growth inhibition of murine Ehrlich carcinoma and B16 melanoma. Int Immunopharmacol 4:355–366.
17. Mallick A, Barik S, Goswami KK, Banerjee S, Ghosh S, et al. (2013) Neem leaf glycoprotein activates CD8(+) T cells to promote therapeutic anti-tumor immunity inhibiting the growth of mouse sarcoma. PLoS One 8:e47434.
18. Barik S, Banerjee S, Mallick A, Goswami KK, Roy S, et al. (2013) Normalization of tumor microenvironment by neem leaf glycoprotein potentiates effector T cell functions and therapeutically intervenes in the growth of mouse sarcoma. PLoS One 8:e66501.
19. Chakraborty T, Bose A, Barik S, Goswami KK, Banerjee S, et al. (2011) Neem leaf glycoprotein inhibits CD4+CD25+Foxp3+ Tregs to restrict murine tumor growth. Immunotherapy 3:949–969.
20. Bose A, Chakraborty K, Sarkar K, Goswami S, Chakraborty T, et al. (2009) Neem leaf glycoprotein induces perforin-mediated tumor cell killing by T and NK cells through differential regulation of IFNgamma signaling. J Immunother 32:42–53.
21. Bose A, Baral R (2007) NK cellular cytotoxicity of tumor cells initiated by neem leaf preparation is associated with CD40-CD40L mediated endogenous production of IL-12. Human Immunol 68:823–831.
22. Goswami S, Bose A, Sarkar K, Roy S, Chakraborty T, et al. (2010) Neem leaf glycoprotein matures myeloid derived dendritic cells and optimizes anti-tumor T cell functions. Vaccine 28:1241–1252.
23. Roy S, Goswami S, Bose A, Chakraborty K, Pal S, et al. (2011) Neem leaf glycoprotein partially rectifies suppressed dendritic cell functions and associated

T cell efficacy in patients with stage IIIB cervical cancer. Clin Vaccine Immunol 18:571–579.
24. Goswami KK, Barik S, Sarkar M, Bhowmick A, Biswas J, et al. (2014) Targeting STAT3 phosphorylation by neem leaf glycoprotein prevents immune evasion exerted by supraglottic laryngeal tumor induced M2 macrophages. Mol Immunol 59:119–127.
25. Bose A, Chakraborty K, Sarkar K, Goswami S, Haque E, et al. (2009) Neem leaf glycoprotein directs T-bet-associated type 1 immune commitment. Hum Immunol 70:6–15.
26. Chakraborty K, Bose A, Chakraborty T, Sarkar K, Goswami S, et al. (2010) Restoration of dysregulated CC chemokine signaling for monocyte/macrophage chemotaxis in head and neck squamous cell carcinoma patients by neem leaf glycoprotein maximizes tumor cell cytotoxicity. Cell Mol Immunol 7:396–408.
27. Barik S, Bhuniya A, Banerjee S, Das A, Sarkar M, et al. (2013) Neem leaf glycoprotein is superior than Cisplatin and Sunitinib malate in restricting melanoma growth by normalization of tumor microenvironment. Int Immunopharmacol 17:42–49.
28. Barik S, Banerjee S, Sarkar M, Bhuniya A, Roy S, et al. (2013) Neem leaf glycoprotein optimizes effector and regulatory functions within tumor microenvironment to intervene therapeutically the growth of B16 melanoma in C57BL/6 mice. Trials in Vaccinology, e-pub on Dec 6, 2013.
29. Haque E, Baral R (2006) Neem (Azadirachta indica) leaf preparation induces prophylactic growth inhibition of murine Ehrlich carcinoma in Swiss and C57BL/6 by activation of NK cells and NK-T cells. Immunobiology 211:721–731.
30. Chatterjee S, Heukamp LC, Siobal M, Schöttle J, Wieczorek C, et al. (2013) Tumor VEGF:VEGFR2 autocrine feed-forward loop triggers angiogenesis in lung cancer. J Clin Invest 123:1732–1740.
31. Daniel WM, Vosseler S, Mirancea N, Hicklin DJ, Bohlen P, et al. Rapid Vessel Regression, Protease Inhibition, and Stromal Normalization upon Short-Term Vascular Endothelial Growth Factor Receptor 2 Inhibition in Skin Carcinoma Heterotransplants. Am J Pathol 167:1389–1403.
32. Vosseler S, Mirancea N, Bohlen P, Mueller MM, Fusenig NE (2005) Angiogenesis inhibition by vascular endothelial growth factor receptor-2 blockade reduces stromal matrix metalloproteinase expression, normalizes stromal tissue, and reverts epithelial tumor phenotype in surface heterotransplants. Cancer Res 65:1294–1305.
33. Facciabene A, Motz GT, Coukos G (2012) T-regulatory cells: key players in tumor immune escape and angiogenesis. Cancer Res 72: 2162–2171.
34. Kujawski M, Kortylewski M, Lee H, Herrmann A, Kay H, et al. (2008) Stat3 mediates myeloid cell–dependent tumor angiogenesis in mice. J Clin Invest 118:3367–3377.
35. Bose A, Haque E, Baral R (2007) Neem leaf preparation induces apoptosis of tumor cells by releasing cytotoxic cytokines from human peripheral blood mononuclear cells. Phytother Res 21: 914–920.
36. Wang D, Stockard CR, Harkins L, Lott P, Salih C, et al. (2008) Immunohistochemistry for the evaluation of angiogenesis in tumor xenografts. Biotech Histochem 83:179–189.
37. Kim H, Cho HJ, Kim SW, Liu B, Choi YJ, et al. (2010) CD31+ cells represent highly angiogenic and vasculogenic cells in bone marrow novel role of nonendothelial CD31+ cells in neovascularization and their therapeutic effects on ischemic vascular disease. Circ Res 107:602–614.
38. Goel S, Wong AH, Jain RK (2012) Vascular normalization as a therapeutic strategy for malignant and nonmalignant disease. Cold Spring Harb Perspect Med 2:a006486. doi: 10.1101/cshperspect.a006486.
39. Dudley AC (2012) Tumor endothelial cell. Cold Spring Harb Perspect Med 2:a006536.
40. Jain RK (2005) Normalization of tumor vasculature: an emerging concept in antiangiogenic therapy. Science 307:58–62.
41. Batchelor TT1, Sorensen AG, di Tomaso E, Zhang WT, Duda DG, et al. (2007) AZD2171, a pan-VEGF receptor tyrosine kinase inhibitor, normalizes tumor vasculature and alleviates edema in glioblastoma patients. Cancer Cell 11:83–95.

42. Kaigler D, Krebsbach PH, Polverini PJ, Mooney DJ (2003) Role of vascular endothelial growth factor in bone marrow stromal cell modulation of endothelial cells. Tissue Engineering 9:95-103.

43. Guillem EB, Nyhus JK, Wolford CC, Friece CR, Sampsel JW (2002) Vascular endothelial Growth factor secretion by tumor-infiltrating macrophages essentially supports tumor angiogenesis and IgG immune complexes potentiate the process. Cancer Res 62:7042–7049.

44. Niethammer AG, Xiang R, Becker JC, Wodrich H, Pertl U, et al. (2002) A DNA vaccine against VEGF receptor 2 prevents effective angiogenesis and inhibits tumor growth. Nat Med 8: 1369–1375.

45. Rafiee P, Heidemann J, Ogawa H, Johnson NA, Fisher PJ, et al. (2004) Cyclosporin A differentially inhibits multiple steps in VEGF induced angiogenesis in human microvascular endothelial cells through altered intracellular signaling. Cell Commun Signal 2:3.

46. Hernández GL, Volpert OV, Iñiguez MA, Lorenzo E, Martínez-Martínez S, et al. (2001) Selective inhibition of vascular endothelial growth factor-mediated angiogenesis by cyclosporin A: roles of the nuclear factor of activated T cells and cyclooxygenase 2. J Exp Med 193:607–620.

47. Duraiswamy J, Kaluza KM, Freeman GJ, Coukos G (2013) Dual blockade of PD-1 and CTLA-4 combined with tumor vaccine effectively restores T-cell rejection function in tumors. Cancer Res 73: 3591–3603.

48. Zhou H, Luo Y, Mizutani M, Mizutani N, Reisfeld RA, et al. (2005) T cell-mediated suppression of angiogenesis results in tumor protective immunity. Blood 106:2026–2032.

49. Qin Z, Schwartzkopff J, Pradera F, Kammertoens T, Seliger B, et al. (2003) A Critical Requirement of Interferon γ-mediated Angiostasis for Tumor Rejection by CD8+ T Cells. Cancer Research 63:4095–4100.

50. Abdollahi A, Folkman J (2010) Evading tumor evasion: current concepts and perspectives of anti-angiogenic cancer therapy. Drug Resist Update 13:16–28.

51. Itasaka S, Komaki R, Herbst RS, Shibuya K, Shintani T, et al. (2007) Endostatin improves radioresponse and blocks tumor revascularization after radiation therapy for A431 xenografts in mice. Int J Radiat Oncol Biol Phys 7:870–878.

52. Cirone P, Bourgeois JM, Shen F, Chang PL (2004) Combined immunotherapy and antiangiogenic therapy of cancer with microencapsulated cells. Hum Gene Ther 15:945–959.

53. Shi S, Wang R, Chen Y, Song H, Chen L, et al. (2013) Combining Antiangiogenic Therapy with Adoptive Cell Immunotherapy Exerts Better Antitumor Effects in NonSmall Cell Lung Cancer Models. PLoS One 8: e65757.

54. Baral R, Mandal I, Chattopadhyay U (2005) Immunostimulatory neem leaf preparation acts as an adjuvant to enhance the efficacy of poorly immunogenic B16 melanoma surface antigen vaccine. Int Immunopharmacol 5:1343–1352.

55. Chakraborty K, Bose A, Pal S, Sarkar K, Goswami S, et al. (2008) Neem leaf glycoprotein restores the impaired chemotactic activity of peripheral blood mononuclear cells from head and neck squamous cell carcinoma patients by maintaining CXCR3/CXCL10 balance. Int Immunopharmacol 8:330–340.

56. Bailey JL (1967) Miscelleneous analytical methods. In: Bailey JL (ed) Techniques in Protein Chemistry, Elsevier Science, NY, USA.

10

Loss of Sirt3 Limits Bone Marrow Cell-Mediated Angiogenesis and Cardiac Repair in Post-Myocardial Infarction

Heng Zeng, Lanfang Li, Jian-Xiong Chen*

Department of Pharmacology and Toxicology, University of Mississippi Medical Center, Jackson, Mississippi, United States of America

Abstract

Sirtuin-3 (Sirt3) has a critical role in the regulation of human aging and reactive oxygen species (ROS) formation. A recent study has identified Sirt3 as an essential regulator of stem cell aging. This study investigated whether Sirt3 is necessary for bone marrow cell (BMC)-mediated cardiac repair in post-myocardial infarction (MI). *In vitro*, BMC-derived endothelial progenitor cells (EPCs) from wild type (WT) and Sirt3KO mice were cultured. EPC angiogenesis, ROS formation and apoptosis were assessed. *In vivo*, WT and Sirt3 KO mice were subjected to MI and BMCs from WT and Sirt3 KO mice were injected into ischemic area immediately. The expression of VEGF and VEGFR2 was reduced in Sirt3KO-EPCs. Angiogenic capacities and colony formation were significantly impaired in Sirt3KO-EPCs compared to WT-EPCs. Loss of Sirt3 further enhanced ROS formation and apoptosis in EPCs. Overexpression of Sirt3 or treatment with NADPH oxidase inhibitor apocynin (Apo, 200 and 400 microM) rescued these abnormalities. In post-MI mice, BMC treatment increased number of $Sca1^+/c-kit^+$ cells; enhanced VEGF expression and angiogenesis whereas Sirt3KO-BMC treatment had little effects. BMC treatment also attenuated NADPH oxidase subunits $p47^{phox}$ and $gp91^{phox}$ expression, and significantly reduced ROS formation, apoptosis, fibrosis and hypertrophy in post-MI mice. Sirt3KO-BMC treatment did not display these beneficial effects. In contrast, Sirt3KO mice treated with BMCs from WT mice attenuated myocardial apoptosis, fibrosis and improved cardiac function. Our data demonstrate that Sirt3 is essential for BMC therapy; and loss of Sirt3 limits BMC-mediated angiogenesis and cardiac repair in post-MI.

Editor: Guo-Chang Fan, University of Cincinnati, College of Medicine, United States of America

Funding: This study was supported by grants from the National Institutes of Health (NIH grant HL102042 to J.X. Chen). The funders had no role in study design, data collection and analysis, decision to publish, or preparation of the manuscript.

Competing Interests: The authors have declared that no competing interests exist.

* Email: JChen3@umc.edu

Introduction

Sirtuins belong to a highly conserved family (Sirtuin 1–7) of histone/protein deacetylases and its activity is closely associated with the prolong lifespan of organisms such as yeast, worms and flies as well as mammalian [1]. Sirtuins mediate histone protein post-translational modification by coupling lysine deacetylation to NAD^+ hydrolysis [2,3]. Sirtuins have critical roles in the regulation of various cell functions, including cardiomyocytes and endothelial cells [4–7]. Sirtuins have been shown to involve in biological functions related to cell growth, aging, stress tolerance as well as cell metabolism [1,8]. Accumulating evidence indicates an important role of Sirt3 in the genetic control of human aging. Older individuals have about 40% reduced Sirt3 levels when compared with younger subjects, and the health benefits of older patients are accompanied by the elevation of Sirt3 levels [9]. Further, increased levels of Sirt3 are associated with an extended lifespan of man [10,11]. Calorie restriction has been shown to increase Sirt3 expression and improve cardiovascular function [12]. Moreover, Sirt3 KO mice are resistant to the protective effects of calorie restriction against oxidative damage [13]. In contrast, overexpression of Sirt3 blocks cardiac hypertrophy by

suppressing reactive oxygen species (ROS) formation. Knockout of Sirt3 in mice promotes angiotensin II-induced cardiac hypertrophy [14,15].

Myocardial infarction (MI) has been shown to induce rapid mobilization of bone marrow derived cells (BMCs) such as endothelial progenitor cells (EPCs), mesenchymal stromal cells and pluripotent very small embryonic-like cells into circulation and home to sites of ischemic area, and promote neovascularization [16,17]. BMC treatment has been shown to lead to a reduction of infarct size and improvement of cardiac function in post-MI [18]. BMCs have been identified as promising candidates for use as cellular therapies for cardiac regeneration and repair in post-MI. Sirt3 is a key regulator of mitochondria ROS formation and telomere length [14,19]. Recent studies highlight the important role of Sirt3 in BMC-derived stem cells [20,21]. Sirt3 expression is significantly reduced in aged hematopoietic stem cells (HSCs). Moreover, upregulation of Sirt3 expression improves their regenerative capacity in aged HSCs [21]. Consistent with these findings, our recent study also shows that loss of Sirt3 attenuates apelin-overexpressing BMC-mediated improvement of cardiac repair and function in post-MI [20]. However, the direct roles of

Sirt3 in the stem cell therapy-mediated cardiac repair and functional recovery in post-MI remain undefined. In this study, we tested our hypothesis that Sirt3 in the BMCs is essential for the stem cell therapy-mediated angiogenesis and cardiac repair in post-MI.

Using BMCs and EPCs from wild type (WT) mice and Sirt3 knockout (Sirt3KO) mice, this study was to determine: (1) whether loss of Sirt3 in EPCs reduces angiogenic growth factor expression and blunts their proangiogenic and anti-apoptotic capacities; (2) whether loss of Sirt3 in BMCs dampens BMC-mediated angiogenesis and cardiac repair in post-MI mice.

Materials and Methods

Ethics Statement

All procedures conformed to the Institute for Laboratory Animal Research Guide for the Care and Use of Laboratory Animals and were approved by the University of Mississippi Medical Center Animal Care and Use Committee (Protocol ID: 1280). The investigation conforms to the Guide for the Care and Use of Laboratory Animals published by the US National Institutes of Health (NIH Publication No. 85–23, revised 1996).

Surgical procedures

Global Sirt3 knockout mice and wild type control of Sirt3 mice (WT) was purchased from Jackson laboratory (Bar Harbor, ME) and breeding by our laboratory. Male Sirt3KO and WT mice at age 12 weeks were used for the experiments. Male mice were anesthetized with ketamine (100 mg/kg) plus xylazine (15 mg/kg), intubated, and artificially ventilated with room air. Adequate anesthesia was monitored by toe pinch. Myocardial infarction was achieved by ligation of the left anterior descending coronary artery (LAD). Sham controls underwent surgery without the LAD [22,23,24]. After induction of myocardial ischemia (IS), mice were intramyocardial injected with fresh donor bone marrow–derived mononuclear cells (1×10^7 cells) immediately [20]. Two weeks after myocardial infarction, mice were sacrificed by cervical dislocation under anesthesia with isoflurane.

Analysis of APJ$^+$/Sca1$^+$/c-kit$^+$ cells in the heart

Heart tissue sections (8 μm) from injected area of ischemia were incubated with Sca1 and c-kit (1:200 Santa Cruz, CA) antibodies overnight. Sca1 was visualized using FITC labeled goat anti-mouse IgG antibodies; c-kit was visualized with Fluorolink Cy3 labeled goat anti-mouse IgG antibodies. Myocardial Sca1$^+$/c-kit$^+$ cells in the injected area were assessed by counting the number of positive cells per 100 nuclei [22,25].

Western analysis of Sirt3, VEGF, VEGFR2, eNOS, Akt, p47^{phox}, gp91^{phox}, CXCR4, beclin-1 and LC3-I/II expression

The hearts or EPCs were harvested and homogenized in lysis buffer for Western blot analysis. Total protein concentrations were determined using a BCA protein assay kit (Pierce Co, IL). Fifteen μg of protein were subjected to SDS-PAGE on 10% polyacrylamide gels and transferred to a nitrocellulose membrane. The blot was probed with Sirt3, VEGFR2, Akt and eNOS (1:1000, Cell Signaling, MA), VEGF, CXCR-4, gp91^{phox}, p47^{phox}, LC3-I/II and beclin-1 (1:1000, Santa Cruz, CA) antibodies. The membranes were then washed and incubated with a secondary antibody coupled to horseradish peroxidase and densitometric analysis was carried out using image acquisition and analysis software (TINA 2.0).

Analysis of myocardial capillary and arteriole densities

Eight-micrometer sections were cut and incubated with fluorescein-labeled Isolectin B4 (1:200; IB4, Molecular Probe, Invitrogen, OR) and Cy3-conjugated anti-α smooth muscle actin (SMA) (1:100; Sigma). The number of capillaries (IB4-positive EC) in the border zone area was counted and expressed as capillary density per square millimeter (mm^2) of tissue. Myocardial arteriole density was measured using image analysis software (Image J, NIH, MD) [22,24].

Myocardial apoptosis and ROS formation

Heart tissue sections were stained with transferase deoxyuridine nick end labeling (TUNEL) following the manufacturer's instructions (Promega, WI). Apoptosis was indexed by counting TUNEL positive cells per 100 nuclei in the infarcted area [22,23]. ROS formation in the infarcted area was measured and quantified by staining with DHE as previously described [26].

Hemodynamic measurements

Experimental mice were anesthetized with ketamine (100 mg/kg) plus xylazine (15 mg/kg), intubated and artificially ventilated with room air. A 1.4-Fr pressure–conductance catheter (SPR-839, Millar Instrument, TX) was inserted into the left ventricle (LV) to record baseline cardiac hemodynamics of the hearts [22,25].

Heart weight to body weight ratio (HW/BW) and fibrosis

Cardiac hypertrophy was assessed by measuring heart-to-body weight ratio at 14 days post-myocardial ischemia. Cardiac β-myosin heavy chain (β-MHC) (1:1000, abcam, MA) and atrial natriuretic peptide (ANP) (1:1000, Santa Cruz, CA) expression were examined by western blot analysis. Cardiac fibrosis was stained with Masson's trichrome (MT, Sigma, MO) and quantified by measuring the blue fibrotic area [24].

Cultured EPC proliferation, tuber formation and apoptosis

Wild type (WT) mice and Sirt3 knockout mice were sacrificed by cervical dislocation under anesthesia with isoflurane. BM–derived EPC were obtained by flushing the tibias and femurs with 10% FBS EGM. EPC was isolated and cultured from femur and tibia bone marrow of WT and Sirt3KO mice as described previously [22,23]. Two EPC markers, IB4 (1:50 dilute) and CD34 (1:200 dilute), were used for EPC identification by immunohistochemistry. Deficiency of Sirt3 in the EPCs was verified by western blot analysis. For the cell proliferation measurement, EPCs were cultured in 10%FBS EGM for 72 hours. The proliferative capacity of cultured EPCs was assayed using a cell proliferation (MTT) kit according to the manufacturer's instructions (Roche Diagnostic Corp., IN, USA) [27,28]. In the apoptosis study, EPCs apoptosis was induced by exposure of cultured EPCs to serum-free medium for 48 hours. The number of apoptotic cells was then examined by counting TUNEL positive cells per 100 nuclei in cultured EPCs.

Measurement of intracellular ROS formation in cultured EPCs

Intracellular ROS were determined by oxidative conversion of cell permeable chloromethyl-2′,7′-dichlorodihydrofluorescein diacetate (CM-H$_2$DCFDA, Molecular Probes, OR) to fluorescent dichlorofluorescein (DCF). Briefly, BMCs cultured in 2 well chamber slides were incubated with 10 μM CM-H$_2$DCFDA in PBS for 30 minutes. DCF fluorescence was measured over the whole field of vision using an EVOS fluorescence microscope connected to an imaging system as previously described [29,30].

BM colony-forming cell assay

BM–derived mononuclear cells were isolated from WT and Sirt3 KO mice. BMCs (105 cells per dish) were then seeded in 2% methylcellulose medium. After 7 days of incubation, BMC colony formation and colony number were scored under phase-contrast microscopy [31].

Statistical analysis

The results were expressed as the mean $\pm$ SD. Statistical analysis was performed using one way ANOVA followed by post hoc multiple comparisons test. Significance was set at $P<0.05$.

Results

Loss of Sirt3 in BMCs reduces c-kit$^+$/Sca1$^+$ cells in post-MI mice

We first examined whether Sirt3 expression is altered in the hearts of post-MI mice. As shown in Fig 1A, there was a significant reduction of Sirt3 expression in the hearts of post-MI mice. Interestingly, BMC treatment led to a significant increase in Sirt3 expression in post-MI mice when compared with control post-MI mice (**Fig 1A**). Treatment with Sirt3 KO-BMCs also increased Sirt3 expression in the ischemic hearts of WT mice, but it was significantly less than WT-BMC treatment (Fig 1A).

We next examined whether BMC treatment increases vascular progenitor cells in the infarcted hearts. The number of c-kit$^+$/Sca1$^+$ cells was evaluated at 14 days after BMC intramyocardial injection. As shown in **Fig 1 B and C**, the number of c-kit$^+$/Sca1$^+$ cells was increased in the mouse infarcted heart after 14 days of MI, however, no c-kit$^+$/Sca1$^+$ cell was detected in the non-ischemic sham control mice. BMC treatment significantly increased the number of c-kit$^+$/Sca1$^+$ cells compared to saline treatment (**Fig 1 B and C**). Injection with Sirt3KO-BMCs had a significant lower number of c-kit$^+$/Sca1$^+$ cells in infarcted hearts in comparison with BMC treated mice (**Fig 1 B and C**). To

determine whether the increased c-kit$^+$/Sca1$^+$ cells came from the donor or the recipient, mice were intramyocardial injected with GFP$^+$-BMCs or GFP$^+$-Sirt3KO-BMCs. No GFP$^+$-BMCs or GFP$^+$-Sirt3KO-BMCs were found in hearts of post-MI mice after 14 and 28 days of BMC treatment (data not shown), indicating these cells may came from recipient but not from donor.

Loss of Sirt3 increases ROS formation and apoptosis in EPCs

Knockout of Sirt3 in BM-derived HSCs has been reported to lead to a 50% reduction in self- renewal compared to WT mice after serial transplantations [21]. We then examined whether loss of Sirt3 affected EPCs function in vitro. Our western blot analysis confirmed that Sirt3 expression was absent in EPCs isolated from Sirt3KO mice (**Fig 2A**). In cultured EPCs, there was a significant increase in ROS formation in Sirt3KO-EPCs when compared with WT-EPCs (**Fig 2 B and C**). Moreover, knockout of Sirt3 in EPCs resulted in a significant increase in stress-induced cell apoptosis. Overexpression of Sirt3 significantly reduced stress-induced EPC apoptosis (**Fig 2 D**). Moreover, treatment of Sirt3KO-EPCs with NADPH oxidase inhibitor apocynin (Apo, 200 and 400 microM) attenuated EPC apoptosis in a dose-dependent manner (**Fig 2E**). Interestingly, autophagy marker LC3-I/II was reduced in Sirt3KO-EPCs. Treatment of Sirt3KO-EPCs with Apo (200 and 400 microM) resulted in an increase in LC3-II levels. Furthermore, overexpression of Sirt3 rescued impairment of LC3-II expression in Sirt3KO-EPCs (**Fig 2F**).

Loss of Sirt3 reduces angiogenic growth factor expression and angiogenesis in EPCs

Similarly, the proliferation of EPCs was significantly reduced in Sirt3KO-EPCs compared with WT-EPCs (**Fig 3A**). Loss of Sirt3 in EPCs resulted in a significant decrease in tube formation when compared with WT-EPCs. In contrast, overexpression of Sirt3 in WT-EPCs significantly enhanced EPC tube formation (**Fig 3B**). EPC colony formation was significantly lower in Sirt3KO-EPCs than WT-EPCs (**Fig 3C**). In addition, VEGF and VEGFR2 levels

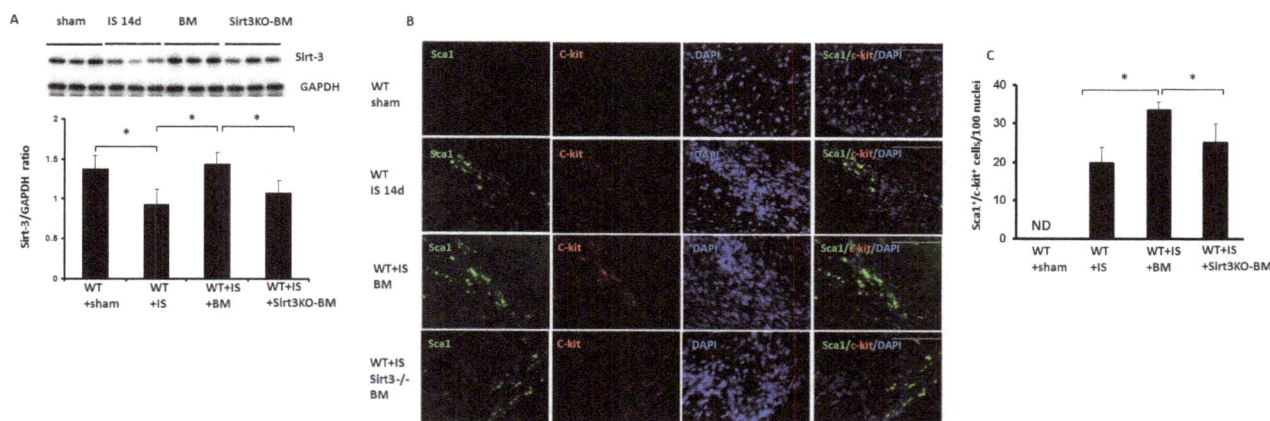

Figure 1. Loss of Sirt3 reduces c-kit$^+$/Sca1$^+$ cell in post MI mice. A. Western blot analysis revealing that Sirt3 expression was significantly reduced in post-MI mice. BMC treatment significantly increased Sirt3 expression compared to post-MI mice. Loss of Sirt3 blunted BMC-mediated upregulation of Sirt3. n = 6 mice, *p<0.05. **B.** Immunofluorescence images showing co-localization of Sca1 and c-kit in the border zone of ischemic mouse hearts. Sca1 was stained with mouse Sca1 antibody (green, 10X). c-kit was stained with rabbit c-kit antibody (red, 10X) and nuclei were stained with DAPI (blue, 10X). **C.** Quantitative analysis of Sca1$^+$/c-kit$^+$ cells demonstrating that the number of Sca1$^+$/c-kit$^+$ cells was increased at 14 days of post-MI mice. BMCs significantly increased Sca1$^+$/c-kit$^+$ cells compared to saline treatment. Treatment with Sirt3KO-BMC had a significant lower number Sca1$^+$/c-kit$^+$ cells in infracted heart compared to the BMC treated mice. All data represent mean $\pm$ SD; n = 5, *p<0.05. ND = not detected.

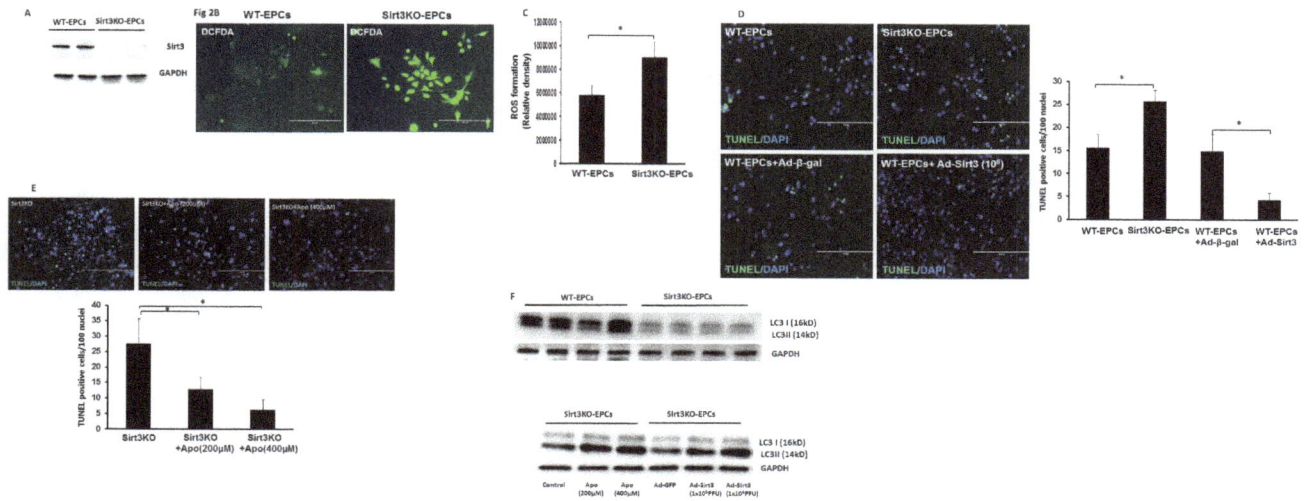

Figure 2. Loss of Sirt3 increases ROS formation and apoptosis in EPCs. A. Western blot analysis showing that Sirt3 expression was absent in EPCs isolated from Sirt3KO mice. n = 2 mice. **B and C**. Representative images and quantification of intracellular ROS formation measured by CM-H_2DCFDA staining in cultured EPCs. ROS formation was significantly increased in cultured EPCs of Sirt3KO mice when compared with that of WT mice (n = 4 mice, *p<0.05). **D and E**. Representative images and quantification of TUNEL positive cell in cultured EPCs. Apoptotic cells were identified by TUNEL staining (green, 20x). Cell apoptosis was significantly increased in cultured EPCs of Sirt3KO mice compared to that of WT mice. Infection of WT-EPC with Ad-Sirt3 (10^6 PFU) significantly reduced EPC apoptosis (n = 6 mice, *p<0.05). Treatment of Sirt3KO-EPC with NADPH oxidase inhibitor apocynin (Apo, 200 and 400 μM significantly reduced EPC apoptosis (n = 6 mice, *p<0.05). **F**. Western blot analysis showing that the basal levels of autophagy gene LC3 II expression were dramatic reduced in the Sirt3KO-EPCs when compared with WT-EPCs. Treatment of Sirt3KO-EPCs with Apo 200 and 400 μM or infection of Sirt3KO-EPCs with Ad-Sirt3 resulted in an increase in LC3 II expression (n = 3 mice).

were reduced in Sirt3KO-EPCs; whereas treatment with Apo (200 and 400 microM) or overexpression of Sirt3 rescued impaired VEGF/VEGFR2 expression in Sirt3KO-EPCs (**Fig 3D and E**). Intriguingly, basal levels of CXCR-4, an EPC recruitment factor, were significantly decreased in Sirt3KO-EPCs when compared with WT-EPCs (**Fig 3F**).

Loss of Sirt3 in BMCs increases p47^{phox} and gp91^{phox} expression in the heart of post-MI

To determine whether Sirt3 is involved in BMC-mediated suppression of ROS formation, NADPH oxidase subunits p47^{phox} and gp91^{phox} expression was examined in the hearts of post-MI mice. BMC treatment led to a significant reduction of NADPH oxidase subunits p47^{phox} and gp91^{phox} expression in ischemic hearts (**Fig 4 A and B**). This was accompanied by a significant reduction of ROS formation in post-MI mice (**Fig 4 C**). In contrast, treatment with Sirt3KO-BMCs did not inhibit p47^{phox} and gp91^{phox} expression in post-MI mice (**Fig 4 A and B**). ROS formation was significantly elevated in Sirt3KO-BMCs + MI mice when compared to WT-BMCs + MI mice (**Fig 4C**).

Loss of Sirt3 in BMCs impairs angiogenesis in post-MI

To elucidate whether Sirt3 in the BMCs is necessary for the myocardial angiogenesis, VEGF, capillary and arteriole densities were examined in post-MI mice. BMC treatment significantly increased VEGF expression in the hearts of post-MI mice. VEGF expression was significantly decreased in Sirt3KO-BMCs + MI mice compared with WT-BMCs + MI mice (**Fig 5A**). BMC treatment further significantly increased capillary and arteriole densities in the border zone of ischemic hearts. However, myocardial capillary and arteriole densities were not significantly increased in Sirt3KO-BMCs + MI mice when compared with post-MI mice (**Fig 5 B-E**).

Sirt3 is necessary for BMC-mediated anti-apoptosis in ischemic hearts

To further elucidate whether Sirt3 in the BMCs is also necessary for the cardiac repair of BMC therapy, myocardial autophagy gene expression, apoptosis, fibrosis and hypertrophy were examined in post-MI mice. Treatment with BMCs led to a significant increase in autophagy gene beclin-1 expression and elevation of LC3-II/I ratio in post-MI mice (**Fig 6A and B**). Beclin-1 expression and LC3-II/I ratio was significantly decreased in Sirt3KO-BMCs+MI mice when compared with WT-BMCs + MI mice. BMC treatment significantly elevated phosphorylation levels of Akt and eNOS in post-MI mice (**Fig 6C and D**). The phosphorylation levels of Akt and eNOS were significantly reduced in Sirt3KO-BMCs + MI mice compared to BMCs+ MI mice. BMC treatment furthermore significantly reduced cardiac apoptosis, but Sirt3KO-BMC treatment did not affect cell apoptosis in post-MI mice (**Fig 6 E and F**).

Loss of Sirt3 in BMCs limits BMC-mediated cardiac repair and functional recovery

In comparison with control post-MI mice, the HW/BW ratio and expression of hypertrophic gene β-MHC and ANP were significantly reduced in the BMCs + MI mice (**Fig 7 A, B, C**). Sirt3KO-BMC treatment did not suppress cardiac hypertrophy compared with BMC treatment (**Fig 7 A, B, C**). BMC treatment also significantly suppressed cardiac fibrosis formation whereas Sirt3KO-BMC treatment had little effects (**Fig 7D**).

After 28 days of myocardial ischemia, post-MI mice exhibited a significant elevation of end-systolic volume (ESV) and reduction of end-systolic pressure (ESP) (**Fig 7E**). The post-MI mice also showed a significant decline in +dp/dtmax and -dp/dtmin pressures compared to non-ischemic sham controls (**Fig 7F**). BMC treatment resulted in a significant decrease in ESV and a dramatic improvement of ESP, +dp/dtmax and -dp/dtmin

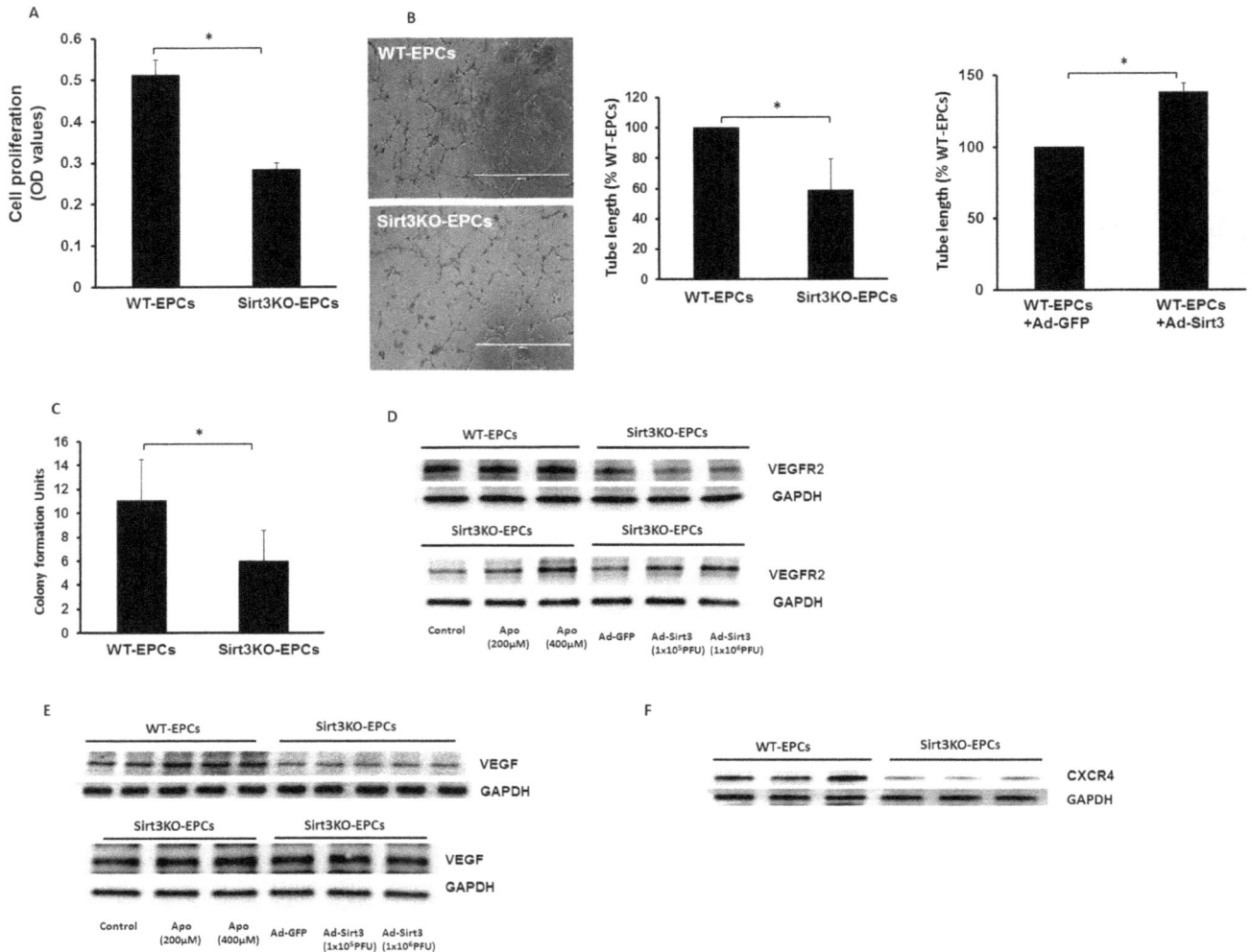

Figure 3. Loss of Sirt3 impairs VEGF/VEGFR2 expression and angiogenesis in EPCs. A. Cell proliferation was measured by MTT assay. The proliferative rate of EPCs was significantly reduced in cultured EPCs of Sirt3KO mice compared to that of WT mice (n = 4 mice, *p<0.05). **B.** EPC tube formation was significantly reduced in EPCs lack of Sirt3 when compared with control EPCs. Overexpression of Sirt3 significantly increased EPC tube formation (n = 4–6 mice, *p<0.05). **C.** BMC colony formation units. EPC colony formation was significantly reduced in Sirt3KO-EPCs when compared with WT-EPCs (n = 6 mice, *p<0.05). **D and E.** Western blot analysis showing that the basal levels of VEGF and VEGFR2 were significantly reduced in Sirt3KO-EPCs (n = 3 mice). Treatment of Sirt3KO-EPCs with NADPH oxidase inhibitor apocynin 200 and 400 μM or infection of Sirt3KO-EPCs with Ad-Sirt3 increased levels of VEGF and VEGFR2 expression (n = 3 mice). **F.** Western blot analysis showing that the basal levels of CXCR-4 expression were dramatic reduced in the Sirt3KO-EPCs (n = 3 mice).

pressures in post-MI mice. Sirt3KO-BMC treatment had little effects on the improvement of these parameters when compared with WT-BMC treatment (**Fig 7E and F**). In contrast, treatment of Sirt3KO post-MI mice with WT-BMCs resulted in a significant reduction of cardiac apoptosis and cardiac fibrosis formation (**Fig 7 G and H**). This was accompanied by a significant improvement of cardiac function in Sirt3KO post-MI mice (**Fig 7I**).

Discussion

Our present study demonstrates that loss of Sirt3 in EPCs reduced angiogenic growth factor expression and angiogenic capacity. Loss of Sirt3 in EPCs increased ROS formation and promoted cell apoptosis *in vitro*. Furthermore, loss of Sirt3 in BMCs abolished BMC therapy mediated protective effects and limited cardiac repair in post-MI mice. Our study suggests that

Sirt3 in BMCs is necessary for the protective effects of stem cell therapy in post-MI.

Sirt3 has been reported to be a major mitochondrial deacetylase in human [2,32,33]. Previous studies show that Sirt3 exists in the mitochondria of the heart [34,35]. Our recent study indicates a critical role of Sirt3 in apelin-overexpressing BMC-mediated improvement of angiogenesis and cardiac function in post-MI mice [20]. In present study, we show that treatment with BMCs resulted in a significant increase in Sirt3 expression in post-MI mice. We then further investigated if BMC treatment improved Sca1$^+$/c-kit$^+$ progenitor cells in ischemic hearts. Our data demonstrated that the number of Sca1$^+$/c-kit$^+$ progenitor cells in ischemic hearts was increased at 14 days of post-MI. Injection of BMCs significantly increased the number of Sca1$^+$/c-kit$^+$ cells and promoted cardiac repair at ischemic area in post-MI mice. Intriguingly, the number of Sca1$^+$/c-kit$^+$ cells was significantly reduced in Sirt3KO-BMC treatment. This was accompanied by a

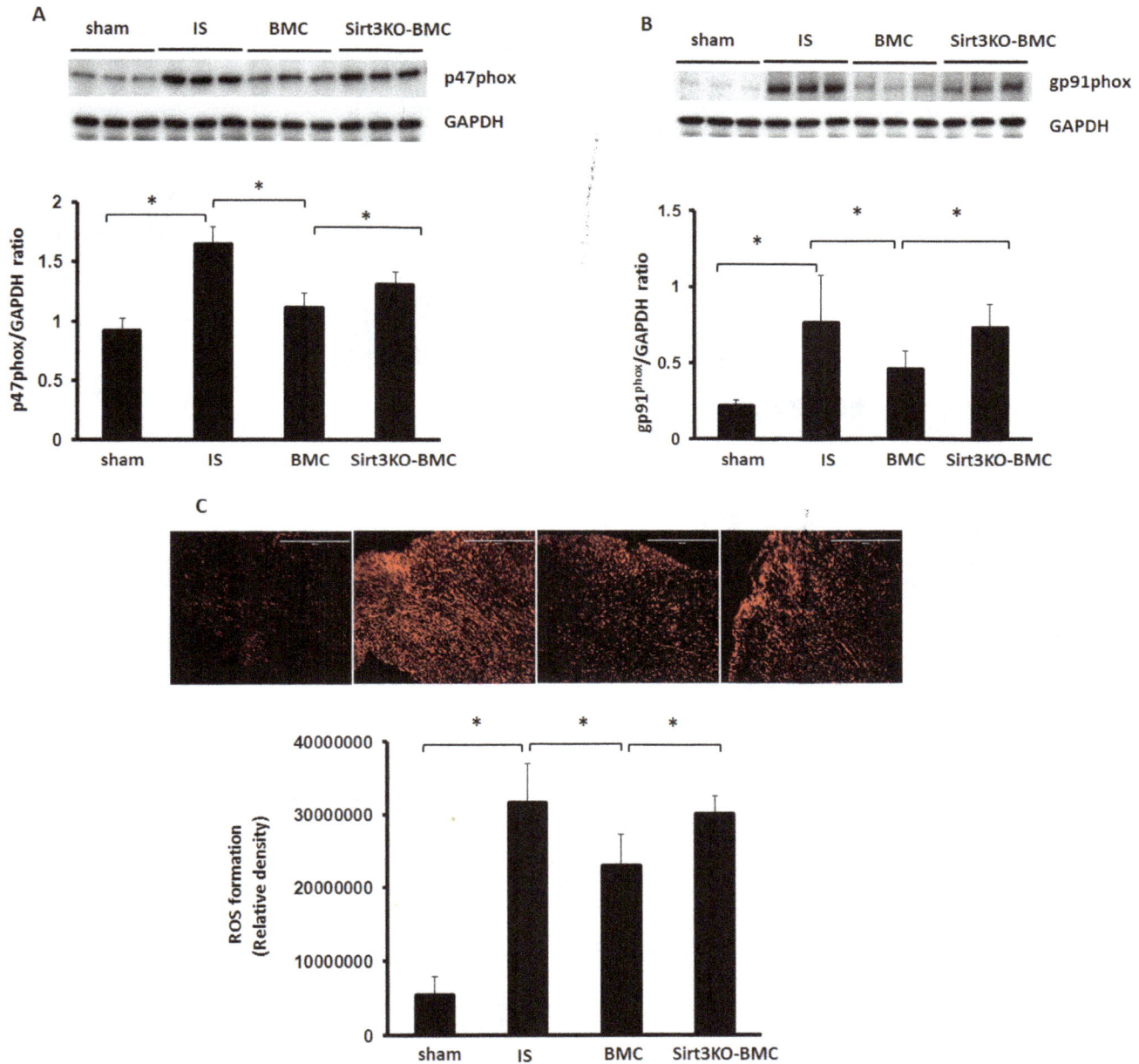

Figure 4. Loss of Sirt3 in BMCs increases ROS formation in post-MI mice. A and B. Western blot analysis revealing that BMC treatment resulted in a significant downregulation of p47^{phox} (A) and gp91^{phox} (B) expression compared to post-MI mice. Sirt3KO-BMC treatment did not inhibit expression of p47^{phox} and gp91^{phox} compared to BMC treatment. n = 6 mice, *p<0.05. **C**. Quantitative analysis of ROS formation by DHE staining revealing that BMC treatment resulted in a significant suppression of ROS formation compared to post-MI mice. Myocardial ROS formation was significantly higher in Sirt3KO-BMC treated mice than BMC treated mice. n = 5 mice; *p<0.05.

significant decline of cardiac function in post-MI mice. A recent study demonstrated that there was no difference in the number of BM derived HSCs (Lin$^-$, c-kit$^+$, sca1$^+$) between WT and Sirt3 KO mice [21]. Consistent with this study, we did not found any GFP$^+$-BMCs or GFP$^+$-Sirt3KO-BMCs in hearts of post-MI mice after 14 and 28 days of BMC treatment, suggesting that injected BMCs had not differentiated into Sca1$^+$/c-kit$^+$ cells in ischemic hearts and Sca1$^+$/c-kit$^+$ cells was not coming from injected BMCs. CXCR-4 has been identified as a key mediator that regulates vascular progenitor cell homing into the ischemic area and contributes to improvement of cardiac function after MI [36].

CXCR-4 has been shown to protect the heart after myocardial infarction via promoting stem cell recruitment [36–38]. We therefore speculated that these increased Sca1$^+$/c-kit$^+$ cells may be recruited to ischemic area due to releasing CXCR-4 after BMC treatment. This notion was confirmed by our data that the basic levels of CXCR-4 were significantly reduced in Sirt3KO-EPCs. Our data suggest that impairment of CXCR-4 expression in EPCs and reduction of number of Sca1$^+$/c-kit$^+$ stem cell in infarcted area may be responsible for impairment of cardiac repair in Sirt3KO-BMC treatment in post-MI mice.

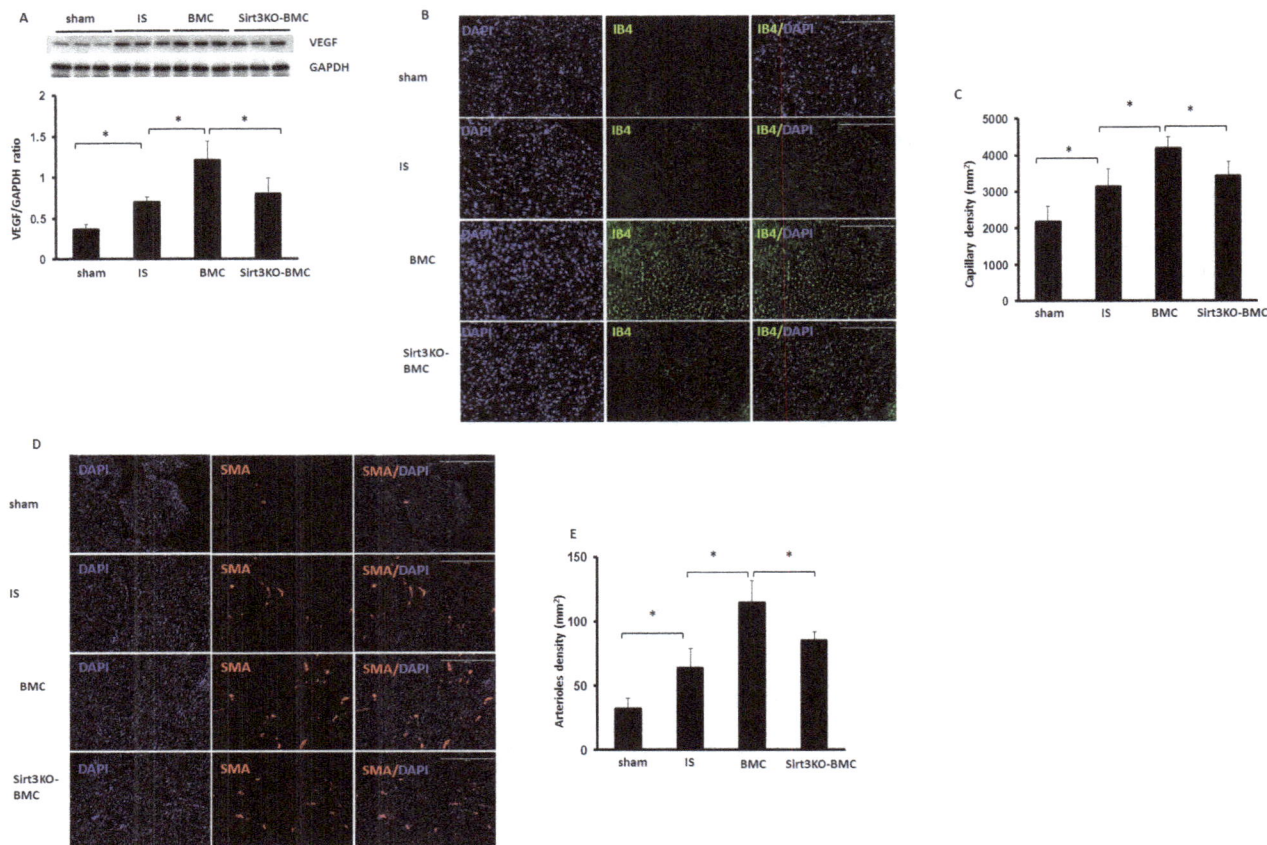

Figure 5. Loss of Sirt3 blunts BMC-induced VEGF expression and angiogenesis. A. Western blot analysis showing that VEGF expression was significantly reduced in Sirt3KO-BMC treated mice compared to BMC treated mice. n = 6 mice; *p<0.05. **B and C**. Myocardial ischemia significantly increased myocardial capillary density by IB4 staining (green, 10x). BMC treatment significantly increased capillary formation compared to post-MI mice. Myocardial capillary density was significant reduced in Sirt3KO-BMC treated mice compared to BMC treated mice. n = 5 mice; *p<0.05. **D and E**. BMC treatment significantly increased myocardial arteriole density by SMA staining (Red, 10x) in post-MI mice. Myocardial arteriole density was significantly decreased in post-MI mice treatment with Sirt3KO-BMCs compared to mice treated with BMCs. n = 5 mice; *p<0.05.

The present study provides evidence that basal Sirt3 activity in EPC is required for the protective effects afforded by BMC therapy in post-MI. Myocardial ischemia has been shown to induce rapid mobilization of bone marrow derived vascular progenitor cells from the bone marrow niches [39,40]. BMCs are recruited into the sites of infarcted area and promote cardiac repair in the infarcted hearts [16,17]. BMCs have been shown to promote cardiac repair and improve functional recovery of post-MI; however, the molecular mechanisms by which BMCs promotes cardiac repair are incompletely understood. Our data, for the first time, showed that Sirt3 levels were reduced in ischemic hearts. Recently studies have directly linked loss of Sirt3 contributing to the ROS formation. Sirt3-deficient cells subjected to metabolic stress lead to a significant increase in ROS formation [41]. Furthermore, cardiomyocytes cultured from Sirt3KO mice show increased ROS production. Sirt3 protects cardiomyocytes from oxidative stress-mediated cell death [15]. Therefore, reduction of Sirt3 levels in the ischemic hearts may contribute to increased ROS formation and apoptosis. In line with these studies, our present data also showed that loss of Sirt3 in EPCs enhanced ROS formation and increased stress-induced cell apoptosis. Furthermore, treatment with NADPH oxidase inhibitor reduced Sirt3KO-EPC apoptosis *in vitro*. Overexpression of Sirt3 protected EPCs against stress-induced cell apoptosis. Our data further

showed that intramyocardial delivery of BMCs in infarcted area led to a significant increase in Sirt3 expression. Moreover, treatment with BMCs resulted in a significant reduction of NADPH oxidase p47^{phox} and gp91^{phox} expression and ROS formation. In contrast, loss of Sirt3 in BMCs significantly blunted BMC therapy mediated upregulation of Sirt3 and suppression of ROS formation. This was accompanied by a significant increase in myocardial apoptosis in post-MI mice. Taken together, our data suggest that a critical role of Sirt3 in the regulation of ROS formation and apoptosis in the ischemic heart and that increased ROS formation and apoptosis in Sirt3KO-EPCs maybe also contribute, at least in part, to the failure of Sirt3KO-BMC treatment in post-MI.

Aging bone marrow cells have been shown to fail to promote cardiac angiogenesis and improve cardiac function [42]. Both experimental and clinical studies demonstrated that aging interferes with bone marrow derived progenitor cell functions [43–45]. ROS formation is increased in HSCs with age. This is accompanied by an increased HSCs apoptosis and impairment of self-renewal capacity. Sirt3 expression is significantly reduced with the aging in skeletal muscle [9]. A recent study also shows a significant reduction of Sirt3 levels with age or stress in HSCs. Overexpression of Sirt3 in HSCs from old mice improves regenerative capacity of aged HSCs [21]. In this study, we

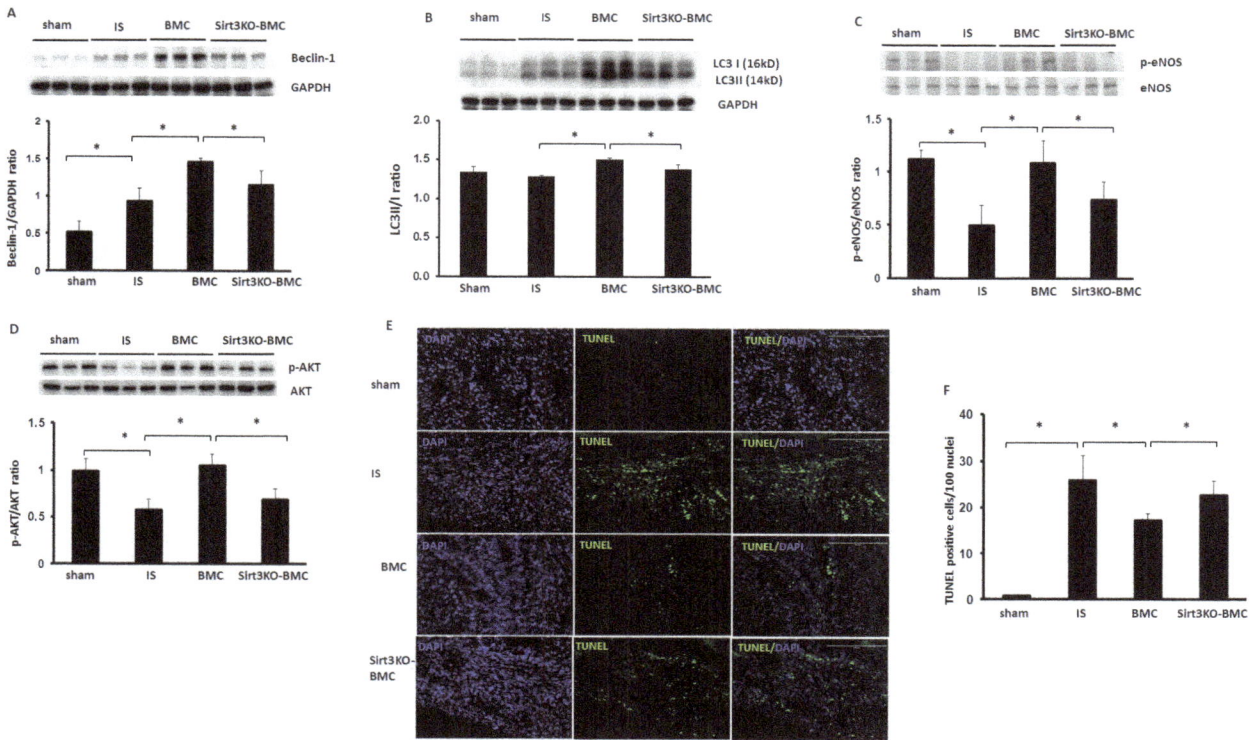

Figure 6. Loss of Sirt3 in BMCs increases apoptosis in post-MI mice. A and B. Western blot analysis demonstrating that treatment of post-MI mice with BMCs resulted in a significant increase in autophagy gene beclin-1 expression (A) and LC3-II/I ratio (B). Beclin-1 expression and LC3-II/I ratio were significantly decreased in Sirt3KO-BMC treated mice compared to BMC treated post-MI mice. n = 6 mice; *p<0.05. **C and D**. Western blot analysis demonstrating that BMC treatment significantly increased phosphorylation levels of eNOS (C) and Akt (D) in post-MI mice. The phosphorylation levels of Akt and eNOS were significantly decreased in Sirt3KO-BMC treated mice compared to BMC treated mice. n = 6 mice; *p< 0.05. **E and F**. Apoptotic cells in the infarcted area of the left ventricle were identified by TUNEL staining (green, 10x). Treatment of post-MI mice with BMCs significantly decreased TUNEL[+] cells in ischemic area. TUNEL[+] cells were significantly increased in Sirt3KO-BMC treated mice when compared with BMC treated mice. n = 5 mice; *p<0.05.

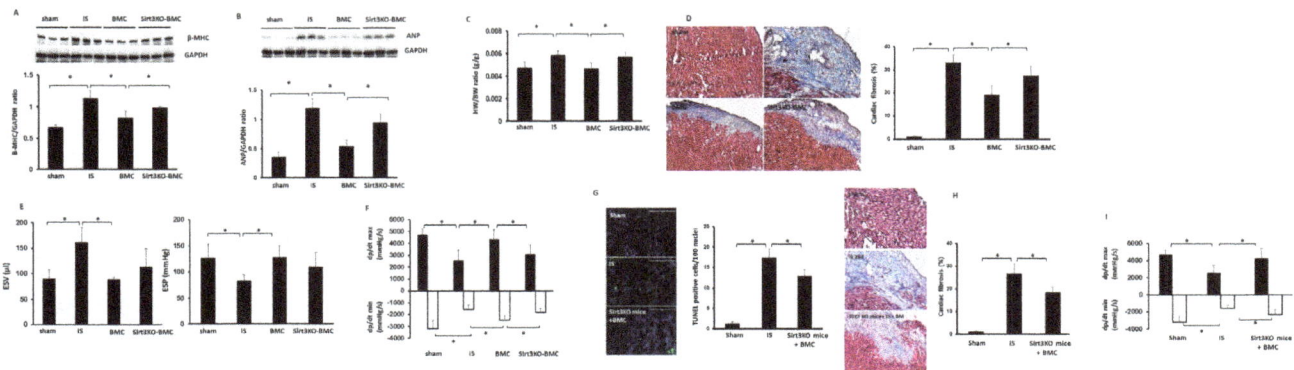

Figure 7. Loss of Sirt3 abolished BMC-mediated cardiac repair in post-MI mice. A and B. Western blot analysis showing that treatment of post-MI mice with BMCs significantly reduced hypertrophic marker β-MHC (A) and ANP (B) expression. Treatment of post-MI mice with Sirt3KO-BMC failed to suppression of β-MHC and ANP expression compared to BMC treated mice. n = 6 mice, *p<0.05. **C**. BMC treatment significantly reduced HW/BW ratio in post-MI mice. Treatment with Sirt3KO-BMCs failed to significant reduction of HW/BW ratio compared to BMC treated mice. n = 6 mice, *p<0.05. **D**. Representative images of cardiac fibrosis in the infarction zone and quantitative analysis of fibrotic area in mice (Masson's trichrome). BMC treatment significantly reduced the area of cardiac fibrosis. Sirt3KO-BMC treatment significantly increased cardiac fibrosis area compared to BMC treated mice. n = 5 mice; *p<0.05. **E**. The end-systolic volume (ESV) was significantly increased in post-MI mice. BMC treatment significantly decreased ESV. The end-systolic pressure (ESP) was decreased in post-MI mice. Treatment with BMCs significantly increased ESP whereas treatment of post-MI mice with Sirt3KO-BMC had little effects on ESV and ESP. n = 5–7 mice, *p<0.05. **F**. BMC therapy led to a significant improvement of maximum +dP/dt and minimum -dP/dt pressures compared to control post-MI mice. Sirt3KO-BMC treatment failed to improve maximum +dP/dt and minimum -dP/dt pressures in post-MI mice. n = 5–7 mice,*p<0.05. **G**. Treatment of Sirt3KO post-MI mice with WT-BMCs significantly reduced TUNEL[+] cells in ischemic area. Apoptotic cells in the infarcted area of the left ventricle were identified by TUNEL staining (green, 10x). n = 6 mice; *p<0.05. **H**. Treatment of Sirt3KO post-MI mice with WT-BMCs significantly reduced the area of cardiac fibrosis (Masson's trichrome). n = 5 mice; *p<0.05. **I**. Treatment of Sirt3KO post-MI mice with WT-BMCs significantly improved maximum +dP/dt and minimum -dP/dt pressures in post-MI mice. n = 5–6 mice,*p<0.05.

hypothesized that loss of Sirt3 in BM stem cells; similar as aged BM derived HSCs, fails to improve angiogenesis and cardiac repair in post-MI. To substantiate this notion, we first compared the expression of angiogenic growth factor and angiogenesis between WT-EPCs and Sirt3KO-EPCs *in vitro*. Our data showed that loss of Sirt3 in EPCs reduced VEGF and VEGFR2 expression. Moreover, treatment with NADPH oxidase inhibitor or overexpression of Sirt3 rescued impaired VEGF and VEGFR2 expression. In addition, the basal proliferation and angiogenic capacities were significantly reduced in Sirt3KO-EPCs. Our study *in vivo* further confirmed that BMC treatment increased VEGF expression and elevated phosphorylation levels of eNOS and Akt. This was accompanied by increased myocardial vascular densities and improved cardiac function in post-MI mice. In contrast, knockout of Sirt3 in BMCs reduced BMC-mediated VEGF expression and neovascularization. Furthermore, loss of Sirt3 in BMCs abolished BMC-mediated cardiac repair and improvement of cardiac function in post-MI mice. These findings indicate that lack of Sirt3 and increased ROS formation in aged EPCs maybe contribute to the failure of aged BMC treatment in post-MI.

Autophagy is a dynamic process of intracellular bulk degradation in which cytosolic proteins and organelles are fused with lysosomes for degradation. Under stressed conditions, autophagy selectively removes damaged mitochondria which prevent activation of apoptotic machinery [46,47]. Overexpression of autophagy gene beclin-1 has been shown to protect cardiac myocyte against ischemia/reperfusion injury [48]. Autophagy has been shown to have a protective role in the heart following myocardial ischemia/reperfusion *in vivo* [49–52]. Our previous study indicates that Sirt3 is necessary for apelin-BMC therapy-mediated upregulation of autophagy. Loss of Sirt3 attenuates apelin-induced autophagy gene marker beclin-1 and LC3-I/II expression [20]. In the present study, we demonstrate that treatment with BMCs led to a significant increase in autophagy gene beclin-1 expression and elevation of LC3-II/I ratio. These are accompanied by a dramatic reduction of cardiac apoptosis. However, treatment with Sirt3KO-BMC had no effect on LC3-II/I ratio and Beclin-1 expression in post-MI mice. This was associated with a significant higher number of apoptotic cells in ischemic hearts. Our studies revealed

a novel molecular mechanism of BMC stem cell therapy which stem cells may attenuate apoptosis via regulation of autophagy in post-MI. Autophagy also has been shown to promote stem cell generation and differentiation. Inhibition of autophagy reduces stem cell self-renewal and differentiation [53–57]. A recent study further underscores the important role of autophagy in EPC survival, proliferation and differentiation. Inhibition of autophagy reduces proliferation and differentiation of EPCs. In contrast, increasing autophagy enhances EPC survival under hypoxic conditions [53]. Our data showed that loss of Sirt3 reduced autophagic gene LC3-II levels whereas overexpression of Sirt3 or treated with NADPH oxidase inhibitor increased LC3-II levels in EPCs. Overexpression of Sirt3 further attenuated EPCs apoptosis. These data suggest that reduction of autophagy may be contributed to the higher apoptosis of Sirt3KO-EPCs. Although Sirt3 has been shown to rejuvenate HSCs [21], so far, it remains unanswered what is necessary for Sirt3 to complete its rejuvenation. In addition, if Sirt3-induced HSCs rejuvenation requires to removing additional damaged organelles such as mitochondria via regulation of autophagy remains unknown. Further studies are warranted to elucidate the molecular mechanisms by which Sirt3 regulates autophagy in stem cell rejuvenation.

In summary, the current study provides evidence that basal levels of Sirt3 in stem cells contribute the therapeutic effects of BMCs in post-MI mice. Since the levels of Sirt3 were reduced in aging and aged stem cells, our findings implicate that reduced levels of Sirt3 may contribute to the failure of BMC therapy in aging patients. Our findings further suggest that augmentation of Sirt3 activity in stem cells may represent a novel therapeutic approach for the improvement of stem cell therapy for the ischemic heart diseases.

Author Contributions

Conceived and designed the experiments: JXC. Performed the experiments: HZ LL. Analyzed the data: HZ LL. Contributed reagents/materials/analysis tools: JXC. Contributed to the writing of the manuscript: JXC.

References

1. Tanno M, Kuno A, Horio Y, Miura T (2012) Emerging beneficial roles of sirtuins in heart failure. Basic Res Cardiol 107: 273. 10.1007/s00395-012-0273-5 [doi].

2. Pillai VB, Sundaresan NR, Jeevanandam V, Gupta MP (2010) Mitochondrial SIRT3 and heart disease. Cardiovasc Res 88: 250–256. cvq250 [pii];10.1093/cvr/cvq250 [doi].

3. Tanno M, Sakamoto J, Miura T, Shimamoto K, Horio Y (2007) Nucleocytoplasmic shuttling of the NAD+-dependent histone deacetylase SIRT1. J Biol Chem 282: 6823–6832. M609554200 [pii];10.1074/jbc.M609554200 [doi].

4. Becatti M, Taddei N, Cecchi C, Nassi N, Nassi PA, et al (2012) SIRT1 modulates MAPK pathways in ischemic-reperfused cardiomyocytes. Cell Mol Life Sci 69: 2245–2260. 10.1007/s00018-012-0925-5 [doi].

5. Donato AJ, Magerko KA, Lawson BR, Durrant JR, Lesniewski LA, et al (2011) SIRT-1 and vascular endothelial dysfunction with ageing in mice and humans. J Physiol 589: 4545–4554. jphysiol.2011.211219 [pii];10.1113/jphysiol.2011.211219 [doi].

6. Sundaresan NR, Pillai VB, Gupta MP (2011) Emerging roles of SIRT1 deacetylase in regulating cardiomyocyte survival and hypertrophy. J Mol Cell Cardiol 51: 614–618. S0022-2828(11)00029-0 [pii];10.1016/j.yjmcc.2011.01.008 [doi].

7. Zu Y, Liu L, Lee MY, Xu C, Liang Y, et al (2010) SIRT1 promotes proliferation and prevents senescence through targeting LKB1 in primary porcine aortic endothelial cells. Circ Res 106: 1384–1393. CIRCRESAHA.109.215483 [pii];10.1161/CIRCRESAHA.109.215483 [doi].

8. Vinciguerra M, Santini MP, Martinez C, Pazienza V, Claycomb WC, et al (2012) mIGF-1/JNK1/SirT1 signaling confers protection against oxidative stress in the heart. Aging Cell 11: 139–149. 10.1111/j.1474-9726.2011.00766.x [doi].

9. Lanza IR, Short DK, Short KR, Raghavakaimal S, Basu R, et al (2008) Endurance exercise as a countermeasure for aging. Diabetes 57: 2933–2942. db08-0349 [pii];10.2337/db08-0349 [doi].

10. Bellizzi D, Rose G, Cavalcante P, Covello G, Dato S, et al (2005) A novel VNTR enhancer within the SIRT3 gene, a human homologue of SIR2, is associated with survival at oldest ages. Genomics 85: 258–263. S0888-7543(04)00308-8 [pii];10.1016/j.ygeno.2004.11.003 [doi].

11. Rose G, Dato S, Altomare K, Bellizzi D, Garasto S, et al (2003) Variability of the SIRT3 gene, human silent information regulator Sir2 homologue, and survivorship in the elderly. Exp Gerontol 38: 1065–1070. S0531556503002092 [pii].

12. Palacios OM, Carmona JJ, Michan S, Chen KY, Manabe Y, et al (2009) Diet and exercise signals regulate SIRT3 and activate AMPK and PGC-1alpha in skeletal muscle. Aging (Albany NY) 1: 771–783.

13. Someya S, Yu W, Hallows WC, Xu J, Vann JM, et al (2010) Sirt3 mediates reduction of oxidative damage and prevention of age-related hearing loss under caloric restriction. Cell 143: 802–812. S0092-8674(10)01138-4 [pii];10.1016/j.cell.2010.10.002 [doi].

14. Pillai VB, Sundaresan NR, Kim G, Gupta M, Rajamohan SB, et al (2010) Exogenous NAD blocks cardiac hypertrophic response via activation of the SIRT3-LKB1-AMP-activated kinase pathway. J Biol Chem 285: 3133–3144. M109.077271 [pii];10.1074/jbc.M109.077271 [doi].

15. Sundaresan NR, Gupta M, Kim G, Rajamohan SB, Isbatan A, et al (2009) Sirt3 blocks the cardiac hypertrophic response by augmenting Foxo3a-dependent antioxidant defense mechanisms in mice. J Clin Invest 119: 2758–2771. 39162 [pii];10.1172/JCI39162 [doi].

16. Isner JM, Asahara T (1999) Angiogenesis and vasculogenesis as therapeutic strategies for postnatal neovascularization. J Clin Invest 103: 1231–1236.

17. Yoon YS, Johnson IA, Park JS, Diaz L, Losordo DW (2004) Therapeutic myocardial angiogenesis with vascular endothelial growth factors. Mol Cell Biochem 264: 63–74.

18. Schachinger V, Assmus B, Britten MB, Honold J, Lehmann R, et al (2004) Transplantation of progenitor cells and regeneration enhancement in acute myocardial infarction: final one-year results of the TOPCARE-AMI Trial. J Am Coll Cardiol 44: 1690–1699.

19. Sack MN (2012) The role of SIRT3 in mitochondrial homeostasis and cardiac adaptation to hypertrophy and aging. J Mol Cell Cardiol 52: 520–525. S0022-2828(11)00470-6 [pii];10.1016/j.yjmcc.2011.11.004 [doi].

20. Li L, Zeng H, Hou X, He X, Chen JX (2013) Myocardial Injection of Apelin-Overexpressing Bone Marrow Cells Improves Cardiac Repair via Upregulation of Sirt3 after Myocardial Infarction. PLoS One 8: e71041. 10.1371/journal.pone.0071041 [doi]; PONE-D-13-05351 [pii].

21. Brown K, Xie S, Qiu X, Mohrin M, Shin J, et al (2013) SIRT3 reverses aging-associated degeneration. Cell Rep 3: 319–327. S2211-1247(13)00012-0 [pii];10.1016/j.celrep.2013.01.005 [doi].

22. Li L, Zeng H, Chen JX (2012) Apelin-13 increases myocardial progenitor cells and improves repair postmyocardial infarction. Am J Physiol Heart Circ Physiol 303: H605–H618. ajpheart.00366.2012 [pii];10.1152/ajpheart.00366.2012 [doi].

23. Tuo QH, Zeng H, Stinnett A, Yu H, Aschner JL, et al (2008) Critical role of angiopoietins/Tie-2 in hyperglycemic exacerbation of myocardial infarction and impaired angiogenesis. Am J Physiol Heart Circ Physiol 294: H2547–H2557.

24. Chen JX, Stinnett A (2008) Ang-1 gene therapy inhibits hypoxia-inducible factor-1alpha (HIF-1alpha)-prolyl-4-hydroxylase-2, stabilizes HIF-1alpha expression, and normalizes immature vasculature in db/db mice. Diabetes 57: 3335–3343.

25. Zeng H, Li L, Chen JX (2012) Overexpression of Angiopoietin-1 Increases CD133+/c-kit+ Cells and Reduces Myocardial Apoptosis in db/db Mouse Infarcted Hearts. PLoS One 7: e35905. 10.1371/journal.pone.0035905 [doi]; PONE-D-11-21968 [pii].

26. Li L, Crockett E, Wang DH, Galligan JJ, Fink GD, et al (2002) Gene transfer of endothelial NO synthase and manganese superoxide dismutase on arterial vascular cell adhesion molecule-1 expression and superoxide production in deoxycorticosterone acetate-salt hypertension. Arterioscler Thromb Vasc Biol 22: 249–255.

27. Chen JX, Stinnett A (2008) Critical role of the NADPH oxidase subunit p47(phox) on vascular TLR expression and neointimal lesion formation in high-fat diet-induced obesity. Lab Invest 88: 1316–28.

28. Chen JX, Tuo Q, Liao DF, Zeng H (2012) Inhibition of protein tyrosine phosphatase improves angiogenesis via enhancing Ang-1/Tie-2 signaling in diabetes. Exp Diabetes Res 2012: 836759. 10.1155/2012/836759 [doi].

29. Chen JX, Zeng H, Tuo QH, Yu H, Meyrick B, et al (2007) NADPH oxidase modulates myocardial Akt, ERK1/2 activation and angiogenesis after hypoxia/reoxygenation. Am J Physiol Heart Circ Physiol 292: H1664–H1674.

30. Chen JX, Zeng H, Lawrence ML, Blackwell TS, Meyrick B (2006) Angiopoietin-1-induced Angiogenesis is Modulated by Endothelial NADPH Oxidase. Am J Physiol Heart Circ Physiol 291: H1563–72.

31. Assmus B, Iwasaki M, Schachinger V, Roexe T, Koyanagi M, et al (2012) Acute myocardial infarction activates progenitor cells and increases Wnt signalling in the bone marrow. Eur Heart J 33: 1911–1919. ehr388 [pii];10.1093/eurheartj/ehr388 [doi].

32. Giralt A, Villarroya F (2012) SIRT3, a pivotal actor in mitochondrial functions: metabolism, cell death and aging. Biochem J 444: 1–10. BJ20120030 [pii];10.1042/BJ20120030 [doi].

33. Liu Y, Zhang D, Chen D (2011) SIRT3: Striking at the heart of aging. Aging (Albany NY) 3: 1–2. 100256 [pii].

34. Sack MN (2011) Emerging characterization of the role of SIRT3-mediated mitochondrial protein deacetylation in the heart. Am J Physiol Heart Circ Physiol 301: H2191–H2197. ajpheart.00199.2011 [pii];10.1152/ajpheart.00199.2011 [doi].

35. Sundaresan NR, Samant SA, Pillai VB, Rajamohan SB, Gupta MP (2008) SIRT3 is a stress-responsive deacetylase in cardiomyocytes that protects cells from stress-mediated cell death by deacetylation of Ku70. Mol Cell Biol 28: 6384–6401. MCB.00426-08 [pii];10.1128/MCB.00426-08 [doi].

36. Askari AT, Unzek S, Popovic ZB, Goldman CK, Forudi F, et al (2003) Effect of stromal-cell-derived factor 1 on stem-cell homing and tissue regeneration in ischaemic cardiomyopathy. Lancet 362: 697–703. S0140-6736(03)14232-8 [pii];10.1016/S0140-6736(03)14232-8 [doi].

37. Hu X, Dai S, Wu WJ, Tan W, Zhu X, et al (2007) Stromal cell derived factor-1 alpha confers protection against myocardial ischemia/reperfusion injury: role of the cardiac stromal cell derived factor-1 alpha CXCR4 axis. Circulation 116:

654–663. CIRCULATIONAHA.106.672451 [pii];10.1161/CIRCULATIO-NAHA.106.672451 [doi].

38. Frederick JR, Fitzpatrick JR, III, McCormick RC, Harris DA, Kim AY, et al (2010) Stromal cell-derived factor-1alpha activation of tissue-engineered endothelial progenitor cell matrix enhances ventricular function after myocardial infarction by inducing neovasculogenesis. Circulation 122: S107–S117. 122/11_suppl_1/S107 [pii];10.1161/CIRCULATIONAHA.109.930404 [doi].

39. Massa M, Rosti V, Ferrario M, Campanelli R, Ramajoli I, et al (2005) Increased circulating hematopoietic and endothelial progenitor cells in the early phase of acute myocardial infarction. Blood 105: 199–206. 10.1182/blood-2004-05-1831 [doi];2004-05-1831 [pii].

40. Wojakowski W, Tendera M (2005) Mobilization of bone marrow-derived progenitor cells in acute coronary syndromes. Folia Histochem Cytobiol 43: 229–232.

41. Kim HS, Patel K, Muldoon-Jacobs K, Bisht KS, Aykin-Burns N, et al (2010) SIRT3 is a mitochondria-localized tumor suppressor required for maintenance of mitochondrial integrity and metabolism during stress. Cancer Cell 17: 41–52. S1535-6108(09)00428-0 [pii];10.1016/j.ccr.2009.11.023 [doi].

42. Edelberg JM, Tang L, Hattori K, Lyden D, Rafii S (2002) Young adult bone marrow-derived endothelial precursor cells restore aging-impaired cardiac angiogenic function. Circ Res 90: E89–E93.

43. Fan M, Chen W, Liu W, Du GQ, Jiang SL, et al (2010) The effect of age on the efficacy of human mesenchymal stem cell transplantation after a myocardial infarction. Rejuvenation Res 13: 429–438. 10.1089/rej.2009.0986 [doi].

44. Khan M, Mohsin S, Khan SN, Riazuddin S (2011) Repair of senescent myocardium by mesenchymal stem cells is dependent on the age of donor mice. J Cell Mol Med 15: 1515–1527. JCMM998 [pii];10.1111/j.1582-4934.2009.00998.x [doi].

45. Zhang H, Fazel S, Tian H, Mickle DA, Weisel RD, et al (2005) Increasing donor age adversely impacts beneficial effects of bone marrow but not smooth muscle myocardial cell therapy. Am J Physiol Heart Circ Physiol 289: H2089–H2096. 289/5/H2089 [pii];10.1152/ajpheart.00019.2005 [doi].

46. Gottlieb RA, Finley KD, Mentzer RM Jr (2009) Cardioprotection requires taking out the trash. Basic Res Cardiol 104: 169–180. 10.1007/s00395-009-0011-9 [doi].

47. Kim I, Rodriguez-Enriquez S, Lemasters JJ (2007) Selective degradation of mitochondria by mitophagy. Arch Biochem Biophys 462: 245–253. S0003-9861(07)00162-2 [pii];10.1016/j.abb.2007.03.034 [doi].

48. Hamacher-Brady A, Brady NR, Gottlieb RA (2006) Enhancing macroauto-phagy protects against ischemia/reperfusion injury in cardiac myocytes. J Biol Chem 281: 29776–29787. M603783200 [pii];10.1074/jbc.M603783200 [doi].

49. Hamacher-Brady A, Brady NR, Gottlieb RA, Gustafsson AB (2006) Autophagy as a protective response to Bnip3-mediated apoptotic signaling in the heart. Autophagy 2: 307–309. 2947 [pii].

50. Hamacher-Brady A, Brady NR, Logue SE, Sayen MR, Jinno M, et al (2007) Response to myocardial ischemia/reperfusion injury involves Bnip3 and autophagy. Cell Death Differ 14: 146–157. 4401936 [pii];10.1038/sj.cdd.4401936 [doi].

51. Kanamori H, Takemura G, Goto K, Maruyama R, Ono K, et al (2011) Autophagy limits acute myocardial infarction induced by permanent coronary artery occlusion. Am J Physiol Heart Circ Physiol 300: H2261–H2271. ajpheart.01056.2010 [pii];10.1152/ajpheart.01056.2010 [doi].

52. Przyklenk K, Undyala VV, Wider J, Sala-Mercado JA, Gottlieb RA, et al (2011) Acute induction of autophagy as a novel strategy for cardioprotection: getting to the heart of the matter. Autophagy 7: 432–433. 14395 [doi].

53. Wang HJ, Zhang D, Tan YZ, Li T (2013) Autophagy in endothelial progenitor cells is cytoprotective in hypoxic conditions. Am J Physiol Cell Physiol 304: C617–C626. ajpcell.00296.2012 [pii];10.1152/ajpcell.00296.2012 [doi].

54. Chen J, Xavier S, Moskowitz-Kassai E, Chen R, Lu CY, et al (2012) Cathepsin cleavage of sirtuin 1 in endothelial progenitor cells mediates stress-induced premature senescence. Am J Pathol 180: 973–983. S0002-9440(11)01102-3 [pii];10.1016/j.ajpath.2011.11.033 [doi].

55. Lee Y, Jung J, Cho KJ, Lee SK, Park JW, et al (2013) Increased SCF/c-kit by hypoxia promotes autophagy of human placental chorionic plate-derived mesenchymal stem cells via regulating the phosphorylation of mTOR. J Cell Biochem 114: 79–88. 10.1002/jcb.24303 [doi].

56. Phadwal K, Watson AS, Simon AK (2013) Tightrope act: autophagy in stem cell renewal, differentiation, proliferation, and aging. Cell Mol Life Sci 70: 89–103. 10.1007/s00018-012-1032-3 [doi].

57. Zhuang W, Li B, Long L, Chen L, Huang Q, et al (2011) Induction of autophagy promotes differentiation of glioma-initiating cells and their radiosen-sitivity. Int J Cancer 129: 2720–2731. 10.1002/ijc.25975 [doi].

11

Role of the Vasohibin Family in the Regulation of Fetoplacental Vascularization and Syncytiotrophoblast Formation

Kaori Suenaga[1,2], Shuji Kitahara[3], Yasuhiro Suzuki[1], Miho Kobayashi[1], Sachiko Horie[1], Junichi Sugawara[2,4], Nobuo Yaegashi[2,4], Yasufumi Sato[1]*

1 Department of Vascular Biology, Institute of Development, Aging, and Cancer, Tohoku University, Aoba-ku, Sendai, Miyagi, Japan, 2 Department of Obstetrics & Gynecology, Tohoku University School of Medicine, Aoba-ku, Sendai, Miyagi, Japan, 3 Department of Anatomy and Developmental Biology, Tokyo Women's Medical University, Shinjuku-ku, Tokyo, Japan, 4 Tohoku Medical Megabank Organization, Tohoku University, Aobaku, Sendai, Miyagi, Japan

Abstract

Vasohibin-1 (VASH1) and vasohibin-2 (VASH2), the 2 members of the vasohibin family, have been identified as novel regulators of angiogenesis. VASH1 ceases angiogenesis, whereas VASH2 stimulates sprouting. Here we characterized their functional role in the placenta. Immunohistochemical analysis of human placental tissue clarified their distinctive localization; VASH1 in endothelial cells and VASH2 in trophoblasts. We then used a mouse model to explore their function. Wild-type, $Vash1^{(-/-)}$, and $Vash2^{(-/-)}$ mice on a C57BL6 background were used in their first pregnancy. As expected, the fetal vascular area was increased in the $Vash1^{(-/-)}$ mice, whereas it was decreased in the $Vash2^{(-/-)}$ mice relative to wild-type. In addition, we noticed that the $Vash2^{(-/-)}$ mice at 18.5dpc displayed thinner villi of the labyrinth and larger maternal lacunae. Careful observation by an electron microscopy revealed that the syncytiotrophoblast formation was defective in the $Vash2^{(-/-)}$ mice. To test the possible involvement of VASH2 in the syncytiotrophoblast formation, we examined the fusion of BeWo cells, a human trophoblastoid choriocarcinoma cell line. The forskolin treatment induced the fusion of BeWo cells, and the knockdown of VASH2 expression significantly inhibited this cell fusion. Conversely, the overexpression of VASH2 by the infection with adenovirus vector encoding *human VASH2* gene significantly increased the fusion of BeWo cells. Glial cell missing-1 and endogenous retrovirus envelope glycoprotein Syncytin 1 and Syncytin 2 are known to be involved in the fusion of trophoblasts. However, VASH2 did not alter their expression in BeWo cells. These results indicate that VASH1 and VASH2 showed distinctive localization and opposing function on the fetoplacental vascularization. Moreover, our study shows for the first time that VASH2 expressed in trophoblasts is involved in the regulation of cell fusion for syncytiotrophoblast formation.

Editor: Tsutomu Kume, Feinberg Cardiovascular Research Institute, Northwestern University, United States of America

Funding: This work was supported by a grant from the Global COE for Conquest of Signal Transduction Diseases with Network Medicine, Tohoku University. The funders had no role in study design, data collection and analysis, decision to publish, or preparation of the manuscript.

Competing Interests: The authors have declared that no competing interests exist.

* Email: y-sato@idac.tohoku.ac.jp

Introduction

The placenta is an organ that connects the fetus to the maternal uterine wall, and it starts to develop upon implantation of the blastocyst into the maternal endometrium. The outer layer of the blastocyst becomes the trophoblast, which forms the outer layer of the placenta. Subsequently, this layer of trophoblast cells is subdivided into the cytotrophoblast and syncytiotrophoblast layers. Cytotrophoblasts proliferate and invade the endometrial tissue to form placental villi. The multinucleate cell layer of syncytiotrophoblasts is formed by the cell fusion of cytotrophoblasts and covers the entire surface area of the placenta [1].

The placenta is a highly vascularized organ that allows for nutrient uptake, waste elimination, and gas exchange for the developing fetus. The placental circulation brings the fetal and maternal vascular systems into close relationship, and multiple steps of vascular development and/or remodeling on both fetal

and maternal sides are required for acquisition of this relationship. These steps include (i) invasion by trophoblast cells, (ii) vascularization within the trophoblast layer to establish and maintain the fetoplacental vasculature, and (iii) subsequent maternal vascular remodeling to gain the uteroplacental circulation [2,3].

The fetoplacental vasculature is formed by vasculogenesis and angiogenesis, and multiple regulatory systems are reported to regulate these processes. They include the vascular endothelial growth factor (VEGF)/VEGF receptor (VEGFR) system, angiopoietin/TIE receptor system, platelet-derived growth factor (PDGF)/PDGF receptor system, and transforming growth factor ß (TGF- ß)/TGF- ß receptor system [4]. Among them, VEGF-A, a prototype of the VEGF family, is considered to be the most important factor that promotes vasculogenesis and angiogenesis in the entire body including the placenta. VEGF-A is intensively expressed in cytotrophoblasts, particularly in the early developmental stage of the placenta. VEGFR2 is the major mediator of

VEGF-A-driven responses in vascular ECs. VEGFR1, on the other hand, has higher affinity for VEGF-A but weaker tyrosine kinase activity. Soluble VEGFR1 (sVEGFR1), a splicing variant of VEGFR1, is highly expressed in trophoblasts and traps VEGF-A by acting as a decoy receptor. Placenta growth factor (PlGF), another member of the VEGF family, is also highly expressed in trophoblasts, but the function of PlGF in the development of placenta has not yet been well characterized [5,6].

Vasohibin-1 (VASH1) was isolated as a negative-feedback regulator of angiogenesis induced in ECs by angiogenesis stimulators such as VEGF and FGF-2 [7]. Subsequently, a gene homologous to VASH1 was identified and named vasohibin-2 (VASH2) [8]. The amino acid sequence of the human VASH2 protein is 52.5% homologous to that of human VASH1, and both VASH1 and VASH2 are highly conserved among species [9]. Although vasohibins lack classical signal sequence for their secretion, they bind to small vasohibin binding protein (SVBP) within a cell and that facilitates the secretion of vasohibins [10].

Expression and function of VASH1 and VASH2 have been examined by the use of hypoxia-induced subcutaneous angiogenesis in mice, and the results revealed that VASH1 is mainly expressed in ECs in the termination zone to halt angiogenesis, whereas VASH2 is mainly expressed in mononuclear cells mobilized from the bone marrow in the sprouting front to stimulate angiogenesis [11]. Thus, these 2 vasohibin family members regulate angiogenesis in a contradictory manner.

As mentioned above, angiogenesis regulators are involved in the regulation of placental morphogenesis, but little is known about the function of vasohibin family in this regulation. Hence, in this present study we characterized the localization of these vasohibins in the human placenta and their expression and function in the murine placenta.

Materials and Methods

Immunohistochemistry for human placenta

The Ethics Committee at Tohoku University approved this study. Human placenta was obtained from normal pregnant women (38~40 weeks of gestation) who provided their written consent to participate in this study at Tohoku University Hospital. The Ethics Committee at Tohoku University approved this consent procedure. Samples were dissected into $2 \times 2 \times 2$ cm cubes, fixed at $4°C$ in 4% paraformaldehyde (Wako, Osaka, Japan) for 2 days, and then embedded in paraffin. Sections (5 μm) were prepared and then deparaffinized, after which endogenous peroxidase activity was blocked by immersion in 3% H_2O_2 (Santoku, Tokyo, Japan)/methanol for 10 min. The sections were then autoclaved for 5 min at $121°C$ in Target Retrieval Solution, pH 6 (Dako, CA) and then blocked for 30 min with 1% bovine serum albumin (BSA, Sigma-Aldrich, MO) diluted in phosphate-buffered saline (PBS) containing 0.1% Tween20 (Sigma-Aldrich). Next, the sections were incubated overnight at $4°C$ with 1st antibodies, anti-human VASH1 mAb (4E12) [7] and anti-human VASH2 mAb (5E3) [8]. On the next day, they were washed with PBS and then incubated with N-histofine simple stain Mouse Max PO (Nichirei, Tokyo, Japan) for 30 min. After having been washed with PBS, the sites of immunoreactivity in the sections were visualized with diaminobenzidine (DAB tablet, Wako).

Animal model of placentation

All of the animal studies were approved by the Center for Laboratory Animal Research of Tohoku University. Nine- to twelve-week-old wild-type (WT), $Vash1^{(-/-)}$ or $Vash2^{(-/-)}$ mice on a C57BL/6 background [9] were mated and used in their first

pregnancy for the present study. The day when the vaginal plug was observed was defined as day 0.5 of gestation. Mice were sacrificed on 12, 16, and 18 day post-coitum (dpc). Both fetal and maternal body and organ weights were recorded. Some of the mice were snap frozen in liquid nitrogen for subsequent analysis.

Immunohistochemistry of mouse placenta

Intravascular perfusion with fluorescein lycopersicon esculentum (TOMATO) lectin (Vector Laboratories, CA) was performed to label vessels for maternal blood circulation as described previously [12]. Briefly, mice were injected intravenously with 100 μl of TOMATO lectin; and 10 min later their thorax was opened and the aorta perfused with 4% PFA (Wako) in 0.1 M PBS at a pressure of 100–120 mm Hg for 5 min, followed by perfusion with PBS for 5 min via the left ventricle. After perfusion, the tissues were processed for subsequent analyses. These tissues were kept overnight at $4°C$ in 30% sucrose in PBS, and the next day they were embedded in O.C.T compound (Sakura Finetek, CA). Subsequently, they were frozen and stored at $-80°C$ in a deep freezer until use. Cryosections (20 μm) were prepared and washed in PBS, after which the endogenous peroxidase activity was quenched for 10 min by immersion in 3% H_2O_2/methanol. The blocking of non-specific binding sites was performed for 30 min by incubation in PBS containing 1% BSA and 0.1% Tween20. First antibodies, which were purified rat anti-mouse CD31 (BD Biosciences, CA), biotinylatead anti-mouse HAI-1 antibody (R&D systems, MN) and anti-type IV collagen (ab6586, Abcam, MA) were diluted 1:200 in PBS containing 1% BSA and 0.1% Tween20. After removal of the blocking buffer, the sections were reacted with the 1st antibodies at $4°C$ overnight. On the next day, after a wash with PBS the sections were incubated for 30 min at RT with fluorescent secondary antibodies, i.e., Alexa Fluor 633-conjugated goat anti-rat IgG (Molecular Probes, Eugene, OR) and Alexa Fluor 555-conjugated donkey anti-rabbit IgG (Molecular Probes), which had been diluted 1:200 in PBS. Finally, the specimens were mounted with fluorescent mounting medium (Dako, CA). Ten fields per section were randomly selected and observed under a fluorescence microscope, and the fetal vascular area was calculated by using software (BZ-9000, Keyence, Osaka, Japan), and the maternal vascular area was calculated by using imageJ 1.48v, an open source Java image processing program.

Enzyme linked immunosorbent assay (ELISA)

Serum samples were collected for the determination of the levels of murine VEGF, soluble VEGFR1, and PlGF. ELISA kits for murine VEGF, solubleVEGFR1, and PlGF were purchased from R&D Systems. ELISA was performed according to the manufacturer's instructions.

Transmission electron microscopy

After perfusion with 4% PFA, some samples of the mouse placenta with uterus were cut into small blocks and incubated in 2% glutaraldehyde in 0.1 M PB for 2 hours. The samples were subsequently incubated with a 1% solution of OsO_4 for 1 hour at $4°C$, dehydrated by passage through a graded series of ethanol followed by propylene oxide, and embedded in epoxy resin. Ultrathin sections (70 nm) were stained with lead citrate and examined with an H-7000 electron microscope (Hitachi, Tokyo, Japan).

Reverse transcriptase-polymerase chain reaction (RT-PCR)

Total RNA was prepared from the placenta of 12.5-, 16.5-, and 18.5-dpc mice by using ISOGEN (Nippon Gene, Toyama, Japan) according to the manufacturer's instructions. Single-stranded cDNA was synthesized by using ReverTra Ace (TOYOBO, Osaka, Japan). RT-PCR was performed with a thermal cycler system (CFX-96 Real-Time system, C1000 Thermal Cycler, Bio-Rad, Tokyo, Japan) and SYBR Premix Ex Taq (TaKaRa). The primer pairs used were as follow: mouse GAPDH, 5'-TGAACGGGAAGCTCACTGG-3' (forward) and 5'-TCCACCACCCTGTTGCTGTA-3' (reverse); mouse Gcm-1, 5'-TCCAACTCCTTACGGATGAA-3' (forward) and 5'- GGGCGTTAGCTATTAAAGGTG-3' (reverse); Syncytin-B, 5'-TCTCACTGGCACTTCATTCC-3' (forward) and 5'- TC-AGGTTATGAGGTGAGAGG-3' (reverse); Syncytin-A, 5'- TT-GGTTGACTTCCCTCATGG-3' (forward) and 5'-AGCAGAAG-GATCTTGTCCAC -3' (reverse).

Cell-cell fusion analysis in vitro

Cells of the human choriocarcinoma cell line BeWo, obtained from RIKEN BioResource Center (Ibaraki, Japan), were cultured in Ham's F10 (Sigma-Aldrich) supplemented with 10% fetal bovine serum(FBS; BioWest S.A.S, Nuaillé, France)and treated with 20 μM forskolin (FK, Sigma-Aldrich) or vehicle (dimethyl sulfoxide; DMSO, Sigma-Aldrich) for 48 hours. Thereafter, immunohistochemistry was performed to detect cell-cell fusion. The cells were first fixed with 3% formaldehyde (Wako) for 10 min at RT. They were then incubated for 10 min with 0.3% Triton-X in TBS and subsequently washed with Tris- buffered saline (TBS, TaKaRa). After blockage of non-specific binding sites for 30 min with 5% BSA in TBS anti-E cadherin at 10 μg/ml (M108, TaKaRa), as 1st antibody, was applied overnight at 4°C. On the next day, the 2nd antibody reaction was performed for 45 min at RT with Alexa 488-conjugated rat IgG (Molecular Probes) at a 1:200 dilution and DAPI at a 1:10,000 dilutions (Invitrogen Life Technologies, Carlsbad, CA). The cells in 10 randomly selected fields per culture dish were observed with a fluorescence microscope (BZ-9000, Keyence) at 400-power magnification. Cell fusion was detected by the loss of E-cadherin between cells, and the number of fused cells (syncytia) was counted. Adobe Photoshop CS6 was used to calculate the fusion index: $[(N-S)/T] \times 100\%$.(N; the number of nuclei in the syncytia, S; the number of syncytia, T; the total number of nuclei counted) [13,14].

For the knockdown of VASH2, BeWo cells were transfected with a non-targeting control small interfering RNA (siRNA) or human VASH2 siRNA by using Lipofectamine RNAiMax (Invitrogen) with Opti-MEM at a final concentration of 25 nmol/L according to the manufacturer's instructions. The siRNA used for human VASH2, were designed and purchased from Invitrogen Life Technologies, and their sequences was 5'-CACUCUGAAUGAA-GUGGGCUAUCAA -3' (sense) and 5'-UUGAUAGCCCACUU-CAUUCAGAGUG -3' (antisense). Non-specific StealthRNAi Negative Control Medium GC Duplex #2 was used as control, was also purchased from Invitrogen. After a 24-h incubation, the cells were treated with 20 μM FK. Forty-eight hours later, cell fusion was determined by immunostaining with anti-E-cadherin as indicated above, and specific gene silencing was verified by RT-PCR as described above. The primer pairs used were as follow: Human β-actin, 5'-ACAATGAGCTGCGTGTGGCT-3' (forward) and 5'-TCTCCTTAATGTCACGCACGA-3' (reverse); human VASH2, 5'-ACGTCTCAAAGATGCTGAGG-3' (forward) and 5'-TTCTCACTTGGGTCGGAGAG-3' (reverse); human Gcm-1, 5'-GCTGGGACTTGAACCAGCAGTAA-3' (forward) and 5'-CTCAAGCACCTTGGACCAGGA-3' (reverse); Syncytin-1, 5'-CGCCTGCTCTTCAAACAA-3' (forward) and 5'-GGCCATGGGGATTTATGATT-3' (reverse); Syncytin-2, 5'-TCGGATACCTTCCCTAGTGC-3' (forward) and 5'-TGT-ATTCCGGAGCTGAGGTT-3' (reverse).

For the overexpression of VASH2, BeWo cells were infected with non-proliferative adenovirus vectors encoding *human VASH2 gene* (AdVASH2) [11] or LacZ (AdLacZ) as control. Accordingly, BeWo cells were plated in 6 cm dishes at 1.5×10^5 cells/ml. On the following day, medium was replaced by fresh ones containing AdVASH2 or AdLacZ at a final multiplicity of infection (MOI) of 10, and the cells were incubated for another 48 hours. Thereafter, cell fusion and the expression of Gcm-1, syncytin-1 and syncytin-2 were evaluated as described above.

Calculations and statistical analysis

The data were analyzed as the mean and standard deviation, except in the case of the maternal body weight and fetus number of fetuses per dam (mean and standard error). For evaluation of the difference in placental mRNA expression between wild type and $Vash2^{(-/-)}$, Welch's t test was used. The statistical significance of differences among 3 groups (WT, $Vash1^{(-/-)}$ and $Vash2^{(-/-)}$) was evaluated by the use of Steel-Dwass test. The significance levels were taken as p<0.001, p<0.05, and p<0.01.

Results

Differential localization of VASH1 and VASH2 in the placenta

In order to identify the localization of VASH1 and VASH2 proteins in the placenta, we performed an immunohistochemical analysis of human placental tissue taken at term pregnancy. We previously showed the selective localization of VASH1 protein in ECs in the human placenta [7]. The present analysis confirmed this previous observation, and further revealed that its expression tended to be more intense at the villous stem (Fig. 1A). In contrast, the localization of VASH2 protein in the placenta had not been determined previously. Here we revealed for the first time that VASH2 protein was selectively localized in the trophoblasts (Fig. 1B).

Opposing role of VASH1 and VASH2 in fetoplacental vascularization

To disclose the function of VASH1 and VASH2 in the placenta, we evaluated the course of pregnancy in WT, $Vash1^{(-/-)}$ and $Vash2^{(-/-)}$ mice. The maternal weight before pregnancy (Fig. 2A) and the number of neonates per dam (Fig. 2B) were not significantly different among WT, $Vash1^{(-/-)}$, and $Vash2^{(-/-)}$ mice. The blood pressure was low in both $Vash1^{(-/-)}$ and $Vash2^{(-/-)}$ mice (Fig. 2C). Interestingly, the weight of the placenta in $Vash2^{(-/-)}$ mice at 18.5 dpc was significantly lower than that in WT mice (Fig. 2D).

As VASH1 and VASH2 regulate angiogenesis in a contradictory manner [10], we assumed that the placental vasculature of $Vash1^{(-/-)}$ mice and $Vash2^{(-/-)}$ mice might be altered. To characterize the difference in vascular structure, we performed triple staining with tomato lectin (green) and antibodies against CD31 (blue) and type IV collagen (red). The area covered by CD31 indicated the fetal vascular area; and that by tomato lectin the maternal blood space (Fig. 3 upper panels). The fetal vascular area was significantly increased in $Vash1^{(-/-)}$ mice and decreased in $Vash2^{(-/-)}$ mice, whereas the maternal vascular area was significantly increased in $VASH2^{(-/-)}$ mice (Fig. 3 lower panels). We assumed that the increased maternal vascular area in $VASH2^{(-/-)}$ mice might be due to the poorly developed villi.

We further determined the serum levels of VEGF-A and its related proteins, PlGF and sVEGFR1, all of which are closely associated with pregnancy. Interestingly, the serum VEGF-A was significantly low in $Vash1^{(-/-)}$ mice at 12.5 dpc, and was

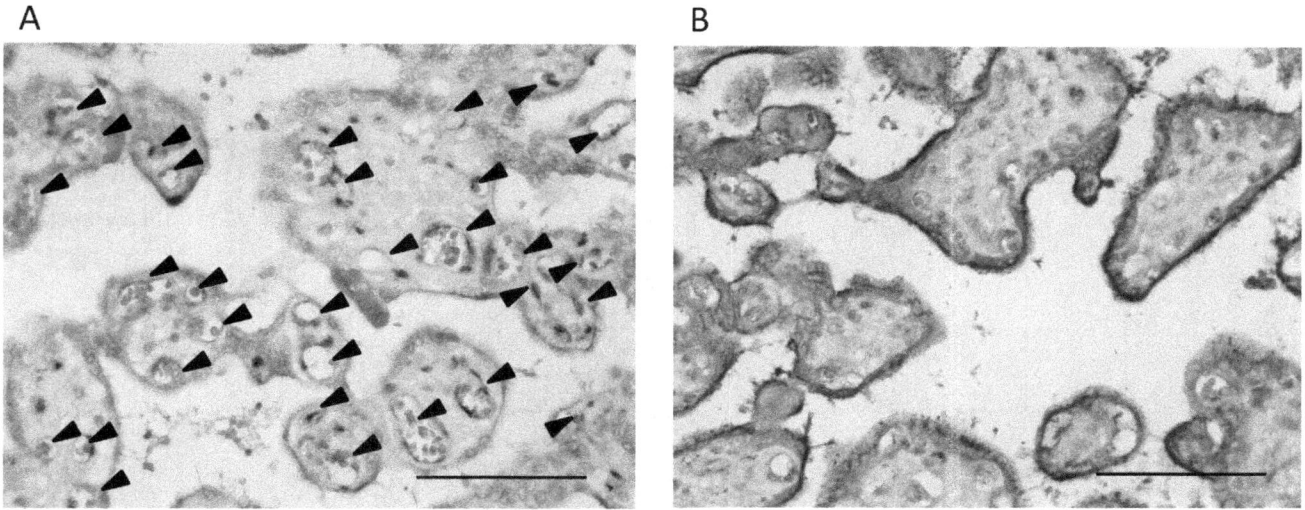

Figure 1. Localization of VASH1 and VASH2 in human placenta. Immunohistochemical analysis for the localization VASH1 (A) and VASH2 (B) in the human placenta was performed. Arrowheads indicate VASH1 vessels (A). Bar = 100 μm.

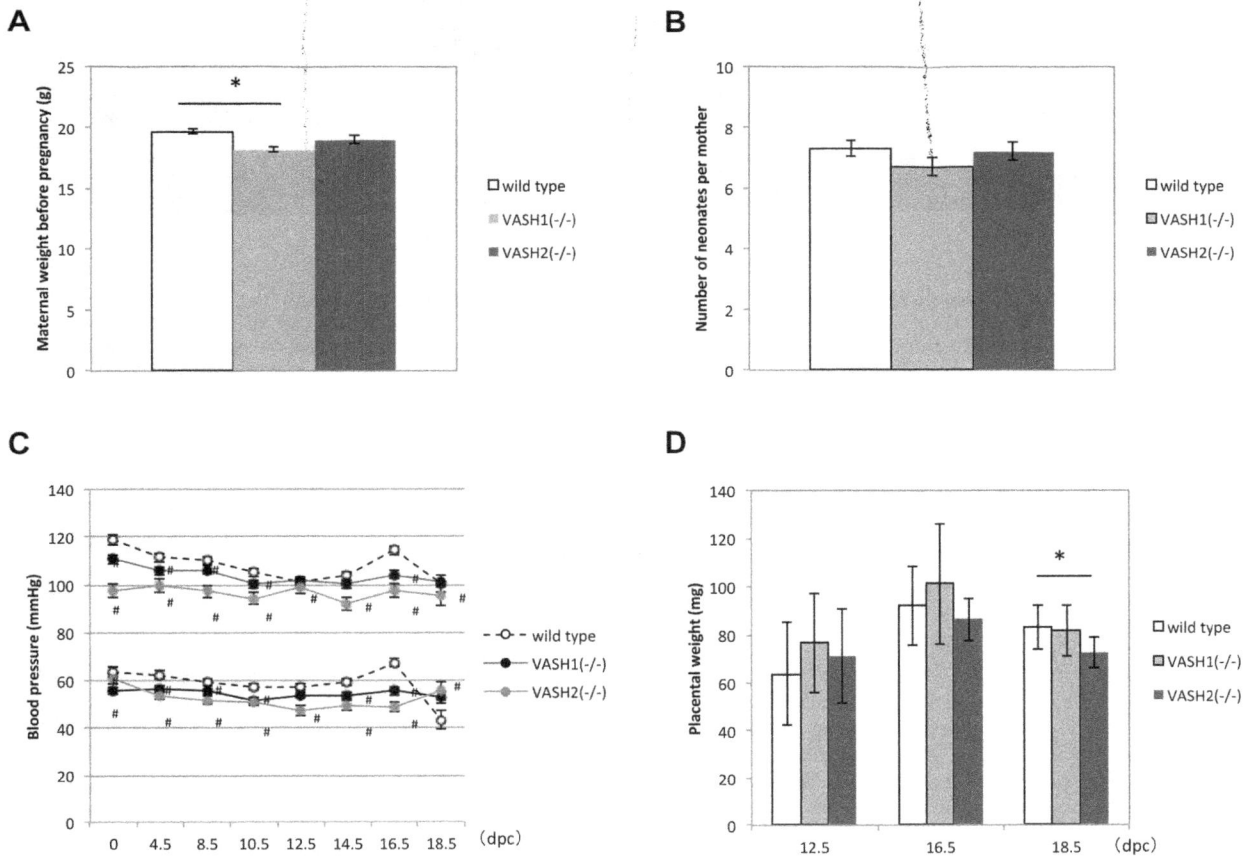

Figure 2. Course of pregnancy in WT, Vash1$^{(-/-)}$ and Vash2$^{(-/-)}$ mice. A: Comparison of maternal weights of WT (N = 30), Vash1$^{(-/-)}$ (N = 45), and Vash2$^{(-/-)}$ (N = 20) mice. *P<0.01. B: Comparison of number of neonates per WT (N = 32), Vash1$^{(-/-)}$ (N = 45), and Vash2$^{(-/-)}$ (N = 20) dams. C: Blood pressure of WT (N = 16), Vash1$^{(-/-)}$ (N = 15), and Vash2$^{(-/-)}$ (N = 7) dams measured at 0, 4.5, 8.5,10.5, 12.5, 14.5, 16.5, and 18.5 dpc. #P<0.05. D: Wet weight of WT (N = 37), Vash1$^{(-/-)}$ (N = 37), and Vash2$^{(-/-)}$ (N = 19) placentas. *P<0.01.

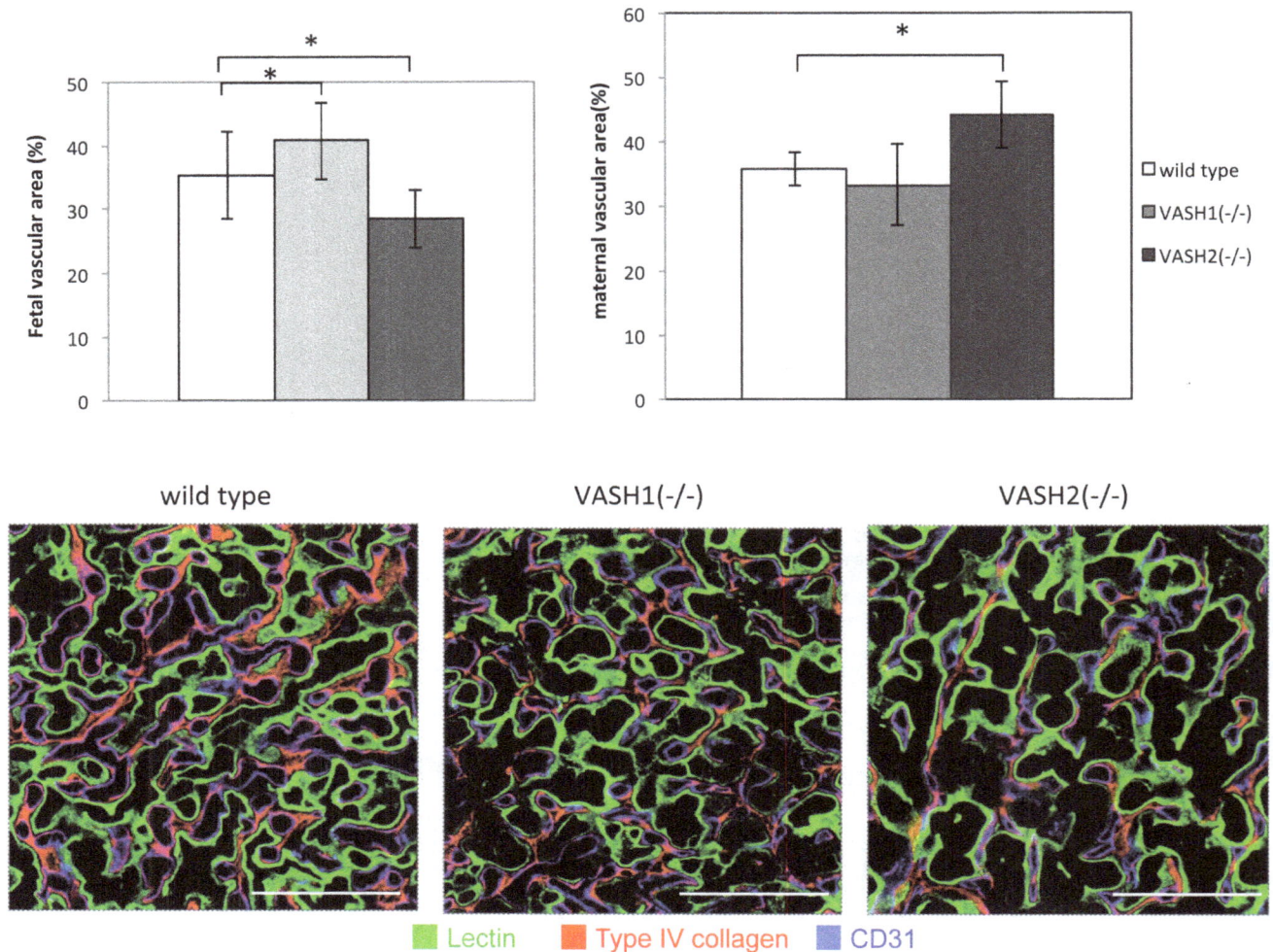

🟩 Lectin   🟥 Type IV collagen   🟦 CD31

Figure 3. Vascularization of placenta in WT, *Vash1*$^{(-/-)}$, and *Vash2*$^{(-/-)}$ mice. Upper panels show vascular morphogenesis. The triple staining with tomato lectin (green), anti-CD31 (blue), and anti-type IV collagen (red) was performed as described in Materials and Methods. Tomato lectin identified the maternal blood vessels; and CD31-positive structures, the fetal blood vessels. The presence of type IV collagen indicated the basement membrane. Bar = 50 μm. Lower graph on the left show the fetal vascular area, and that on the right shows the maternal vascular area determined for WT (N = 5), *Vash1*$^{(-/-)}$ (N = 3), and *Vash2*$^{(-/-)}$ (N = 3) placentas. Ten 400× fields per placenta were used for quantification. *P<0.01.

significantly high in *Vash2*$^{(-/-)}$ mice at 18.5 dpc (Fig. 4A). We could not find any significant differences in the serum levels of sVEGFR1 and PlGF (Fig. 4B and C).

VASH2 expressed in trophoblasts regulates cell fusion for syncytiotrophoblast formation

We further clarified the morphological changes in the placenta of the 3 types of mice. Electron microscopic observation of semi-thin sections showed that the fetal vascular area containing red blood cells within the labyrinth layer was increased in *Vash1*$^{(-/-)}$ mice and decreased in *Vash2*$^{(-/-)}$ mice (Fig. 5, A). These observations correlated well with the immunohistochemical findings shown in Fig. 3. However, a more striking change that we noticed was the thin and poorly developed villi in the *Vash2*$^{(-/-)}$ mice. As a result, the placenta was more porous having larger maternal lacunae in the *Vash2*$^{(-/-)}$ mice. This may explain the reduced weight of placenta in the *Vash2*$^{(-/-)}$ mice (Fig. 2D). The mouse placenta has 2 distinct syncytiotrophoblast layers, ST-I and ST-II. Our careful observation by the electron microscopy revealed that the cell fusion of ST-II was incomplete in the *Vash2*$^{(-/-)}$ mice (Fig. 5B). Murine endogenous retrovirus (ERV) envelope glycoprotein syncytin-A (Syn-A) and syncytin-B (Syn-B) are expressed in trophoblasts and regulates their fusion [15,16]. The transcription factor glial cells missing-1 (Gcm-1) regulates the expression of Syn-A [17]. We therefore compared the mRNA expression of Gcm-1, Syn-A, and Syn-B in the placenta, and found that only the expression of Syn-B was down-regulated in the *Vash2*$^{(-/-)}$ mice (Fig. 5 C–E).

To examine the role of VASH2 more directly, we used BeWo cells a human trophoblastoid choriocarcinoma cell line, in culture. As it is previously reported [18,19], the FK treatment induced cell fusion in BeWo cells (Fig. 6A) When the VASH2 expression in BeWo cells was knocked-down by siRNA (Fig. 6B), we observed a significant decrease in cell fusion (Fig. 6A and C). Human ERV envelope glycoproteins, Syn-1 and Syn-2 have been identified to regulate the fusion of trophoblasts [18–22]. They are not orthologous to murine Syn-A and Syn-B, but Gcm-1 regulates the expression of Syn-1 [19]. We therefore examined the expression of Gcm-1, Syn-1 and Syn-2 in BeWo cells, and found that it was not altered by the knock-down of VASH2 (Fig. 6D–F). To further clarify the role of VASH2 in the cell fusion, we

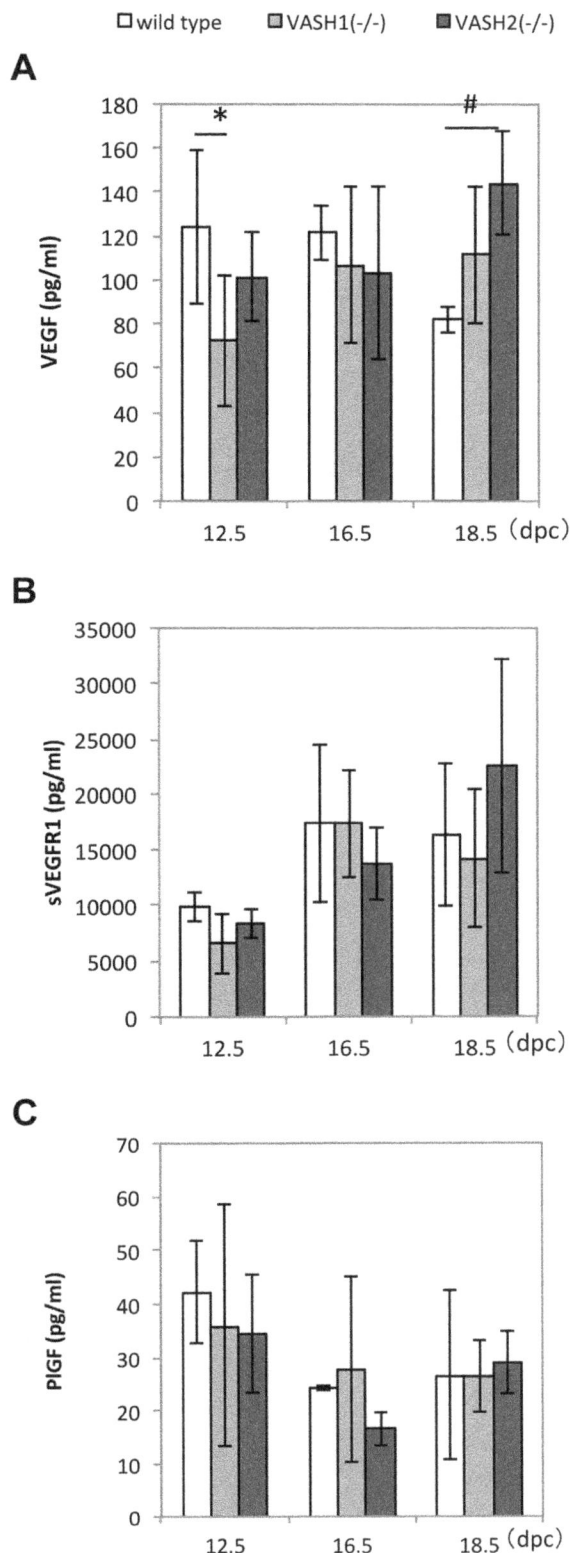

Figure 4. Serum levels of VEGF, sVEGFR1, and PlGF in WT, Vash1$^{(-/-)}$, and Vash2$^{(-/-)}$ dams. A: Serum levels of VEGF-A at 12.5, 16.5, and 18.5 dpc. The respective numbers of WT dams at these time points were 6, 3 and 4; of Vash1$^{(-/-)}$ ones, 7, 10 and 22; and of Vash2$^{(-/-)}$ dams, 4, 4 and 8. $^{#}P<0.05$, $^{*}P<0.01$. B: Serum levels of sVEGFR1 at 12.5, 16.5, and 18.5 dpc. The respective numbers of WT dams at these time points were 5, 4, and 5; of Vash1$^{(-/-)}$ ones, 6, 8 and 17; and of Vash2$^{(-/-)}$ dams, 4, 4, and 5. C: Serum levels of PlGF at 12.5, 16.5, and 18.5 dpc. Respective numbers of WT dams at these stages were 4, 2 and 2; of Vash1$^{(-/-)}$ ones, 5, 5, and 5; and of Vash2$^{(-/-)}$ dams, 3, 3, and 4.

overexpressed human VASH2 in BeWo cells. AdVASH2 infection significantly increased the expression of VASH2 and cell fusion of BeWo cells (Fig. 7A and B). Importantly, the AdVASH2 infection did not alter the expression of Gcm-1, Syn-1 and Syn-2 in BeWo cells (Fig. 7 C–E).

Discussion

The vasohibin family comprises 2 proteins, the anti-angiogenic VASH1 and the pro-angiogenic VASH2. It was previously shown that the VASH1 protein is selectively localized in ECs at the site of angiogenesis associated with various pathophysiological conditions and at that occurring in the human placenta [7,23–28]. Here we confirmed its selective localization in ECs in the placenta. The localization of VASH2 protein in the placenta had not been previously examined. Our present study revealed for the first time that VASH2 was selectively localized in trophoblasts in the placenta. The distinctive expression and localization of VASH2 from those of endothelial VASH1 were shown previously. For example, VASH2 is expressed in infiltrating CD11b^{+} monocyte/macrophage lineage cells that infiltrate the dermis in hypoxia-induced angiogenesis [11]. In addition, VASH2 is expressed in ovarian or hepatocellular carcinoma cells [29,30]. The present study disclosed another instance of such distinctive localization of VASH2 from that of endothelial VASH1, i.e., in the placenta.

When we evaluated the role of VASH1 and VASH2 in the vascularization of placenta, our analysis revealed that the fetal vascular area was significantly increased in the Vash1$^{(-/-)}$ mice and decreased in the Vash2$^{(-/-)}$ ones. These results correlate well with the anti-angiogenic function of VASH1 and pro-angiogenic function of VASH2. Moreover, their differential expressions further suggest that VASH1 acts as an autocrine factor whereas VASH2 acts as a paracrine factor. Interestingly, the serum level of VEGF-A was significantly low in Vash1$^{(-/-)}$ mice at E12.5, and significantly high in Vash2$^{(-/-)}$ mice at E18.5. We assumed that those changes in VEGF-A were due to biological adaptation; i.e., when the angiogenesis inhibitor VASH1 was defective, angiogenic VEGF-A was decreased, and when angiogenesis stimulator VASH2 was defective, angiogenic VEGF-A was increased. These adaptations would be expected to minimize the change of vascularization in Vash1$^{(-/-)}$ and Vash2$^{(-/-)}$ mice.

Here we disclosed the novel function of VASH2, namely, its involvement in trophoblast fusion. A neutralizing anti-human VASH2 monoclonal antibody inhibited the FK-induced fusion of HUVECs (Suenaga et al. unpublished observation). Thus, this effect of VASH2 is mediated via the autocrine/paracrine manner. The syncytiotrophoblast layer is formed by the fusion of trophoblasts. The mouse placenta has 2 distinct and highly specialized syncytiotrophoblast layers, ST-I and ST-II; whereas the human placenta has a single layer. The known regulators of trophoblast fusion are ERV envelope glycoproteins, Syn-A and Syn-B in mice and Syn-1 and Syn-2 in humans [15–22]. Among them, Syn-A and Syn-1 are the target of Gcm-1. We observed that Vash2$^{(-/-)}$ mice displayed impaired cell fusion of trophoblasts only in ST-II. The defect in trophoblasts in Vash2$^{(-/-)}$ mice might not severely affect the function of placenta, because the number of neonates was not impaired in Vash2$^{(-/-)}$ mice (Fig. 2B).

This defect of ST-II resembles that of Syn-B$^{(-/-)}$ mice [31–33]. Interestingly, the expression of Syn-A was unchanged but that of

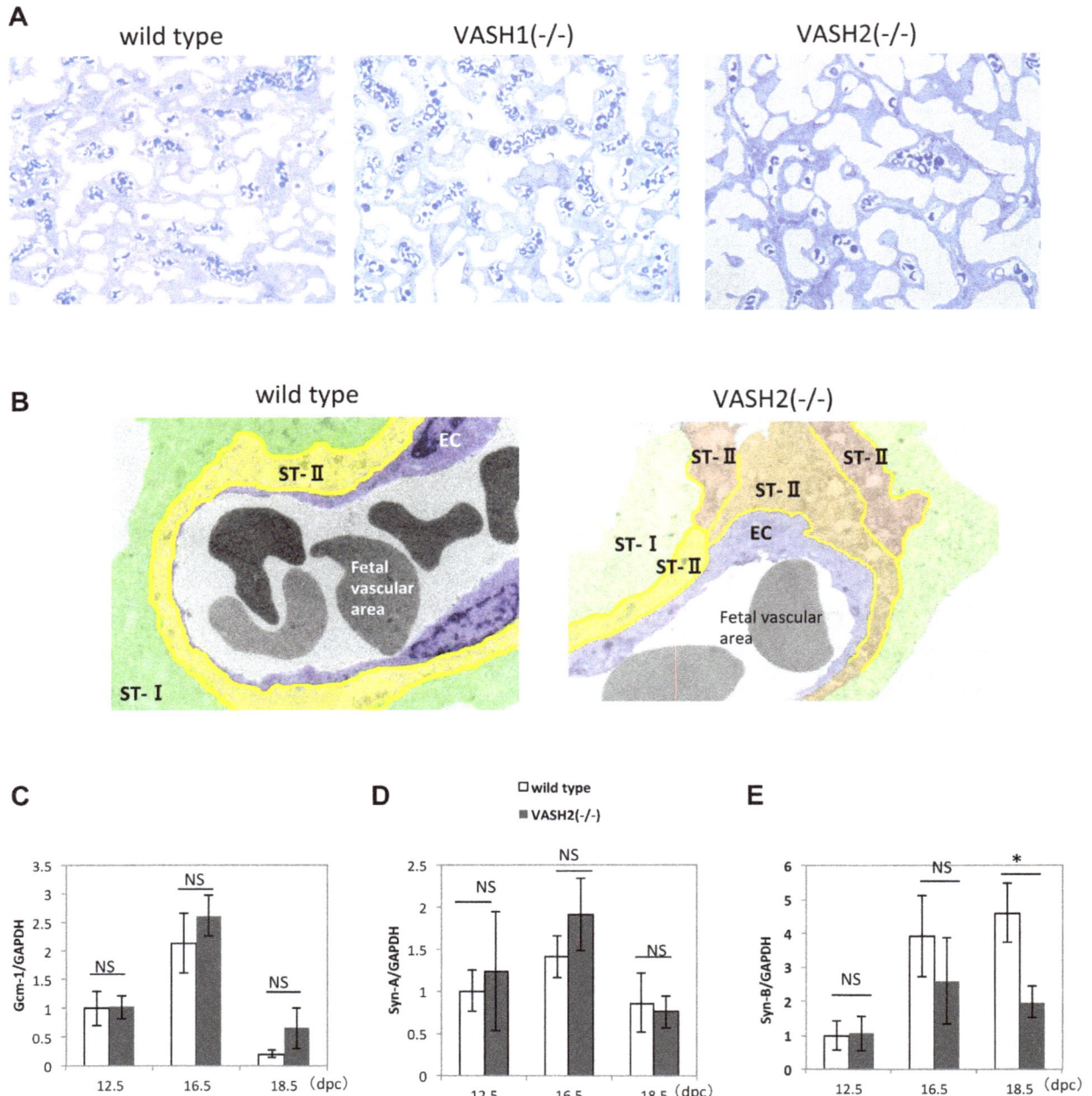

Figure 5. Labyrinth and syncytiotrophoblast layers of WT, *Vash1*$^{(-/-)}$ and *Vash2*$^{(-/-)}$ mice. A: Semi-thin sections of the labyrinth layer of WT, *Vash1*$^{(-/-)}$, and *Vash2*$^{(-/-)}$ placentas. Bar = 20 μm. B: Electron microscopic pictures of WT and *Vash2*$^{(-/-)}$ placentas. Purple indicates ECs; green, ST-I; and yellow, ST-II. Bar = 5 μm. C–E: Expression of Gcm-1, Syn-B, and Syn-A in WT, *Vash1*$^{(-/-)}$ and *Vash2*$^{(-/-)}$ placentas at the indicated dpc, was determined by qRT-PCR. At 12.5, 16.5, and 18.5 dpc, the respective placenta numbers were 7, 6, and 5 for WT; 7, 7, and 7 for *Vash1*$^{(-/-)}$; and 5, 7, and 6 for *Vash2*$^{(-/-)}$. *P<0.01, NS; not significant.

Syn-B was down-regulated in the *Vash2*$^{(-/-)}$ placenta. These observations may explain the reason why the impaired cell fusion was only observed in ST-II of the *Vash2*$^{(-/-)}$ placenta, and thus suggest a possible interaction between VASH2 and Syn-B for the formation of ST-II in mice. Nonetheless, the interaction of VASH2 and ERV envelope glycoproteins cannot be applied to the human system. FK induced the fusion of human BeWo cells, and this fusion was inhibited by the knockdown of VASH2. In this situation, the expression of Gcm-1, Syn-1, and Syn-2 was unchanged. Conversely, the overexpression of VASH2 by the AdVASH2 infection augmented the fusion of BeWo cells without any changes in the expression of Gcm-1, Syn-1, and Syn-2. Thus, the role of VASH2 in the fusion of trophoblasts is independent of Gcm-1 and ERV envelope glycoproteins at least in the human system.

Cell fusion is a phenomenon that is seen not only in placentation but also in various physiological/pathophysiological conditions such as fertilization, development of skeletal muscle and

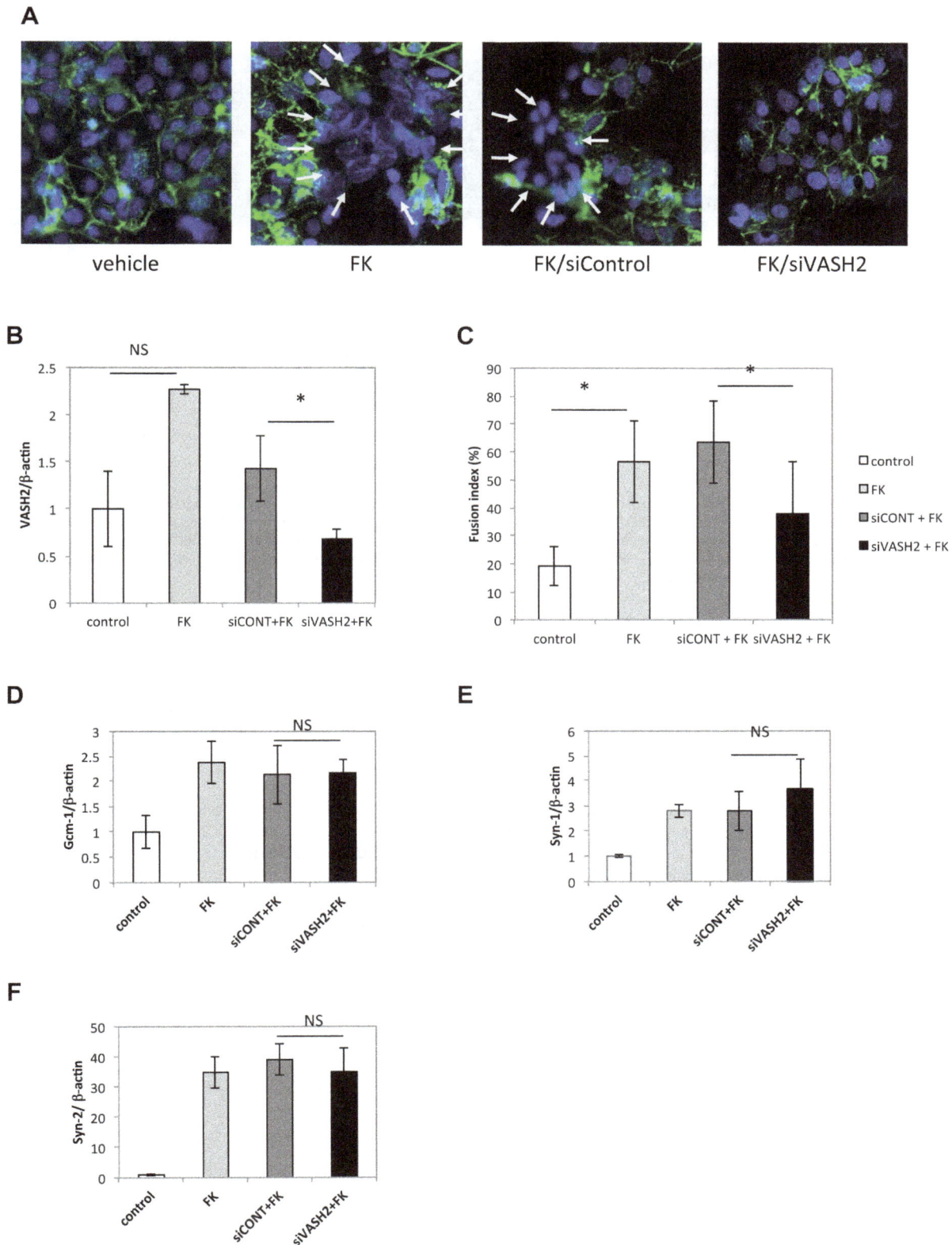

Figure 6. Knockdown of VASH2 inhibited the forskolin-induced fusion of BeWo cells. A: BeWo cells with or without siRNA treatment were stimulated with FK, and cell fusion was observed as described in Materials and Methods. Bar = 100 μm. Arrows indicate fused cells with multiple nuclei. B: Expression of human VASH2 was quantified (N = 3). *P<0.01, NS; not significant. C: Cell fusion was quantified as described in Materials and Methods (N = 2, 10 fields each). *P<0.01. D–F: Expression of Gcm-1, Syn-2, and Syn-1 in BeWo cells with each treatment (N = 3) was determined by qRT-PCR. NS; not significant.

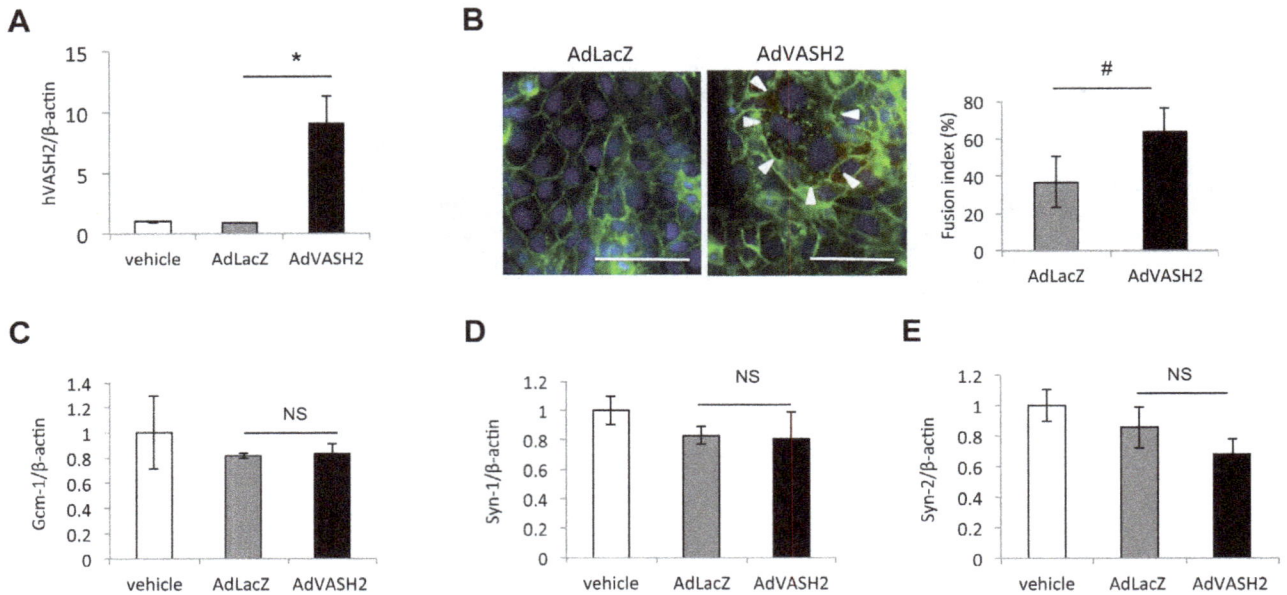

Figure 7. The overexpression of VASH2 augmented the fusion of BeWo cells. A: BeWo cells were infected with adenovirus vectors. Expression of human VASH2 was quantified by qRT-PCR (N = 3). B: Cell fusion was observed as described in Materials and Methods. Bar = 100 μm. Arrowheads indicate a fused cell with multiple nuclei. Cell fusion was quantified as described in Materials and Methods (N = 3, 5 fields each). # < P0.05. C: Expression of Gcm-1 was quantified by qRT-PCR (N = 3). D: Expression of Syn-1 was quantified by qRT-PCR (N = 3). E: Expression of Syn-2 was quantified by qRT-PCR (N = 3). NS; not significant.

bone, removal of apoptotic cells by macrophage, and the development and progression of cancers; but the commonality of the mechanism of cell fusion in those conditions is currently unknown [34,35]. The expression of VASH2 is scarce and limited, but our earlier observations showed this expression in cancer cells [28,29] and cells of the macrophage lineage [11]. The present study revealed its expression in trophoblasts. We also have detected the expression of VASH2 in skeletal muscle (unpublished data). These circumferential lines of evidence may suggest a role for VASH2 in cell fusion. This hypothesis needs to be investigated in a future study.

In summary, we disclosed the role of vasohibin family proteins in placental morphogenesis. As expected, VASH1 in ECs acted as an angiogenesis inhibitor and VASH2 in trophoblasts acted as an angiogenesis stimulator, in the placenta. However, perhaps the most intriguing finding was that VASH2 in trophoblasts played the role in the cell fusion for syncytiotrophoblast formation. Our present study provides innovative information on the function of VASH2 beside the stimulation of angiogenesis. Further study is currently underway to clarify the mechanism as to how VASH2 regulates the fusion of trophoblasts

Acknowledgments

We thank Ms. Miki Nakagawa for her excellent technical assistance.

Author Contributions

Conceived and designed the experiments: JS NY Y. Sato. Performed the experiments: KS SK. Analyzed the data: KS SK. Contributed reagents/materials/analysis tools: Y. Suzuki MK SH. Contributed to the writing of the manuscript: KS Y. Sato.

References

1. Pötgens AJ, Drewlo S, Kokozidou M, Kaufmann P. (2004) Syncytin: the major regulator of trophoblast fusion? Recent developments and hypotheses on its action. Hum Reprod Update 10: 487–496.
2. Wang A, Rana S, Karumanchi SA. (2009) Preeclampsia: the role of angiogenic factors in its pathogenesis. Physiology (Bethesda) 24: 147–158.
3. Bulmer JN, Innes BA, Levey J, Robson SC, Lash GE. (2012) The role of vascular smooth muscle cell apoptosis and migration during uterine spiral artery remodeling in normal human pregnancy. FASEB J 26: 2975–2985.
4. Burton GJ, Charnock-Jones DS, Jauniaux E. (2009) Regulation of vascular growth and function in the human placenta. Reproduction 138: 895–902.
5. Arroyo JA, Winn VD. (2008) Vasculogenesis and angiogenesis in the IUGR placenta. Semin Perinatol 32: 172–177.
6. Barut F, Barut A, Gun BD, Kandemir NO, Harma MI, et al. (2010) Intrauterine growth restriction and placental angiogenesis. Diagn Pathol 5: 24.
7. Watanabe K, Hasegawa Y, Yamashita H, Shimizu K, Ding Y, et al. (2004) Vasohibin as an endothelium-derived negative feedback regulator of angiogenesis. J Clin Invest 114: 898–907.
8. Shibuya T, Watanabe K, Yamashita H, Shimizu K, Miyashita H, et al. (2006) Isolation and characterization of vasohibin-2 as a homologue of VEGF-inducible endothelium-derived angiogenesis inhibitor vasohibin. Arterioscler Thromb Vasc Biol 26: 1051–1057.

9. Sato Y. (2013) The vasohibin family: a novel family for angiogenesis regulation. J Biochem 153: 5–11.
10. Suzuki Y, Kobayashi M, Miyashita H, Ohta H, Sonoda H, et al. (2010) Isolation of a small vasohibin-binding protein (SVBP) and its role in vasohibin secretion. J Cell Sci 123: 3094–4101.
11. Kimura H, Miyashita H, Suzuki Y, Kobayashi M, Watanabe K, et al. (2009) Distinctive localization and opposed roles of vasohibin-1 and vasohibin-2 in the regulation of angiogenesis. Blood 113: 4810–4818.
12. Kitahara S, Morikawa S, Shimizu K, Abe H, Ezaki T. (2010) Alteration of angiogenic patterns on B16BL6 melanoma development promoted in Matrigel. Med Mol Morphol 43: 26–36.
13. Yoshie M, Kaneyama K, Kusama K, Higuma C, Nishi H, et al. (2010) Possible role of the exchange protein directly activated by cyclic AMP (Epac) in the cyclic AMP-dependent functional differentiation and syncytialization of human placental BeWo cells. Hum Reprod 25: 2229–2238.
14. Matsuura K, Jigami T, Taniue K, Morishita Y, Adachi S, et al. (2011) Identification of a link between Wnt/β-catenin signalling and the cell fusion pathway. Nat Commun 2: 548.
15. Simmons DG, Natale DR, Begay V, Hughes M, Leutz A, et al. (2008) Early patterning of the chorion leads to the trilaminar trophoblast cell structure in the placental labyrinth. Development 135: 2083–2091.

16. Dupressoir A, Lavialle C, Heidmann T. (2012) From ancestral infectious retroviruses to bona fide cellular genes: role of the captured syncytins in placentation. Placenta 33: 663–671.

17. Schubert SW, Lamoureux N, Kilian K, Klein-Hitpass L, Hashemolhosseini S. (2008) Identification of integrin-alpha4, Rb1, and syncytin a as murine placental target genes of the transcription factor GCMa/Gcm1. J Biol Chem 283: 5460–5465.

18. Mi S, Lee X, Li X, Veldman GM, Finnerty H, et al. (2000) Syncytin is a captive retroviral envelope protein involved in human placental morphogenesis. Nature 403: 785–789.

19. Chen CP, Chen LF, Yang SR, et al. Functional characterization of the human placental fusogenic membrane protein syncytin 2. Biol Reprod 2008;79:815–23.

20. Yu C, Shen K, Lin M, Chen CY, Ko CC, et al. (2002) GCMa regulates the syncytin-mediated trophoblastic fusion. J Biol Chem 277: 50062–50068.

21. Frendo JL, Olivier D, Cheynet V, Blond JL, Bouton O, et al. (2003) Direct involvement of HERV-W Env glycoprotein in human trophoblast cell fusion and differentiation. Mol Cell Biol 23: 3566–3574.

22. Holder BS, Tower CL, Abrahams VM, Aplin JD. (2012) Syncytin 1 in the human placenta. Placenta33: 460–466.

23. Yamashita H, Abe M, Watanabe K, Shimizu K, Moriya T, et al. (2006) Vasohibin prevents arterial neointimal formation through angiogenesis inhibition. Biochem Biophys Res Commun 345: 919–925.

24. Yoshinaga K, Ito K, Moriya T, Nagase S, Takano T, et al. (2008) Expression of vasohibin as a novel endothelium-derived angiogenesis inhibitor in endometrial cancer. Cancer Sci 99: 914–919.

25. Wakusawa R, Abe T, Sato H, Yoshida M, Kunikata H, et al. (2008) Expression of vasohibin, an antiangiogenic factor, in human choroidal neovascular membranes. Am J Ophthalmol 146: 235–243.

26. Tamaki K, Moriya T, Sato Y, Ishida T, Maruo Y, et al. (2009) Vasohibin-1 in human breast carcinoma: a potential negative feedback regulator of angiogenesis. Cancer Sci 100: 88–94.

27. Sato H, Abe T, Wakusawa R, Asai N, Kunikata H, et al. (2009) Vitreous levels of vasohibin-1 and vascular endothelial growth factor in patients with proliferative diabetic retinopathy. Diabetologia 52: 359–361.

28. Hosaka T, Kimura H, Heishi T, Suzuki Y, Miyashita H, et al. (2009) Vasohibin-1 expression in endothelium of tumor blood vessels regulates angiogenesis. Am J Pathol 175: 430–439.

29. Takahashi Y, Koyanagi T, Suzuki Y, Saga Y, Kanomata N, et al. (2012) Vasohibin-2 expressed in human serous ovarian adenocarcinoma accelerates tumor growth by promoting angiogenesis. Mol Cancer Res 10: 1135–1146.

30. Xue X, Gao W, Sun B, Xu Y, Han B, et al. (2013) Vasohibin 2 is transcriptionally activated and promotes angiogenesis in hepatocellular carcinoma. Oncogene 32: 1724–1734

31. Dupressoir A, Vernochet C, Harper F, Guégan J, Dessen P, et al. (2011) A pair of co-opted retroviral envelope syncytin genes is required for formation of the two-layered murine placental syncytiotrophoblast. Proc Natl Acad Sci U S A 108: E1164–1173.

32. Dupressoir A, Marceau G, Vernochet C, Bénit L, Kanellopoulos C, Sapin V, et al. (2005) Syncytin-A and syncytin-B, two fusogenic placenta-specific murine envelope genes of retroviral origin conserved in Muridae. Proc Natl Acad Sci U S A 102: 725–730.

33. Lavialle C, Cornelis G, Dupressoir A, Esnault C, Heidmann O, et al. (2013) Paleovirology of 'syncytins', retroviral env genes exapted for a role in placentation. Philos Trans R Soc Lond B Biol Sci 368: 20120507.

34. Larsson LI, Bjerregaard B, Talts JF. (2008) Cell fusions in mammals. Histochem Cell Biol 129: 551–561.

35. Dittmar T, Nagler C, Niggemann B, Zänker KS. (2013) The dark side of stem cells: triggering cancer progression by cell fusion. Curr Mol Med 13:735–750.

12

Lack of Involvement of CEP Adducts in TLR Activation and in Angiogenesis

John Gounarides[1], Jennifer S. Cobb[1], Jing Zhou[1], Frank Cook[1], Xuemei Yang[1], Hong Yin[1], Erik Meredith[2], Chang Rao[1], Qian Huang[3], YongYao Xu[3], Karen Anderson[4], Andrea De Erkenez[4], Sha-Mei Liao[4], Maura Crowley[4], Natasha Buchanan[4], Stephen Poor[4], Yubin Qiu[4], Elizabeth Fassbender[4], Siyuan Shen[4], Amber Woolfenden[4], Amy Jensen[4], Rosemarie Cepeda[4], Bijan Etemad-Gilbertson[4], Shelby Giza[4], Muneto Mogi[2], Bruce Jaffee[4], Sassan Azarian[4]*

1 Analytical Sciences, Novartis Institutes for Biomedical Research, Cambridge, MA, United States of America, 2 Global Discovery Chemistry, Novartis Institutes for Biomedical Research, Cambridge, MA, United States of America, 3 Developmental and Metabolic Pathways, Novartis Institutes for Biomedical Research, Cambridge, MA, United States of America, 4 Ophthalmology, Novartis Institutes for Biomedical Research, Cambridge, MA, United States of America

Abstract

Proteins that are post-translationally adducted with 2-(ω-carboxyethyl)pyrrole (CEP) have been proposed to play a pathogenic role in age-related macular degeneration, by inducing angiogenesis in a Toll Like Receptor 2 (TLR2)-dependent manner. We have investigated the involvement of CEP adducts in angiogenesis and TLR activation, to assess the therapeutic potential of inhibiting CEP adducts and TLR2 for ocular angiogenesis. As tool reagents, several CEP-adducted proteins and peptides were synthetically generated by published methodology and adduction was confirmed by NMR and LC-MS/MS analyses. Structural studies showed significant changes in secondary structure in CEP-adducted proteins but not the untreated proteins. Similar structural changes were also observed in the treated unadducted proteins, which were treated by the same adduction method except for one critical step required to form the CEP group. Thus some structural changes were unrelated to CEP groups and were artificially induced by the synthesis method. In biological studies, the CEP-adducted proteins and peptides failed to activate TLR2 in cell-based assays and in an *in vivo* TLR2-mediated retinal leukocyte infiltration model. Neither CEP adducts nor TLR agonists were able to induce angiogenesis in a tube formation assay. *In vivo*, treatment of animals with CEP-adducted protein had no effect on laser-induced choroidal neovascularization. Furthermore, *in vivo* inactivation of TLR2 by deficiency in Myeloid Differentiation factor 88 (Myd88) had no effect on abrasion-induced corneal neovascularization. Thus the CEP-TLR2 axis, which is implicated in other wound angiogenesis models, does not appear to play a pathological role in a corneal wound angiogenesis model. Collectively, our data do not support the mechanism of action of CEP adducts in TLR2-mediated angiogenesis proposed by others.

Editor: Michael E. Boulton, Indiana University College of Medicine, United States of America

Funding: This study was funded by the Novartis Institutes for Biomedical Research. The funder provided support in the form of salaries for all authors, but did not have any additional role in the study design, data collection and analysis, decision to publish, or preparation of the manuscript. The specific roles of these authors are articulated in the 'author contributions' section.

Competing Interests: The authors were all full-time employees of the Novartis Institutes of Biomedical Research, which funded this study, at the time this work was completed. There are no patents, products in development or marketed products to declare.

* Email: Sassan.Azarian@novartis.com

Introduction

Age-related macular degeneration (AMD) is a major cause of legal blindness in the elderly. The macula is a specialized area of the central retina that is enriched in photoreceptor cells and is responsible for high acuity vision. In AMD, progressive macular degeneration can impair critical daily functions such as reading, driving, and face recognition. Thus AMD can have a profound impact on quality of life. There are two forms of advanced AMD: dry and wet (neovascular) AMD [1]. AMD is thought to be a disease of the retinal pigment epithelium (RPE) cells, which provide critical support functions to adjacent photoreceptors [1]. In the early stage of disease, AMD retinas show progressive accumulation of extracellular deposits, drusen, as well as intracellular deposits, lipofuscin, at the level of the RPE. These deposits initially tend to accumulate in the macular area. Over time, RPE cells show pigmentary changes and begin to degenerate. In advanced stages, dry AMD patients exhibit substantial delineated areas of RPE atrophy, or geographic atrophy. Advanced wet AMD patients exhibit leaky blood vessels in the macula, in many cases emanating from the choriocapillaris [1].

Currently there are no treatments for dry AMD. In the Age-Related Eye Disease Study 1 (AREDS 1), dietary supplements comprised of anti-oxidants and select minerals reduced the risk of progression to advanced AMD by 25% [1]. Several therapeutic approaches are being tested in clinical trials [2] but there are no FDA-approved treatments in practice at this point. For wet AMD, anti-angiogenic treatments have been clinically proven to be efficacious [3]. However, not all patients respond to treatment and the burden of treatment is still relatively high. Thus there is a great medical need for novel treatments for AMD. The molecular details of pathogenesis in AMD are not fully established but several pathogenic mechanisms have been implicated [1]. For example, human molecular genetic data indicate the involvement of the alternative complement pathway. Another potential cause is proposed to be cumulative oxidative stress, based on preclinical studies and on the AREDS1 trial. One manifestation of oxidative stress is proposed to be the formation of CEP adducts, which are a type of advanced glycation end products [4].

Photoreceptor cells are highly enriched in docosahexaenoic acid (DHA), a labile fatty acid that is susceptible to breakdown by photo-oxidation and other forms of oxidative stress. The breakdown products include a reactive aldehyde, 4-hydroxy-7-oxohept-5-enoic acid, which can condense with primary amines to form a Schiff base. In the case of proteins, 4-hydroxy-7-oxohept-5-enoic acid condenses with lysineε-amines. Subsequent reactions result in a covalently attached CEP moiety, yielding a stable CEP adduct [4]. In previous reports, antibodies raised against synthetic CEP reagents were used to identify, localize, and quantify CEP adducts by various immunological assays [5]. Elevated levels of CEP adducts were initially reported in proteomic studies of AMD donor eyes [5] and subsequently in AMD plasma [6,7]. Thus CEP adducts were implicated in AMD [5–7]. In later studies CEP adducts were reported to be pro-angiogenic, both *in vitro* and *in vivo*. These *in vivo* studies utilized the micropocket corneal neovascularization (CoNV) and the laser-induced choroidal neovascularization (CNV) models [8]. More recently, Toll-like receptor 2 (TLR2) was reported to mediate the CEP adduct-induced angiogenesis [9]. The angiogenic activity was reported to be independent of the vascular endothelial growth factor (VEGF) pathway [8,9].

There is a medical need for novel treatments for both wet and dry AMD. CEP adducts are implicated in both forms of AMD and represent an attractive potential target for drug discovery. Thus we initiated validation studies to assess the therapeutic potential of inhibiting CEP adducts.

Results

Synthesis of Tool Reagents

Several synthetic CEP adducts were generated according to reported procedures [10]. These tool reagents included protein (e.g. human serum albumin-CEP, or HSA-CEP), peptide (e.g. Ac-Gly-Lys-OMe-CEP, or dipeptide-CEP), and phospholipid (e.g. phosphatidyl ethanolamine-CEP, or PE-CEP) adducts, as listed in **Table S1**. The presence of CEP adducts and the stoichiometry of adduction was confirmed by ^{1}H-NMR and LC-MS/MS (**Figure S1 and Figure S2**). Invariably the presence of CEP moiety was established in the adducted samples and was never detected in the controls. CEP adduction was deemed successful by several measures. For example, ^{1}H-NMR analysis indicated the expected molecular signature of the CEP group in dipeptide-CEP but not the untreated dipeptide (**Figure S1B**). Likewise, LC-MS/MS analysis of enzymatic hydrolyzed adducted proteins detected lysine-CEP in HSA-CEP and MSA-CEP (mouse serum albumin-CEP) but not the respective controls (**Figure S1C**). For protein adducts, two controls were used: CTL1, which represents untreated protein; and CTL2, which represents treated unadducted protein. The latter control was treated exactly the same way as the corresponding CEP adduct except for one step, to prevent adduction (see Materials and Methods). No CEP moiety was detected in HSA-CTL2 or MSA-CTL2. There are a total of 59 lysines in HSA (UnitPro P02768) and 50 lysines in MSA

(UnitPro P07724). We identified 14 lysine-CEP sites in HSA-CEP and 40 lysine-CEP sites in MSA-CEP (**Figure S2**). These values are in fair agreement with the reported stoichiometries: 6 or 17 CEP-modified lysines for HSA-CEP [10,11], and 15 for MSA-CEP [10].

Does CEP-Adduction Affect Protein Structure?

When we analyzed HSA-CEP, HSA-CTL2, and HSA-CTL1 in structural studies we observed significant structural alterations in HSA-CEP in comparison with HSA-CTL1. However, HSA-CTL2 also incurred significant alterations, similar to but less extensive than HSA-CEP. On SDS-PAGE gels HSA-CEP and HSA-CTL2 but not HSA-CTL1 appeared to form oligomers in a ladder-like fashion (**Figure 1A**). Comparison of size exclusion chromatography (SEC) profiles indicated progressive loss of the HSA monomer in the order of HSA-CTL1 > HSA-CTL2 > HSA-CEP (**Figure 1B**). Circular dichroism (CD) also indicated a significant loss in secondary structure in HSA-CTL2 and HSA-CEP compared to HSA-CTL1 (**Figure 1C**).

Collectively these data show that our synthetic CEP adducts can incur two kinds of structural changes: a) CEP-independent changes and b) CEP-dependent changes. Comparison of our HSA-CTL1 and HSA-CTL2 illustrates the CEP-independent changes in protein structure, which indicate artificial changes introduced by the procedure for generating synthetic adducts. Comparison of our HSA-CTL2 and HSA-CEP illustrates the CEP-dependent changes that occur as a result covalent CEP groups in HSA-CEP, beyond the CEP-independent changes in HSA-CTL2.

Is TLR2 Activated By CEP Adducts?

We tested several CEP adducts in a cell-based TLR2 assay, essentially as described [9]. Pam3CSK4, a known TLR2 agonist, showed dose-dependent activation of TLR2 as monitored by production of NF-κB or IL-8 in cellular assays (**Figure 2**, top and middle panels). However, no TLR2 activation was detected by HSA-CEP (**Figure 2**), or several other CEP adducts tested: MSA-CEP, dipeptide-CEP, or PE-CEP (not shown). None of these adducts showed any cytotoxicity, as measured with CellTiter-Glo (CTG) kit (**Figure 2**). Next we used THP-1 cells, which naturally express several TLRs, including TLR2. While positive controls showed specific activation of the corresponding TLR, CEP adducts failed to activate TLR2 or any other TLR that was monitored (**Figure 2**, bottom panel). *In vivo*, CEP adducts did not induce biological effects that are mediated by TLR2. As **Figure 3A** shows, treatment of mice with Pam3CSK4 induced infiltration of neutrophils and macrophages in the retina. However, neither dipeptide-CEP nor MSA-CEP (not shown) induced retinal infiltration in the same assay. Representative images of this experiment are shown in **Figure 3B**. These results suggest that CEP adducts do not activate TLRs, including TLR2.

Are CEP Adducts or TLR2 Involved in Angiogenesis?

We used the tube formation *in vitro* assay to determine if CEP adducts are angiogenic, similar to a previously reported assay [9]. VEGF induced significant tube formation; however, neither CEP adducts nor Pam3CSK4 affected tube formation (**Table 1**). In addition, poly (I:C) (a TLR3 agonist) and LPS (a TLR4 agonist) failed to show any effect. Representative images of the tube formation assay are shown in **Figure 4**.

The CEP adducts were further evaluated in the laser-induced choroidal neovascularization (CNV) model, as was reported earlier [8]. Initial laser CNV studies were performed with C57BL/6N mice, which showed no effect of MSA-CEP (**File S1**). In light of

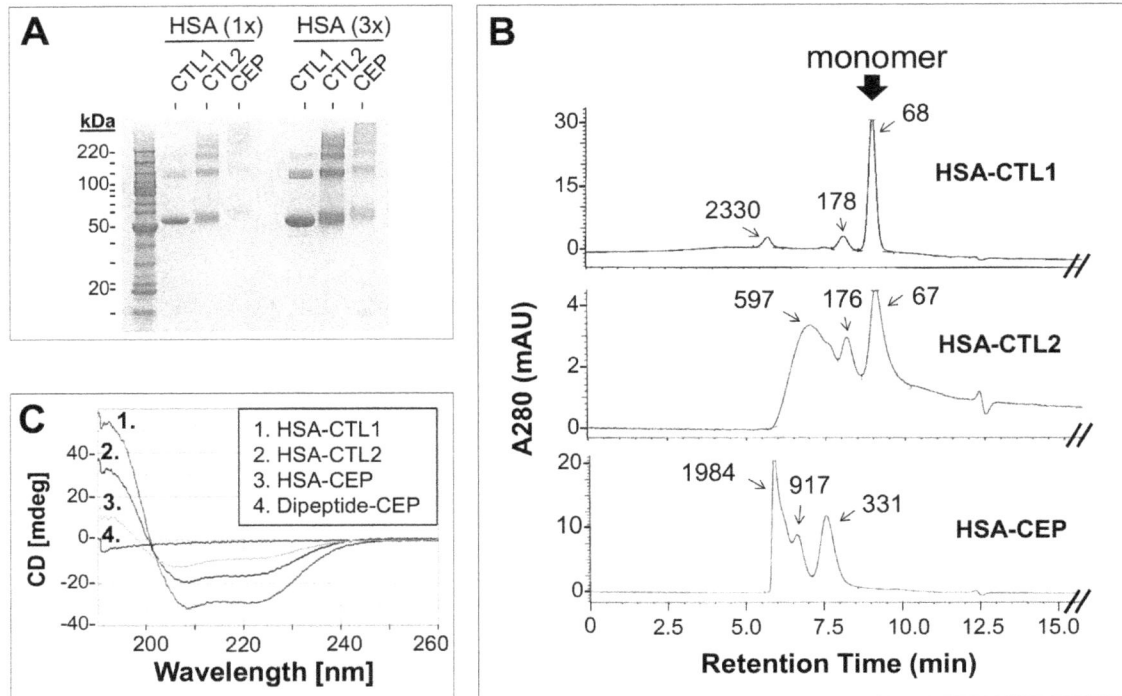

Figure 1. Structural Analyses of CEP Adducts. A) *SDS-PAGE analysis.* Aliquots of HSA-CTL1 (untreated), HSA-CTL2 (treated but unadducted) and HSA-CEP were subjected to reducing SDS-PAGE on 4–10% gels. Compared to HSA-CTL1, both HSA-CTL2 and HSA-CEP showed an increase in high-MW bands. B) *Size exclusion chromatography.* SEC under non-denaturing conditions indicated an increase in faster-eluting peaks in HSA-CTL2 and HSA-CEP compared to HSA-CTL1. C) *Circular dichroism.* CD analysis revealed a loss of secondary structure in HSA-CTL2 and HSA-CEP compared to HSA-CTL1.

the *rd8* mutation in the *Crb1* gene reported in this strain [12], we repeated the study with C57BL/6J mice which are wildtype for *Crb1* [12] and were used in the previously reported study [8]. We observed the same results with 2 experiments in each strain. Subretinal injection of VEGF significantly exacerbated CNV, while a VEGF-neutralizing antibody inhibited CNV (**Figure 5A and File S1**). This is consistent with VEGF being a major pro-angiogenic factor in CNV. However, subretinally administered MSA-CEP, at a dose nearly identical to that used in the previous report [8], had no effect in this model (**Figure 5A and File S1**). Representative images of the experiments in Figure 5A are shown in **Figure 5B**.

In studies with a corneal neovascularization (CoNV) mouse model, we observed that *Myd88*-deficiency had no significant effect on CoNV (**Figure 6**) when compared with similarly treated wild-type mice. Since *Myd88* deficiency abolishes TLR2 activity, this indicates that TLR2 is not required for angiogenesis in the abrasion-induced CoNV model. In contrast, CoNV is greatly dependent on VEGF-A: a) qPCR analysis showed a 30-fold increase in *VEGF-A* mRNA expression and b) treatment of abraded mice with VEGF-A neutralizing antibody showed significant reduction in CoNV area (**Figure S3**).

Discussion

Summary

Here we performed validation studies for the proposed CEP-TLR2 axis to assess the therapeutic potential for wet AMD treatment. Following a published procedure we generated synthetic CEP adducts and confirmed the presence of covalent

CEP groups. Structural analyses of a CEP adduct indicated changes in tertiary structure that were not observed in the naïve protein; however, similar structural changes were observed in the treated, unadducted control. Thus the physiological relevance of the observed structural changes is uncertain. Next we attempted to reproduce some of the reported biological effects of synthetic CEP adducts. When we tested our synthetic CEP adducts in *in vitro* and *in vivo* assays, we observed neither TLR2 activation nor pro-angiogenic activity. We conclude that our data do not support the CEP-TLR2 hypothesis.

Structural Changes in CEP Adducts

In our hands the published protocol for generating CEP adducts worked successfully, by the criterion of the presence of covalently-linked CEP groups in the adduct. This protocol worked robustly with all classes of reagents tested, including proteins, dipeptide, and lipid. Furthermore, the stoichiometry of adduction of each reagent was in fair agreement with the corresponding published stoichiometry.

In our attempt to understand the biological consequences of CEP adduction we initiated protein structural studies with HSA-CEP. Since the conversion of a significant number of positively-charged lysine side chains to negatively charged CEP groups (from the carboxylate group) would greatly alter its surface electrostatic potential, we anticipated and indeed observed structural changes in HSA-CEP in comparison to untreated HSA control (HSA-CTL1). We were surprised, however, to detect similar changes in HSA-CTL2, the treated unadducted control (**Figure 1**). Our interpretation is that two kinds of structural alterations can occur in synthetic CEP adducts: a) alterations that do not involve the

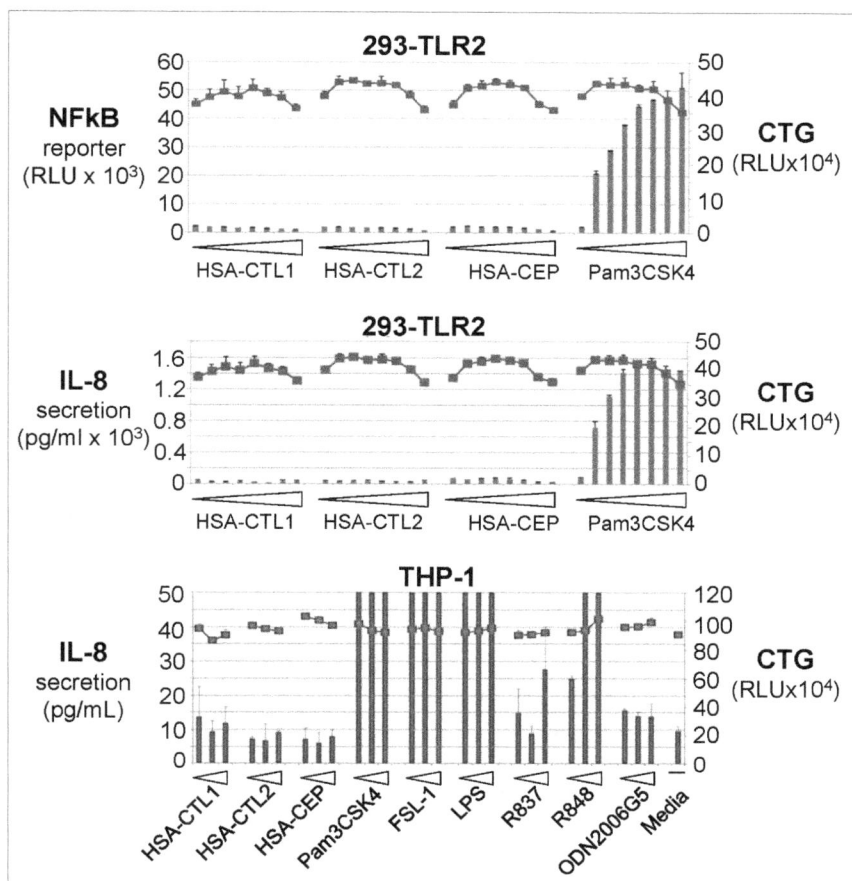

Figure 2. Cell-Based TLR Activation Assays. Various CEP adducts and TLR agonists were tested in HEK293 or THP-1 cells. Readouts were NFkB reporter signal or IL-8 secretion (columns), as indicated. In addition, the same wells were analyzed for viability with the CellTiter-Glo kit (axis on right; square symbols) to ensure that any lack of activation was not due to cell toxicity. HEK293 cells were treated with the following reagents: HSA-CTL1, HSA-CTL2, or HSA-CEP: 0, 3.9, 7.8, 15.6, 32.6, 62.5, and 125 and 250 µg/ml; Pam3CSK4: 0, 1.5, 3.2, 6.3, 12.5, 25, 50, 100 ng/mL. THP-1 cells were treated with the following reagents: HSA-CTL1, HSA-CTL2, or HSA-CEP: 62.5, 125, and 250 µg/mL; Pam3CSK4: 4, 20, and 100 ng/mL; FSL-1:0.4, 2, and 10 ng/mL; LPS: 4, 20, and 100 ng/mL; R837 or R848:0.4, 2, and 10 µM; ODN2006G5:0.2, 1, and 5 µM.

CEP group and were observed when comparing HSA-CTL2 to HSA-CTL1; and b) alterations that occur as a result of covalently-linked CEP groups and were observed when comparing HSA-CEP to HSA-CTL2. It is not clear which step(s) or reagents in the published adduction procedure led to the CEP-independent changes in HSA-CTL2. A candidate culprit is the organic solvent, dimethylformamide; organic solvents are known to affect the structure of some proteins. The adduction procedure entails exposure of protein to 30% dimethylformamide/PBS solution for 4 days at 37°C [10]. In searching the literature we found similar significant structural alteration in a CEP adduct published by another laboratory. A synthetic MSA-CEP adduct appeared to migrate as a continuous smear on denaturing SDS-PAGE and immunoblot, whereas the untreated MSA (the equivalent of MSA-CTL1) migrated as one predominant electrophoretic band (Figure 1 in [13]). A treated unadducted control, the equivalent of our MSA-CTL2, was not included in the report [13]. However since we used similar procedures for generating CEP adducts, in all likelihood the published MSA-CEP incorporated both CEP-independent and -dependent changes.

Thus far, no endogenous CEP adducts have been isolated directly from any biological sources and none have been characterized in the literature. For example, the stoichiometry of

CEP adduction (moles CEP per mole protein) and structural properties have not been reported for any endogenous CEP adducts. Hence at this point it would not be possible to verify that any synthetic CEP adduct is representative of endogenous ones with respect to protein structure. This caveat notwithstanding, we proceeded with biological studies to see if we could reproduce the biological effects of CEP adducts with regards to TLR2 activation and angiogenesis. In our approach we included HSA-CTL2 and MSA-CTL2 in the biological assays of the corresponding CEP adducts, so we might discern biological effects that are specific to the CEP group.

TLR2 Activation by CEP Adducts

We tested CEP-adducted protein or dipeptide in two cell-based assays: a) HEK293-TLR2 cells that specifically expressed TLR2 and, b) THP-1 cells that express multiple TLRs, including TLR2. In both assays, TLR2 activation was observed with a synthetic TLR2 agonist, Pam3CSK4, but not with synthetic CEP adducts. Specifically, we did not detect any effect of HSA-CEP in TLR2-expressing HEK293 cells, as was reported (Figure S14 in [9]). Not surprisingly the controls for our CEP adducts did not have any effects, either. Our cellular assays also did not register any effect of

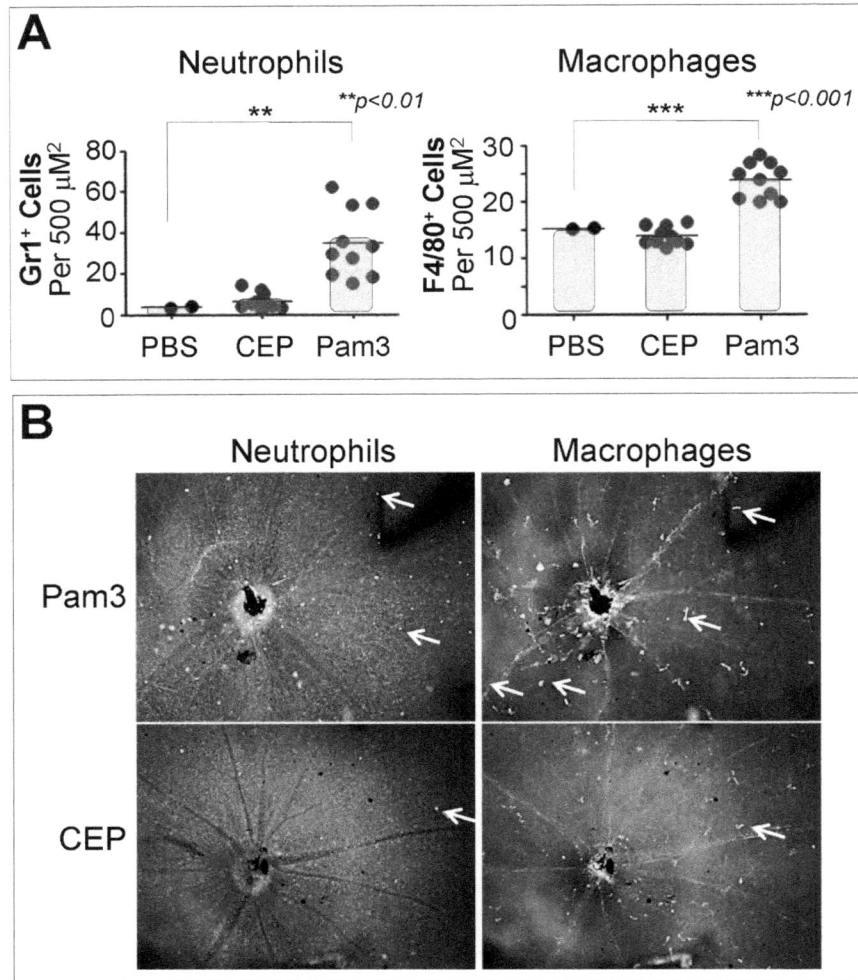

Figure 3. Retinal Leukocyte Infiltration Assay. A) Mice were injected intraperitoneally with either PBS, Pam3CSK4 (25 μg per animal, in PBS), or dipeptide-CEP (400 μg per animal, in PBS) and the retinas were analyzed 8 hours later. Retinal infiltration by neutrophils (Gr1+ cells) or macrophages (F4/80+ cells) was assessed by immunostaining with the respective markers and quantitated with Axiovision, as described in Materials and Methods. Statistical analysis was performed using the Student t-test. Only statistically significant differences are indicated in the graph. B) Shown are representative images of the experiment in **Figure 3A**. Arrows indicate examples of macrophages or neutrophils in the corresponding images. *CEP*, Dipeptide-CEP; *Pam3*, Pam3CSK4.

the dipeptide-CEP, which was reported to be pro-angiogenic in several cellular and *in vivo* assays in a TLR2-dependent manner [9]. However, this dipeptide-CEP was not tested in the same cell-based TLR assay used for HSA-CEP [9], so a direct comparison with our cell-based data is not possible.

We also evaluated CEP adducts in an *in vivo* model for TLR2 activation. In this model, treatment with Pam3CSK4 induced retinal leukocyte infiltration in wild-type mice, but not in *Myd88−/−* nor *TLR2−/−* mice (not shown). However, treatment of wild-type mice with CEP adducts did not result in measurable retinal leukocyte infiltration, indicating that TLR2 was not activated by CEP adducts *in vivo*.

CEP-TLR2 in Angiogenesis Assays

In vitro, neither HSA-CEP nor Pam3CSK4 (TLR2 agonist) showed any pro-angiogenic effect in the tube formation assay with human umbilical vein endothelial cells (HUVECs). Likewise, agonists to other TLRs (LPS, poly (I:C)) were not pro-angiogenic, whereas VEGF was.

In vivo, synthetic MSA-CEP did not exacerbate laser-induced CNV in a mouse model as reported [8]. This was the case with two substrains of C57BL/6 mice. In the initial two laser CNV studies we used C57BL/6N mice. Subsequently, it was reported that this substrain carries the *rd8* mutation in the *Crb1* gene [12]. We then performed two additional laser CNV studies with the C57BL/6J substrain, which has the wild-type *Crb1* gene [12]. The C57BL/6J substrain is the same one used in the previously published laser CNV study [8]. We observed similar results in all four laser CNV studies: CNV was exacerbated with exogenous VEGF, ameliorated with a VEGF-neutralizing antibody, and unaffected with MSA-CEP. Collectively, these data are consistent with a major angiogenic role for the VEGF pathway, but not for CEP adducts, in the laser-induced CNV model.

As an alternative *in vivo* model of ocular angiogenesis for exploring the CEP-TLR2 hypothesis, we used an abrasion-induced corneal neovascularization model (CoNV). This CoNV model is different from that used earlier with CEP adducts: in the corneal pocket CoNV model, a pellet containing synthetic HSA-

Table 1. Evaluation of CEP Adducts and TLR Agonists in the Tube Formation Assay.

	Reagent	Concentration	Average Tube Length (mm/mm²)	Std Dev	P value[a]
Experiment 1	untreated	–	1.97	+/−0.35	–
	LPS	10 ng/mL	3.38	+/−0.59	0.0072
	Poly (I:C)	10 µg/mL	0.16	+/−0.09	0.0005
	Pam3CSK4	500 nM	2.13	+/−0.24	0.9997
	VEGF[b]	3.1 ng/mL	10.61	–	<0.0001
Experiment 2	untreated	–	1.85	+/−0.27	–
	HSA-CEP	2 µg/mL	1.18	+/−0.32	0.1079
	HSA-CTL2	2 µg/mL	2.32	+/−0.45	0.3594
	VEGF	4 ng/mL	9.00	+/−1.64	<0.0001

GFP-transfected HUVEC, co-cultured with human fibroblasts, were treated on days 1, 2, 5, 7 and 9 with VEGF, TLR agonists, HSA-CEP, or HSA-CTL2. Control wells ("untreated") received media alone. Average tube length (mm/mm²) was determined by fluorescence measurements as described in Materials and Methods. Representative images from these two experiments are shown in **Figure 3**.
[a]One way ANOVA with Dunnett's multiple comparison test, compared to untreated sample.
[b]This VEGF control was measured in duplicate and not in triplicate, therefore no Std Dev is presented.

CEP was implanted in the cornea [8]. Since our synthetic CEP adducts were biologically inactive in all assays so far, we aimed to use a model where endogenous -not synthetic- CEP adducts might play a role. In the abrasion-induced CoNV model, angiogenesis occurs as part of the wound healing process, induced by mechanical abrasion of the cornea. Furthermore, it has been shown that macrophages are recruited to the cornea during early stages of neovascularization [14]. This resembles the back punch model, in which wound angiogenesis entails recruitment of macrophages [9]. CEP adducts were reported to be transiently present during this time, detected by immunocytochemistry with an antibody against synthetic CEP adducts. By immunolabeling, a substantial portion of CEP adducts was present in the recruited F4/80+ macrophages [9]. Treatment with dipeptide-CEP in this model accelerated wound closure and vascularization in a TLR2-

dependent manner, as shown by the comparison of *TLR2−/−* and *TLR2+/+* mice. In the same vein, we used the abrasion-induced CoNV model and compared littermate *Myd88−/−* and *Myd88+/+* mice. (Myd88 is required for TLR2 function.) We found no difference in CoNV area between the two groups. This indicates that, in the abrasion-induced CoNV model, TLR2 and other Myd88-dependent TLRs are not involved in angiogenesis. It is not known whether endogenous CEP adducts are present in the abrasion-induced CoNV model. We also tested topical treatment with synthetic HSA-CEP, but observed no effect on CoNV (not shown). It seems therefore the CEP-TLR2 axis proposed for other wound angiogenesis models [9] does not apply to corneal abrasion-induced wound angiogenesis model tested here.

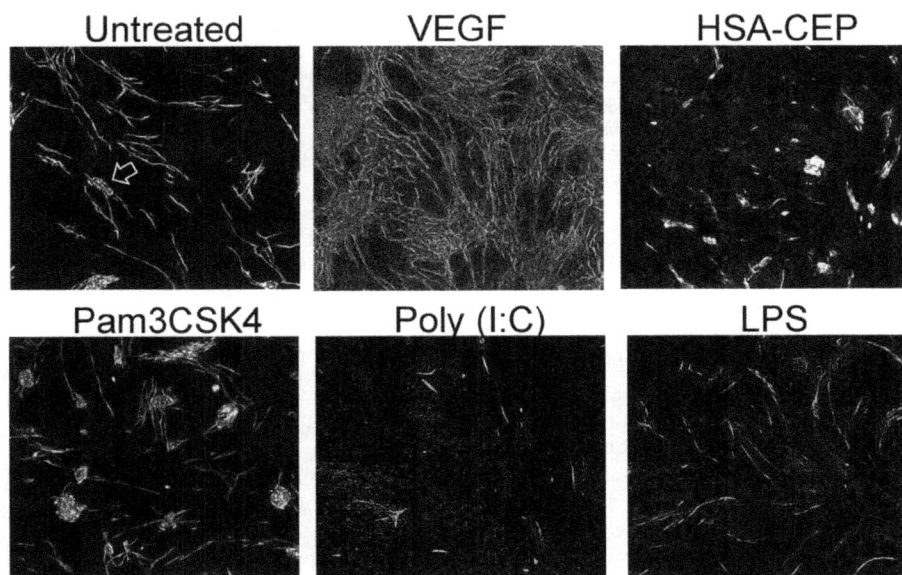

Figure 4. Tube Formation Assay. Shown are representative images of the experiments in presented numerically in **Table 1**. The figure shows images for untreated negative control (untreated), positive control (VEGF 165, 4 ng/mL), HSA-CEP (2 µg/mL), Pam3CSK4 (500 nM), LPS (10 ng/mL), poly (I:C) (10 µg/mL). The arrow in the untreated image shows an example of an island of unmigrated HUVEC cells, which is also seen in other images.

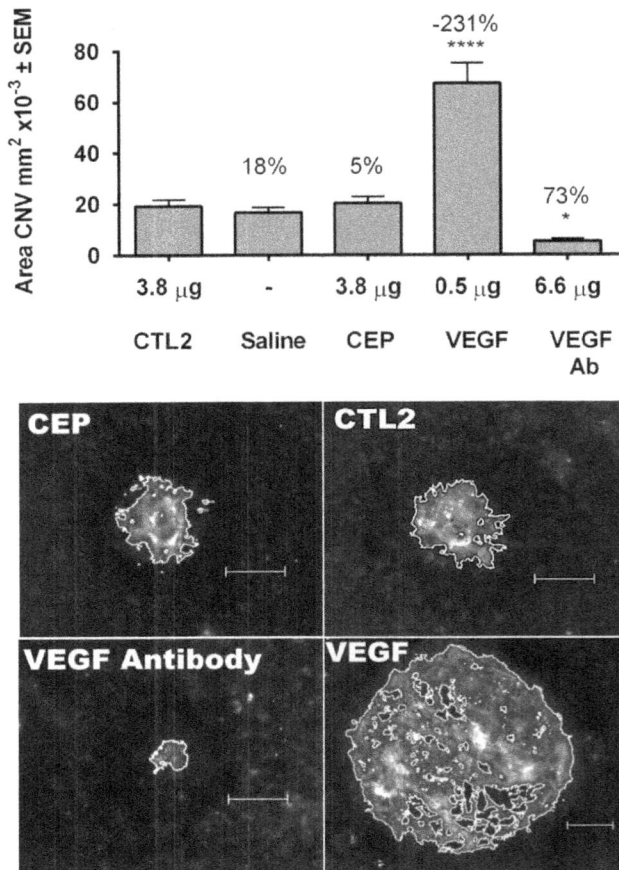

Figure 5. Mouse Laser-Induced CNV Assay. (A) Subretinal injection of MSA-CEP does not increase CNV area compared to mice injected with saline or MSA-CTL2. Bar graph shows mean area of CNV +/− SEM from first experiment evaluating the effect of subretinal injection of saline, 0.5 µg of rhVEGF165, 3.8 µg of MSA-CTL2, 3.8 µg of MSA-CEP, or 6.6 µg of 4G3 (an anti-mVEGF antibody) on laser-induced CNV in C57BL/6J mice. The number above each bar is the percentage inhibition relative to average CNV area in mice injected with MSA-CTL2. Subretinal injection of VEGF increases CNV area and subretinal injection of an anti-mVEGF antibody inhibits CNV area. * p<0.05, **** p<0.0001 by ANOVA with a Dunnett's post hoc analysis. (B) Representative fluorescent images of CNV lesions 7 days after laser from mice injected in the subretinal space with MSA-CEP, MSA-CTL2, VEGF or a VEGF Antibody as described above. Scale bar = 100 microns. *CTL2*, MSA-CTL2; *CEP*, MSA-CEP.

Figure 6. Mouse CoNV Assay. A) Adult *Myd88−/−* (KO) and littermate *Myd88+/+* (WT) mice (N = 7 to 8 animals/group) were subjected to corneal abrasion on Day 0. On Day 21 post-abrasion animals were euthanized and CoNV area (+/− SEM) was measured by fluorescence microscopy, as described in Materials and Methods. Statistical analysis was performed using two-way ANOVA. Within each genotype, the abraded group was significantly different from the naïve group (p<0.0001). However, comparison between the two genotypes showed no significant effect of the *Myd88* deficiency on CoNV area in response to abrasion. B) Representative images of the 4 groups shown in **Figure 6A**.

Synthetic vs. Endogenous CEP Adducts

It has been proposed that the biological effects of CEP adducts depend solely on the presence of CEP groups and not the host carrier [9]. This was not the case in our study: neither protein CEP adducts nor dipeptide CEP adducts produced any of the published biological effects [8,9] that were tested here. Our synthetic reagents were verified for the presence of covalently-attached CEP groups. There is no obvious explanation for these discrepancies. As innate immune receptors, TLRs recognize structures and patterns so it is conceivable that changes in structure, even if artificial, could elicit TLR activation. Thus one possibility is that there are structural differences between our synthetic CEP adducts and those used in previous studies, as the reagents were prepared at different laboratories.

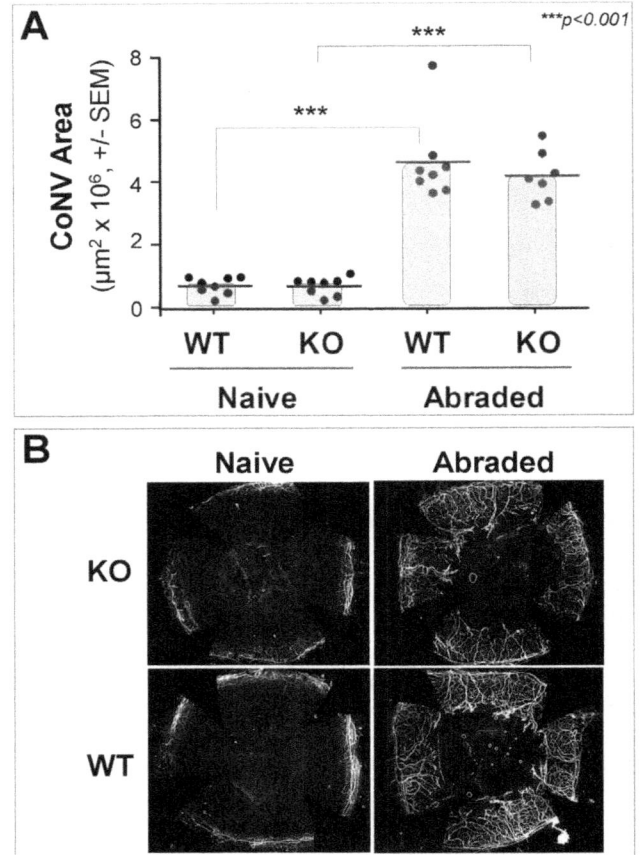

So far endogenous CEP adducts from any biological systems have not been isolated and therefore none have been characterized in structural studies. Furthermore, the abnormal electrophoretic patterns seen with synthetic CEP adducts reported here or by others [13] do not seem to resemble those of *in vivo* CEP adducts detected on immunoblots, reported either in human donor material (e.g. Figure 3 in [5]) or in the light-induced rat retinal degeneration model (e.g. Figure 1 in [15]). It is therefore uncertain which synthetic CEP adducts are representative of endogenous ones; perhaps none. The final answer awaits the isolation of endogenous CEP adducts and their characterization.

By extension, the biological effects reported with synthetic CEP adducts also need to be confirmed with endogenous CEP adducts. Our HSA-CTL2 did not show any biological activity, but neither did our HSA-CEP; hence in our study there was no concern about non-physiological biological effects, which HSA-CTL2 was intended for as a control. However, a treated unadducted control would be critically important when biological activity with a synthetic CEP adduct is observed. This is exemplified in a recent publication where the unadducted control, "sham-MSA", showed biological activity in some assays. In BALB/c macrophages, sham-MSA induced the upregulation of M1 markers and of an inflammatory gene, *KC*, 2 to 5 fold above that of control levels (Figures 1A and S2, respectively, in [16]). In some cases the sham-MSA effect represented 30%–40% in magnitude of the MSA-CEP effect: (*IL-1β, TNFα*, and *KC*), despite the absence of CEP groups in sham-MSA [16].

Treated unadducted controls were not used in earlier studies that reported a role for synthetic CEP adducts in TLR2 activation and in angiogenesis [8,9]. If it is possible that our CEP adducts are different from those used by others, it is also possible that our treated unadducted controls are different. The fact that our treated, unadducted controls (HSA-CTL2, MSA-CTL2) were biologically inactive does not necessarily apply to other studies in literature, as the example above illustrates. Thus the physiological relevance of synthetic CEP adducts is unclear, especially when untreated proteins were used as the only controls in the biological assays.

Polyclonal and monoclonal antibodies raised to synthetic CEP adducts have been reported to immunolabel biological samples from AMD patients in Western blots, immunohistochemical sections, and ELISAs [5–7,11]. The same antibodies reportedly immunolabelled biological samples in animal studies, e.g. [15,17]. However, the immunolabelled proteins were not confirmed to have any CEP moieties, by other independent assays that do not use antibodies (e.g. LC-MS/MS); i.e. the immunolabelled proteins were not confirmed to be bona fide CEP adducts. For example, several candidate CEP adducts were immunolabelled on Western blots of patient donor material and subsequently identified by LC-MS/MS analysis, however the presence of covalently-linked CEP groups was not confirmed by LC-MS/MS or other assays [5]. The fact that a synthetic CEP adduct (used a control) was immuno-labelled on the same western blot is not a surprise, as CEP antibodies were raised against a synthetic CEP adduct [5]. At this point, the antibodies against synthetic CEP adducts [5] have not yet been validated for detection of endogenous CEP adducts. This is underscored by the electrophoretic changes in synthetic CEP adducts that do not seem to resemble those of endogenous CEP adducts, as explained above. Data generated by other (non-immunological) assays is needed to validate CEP antibodies.

Arguably the *in vivo* existence of CEP adducts requires confirmation, as well, since all evidence so far has been generated with these antibodies. For example, a proteomics study of AMD patient samples identified and quantified hundreds of proteins by LC-MS/MS [18]. Yet the same study reported that CEP adducts were below detection limits and "none were reliably identified" (supplemental information in [18]). On a promising note, an improved LC-MS/MS assay has been reported, with a sensitivity of 1 pmol or less of CEP-lysine in enzymatically-digested patient plasma samples [19]. According to ELISA data [7] the average levels of CEP adducts in AMD plasma is 37 pmol/mL, thus hopefully the improved LC-MS/MS assay can confirm the presence of CEP adducts *in vivo*.

In conclusion, our studies of synthetic CEP adducts did not validate the CEP-TLR2 axis in angiogenesis as proposed [8,9]. While the cause of the discrepancies is not clear, it does seem clear that the mere presence of CEP groups is not sufficient to elicit the reported biological responses. More data, ideally with endogenous CEP adducts, is needed to understand what properties of CEP adducts, if any, can lead to TLR2 activation and to angiogenesis. In light of the prevalence of AMD and the unmet medical needs, more research into the pathophysiology of CEP adducts is warranted.

As a postscript, after submission of our manuscript an independent report [20] also showed that CEP adducts alone do not induce TLR2 signalling nor related biological effects (e.g. Figures 1A and 1B), as we have reported here. Rather, the report claims that CEP adducts potentiate the effect of a synthetic TLR2 agonist, Pam3CSK4, in cultured murine bone-marrow derived macrophages [20].

Materials and Methods

Synthesis and Verification of CEP Adducts

Synthesis. All CEP adducts were synthesized as described [10]. The dipeptide, Ac-Gly-Lys-OMe, was obtained from BACHEM; HSA from AlbuminBio; MSA from AlbuminBio or Sigma; phosphatidyl ethanolamine was from Sigma. Controls for protein CEP adducts included untreated protein (CTL1) and treated unadducted protein (CTL2). The latter control was processed in the same synthesis procedure as that for CEP adducts, except 4,7-dioxoheptanoic acid 9-fluorenylmethyl ester was left out to avoid the covalent addition of CEP moiety. Protein CEP adducts, after final dialysis in PBS, were quantified by the Bradford assay and tested for endotoxins with the Endosafe-PTS kit (Charles River). For storage, samples were filtered through 0.2 μm, divided aseptically in 1-mL aliquots, and stored at −80 C.

Amino acids complete digestion. Enzymatic hydrolysis was adapted from [21]. An aliquot of 100 μg of protein is dissolved in 25 μl of PBS buffer (pH 7.4). Pronase E (Sigma, Cat. # P5147) (2 mg/ml in 10 mM potassium phosphate buffer, pH 7.4, 5 μl) was added. The sample was incubated at 37°C for 24 hours. Prolidase (Sigma, Cat. # P6675) and aminopeptidase (Sigma, Cat. # A8200) (both 2 mg/ml in 10 mM potassium phosphate buffer, pH 7.4, 5 μl) were added. The sample was incubated at 37°C for 48 hours. Amino acids from enzymatic hydrolysate (10 μl) was derivatized by Waters AccQ•Fluor (Waters, Cat.# WAT052880). Then 2 μl of derivatized samples was analyzed by Xevo-G2QTOF with Waters BEH C18 2.1 × 50 mm 1.7 μm column at 50°C at 1.0 mL/min, 0.1% formic acid in water, 0.04% formic acid in acetonitrile, 3–98% B in 9 min. An aliquot of 100 μg of protein is dissolved in 25 μl of PBS buffer (pH 7.4). Pronase E (Sigma, Cat. # P5147) (2 mg/ml in 10 mM potassium phosphate buffer, pH 7.4, 5 μl) was added. The sample was incubated at 37°C for 24 hours. Aminopeptidase (Sigma, Cat. # P6675) and prolidase (Sigma, Cat. # A9934) (both 2 mg/ml in 10 mM potassium phosphate buffer, pH 7.4, 5 μl) were added. The sample was incubated at 37°C for 48 hours. Amino acids from enzymatic hydrolysate (10 μl) was derivatized by Wasters AccQ Fluor (Waters, Cat.# Wat052880). Then 2 μl of derivatized samples was analyzed by Xevo-G2QTOF with Waters BEH C18 2.1 × 50 mm 1.7 μm column at 50°C at 1.0 mL/min, 0.1% formic acid in water, 0.04% formic acid in acetonitrile, 3–98% B in 9 min.

NMR of protein hydrolysate samples. Hydrolyzed protein samples were prepared for NMR analysis by the addition of 5 μL of D2O (CIL) to 15 μL of Hydrolysate solutions. Sodium 3-trimethylsilyl [2,2,3,3-d4]propionate (TMSP) as added as an internal chemical shift and quantitation reference. High-resolution ^{1}H-NMR spectra were acquired at 300±1 K, using a standard (D-90°-acquire) pulse sequences on a Bruker-600 Avance spectrometer (^{1}H frequency of 600.26 MHz). ^{1}H-NMR spectra were acquired with 256 free induction decays, 65,536 complex data points, a spectral width of 7.2 kHz, and a relaxation delay of 5 s. All spectra were processed by multiplying the FID by an exponential weighting function corresponding to a line broadening of 0.3 Hz. The CEP pyrrole resonances at ^{1}H$_δ$ 6.8 ppm, ^{1}H$_δ$

6.1 ppm and $^1H_\delta$ 5.9 ppm were integrated relative to the aromatic resonance of phenylalanine and tyrosine using the ACD 10.0 package (Advanced Chemistry Development, Toronto, Canada).

LC-MS/MS confirmation of CEP-lysine adduct. Carboxyethylpyrrole (CEP) adduct presence in CEP-conjugated murine serum albumin (MSA) and human serum albumin (HSA) has been confirmed by LC-MS/MS methodologies. CEP-MSA and CEP-HSA were hydrolyzed using protease cocktails (descriptions in above, AA complete digestion), followed by Accq-Tag Ultra derivatization (Catalog number 186003836, Waters Corporation, Milford, MA). Accq-Tagged CEP-lysine ionizes in electrospray positive mode and gives a protonated molecular ion of 439.1981, which can fragment and gives a characteristic 171.1 daughter ion from the Accq-Tag and a daughter ion of 206.1 from the carboxyethylpyrrole moiety. We employed multiple reaction monitoring, 206.1 precursor scan on a Triple Quadrupole mass spectrometer. Strong signal of 439.2 → 171.1 and 439.2 → 206.1 were observed using AB Sciex API4000 Triple Quad. Precursor ion of 439.2 was observed for 206.1 daughter ion in a precursor ion scan on the same API4000. Waters Xevo G2 Q-TOF mass spectrometer was employed for its high resolution power to further confirm the presence of CEP-lysine adducts. The molecular species of 439.1981 was observed in MS scan with 5 ppm mass accuracy across the chromatographic peak; the daughter ion 206.1181 was observed in the MS/MS scan with 10 ppm mass accuracy in the MSE approach.

Peptide Mapping for CEP Modification Location

Sample preparation. All solvents (HPLC grade) and chemicals were purchased from Sigma-Aldrich (St. Louis, MO) unless otherwise stated. MSA-CEP and MSA-CTL2 (50 ug each) were denatured with 6 M guanidine hydrochloride (GuHCl), reduced with 25 mM dithiothreitol (DTT), alkylated with 50 mM iodoacetamide, dialyzed against 50 mM ammonium bicarbonate using 10 kDa MWCO Slide-A-Lyzer cassettes (Thermo Scientific, Rockford, IL). Protein was digested 1 to 50 enzyme to protein with trypsin, chymotrypsin, and trypsin/Glu-C overnight at 37°C; note all enzymes purchased from Roche Diagnostics GMBH, Germany. For HSA-CEP and HSA-CTL1 digestions, 125 µg protein was denatured using ProteaseMAX surfactant (Promega, Madison, WI), reduced with 5 mM DTT, alkylated with 15 mM iodoacetamide and digested with 1 to 50 trypsin to protein overnight at 37°C.

Reverse phase LC-MS/MS analysis. Resulting peptides from MSA-CEP and MSA-CTL2 were analyzed by LC-ESI MS/MS on a Thermo Velos Orbitrap coupled to a Waters nanoACQUITY UPLC (Milford, MA). 70 pmol of digested MSA-CEP and MSA-CTL2 were HPLC separated on column (Waters Acquity HSS T3 1.8 µm beads, 1 × 100 mm at 40°C) at 15 µL/min. The 55 min gradient started 0–3 min, 3% B (B = acetonitrile, 0.1% formic acid), increased to 97% B at 35 min, then 95% B at 37 min, followed by washing and column equilibration. Mass spectrometer parameters included a full scan event using the FTMS analyzer at 100000 resolution from m/z 300–2000 for 10 ms. Collision induced dissociation (CID) MS/MS was conducted on the top seven intense ions (excluding 1+ ions) in the ion trap analyzer, activated at 500 (for first event) and 2000 (for remaining events) signal intensity for 10 ms.

For HSA-CEP and HSA-CTL1 digestion, resulting peptides were analyzed by LC-ESI MS/MS on a Thermo LTQ Orbitrap Discovery coupled to Agilent CapLC (Santa Clara, CA). 10 pmol of digested HSA-CEP and HSA-CTL1 were HPLC separated on column (Waters Acuity BEH C18, 1.7 µm, 1 × 100 mm column at 40°C) at 10 µL/min. The 80 min gradient started 0–1 min, 4%

B, increased to 7% B at 1.1 min, 45% B at 55 min, then 95% B at 63 min, followed by washing and column equilibration. Mass spectrometer parameters included a full scan event using the FTMS analyzer at 30000 resolution from m/z 300–2000 for 30 ms. CID MS/MS was conducted on the top seven intense ions (excluding 1+ ions) in the ion trap analyzer, activated at 500 (for all events) signal intensity for 30 ms.

Data analysis and database searching. All mass spectra were processed in Qual Browser V 2.0.7 (Thermo Scientific). Mascot generic files (mgf) were generated with MS DeconTools (R.D. Smith Lab, PPNL) and searched using Mascot V2.3.01 (Matrix Science Inc., Boston, MA) database search against the SwissProt database, V57, with 513,877 sequences. Search parameters included: enzyme: semitrypsin, chymotrypsin, none, or trypsin/Glu-C, allowed up to two missed cleavages; fixed modification carbamidomethyl on cysteines (when applicable); variable modifications searched: Arg-CEP on arginines, Gln->pyro-Glu (at N-term glutamine), Lys-CEP on lysines, oxidation on methionine; peptide tolerance: ±25 ppm; MS/MS tolerance: ±0.6 Da. Sequence coverage and CEP modification assessments were evaluated on peptide scores with >95% confidence. High-scoring peptide ions were then selected for manual MS/MS analysis using Qual Browser.

Structural Analyses of CEP Adducts

SDS-PAGE analysis. After boiled for 5 min, 5 µg of total protein mixed with 4X sample buffer (Invitrogen, cat. # NP0007) was loaded on 4–12% NuPAGE Bis-Tris gel (Invitrogen, Cat. # NP0321BOX) with NuPAGE MOPS running buffer (Invitrogen, Cat. # NP0001). SeeBlue Plus2 Protein Ladder (Invitrogen, cat. # LC5925) or BenchMark Protein Ladder (Invitrogen, Cat. # 10747-012) was used to estimate the protein size. Gel was stained with SimpleBlue SafeStain (Invitrogen, Cat. # LC6060) for overnight at 4°C and destained with HPLC water. The gel image was taken by Bio-Rad ChemiDoc XRS+ Imaging System.

Size exclusion chromatography (SEC). Human Serum Albumin (HSA) samples (20 µg) were injected on Shodex KW-803 column with 1 mL/min flow rate, 20 mM Tris, 200 mM NaCl, 0.25 mM TCEP, 3 mM NaN3, pH 7.5 as mobile phase on Agilent 1200 HPLC. UV signal was recorded at 280 nm by Agilent 1260 DAD detector. Mouse Serum Albumin (MSA) samples (50 µg) were injected on a Large S200 Column with GE Superdex 200 10/300GL and at 500 µL/min flow rate, 150 mM NaCl and 0.02% NaN3 in Dulbecco's PBS as mobile phase on Agilent 1260 BioInert HPLC. UV signal was measured at 280 nm by Wyatt TREOS/OptiLab Rex.

Circular dichroism (CD). Protein samples were diluted in 10X diluted PBS (pH 7.4) to achieve similar concentration. Baseline was blanked by 10X diluted PBS (pH 7.4). The CD spectra (average of five scans) of protein samples were collected from 260 nm to 190 nm on a Jasco J-815 CD Spectrometer with 0.02-cm path length quartz cell at 10°C.

In Vitro Assays

Cell-based TLR assays. HEK293 cells expressing TLR2 and NFKB luciferase reporter (gift from Novartis Vaccine, Siena, Italy) were seeded at 30000 per well the night before. HSA-CEP was added and incubated for either 6 hr or 24 hr. Supernatant was collected for IL-8 ELISA (R&D, cat# DY208). NFkB luciferase activity was assayed on remaining cells, using Bright-Glo (Promega, cat# E2610). HEK293 cells in a separate plate with the same treatment were used for cell viability measurement using CellTiter-Glo (Promega, cat# G7570), according to manufacturer's instruction.

Thp1 (ATCC, cat# TIB-202) was primed with 0.5% DMSO for overnight, at 100,000/well, then incubate with HSA-CEP for 24 hr, with TLR ligands (Pam3CSK4, FSL1, R837 and R848 were all from Invivogen; LPS was purchased from Sigma) as controls. Supernatant was collected for IL-8 ELISA (R&D), and the remaining cells were used for cell viability measurement using CellTiter-Glo.

In vitro tube formation assay. The CellPlayer GFP Angiokit-96 by Essen BioScience (Ann Arbor, MI) was used to measure tube formation in vitro. Briefly, GFP-transfected HU-VEC were co-cultured with human fibroblasts in a specially designed medium for 11 days in a 96-well format. Cells were treated on days 1, 2, 5, 7 and 9 with VEGF, TLR agonists, or CEP-adducted or control-treated proteins. Fluorescence measurements (IncuCyte, Essen BioScience) were taken kinetically every 12 hours for the duration of the experiment and average tube length (mm/mm^2) was quantified on the last day of the experiment according to the manufacturer's instructions. Control wells received media alone. Reagents were obtained from the following sources: Human VEGF 165– Peprotech; Pam3CSK4– InvivoGen; LPS -Sigma-Aldrich; Poly (I:C) –InVivoGen.

In Vivo Assays

Animals. All animal experiments were approved by the Animal Care and Use Committee at the Novartis Institutes for Biomedical Research. Upon arrival at the vivarium, mice were acclimated for at least 4 days before any studies were initiated. The animals were fed standard laboratory chow and sterile water ad libitum. Genotyping was performed on genomic DNA obtained from tail snips by standard procedures. All mouse strains were genotyped for the *Crb1* gene, to determine if they carried the *rd8* mutation.

C57BL/6N mice were obtained from Taconic; the *rd8* mutation was present in these mice. C57BL/6J mice were obtained from Jackson; the *rd8* mutation was absent in these mice. *Myd88*-deficient mice lacking exons 2–5 were generated at Novartis Institutes for Biomedical Research. Mice were back-crossed to C57BL/6J mice for at least 10 generations; the *rd8* mutation was absent in these mice. Heterozygous breeding generated littermate pups of each genotype, identified by PCR genotyping. *Myd88* deficiency was also functionally confirmed by the *in vivo* retinal infiltration assay below: mutant vs. littermate *wt* mice with treated with either TLR2 agonists and with TLR4 agonists and the retinal infiltration was measured as described (not shown).

Laser-induced choroidal neovascularization (CNV). CNV was induced by laser injury in age and sex matched on a) C57BL/6N mice and b) C57BL/6J mice. Two in vivo experiments were performed with each mouse strain. After pupil dilation with 1% cylate and 10% phenylephrine, the mice were anesthetized and the retinas were visualized with a slit lamp microscope and a cover slip. The laser (Iridex Oculight GLx 532 nm green laser) was applied at 3 locations with a successful laser shot inducing a vaporization bubble. Laser pulses are applied to both eye yielding 6 CNV area data points per mouse and with 10 mice per group yielding 60 CNV area data points per test condition. Immediately after laser 2.0 µl of test article was injected into the subretinal space of both eyes. A sclerotomy was first made with a 30 gauge needle, and then the test article was injected through the same incision with a 33 gauge blunt tipped needle and a 10 µl Hamilton syringe. Injections were visualized under a surgical microscope with direct observation of a small retinal detachment. 7 days post laser, mice were injected i.v. with a vascular label and then euthanized. Mouse eyes were fixed in 4%

paraformaldehyde; RPE-choroid-scleral complexes were isolated and mounted on microscope slides. Fluorescent images of each laser-induced CNV were captured using a Axiocam MR3 camera on a Axio.Image M1 microscope (Zeiss). The CNV lesion sizes were quantified with Axiovision software (Version 4.5 Zeiss). Inter-group differences were analyzed with an ANOVA with a Dunnett's multiple comparison test on GraphPad Prism 6 for Windows software. Data was masked during image acquisition and data analysis.

Recombinant human VEGF165 (Peprotech), IgG2A (R&D, MAB006) and a proprietary anti-mouse VEGF antibody (4G3) were reconstituted in sterile saline (Hospira) to a concentration of 0.05, 0.5, 2.5 or 3.3 mg/ml respectively. 1.4 or 1.9 mg/ml of CEP-MSA and MSA-CTL2 (control 2, mouse serum albumin treated but not adducted) or the other reagents were injected in to the subretinal space on day 0 immediately after a laser as described. After the application of laser burns and subretinal injections of test reagents, antibiotic ointment (Tobramycin or Neomycin ophthalmic ointment depending on availability) was applied to both eyes. The anti-VEGF antibody, 4G3, is a mouse anti-VEGF IgG1 antibody. It binds to mouse VEGF with an EC50 of 0.047 nM in a sandwich ELISA and neutralizes mouse VEGF binding to human VEGFR-2 with an EC50 of 0.15 nM in a binding assay (ELISA MSD).

Corneal neovascularization (CoNV). Acute CoNV was induced in 7- to 9- week old anesthetized mice by complete removal of the corneal epithelium with mechanical abrasion, as detailed [14]. At the end of the studies, mice were humanely euthanized and the area of CoNV was quantitated as described [14]. Animals were randomized prior to treatment and analysis was performed in a masked fashion. N = 5–10 mice/group.

In studies using *Myd88−/−* mice (**Figure 6**), male knockout (KO) and male wild-type littermate controls (WT) were abraded on day 0 and euthanized at the end of the study on day 21 for analysis. *Myd88*-deficient and littermate wild-type mice are on the C57BL6/J background and are described above.

For other CoNV studies (**Figure S3**), C57BL6/N mice were used. The *Crb1* gene product is expressed in the retina, but not in the cornea [22]. In the study presented in **Figure S3C**, animals (N = 10–12 mice/group) were injected i.p. with PBS (200 µl), control antibody (IgG1, 0.5 mg/kg) or anti-VEGF antibody (4G3, 0.5 mg/kg) on days 0, 3 and 5 post-abrasion and eyes were collected on day 6 for analysis.

In vivo TLR2-mediated retinal leukocyte infiltration. TLR2 ligand, Pam3CSK4, was purchased from Invivogen. Female C57BL/6N mice (7 weeks old, Taconic) were treated with either dipeptide-CEP (400 µg per animal, in PBS) or Pam3CSK4 (25 µg per animal, in PBS) via intraperitoneal injection. Control animals received an intraperitoneal injection of sterile PBS. Eight hours after injection, mice were euthanized. Eyes were enucleated and were fixed in 4% paraformaldehyde. For immunostaining, retinas were dissected out. Macrophages was stained using the F4/80-Alexa 488 conjugated antibody (AbD serotec, Oxford, UK). Neutrophils were stained using a biotiny-lated-Gr-1 antibody (San Diego, CA) and an Alexa Fluor 594 conjugated streptavidin secondary antibody (Molecular Probes, Eugene, OR). After retinas were flat mounted onto glass slides, fluorescent images were taken. And F4/80 and Gr-1 positive cells on the retina were counted using Zeiss AxioVision program.

Supporting Information

Figure S1 Confirmation of CEP Adduction By ^{1}H-NMR and LC-MS/MS. A) *Structure for Dipeptide-CEP*. B) *^{1}H-NMR* *of Dipeptide-CEP*. The signature peaks for CEP, lysine, and glycine are indicated. The CEP peaks were not detected in the unadducted dipeptide (not shown). C) *LC-MS/MS of completely hydrolyzed MSA-CEP*. MSA-CEP was enzymatically hydrolyzed and processed for LC-MS/MS analysis. Only MSA-CEP showed a peak corresponding to lysine-CEP; untreated MSA-CTL1 (not shown) and treated but unadducted MSA-CTL2 (lower panel) did not have the CEP peak. D) *^{1}H-NMR of completely hydrolyzed HSA-CEP*. The signature peaks for CEP, Tyr, and Phe are indicated. The resonances corresponding to CEP were absent in HSA-CTL1 and HSA-CTL2 (not shown).

Figure S2 Peptide Mapping of CEP Adduction by LC-MS/MS. A) *LC-MS/MS Analysis of Trypsinized HSA-CEP*. LC-MS/MS of trypsin digested HSA-CEP showed sequence coverage of 65% where bold residues represent observed peptides. In HSA-CEP 14 sites of CEP adduction were identified by this analysis (shown as underlined amino acids). B) *LC-MS/MS Analysis of Trypsinized MSA-CEP*. MSA-CEP was digested with trypsin, chymotrypsin, and trypsin-gluC yielding a sequence coverage of 92% with bold residues representing observed peptides. In MSA-CEP 40 sites of CEP adduction were identified by this analysis (shown as underlined amino acids). The initial signal and propeptides are not observed in the mature, processed protein sequence for HSA and MSA and are shown as italicized residues.

Figure S3 CoNV Model is VEGF-Driven. A) *Progression of Neovascularization*. Adult C57BL/6N mice (N = 5 animals/group) were subjected to corneal abrasion on Day 0 and dissected corneas were analyzed for neovascularization area at different timepoints after abrasion. Neovascularization area progressively increased and plateaued around 2 weeks after abrasion. Statistical analysis was performed using one-way ANOVA with Dunnet's post-test, comparing each time point to Naïve. Only the statistically significant differences between groups are indicated. B) *Upregulation of VEGFA Transcript*. Total RNA was prepared from dissected corneas from naïve mice and or cornea-abraded mice that were euthanized on Day 1 and Day 6 post-abrasion as indicated (N = 5 to 6 animals/group). First-strand cDNA was generated using the High Capacity RNA-to-cDNA Master Mix (Applied Biosystems). Pre-amplification products were generated using the Taqman PreAmp Master Mix Kit (Applied Biosystems)

and a pool of FAM-labelled Taqman assays on demand (Applied Biosystems). qPCR was performed on diluted pre-amplification products using the same Taqman assays on demand in qPCR singleplex reactions. Relative quantification (RQ) performed using $\Delta\Delta$Ct method and data presented as RQ median with error bars as RQ min and RQ max. *VEGFA, PECAM-1*(expressed by vascular endothelial cells), and *β-actin* mRNA expression was normalized by expression of *β-actin* gene and expressed relative to naïve animals. Statistical analysis was performed using one-way ANOVA with Dunnett's post-test. C) *VEGF Ab inhibits CoNV*. Adult C57BL/6N mice (N = 10–12 animals/group) were subjected to corneal abrasion on Day 0 and injected intraperitoneally with the reagents as indicated on Days 0, 3, and 5 post-abrasion. Reagents included PBS (vehicle), control IgG1 Ab, and anti-VEGF antibody (4G3). The antibodies were dosed at 0.5 mg/kg. On Day 6 the animals were euthanized and CoNV area was measured by fluorescence microscopy as described in Materials and Methods. Statistical analysis was performed using one-way ANOVA with Dunnett's post-test.

Acknowledgments

Myd88−/− mice were generated by Mueller M, Wirsching J, Lemaistre M, Doll T, Isken A, Kinzel B (Developmental & Molecular Pathways, NIBR, Basel, Switzerland). Littermate *Myd88−/−* and *Myd88+/+* mice were bred and genotyped by Vanessa Davis and John Halupowski (Transgenic Services, NIBR, Cambridge, USA). Shawn Hanks (Ophthalmology, NIBR, Cambridge, USA) helped with some of the statistical analyses.

Author Contributions

Conceived and designed the experiments: JG EM QH KA S-ML SP BEG MM BJ SA. Performed the experiments: JG JSC JZ FC XY HY EM CR YX ADE MC NB YQ EF SS AW AJ RC SG. Analyzed the data: JG JSC JZ EM QH KA S-ML SP BEG MM BJ SA. Contributed reagents/materials/analysis tools: JG EM QH KA S-ML SP BEG SA. Wrote the paper: JG EM QH KA S-ML SP BEG MM BJ SA.

References

1. Miller JW (2013) Age-related macular degeneration revisited–piecing the puzzle: the LXIX Edward Jackson memorial lecture. Am J Ophthalmol 155: 1–35 e13.
2. Kuno N, Fujii S (2011) Dry age-related macular degeneration: recent progress of therapeutic approaches. Curr Mol Pharmacol 4: 196–232.
3. Nguyen DH, Luo J, Zhang K, Zhang M (2013) Current therapeutic approaches in neovascular age-related macular degeneration. Discov Med 15: 343–348.
4. Salomon RG, Hong L, Hollyfield JG (2011) Discovery of carboxyethylpyrroles (CEPs): critical insights into AMD, autism, cancer, and wound healing from basic research on the chemistry of oxidized phospholipids. Chem Res Toxicol 24: 1803–1816.
5. Crabb JW, Miyagi M, Gu X, Shadrach K, West KA, et al. (2002) Drusen proteome analysis: an approach to the etiology of age-related macular degeneration. Proc Natl Acad Sci U S A 99: 14682–14687.
6. Gu X, Meer SG, Miyagi M, Rayborn ME, Hollyfield JG, et al. (2003) Carboxyethylpyrrole protein adducts and autoantibodies, biomarkers for age-related macular degeneration. J Biol Chem 278: 42027–42035.
7. Gu J, Pauer GJ, Yue X, Narendra U, Sturgill GM, et al. (2009) Assessing susceptibility to age-related macular degeneration with proteomic and genomic biomarkers. Mol Cell Proteomics 8: 1338–1349.
8. Ebrahem Q, Renganathan K, Sears J, Vasanji A, Gu X, et al. (2006) Carboxyethylpyrrole oxidative protein modifications stimulate neovascularization: Implications for age-related macular degeneration. Proc Natl Acad Sci U S A 103: 13480–13484.
9. West XZ, Malinin NL, Merkulova AA, Tischenko M, Kerr BA, et al. (2010) Oxidative stress induces angiogenesis by activating TLR2 with novel endogenous ligands. Nature 467: 972–976.
10. Lu L, Gu X, Hong L, Laird J, Jaffe K, et al. (2009) Synthesis and structural characterization of carboxyethylpyrrole-modified proteins: mediators of age-related macular degeneration. Bioorg Med Chem 17: 7548–7561.
11. Gu J (2009) Biomarkers for Age-Related Macular Degeneration [Electronic Thesis or Dissertation.]. Cleveland, Ohio: Case Western Reserve University. 223 p.
12. Mattapallil MJ, Wawrousek EF, Chan CC, Zhao H, Roychoudhury J, et al. (2012) The Rd8 mutation of the Crb1 gene is present in vendor lines of C57BL/6N mice and embryonic stem cells, and confounds ocular induced mutant phenotypes. Invest Ophthalmol Vis Sci 53: 2921–2927.
13. Hollyfield JG, Bonilha VL, Rayborn ME, Yang X, Shadrach KG, et al. (2008) Oxidative damage-induced inflammation initiates age-related macular degeneration. Nat Med 14: 194–198.
14. Sivak JM, Ostriker AC, Woolfenden A, Demirs J, Cepeda R, et al. (2011) Pharmacologic uncoupling of angiogenesis and inflammation during initiation of pathological corneal neovascularization. J Biol Chem 286: 44965–44975.
15. Renganathan K, Gu J, Rayborn ME, Crabb JS, Salomon RG, et al. (2013) CEP Biomarkers as Potential Tools for Monitoring Therapeutics. PLoS One 8: e76325.
16. Cruz-Guilloty F, Saeed AM, Duffort S, Cano M, Ebrahimi KB, et al. (2014) T cells and macrophages responding to oxidative damage cooperate in

pathogenesis of a mouse model of age-related macular degeneration. PLoS One 9: e88201.

17. Organisciak DT, Darrow RM, Rapp CM, Smuts JP, Armstrong DW, et al. (2013) Prevention of retinal light damage by zinc oxide combined with rosemary extract. Mol Vis 19: 1433–1445.

18. Yuan X, Gu X, Crabb JS, Yue X, Shadrach K, et al. (2010) Quantitative proteomics: comparison of the macular Bruch membrane/choroid complex from age-related macular degeneration and normal eyes. Mol Cell Proteomics 9: 1031–1046.

19. Jang G-F, Zhang L, Hong L, Wang H, Salomon RG, et al. (2012) Quantification Of CEP By LC MS/MS. Investigative Ophthalmology & Visual Science 53: 6478.

20. Saeed AM, Duffort S, Ivanov D, Wang H, Laird JM, et al. (2014) The Oxidative Stress Product Carboxyethylpyrrole Potentiates TLR2/TLR1 Inflammatory Signaling in Macrophages. PLoS One 9: e106421.

21. Ahmed N, Argirov OK, Minhas HS, Cordeiro CA, Thornalley PJ (2002) Assay of advanced glycation endproducts (AGEs): surveying AGEs by chromatographic assay with derivatization by 6-aminoquinolyl-N-hydroxysuccinimidyl-carbamate and application to Nepsilon-carboxymethyl-lysine- and Nepsilon-(1-carboxyethyl)lysine-modified albumin. Biochem J 364: 1–14.

22. Alves CH, Pellissier LP, Wijnholds J (2014) The CRB1 and adherens junction complex proteins in retinal development and maintenance. Prog Retin Eye Res 40: 35–52.

13

Elk3 Deficiency Causes Transient Impairment in Post-Natal Retinal Vascular Development and Formation of Tortuous Arteries in Adult Murine Retinae

Christine Weinl[1], **Christine Wasylyk**[2,3,4,5], **Marina Garcia Garrido**[6], **Vithiyanjali Sothilingam**[6], **Susanne C. Beck**[6], **Heidemarie Riehle**[1], **Christine Stritt**[1], **Michel J. Roux**[2,3,4,5], **Mathias W. Seeliger**[6], **Bohdan Wasylyk**[2,3,4,5], **Alfred Nordheim**[1]*

1 Department of Molecular Biology, Interfaculty Institute for Cell Biology, University of Tuebingen, Tuebingen, Germany, **2** Institut de Génétique et de Biologie Moléculaire et Cellulaire, Illkirch, France, **3** Centre National de la Recherche Scientifique, Illkirch, France, **4** Institut National de la Santé et de la Recherche Médicale, Illkirch, France, **5** Université de Strasbourg, Illkirch, France, **6** Division of Ocular Neurodegeneration, Centre for Ophthalmology, Institute for Ophthalmic Research, University of Tübingen, Tübingen, Germany

Abstract

Serum Response Factor (SRF) fulfills essential roles in post-natal retinal angiogenesis and adult neovascularization. These functions have been attributed to the recruitment by SRF of the cofactors Myocardin-Related Transcription Factors MRTF-A and -B, but not the Ternary Complex Factors (TCFs) Elk1 and Elk4. The role of the third TCF, Elk3, remained unknown. We generated a new *Elk3* knockout mouse line and showed that Elk3 had specific, non-redundant functions in the retinal vasculature. In *Elk3*(−/−) mice, post-natal retinal angiogenesis was transiently delayed until P8, after which it proceeded normally. Interestingly, tortuous arteries developed in *Elk3*(−/−) mice from the age of four weeks, and persisted into late adulthood. Tortuous vessels have been observed in human pathologies, e.g. in ROP and FEVR. These human disorders were linked to altered activities of vascular endothelial growth factor (VEGF) in the affected eyes. However, in *Elk3*(−/−) mice, we did not observe any changes in VEGF or several other potential confounding factors, including mural cell coverage and blood pressure. Instead, concurrent with the post-natal transient delay of radial outgrowth and the formation of adult tortuous arteries, Elk3-dependent effects on the expression of Angiopoietin/Tie-signalling components were observed. Moreover, *in vitro* microvessel sprouting and microtube formation from P10 and adult aortic ring explants were reduced. Collectively, these results indicate that Elk3 has distinct roles in maintaining retinal artery integrity. The *Elk3* knockout mouse is presented as a new animal model to study retinal artery tortuosity in mice and human patients.

Editor: Rudolf Kirchmair, Medical University Innsbruck, Austria

Funding: This work was supported by Hyponet, PLBIO2010 (http://www.e-cancer.fr, BW); Fondation ARC pour la recherche sur le cancer, SF2010 (http://www.recherche-cancer.net, BW); Centre national de la recherche scientifique, institutional funds (BW); Université Strasbourg, institutional funds (http://www.unistra.fr, BW); Deutsche Forschungsgemeinschaft, Se837/6-2 (http://www.dfg.de, MWS); and German Cancer Aid, 109886 (http://www.krebshilfe.de, AN). The funders had no role in study design, data collection and analysis, decision to publish, or preparation of the manuscript.

* Email: alfred.nordheim@uni-tuebingen.de

Introduction

Angiogenesis is an important physiological process in which new blood vessels are generated by sprouting of existing ones. Dysregulated angiogenesis is implicated in many human diseases, including cancer and retinopathies [1,2]. During angiogenesis, endothelial tip cells at the angiogenic front form numerous filopodia and guide vascularization, whereas stalk cells located behind tip cells are involved in proliferation and vessel extension [3]. Angiogenesis can be readily studied using the mouse retina. Many angiogenic events, such as endothelial cell (EC) proliferation, sprouting, recruitment of mural cells and maturation, occur post-natally and can be followed *ex vivo* on two-dimensional retinal flat-mount preparations [4]. At post-natal day 0 (P0), vascularization starts as a ring-shaped vessel around the optic nerve head. By P4, half of the retina is covered by blood vessels, and around P8, the retina is fully vascularized regarding the primary plexus, while sprouts develop to form the additional deep plexus capillary networks [5]. Site-directed mutagenesis of the mouse genome can be used to identify genes involved in murine retinal vessel angiogenesis and physiology.

Murine retinal angiogenesis requires the SRF transcription factor [6,7,8]. SRF is ubiquitously expressed and fulfills many essential functions [9]. Constitutive deletion of *Srf* results in embryonic lethality at E7.5 [10]. Tissue specific, conditional ablation of *Srf* reveals specific functions in skeletal muscle cells, cardiomyocytes, forebrain neurons, hepatocytes, keratinocytes, intestinal smooth muscle cells and endothelial cells (see below) (for review [9]). Tissue and target gene specificity results from differential recruitment of cofactors to SRF [11,12,13]. Recruitment of Ternary Complex

Factor (TCF) family members (Elk1, Elk3 or Elk4) [13,14] can lead to the induction of immediate early genes (IEGs) involved in cell cycle entry, whereas recruitment of Myocardin Related Transcription Factors (MRTF-A and MRTF-B) [15,16,17] induces the transcription of genes involved in adhesion and motility [11,18]. Interestingly, these SRF cofactors have different effects on angiogenesis. Murine endothelial *Srf* depletion results in characteristic phenotypes in early post-natal and adult retinae [7,8], which are mimicked by deletion of *Mrtf-a and Mrtf-b*, but not by single or double deletion of the *Elk1* and *Elk4* genes [8]. The murine phenotypes upon post-natal endothelial depletion of SRF or MRTF-A/-B reflect some pathological features exhibited by human patients suffering from FEVR (familial exudative vitreoretinopathies) and AMD (adult macular degeneration) [8]. Potential contributions to retinal angiogenesis of the third TCF, Elk3, have not yet been reported. Therefore, we have developed a new mouse model for constitutive Elk3 depletion. We show that *Elk3* deletion leads to a distinct retinal phenotype, manifested in transiently delayed post-natal primary plexus formation and lasting tortuous arteries in adult retinae. This does not impair visual function. At the molecular level, *Elk3*(−/−) mice display altered retinal expression of immediate-early genes and angiogenic Tie receptor genes. *Elk3*(−/−) phenotypic features partly resemble human ophthalmologic diseases with tortuous vessels, i.e. retinopathy of prematurity (ROP) [19] and familial exudative vitreoretinopathy (FEVR) [20]. Thus, *Elk3*(−/−) mice promise to be a useful animal model to reveal insufficiently understood pathogenic mechanisms that lead to human retinal vessel tortuousity.

Materials and Methods

Generation of *Elk3* constitutive knockout (KO) mice

A previously used mouse model of Elk3 deficiency expresses a truncated form of the protein (Net δ) [21]. To avoid this confounding factor, a new constitutive Elk3 knockout mouse line was established in a cooperation between the IGBMC and the MCI/ICS (Mouse Clinical Institute (Institut Clinique de la Souris), Illkirch, France; http://www.ics-mci.fr). The targeting vector was constructed as follows. The 5′ (4.3 kb), 3′ (3 kb) and interloxP (3 kb) fragments were PCR amplified on 129sv genomic DNA and sequentially subcloned in an ICS proprietary vector containing the LoxP sites and a Neo cassette flanked by FRT sites (Figure S1). The linearized construct was electroporated in 129S2/SvPas mouse embryonic stem (ES) cells. After selection, targeted clones were identified by PCR using external primers and further confirmed by Southern blotting with 5′ external probe. Two positive ES clones were injected into C57BL/6J blastocysts, and derived male chimeras gave germline transmission. The excision of the neomycin-resistance cassette was performed *in vivo* by breeding the chimeras with a Flp deleter line (C57BL/6J genetic background). The Flp transgene was segregated by breeding the first germ line mice with a wild type C57BL/6J animal. Constitutive KO mice were generated by breeding floxed-allele heterozygotes with a Cre deleter line followed by segregation in a further breeding step.

Experimental animals

To generate *Elk1/Elk4* double knockout (*dKO*) animals, termed *Elk1/Elk4^dKO*, single *Elk1*(−/0) [22] and single *Elk4*(−/−) [23] founder mice were used. These mouse strains were crossed in matings of *Elk1*(−/−)::*Elk4*(+/−) females with *Elk1*(−/0)::*Elk4*(+/−) males [24].

Antibody staining of retinal flat-mounts *in vitro*

Generation of IsolectinB4 stained retinal flat-mounts was performed as described previously [8]. Briefly, eyes were isolated and fixed in 4% PFA for two hours at RT. After 2×5 minutes in PBS, retinae were dissected and incubated in blocking buffer (1% BSA, 0.3% Triton-X, PBS) for 2 h at RT. Incubation with primary antibodies was performed at 4°C in blocking buffer overnight. After washing 3×20 minutes with PBS, retinae were incubated with secondary antibodies in blocking buffer for two hours at RT. After washing 3×20 minutes in PBS, retinae were flat-mounted on coverslides and embedded in Mowiol for fluorescence microscopy.

Primary antibodies: CollagenIV 1:40 (AbD Serotec), Ki67 (SP6 undiluted) (DCS). Secondary antibodies: anti rabbit Alexa 546 1:200 (Molecular Probes), SMA-Cy3 conjugate 1:200 (Sigma Aldrich). Retinal vessels were stained with Isolectin B4 (ILB4) from Griffonia simplicifolia 1:25 (Sigma), detected by Streptavidin-Alexa488 1:100 (Molecular Probes).

RNA isolation, cDNA synthesis and qRT-PCR analysis of brain and retinal tissue

Brains and retinae of post-natal pups or adult animals were dissected and frozen in liquid nitrogen for further use. All tissues were lysed for RNA isolation according to the manufacturer's protocol (Qiagen, RNeasy). cDNA synthesis was performed using random hexamers. qRT-PCR analysis was performed using specific primers (Sigma) and SYBR green technology in an ABI Prism 7000 cycler. Primer mix for one sample included 10 μM forward primer (0.3 μl), 10 μM reverse primer (0.3 μl) and 2.4 μl water. cDNA mix for one sample included 5 μl SYBR green and 2 μl cDNA. For each qRT-PCR reaction, 7 μl of the cDNA mix and 3 μl of the primer mix were combined in the 96-well plates. Primer sequences are listed in Table S1. For description of general methods, see [25]. Amplification protocol: segment 1: 50°C, 2 min., segment 2: 95°C, 10 min., segment 3: 95°C, 15 sec, 60°C, 1 min., 40 cycles.

Western Blot

Retinal tissue was lysed in Iyer-buffer (0.5 M Hepes pH 7.5; 1 M $MgCl_2$; 0.5 M EDTA; 5 M NaCl; in water) [26]. Protein content of cell lysates was determined by Bradford reagent. Separation of bands was performed by SDS-PAGE (12% gel for SMA, 15% for P-Cofilin). Electrotransfer was done at 4°C for 2 h at 100 V and 400 mA. To detect specific bands, membranes were blocked in 5% bovine serum albumin BSA for one hour at RT. Incubation in primary antibodies was performed overnight at 4°C. After three washes with TST (Tris Saline Tween), membranes were incubated in secondary antibodies for one hour at RT. Primary antibodies: GAPDH 1:20000 (Hytest Ltd.), P-Cofilin 1:500 (Cell Signalling), SMA 1:1000 (Sigma Aldrich). Secondary antibodies (1:10000 dilution, GE Healthcare): anti-mouse IgG HRP-conjugated, anti-rabbit IgG HRP-conjugated.

Scanning laser ophthalmoscopy (SLO)

Scanning-laser ophthalmoscopy (SLO) was performed as described previously [27]. Briefly, mice were anaesthetized by subcutaneous injection of ketamine (66.7 mg/kg) and xylazine (11.7 mg/kg). After anaesthesia, pupils were dilated with tropicamide eye drops (Mydriaticum Stulln, Pharma Stulln, Stulln, Germany). SLO imaging was performed using a Heidelberg Retina Angiograph (HRA I) equipped with an argon laser featuring two wavelengths (488 nm and 514 nm) in the short wavelength range and two infrared diode lasers (795 nm and

830 nm) in the long wavelength range. The laser wavelength used for fundus visualization was 514 nm (RF, red-free channel). The 488 nm wavelength was used for fundus autofluorescence (AF) analysis. Additionally, the 488 nm and 795 nm lasers were used for fluorescein angiography (FLA) and indocyanine green angiography (ICGA), respectively. FLA and ICGA were performed using subcutaneous injection of 75 mg/kg body weight fluorescein-Na (University pharmacy, University of Tübingen, Germany), or 50 mg/kg body weight ICG (ICG-Pulsion, Pulsion Medical Systems AG, Munich, Germany), respectively.

Electroretinography (ERG)

Electroretinograms were recorded as described previously [28]. After overnight dark-adaptation, single-flash ERG responses were obtained under scotopic (dark-adapted; no background illumination) and photopic (light-adapted with a background illumination of 30 cd/m^2, starting 10 min before recording) conditions. Single white-flash stimuli ranged from -4 to 1.5 log cd s/m2 under scotopic and from -2 to 1.5 log cd s/m^2 under photopic conditions. Ten responses were averaged with inter-stimulus intervals of 5 s (for -4 to -0.5 log cd s/m^2) or 17 s (for 0 to 1.5 log cd s/m^2).

Hematoxylin/Eosin (H&E) staining of paraffin sections of whole eyes

Eyes were fixed overnight at 4°C in Davidson's fixative (6% formaldehyde, 32% ethanol, 11% acetic acid, 5% sucrose in PBS). Histological examination of the eyes was performed on 4 μm sections of paraffin embedded eyes mounted on Superfrost Plus slides (Langenbrinck, Emmendingen, Germany). Sections were stained with Hematoxylin/Eosin followed by dehydration and mounting in Entellan.

Aortic ring assay

Aortae from P10 or adult Elk3(+/+) control and Elk3(−/−) knockout animals were excised, cut into 1 mm rings and embedded in Matrigel (BD Biosciences) on cleaned coverslips (12 mm diameter) in 4-well plates. Matrigel was polymerized for 10 minutes at RT followed by 30 minutes at 37°C. Embedded rings were covered with 700 μl of HUVEC EGM growth medium with all required supplements added according to the manufacturer's protocol (Lonza). Fresh medium was supplied every other day. Aortic rings from P10 and adult mice were cultivated for two and three weeks, respectively, and microvessel sprouting of each aortic ring was quantified every day using the following score: 0 = no microvessel sprouting, 0.25 = isolated sprouting, 0.5 = 20–50% sprouting, 0.75 = 50–75% sprouting, 1 = 75–100% sprouting, 1.25 = 100% sprouting. A tip cell index for microvessel sprouting was calculated for each day and plotted to reveal the kinetics of microvessel sprouting for each genotype. To stain actin filaments of embedded aortic rings, rings were fixed with 4% PFA, washed 3× with PBS, permeabilized with 10% Triton, blocked with 2% BSA, and incubated with Phalloidin-Texas Red. Rings were washed 3× with PBS and photographed on coverslips, which were removed from the 4-well plates.

Microscopic analysis

For fluorescent staining analysis, a Zeiss Axiovert 200 M microscope equipped with an AxioCam MRm camera and an ApoTome (Zeiss) was used. Retinal overviews (original magnification 5×) are presented as composite images of individual, successively overlapping (5%) images, generated by computer-controlled x-y settings and processed using MosaiX Software.

H&E-stained sections were visualized using Zeiss Axioplan 2 with AxioCamHRc camera. Higher magnifications were obtained with 10× and 20× objectives. % radial outgrowth, a quantitative measure for retinal vascularization, was calculated by dividing the retinal area covered by blood vessels (yellow line in Figure 1A) by the total retinal area (red line in Figure 1A). The percentage of abnormally shaped arteries was calculated by counting both abnormally shaped arteries and the total number of arteries, using SLO imaged retinae and retinal flat-mounts. Mean blood vessel width was calculated as follows: blood vessels were identified by ILB4 staining followed by measuring blood vessel areas and blood vessel lengths. Blood vessel widths (W) were calculated dividing vessel length (L) by area (A), i.e. $W = L/A$. Tortuosity of adult vessels was quantified as shown in Figure S2. A tortuosity factor was calculated by normalizing actual vessel length (red line) over idealized vessel length (yellow line), as measured between common equidistant endpoints. For quantitation of proliferation in arteries and veins, retinal flat-mounts of Elk3(+/+) WT and Elk3(−/−) KO P6 animals were co-stained with ILB4 and Ki67 and photographed at 20× magnification with focus on single arteries and veins. Using these images, Ki67 positive endothelial cells were counted and normalized to 100 μm vessel length. Obtained values are expressed as % of WT values (Table S2).

Statistical analysis

For all quantitative analyses, data are presented as means +/− s.e.m. For comparison of different experiments, values are normalized to the control = 100%. To test significance, Student's t-tests were used, p levels<0.05 were considered significant. Significance is indicated by * p<0.05, ** p<0.01, *** p<0.001 and ns (not significant).

Study approval

All animal experiments were approved by the Regierungspräsidium Tübingen (Tübingen, Germany) permit for SLO angiography of wt and Elk3(−/−) mice (IM 1/13, approved 20th February 2013, valid until 28th February 2016), permit for SLO imaging of wt and Elk1/Elk4^{dko} mice (IZ 1/13, approved 15th August 2013, valid until 31st August 2016), and permit for ERG measurements of wt and Elk3(−/−) mice (IM 3/13, approved 06th December 2013, valid until 15th December 2016).

Results

Generation of Elk3 deficient constitutive knockout mice

Elk3 deficient mice were generated by homologous recombination and subsequent Cre-mediated deletion, as described in Materials and Methods and Figure S1. The Elk3 gene was deleted around the major transcription start and exon 1, from −1720 to + 650 relative to the major transcriptional start site. The deletion decreased Elk3 expression at the RNA level, by at least 99.5% in the retina (see below) and other adult tissues and embryos (E8.5, 10.5, 12.5 and 14.5; data not shown), and at the protein level in E12.5 mouse embryo fibroblasts (data not shown).

General description of phenotypic features of Elk3 knockout mice

The Elk3 homozygous knockout mice displayed impaired viability with variable penetrance (usually around 50% of the expected ratio at P10 for heterozygous crosses in this study). The reasons for this partial lethality were not systematically examined, but chylothorax was observed, as in the previous study with the Net δ mouse [21] (and data not shown). Surviving 8 week old mice were globally phenotyped by the EUMODIC Pipelines 1 & 2 (see

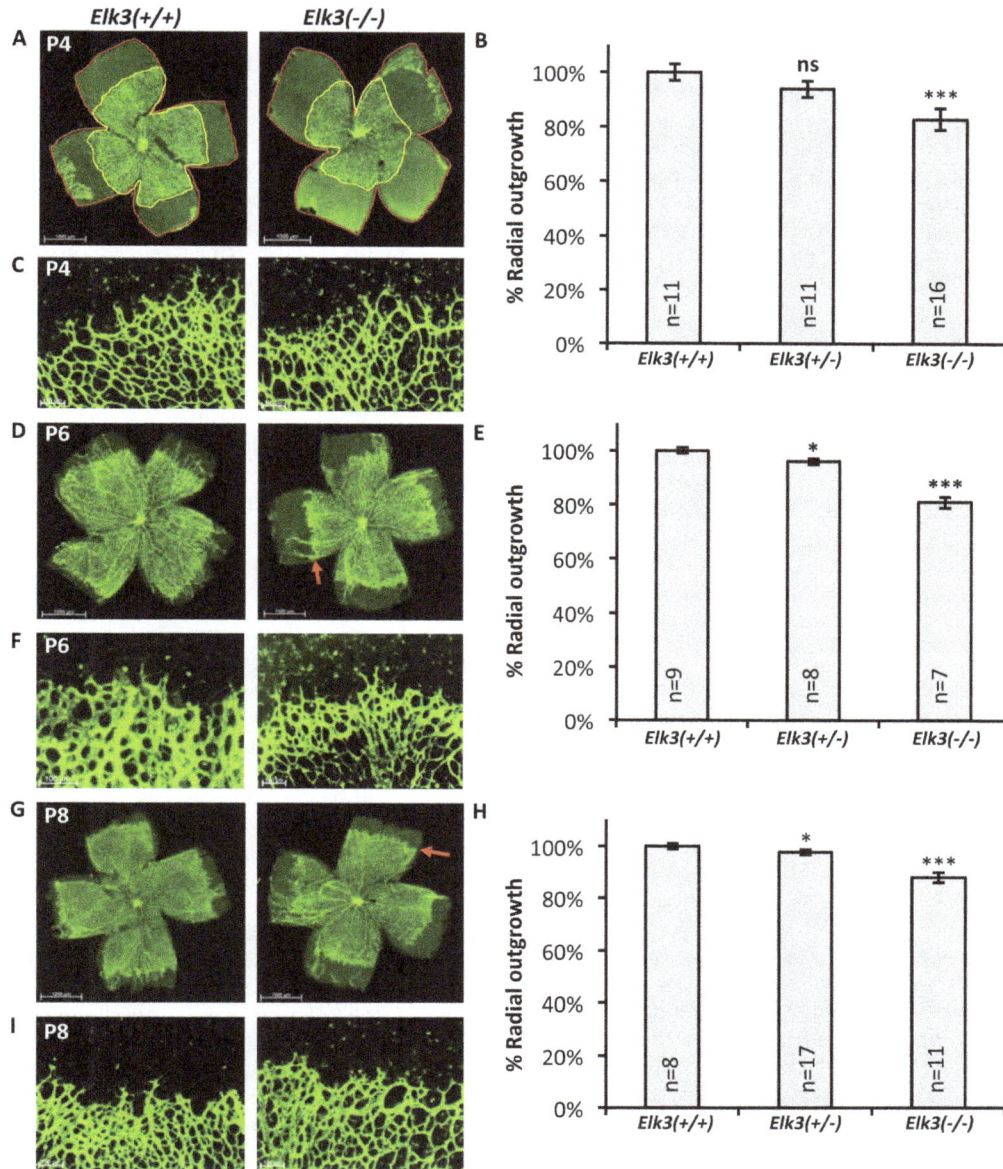

Figure 1. Deletion of *Elk3* leads to delayed retinal angiogenesis during early post-natal stages in *Elk3(−/−)* knockout mice. (A) IsolectinB4 staining of flat-mounts of retinae from P4 *Elk3(+/+)* control and *Elk3(−/−)* knockout mice. The red lines outline the whole retinal area, the yellow lines the areas covered by blood vessels. (B) Quantitation of retinal area covered by blood vessels (% vascularization) at P4. (C) Higher magnification of the angiogenic front in P4 control and *Elk3(−/−)* knockout retinae. (D) IsolectinB4 staining of retinal flat-mounts of a P6 *Elk3(+/+)* control and *Elk3(−/−)* knockout mouse. The red arrow points towards delayed angiogenic front in the *Elk3(−/−)* retina. (E) Quantitation of retinal area covered by blood vessels (% vascularization) at P6. (F) Higher magnification of the angiogenic front in P6 control and *Elk3(−/−)* knockout retinae. (G) IsolectinB4 staining of retinal flat-mounts from P8 *Elk3(+/+)* control and *Elk3(−/−)* knockout mice. The red arrow points towards the delayed angiogenic front in the *Elk3(−/−)* retina. (H) Quantitation of retinal area covered by blood vessels (% vascularization) at P8. (I) Higher magnification of the angiogenic front in P8 control and *Elk3* knockout retinae. All quantitation data are normalized to the control = 100%. The data shown are means +/− s.e.m. Statistical significance using Student's t-test is indicated with * p<0.05 ** p<0.01 *** p<0.001. Scale bar in (A, D, G) 1000 µm, in (C, F, I) 100 µm.

EMPRESS). The most significant (p<0.001) annotation in both Pipelines (PipelinesElk3) was vessel pattern detected by indirect ophthalmoscopy (see below). There was no change in systolic arterial pressure and pulse rate that could be detected by the non-invasive blood pressure tests (Figure S3). These "high throughput" observations suggested that the "retinal vascular structure" defect was a prime candidate for further investigation, especially given the role in this tissue of the Elk3 interacting partner SRF [7,8].

Elk3 deficiency results in reduced vascularization during early post-natal retinal angiogenesis

Guided by the observations obtained after endothelial-specific *Srf* deletion, we analysed the effect of Elk3 depletion on post-natal retinal angiogenesis since, during this period, SRF depletion resulted in reduced vascularization of the retina, formation of distal microaneurysms at the angiogenic front, and absence of deep plexi [8]. Observation of IsolectinB4 stained retinal flat-mounts at post-natal stages P4, 6, and 8 showed that retinal primary plexus vascularization was reduced in *Elk3(−/−)* animals (Figures 1A, D and G; quantifications in Figures 1B, E and H, red arrows point towards delayed angiogenic fronts in P6 and P8 *Elk3(−/−)* retinae). However, higher magnification views of angiogenic fronts did not reveal any abnormalities of tip cell morphology and number and length of tip cell filopodia in *Elk3(−/−)* knockout retinae (Figure 1C, F, I), suggesting that the phenotype is different from *Srf*[iECKO] animals, as well as from *Mrtf-a(−/−)Mrtf-b*[iECKO] animals [8].

Reduced angiogenesis in *Elk3* knockout retinae is transient and is overcome at post-natal day 10

The delay in radial outgrowth of the primary plexus was mild, suggesting that it could be overcome with time. Indeed, the outgrowth at post-natal day 10, observed on IsolectinB4 stained retinal flat-mounts, was indistinguishable in *Elk3(+/+)* control and *Elk3(−/−)* knockout retinae (Figure 2A and quantitation of radial outgrowth in Figure 2D). There were no avascular zones in the primary retinal periphery, and deep plexi formed normally in both control and *Elk3(−/−)* knockout retinae (Figure 2B and 2C). These findings indicated that impaired radial outgrowth at P4/P6/P8 was transient and was overcome by P10 in *Elk3(−/−)* knockout animals.

Scanning laser ophthalmoscopy reveals tortuous arteries in *Elk3* deficient, but not in *Elk1/Elk4* deficient, adult retinae

Adult *Srf*[iECKO] animals have neovascular lesions that connect to the retinal pigment epithelium, which can be detected by *in vivo* SLO imaging of adult eyes and confirmed by subsequent H&E staining of paraffin sections [8]. We therefore studied the effects of Elk3 deficiency using the same techniques. With SLO imaging, we found that arteries of *Elk3(−/−)* animals exhibited an abnormal tortuous morphology, which was not observed in control animals (Figure 3A left; tortuous arteries in the knockout retina are highlighted by red arrowheads). These findings were confirmed on IsolectinB4 stained retinal flat-mounts prepared after completion of *in vivo* imaging (Figure 3A middle). The penetrance of the tortuous arterial phenotype was 100%, i.e. all *Elk3(−/−)* knockout animals showed tortuosity of arteries in their retinae. We studied the effect of age on the proportion of abnormally shaped arteries. Two-week old animals did not have any detectable abnormalities (data not shown). Arterial tortuosity was detected as early as 4 weeks after birth and increased with age (Table 1). Heterozygotes also exhibited this phenotype, which was however less pronounced (Table 1). Tortuosity was quantified by measuring the lengths of arteries and calculation of a tortuosity factor (see Material and Methods, and Figure S2). *Elk3(−/−)* knockout arteries were significantly longer than control *Elk3(+/+)* arteries (Table 2). In contrast, there were no changes in vessel widths (see Material and Methods, and Table 2). Retinal layering and layer thickness, as determined by H&E staining on paraffin sections of whole eyes, were similarly unaffected. In addition, neovascularization was not observed in *Elk3(−/−)* knockout retinae (Figure 3A right), in contrast to adult *Srf*[iECKO] animals [8].

To determine if deficiency of the two other TCFs, Elk1 and Elk4, had similar effects as Elk3 deficiency, we analysed control and *Elk1/Elk4*[dKO] adult animals by the same techniques. No abnormalities were detected in *Elk1/Elk4*[dKO] retinae by *in vivo* imaging and on retinal flat-mounts stained with IsolectinB4

(Figure 3B left and Figure 3B middle). There were no changes in arterial shapes, lengths and widths (Table 2), nor in retinal layering and layer thickness (as judged by H&E staining on paraffin sections of whole eyes, Figure 3B right). Moreover, neovascularizations were not detected in *Elk1/Elk4*[dKO] retinae, in contrast to adult *Srf*[iECKO] animals. Taken together, these data indicate that the *Elk3(−/−)* phenotype of tortuous retinal arteries is distinct from Elk1 and Elk4 deficiencies in the *Elk1/Elk4*[dKO] mice, and SRF deficiency in *Srf*[iECKO] animals. This reveals a specific role of Elk3 in retinal vessel formation, which is non-redundant to the TCF paralogues Elk1 and Elk4. Analysis of visual function by ERG in adult *Elk3(+/+)* control and *Elk3(−/−)* knockout mice did not detect any impairment, suggesting that *Elk3(−/−)* mice can see normally despite their abnormally shaped arteries (Figure S4).

Molecular and cellular defects in post-natal *Elk3* deficient retinae

To study the underlying molecular mechanisms for the observed phenotypes of Elk3 deficient mice, we studied candidate target-gene expression by quantitative RT-PCR. In post-natal brains of *Elk3(−/−)* animals, *Elk3* RNA levels were <0.5% when compared to wild type, and 48% in *Elk3(+/−)* heterozygotes (Figure 4A). There were no changes in *Elk3* knockout brains of the related factors *Srf*, *Elk1* and *Elk4*, or of the potential target genes β-actin and *Vegfr-1* and *Vegfr-2* (Figure 4B).

In P6 retinae from *Elk3* knockouts, *Elk3* levels were greatly decreased (<0.2%, data not shown), the immediate-early genes (IEGs) *Egr-1*, *Egr-2* and *c-fos* were significantly downregulated, and regarding angiogenic factors, *Vegf* and *Vegf-r2* were unchanged, while *Vegfr-1* was slightly downregulated (Figure 4C). These data suggested that decreased IEG expression and possibly reduced proliferation could account for the delay in vascular outgrowth during the early post-natal period. However, when investigating this possibility, we did not detect any differences in width (measured microscopically at P6 and P8) and proliferative activity (measured by Ki67 staining at P6) of either arteries and veins in *Elk(−/−)* compared to control retinae (Table S2).

In *Elk3(−/−)* retinae of the later time point P10, when the transient delay in retinal vascularization was overcome, RNA expression level of *Vegfr-1* was restored to wild-type levels, whereas *Egr-1*, *Egr-2* and *c-fos* were still reduced, similar to P6 (Figure 4C).

To uncover potential causes for the observed delay in vascular outgrowth of *Elk3(−/−)* retinae, we studied RNA expression patterns of the second major class of angiogenic signalling partners, the Angiopoietins and their Tie-receptors Tie1 and Tie2. Interestingly, at P6, both Tie1 and Tie2 were significantly downregulated, whereas the Angiopoietins Ang-1 and Ang-2 were unchanged (Figure 4C). In contrast, at the later stage of P10, only Tie1 was significantly downregulated while Tie2 was restored to wildtype levels (Figure 4C).

We next investigated whether the transiently impaired primary plexus formation in *Elk3(−/−)* retinae was possibly due to impaired migration of astrocytes towards the periphery. We found that astrocytic radial outgrowth, at all stages analysed (P4, P6, P8), was unaffected by the knockout of *Elk3*, as judged by glial fibrillary acidic protein (GFAP) staining on retinal flat-mounts (Figure S5).

Reduced retinal vascularization could be a result of enhanced vessel regression. We therefore performed co-staining of ILB4-positive retinal blood vessels and extracellular collagenIV, using P6 retinal flat-mounts of Elk3 wildtype and knockout mice. Thus we checked for so-called 'empty sleeves' of regressed, previously

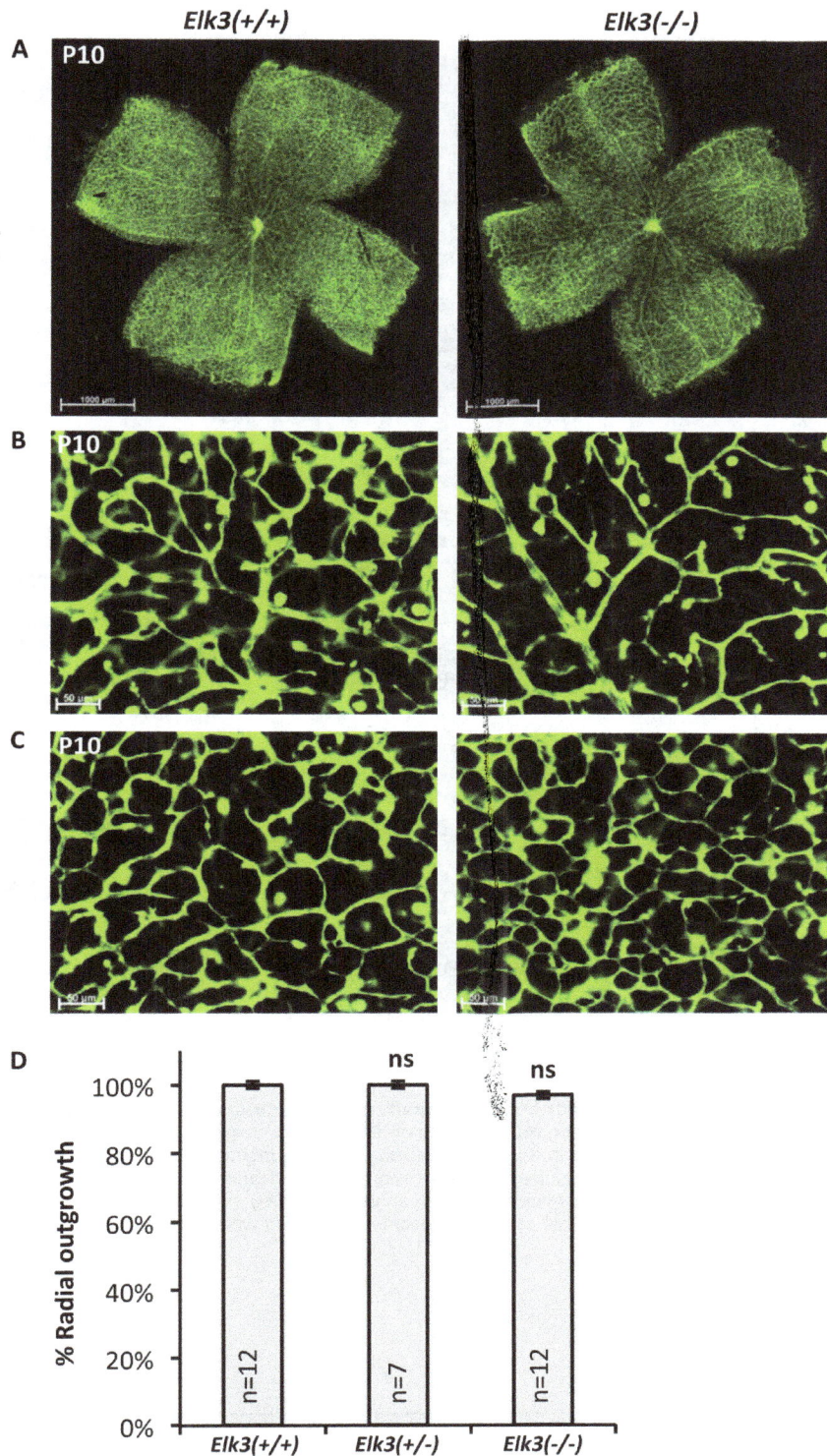

Figure 2. At P10, retinal vascular plexi appear normal in *Elk(−/−)* **knockout mice.** (A) Representative images of IsolectinB4 stained retinal flat-mounts from P10 control and *Elk3(−/−)* knockout mice. (B) Focal plane set on the primary plexus in control and *Elk3(−/−)* knockout retinae. (C) Focal plane set on the deep plexus in control and *Elk3(−/−)* knockout retinae. (D) Quantitation of retinal area covered by blood vessels (% vascularization) at P10. Data are normalized to the control = 100%. The data shown are means +/− s.e.m, ns = not significant. Scale bar in (A) 1000 μm, in (B, C) 50 μm.

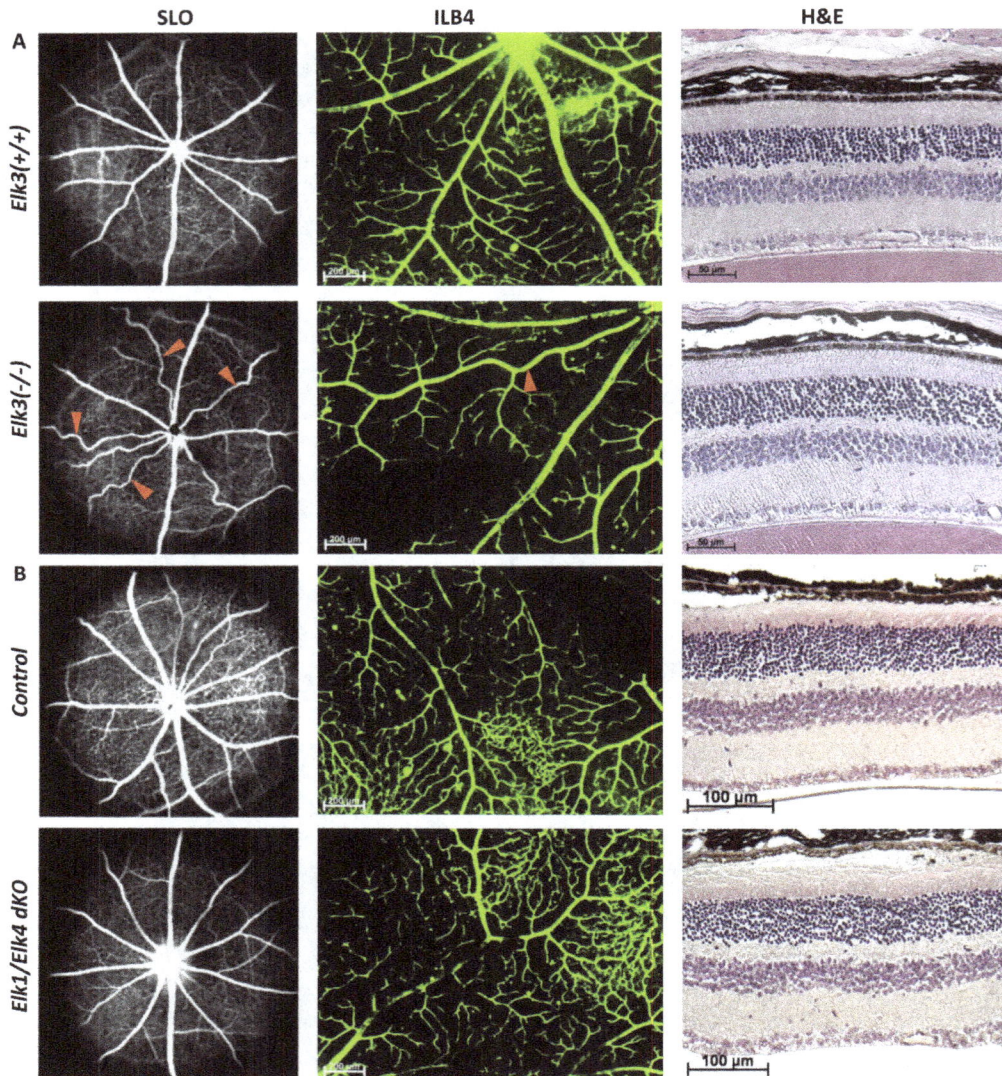

Figure 3. Scanning laser ophthalmoscopy reveals abnormally shaped tortuous arteries in adult *Elk3(−/−)*, but not *Elk1/Elk4*^dKO eyes.
(A) Scanning laser ophthalmoscopy (SLO) of *Elk3(+/+)* control (upper panel) and *Elk3(−/−)* knockout (lower panel) retinae by indocyanin green angiography (left) and a higher magnification of arteries in IsolectinB4 stained retinal flat-mounts of the same retina (middle; tortuous arteries are highlighted by red arrowheads). H&E staining of paraffin embedded whole eyes (right). (B) Scanning laser ophthalmoscopy (SLO) of *Elk1/Elk4* control (upper panel) and *Elk1/Elk4*^dKO (lower panel) retinae by indocyanin green angiography (left) and a higher magnification of arteries in IsolectinB4 stained retinal flat-mounts of the same retina (middle). H&E staining of paraffin embedded whole eyes (right). Scale bar in (middle) 200 μm, in (A right) 50 μm, in (B right) 100 μm.

Table 1. Incidence (%) of tortuous arteries.

Age/months	*Elk3(+/+)* control	*Elk3(+/−)* heterozygotes	*Elk3(−/−)* KO
1	0% (n = 7)	12% (±5%) (n = 8) *	62% (±11%) (n = 5) ***
2	0% (n = 6)	11% (±5%) (n = 8) **	91% (±7%) (n = 5) ***
≥4	3% (±3%) (n = 5)	44% (±9%) (n = 10) ***	85% (±8%) (n = 5) ***
	Elk1/Elk4 control	*Elk1/Elk4* heterozygotes	*Elk1/Elk4* ^dKO
≥4	0% (n = 4)	na	0% (n = 5) ns

(* p<0.05 ** p<0.01 *** p<0.001, na = not analysed, ns = not significant, n = number of retinae analysed).

Table 2. Extent of tortuousity and width of adult arteries.

	Elk3(+/+) control	Elk3(−/−) KO	Elk1/Elk4 control	Elk1/Elk4 dKO
Tortuousity factor	1.0 (±0.003) (n = 9)	1.06 (±0.008) (n = 9) ***	1.0 (±0.001) (n = 6)	0.999 (±0.002) (n = 5) ns
Width of adult arteries	20.5 μm (±1.0) (n = 9)	20.6 μm (±1.0) (n = 9) ns	19.7 μm (±1.0) (n = 6)	20.3 μm (±1.06) (n = 5) ns

(*** p<0.001, ns = not significant, n = number of retinae analysed).

existing vessels, as identified by exclusive collagenIV positivity. At the angiogenic front we did not find any vessel regression (Figure S6). Inside the primary plexus, occasional vessel regression (Figure S6, white arrows) was normalized to plexus area and found not to be significantly different between *Elk3* genotypes (Figure S6; for measurements, see Materials and Methods).

SRF deficiency in neurons of the forebrain results in increased Ser3 phosphorylation of the actin-severing protein cofilin [29]. To analyze whether this indicator of imbalance in actin dynamics was changed in *Elk3(−/−)* knockout retinal ECs compared to controls, similar to *Srf* ^{iECKO} endothelial cells [8], we performed Western blotting using a P-Cofilin antibody on adult retinal lysates (Figure S7A). No change in P-Cofilin levels were detected after quantitation of five pairs of control and knockout samples (Figure S7B) indicating that actin imbalance is not the reason for disturbed retinal vascular development.

Molecular and cellular defects in adult *Elk3* deficient retinae

Various mechanisms could account for the observed formation of tortuous arteries in adult *Elk3(−/−)* animals (see Discussion). We tested for VEGF levels in affected retinae, increased blood pressure, altered coverage of retinal blood vessels with smooth muscle cells and procollagen type IVα1, and expression of the tight junctional components claudin1 and claudin5. Further, since knockout mice of the angiogenic factor Ang-2 displayed arteriolar tortuousity [30], we studied retinal expression of the Ang-1/-2 system, including Tie1 and Tie2 co-receptors.

We did not detect any significant changes of *Vegf* RNA level in adult *Elk3* knockout retinae (Figure 4D). Interestingly, amongst Angiopoietins and cognate Tie receptors, a significant change was observed for Tie1, as was already found at post-natal ages P6 and P10 (compare Figure 4C and 4D). There were no significant changes in systolic blood pressure, measured by the tail cuff method (Non Invasive blood pressure) (Figure S3). We did not detect any differences in smooth muscle actin (SMA) coverage as judged by antibody staining on retinal flat-mounts (Figure 5A) and analysis of SMA levels by Western blot (Figure 5D and quantitation in Figure 5E). Mutations in the mouse *Col4a1* gene, encoding procollagen type IVα1, resulted in tortuous arteries in the C57BL/6J background [31]. However, we did not detect any significant changes by collagenIV antibody staining of adult retinal flat-mounts (Figure 5B) and qRT-PCR of whole retinal adult tissue (Figure 5C). In *Drosophila*, mutation of the *megatrachea* gene, which plays an essential role in the tracheal system of invertebrates, results in elongated and tortuous tracheal branches in mutant embryos [32] reminiscent of the tortuous vessel phenotype in *Elk3(−/−)* knockout mice. *Mega* encodes a transmembrane protein that is located in septate junctions and is thereby similar in structure and function to claudins, the component of tight junctions in vertebrates. We therefore analysed if claudins were changed in adult *Elk3(−/−)* knockout retinae but

did not find any significant changes on RNA levels of claudin1 and claudin5 (data not shown).

Impairment in *in vitro* microvessel sprouting and microtube formation of aortic ring explants derived from post-natal and adult *Elk3* deficient mice

The aortic ring assay is a commonly used assay of angiogenesis. It bridges the gap between *in vivo* and *in vitro* models of angiogenesis, thereby combining advantages of both systems [33]. Endothelial cells first appear at the severed edges of the explants after 2–3 days in culture and subsequently proliferate and migrate thereby resulting in microvessels around the explants. Previous studies using the hypomorphic Net$^{δ/δ}$ mutant mouse line indicated that Elk3 was required for aortic ring sprouting [34]. Using the aortic ring assay, we investigated whether the observed retinal phenotypic abnormalities reflected altered characteristics of endothelial cells in general or represented specific effects of retinal endothelial cells. Aortic rings were embedded in a polymerized extracellular matrix gel supplemented with endothelial growth medium. Microvessel sprouting from *Elk3(−/−)* knockout adult aortic explants was found to be reduced compared to *Elk3(+/+)* control animals (Figure 6A left). A scoring system was used to quantitate and follow the kinetics of microvessel sprouting (see Material and Methods). Sprouting from *Elk3(−/−)* aortic rings was reduced at all time points examined. Sprouting from *Elk3(+/+)* control explants reached a maximum after seven days, whereas *Elk3(−/−)* explants did not reach this level even after 20 days (Figure 6B). Microtube formation after three weeks was robust in *Elk3(+/+)* control explants cultures and greatly reduced in *Elk3(−/−)* cultures (Figure 6A middle). Staining of the cytoskeleton of fixed aortic explants after three weeks *in vitro* was used to study the microtubes. *Elk3(+/+)* control explants had intact interconnections between endothelial tubes and filopodia; whereas *Elk3(−/−)* explants had degenerated endothelial tip cells with retraction bulbs and lacked filopodia (Figure 6A right). Microvessel sprouting from P10 *Elk3(−/−)* aortae was also reduced compared to control animals (Figure 6C). This analysis demonstrates that Elk3 contributes to endothelial cell sprouting and migration.

Discussion

In this study we show that *Elk3(−/−)* mice display a dual retinal phenotype: (i) transient impairment in post-natal development of the superficial vascular plexus, paralleled by (ii) a lasting retinal arterial tortuousity in animals 4 weeks of age and older. Arterial tortuousity is found in the retinae of adult Elk3 deficient mice with 100% penetrance. These phenotypic features are not displayed by knockout animals of the paralogues *Elk1* and *Elk4* (Table 3). This shows that Elk3 has distinct, non-redundant functions relative to Elk1 and Elk4 in retinal vascular development, as was similarly indicated for thymocyte development [23] and adhesion of cultured cells [35].

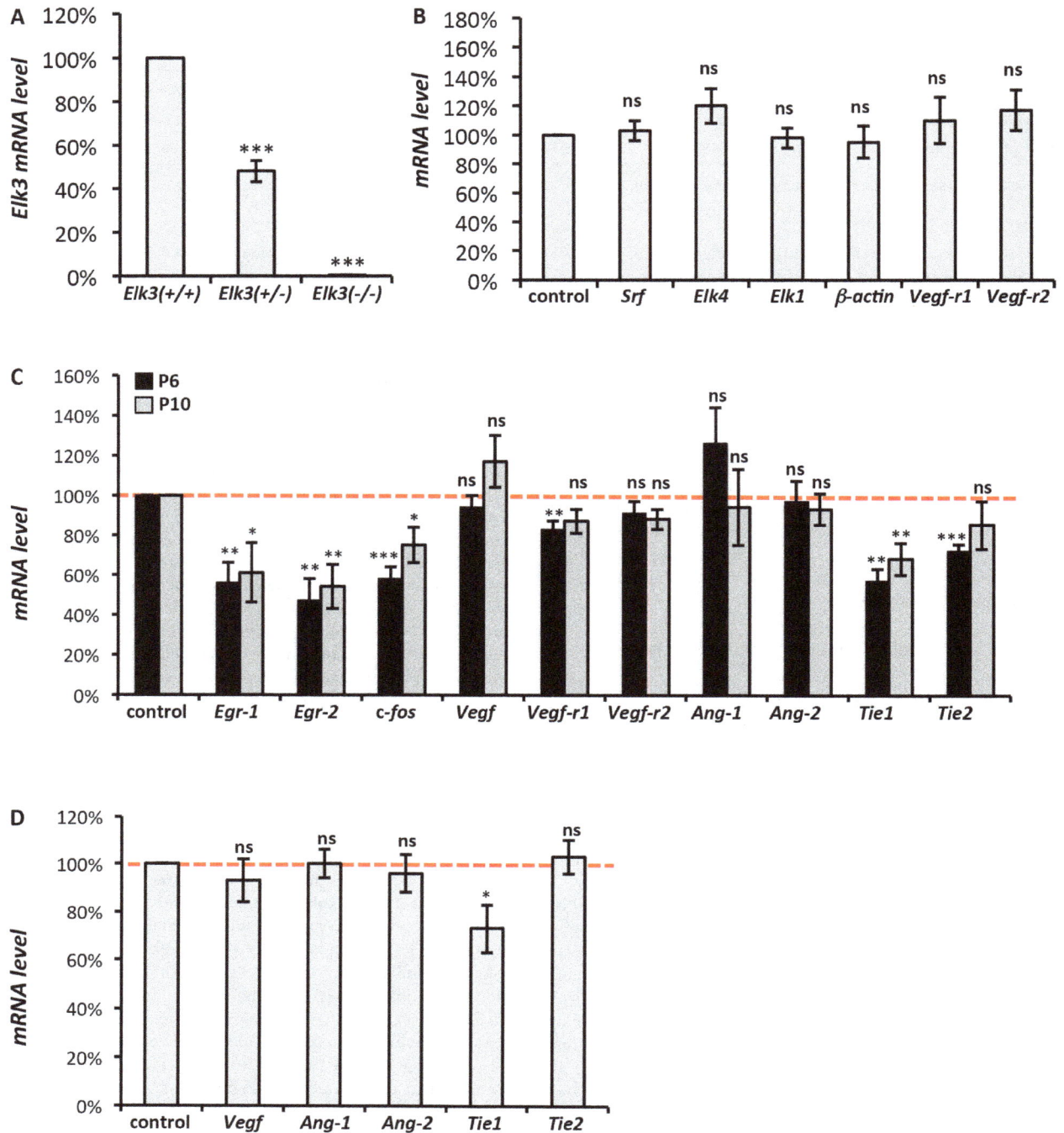

Figure 4. Downregulation of immediate-early genes and the angiogenic Tie1 receptor gene in post-natal Elk3(−/−) retinae. (A) Quantitative RT-PCR analysis of whole brain lysates of Elk3(+/+) control, Elk3(+/−) heterozygote and Elk3(−/−) knockout P4-P10 animals for expression of Elk3 RNA level (n = 9 independent experiments). (B) Semiquantitative RT-PCR analysis of whole brain lysates of Elk3(+/+) control and Elk3(−/−) knockout P6 animals for Srf, Elk1, Elk4, β-actin, Vegfr-1, Vegfr-2 expression level (n = 5 independent experiments). (C) Quantitation of RNA levels in P6 and P10 control and Elk3(−/−) knockout retinae for Vegf, Egr-1, Egr-2, c-fos, Vegfr-1, Vegfr-2, Ang-1, Ang-2, Tie1 and Tie2 (n>5 independent experiments). (D) Quantitation of Vegf, Ang-1, Ang-2, Tie1 and Tie2 RNA levels in adult control and Elk3(−/−) knockout retinae (n>5 independent experiments).

At the molecular level, we find Elk3(−/−) mice to display reduced retinal RNA expression of the angiogenic receptor Tie1, at P6, P10 and adult stage. The co-receptor Tie2 was found to have lower RNA levels at P6 but not P10 or adult retinae, while the cognate ligands Ang-1 and Ang-2 were expressed at normal

RNA levels at all times investigated. These findings correlate with the arterial tortuosity phenotype shared by Elk3(−/−) and Ang-2(−/−) mice [30], indicating in both knockout models an impaired functionality of the Tie/Ang receptor/ligand signalling system. Of note, endothelial Tie1 depletion in conditional

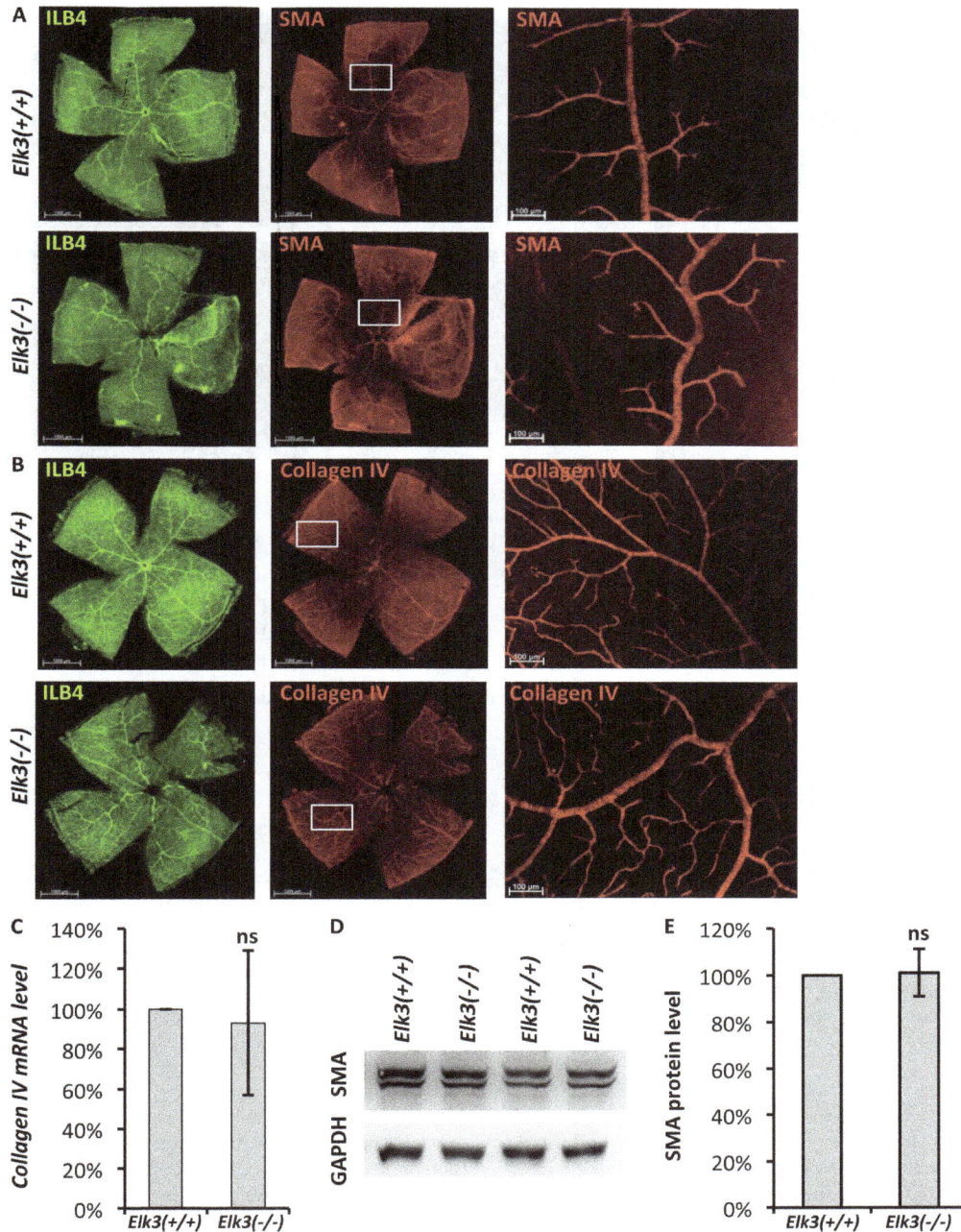

Figure 5. Smooth muscle actin and CollagenIV levels are not altered in *Elk3(−/−)* **knockout retinae.** (A) IsolectinB4 (ILB4) (left) and smooth muscle actin (SMA) (middle and right) staining of retinal flat-mounts of control (upper panel) and *Elk3(−/−)* knockout animals. (B) IsolectinB4 (left) and collagenIV (middle and right) staining of retinal flat-mounts of control (upper panel) and *Elk3(−/−)* knockout animals. (C) Quantitation of collagenIV RNA levels in control and *Elk3(−/−)* knockout retinae (n = 5 independent experiments). (D) Representative pairs of control and *Elk3(−/−)* knockout retinal lysates tested for smooth muscle actin expression in Western Blot analysis. (E) Quantitation of control and *Elk3(−/−)* knockout retinal levels of SMA (n = 5 independent experiments). Scale bar in (A, B left and middle) 1000 μm, in (A, B right) 100 μm.

knockout mice leads to decreased sprouting angiogenesis in the post-natal retinal vasculature [36], similar to *Elk3(−/−)* mice. Interestingly, this conditional phenotype was only seen when *Tie1* deletion was induced directly after birth but not when the deletion was induced between P7 and P9, suggesting a short window for the requirement of Tie1 during initial post-natal retinal angiogenesis, while – at the same time - arguing for Tie1 not being important in subsequent vascular remodelling [36]. Thus, the transient post-

natal requirement for Tie1 in retinal angiogenesis, as revealed by conditional Tie1 depletion [36], is fully congruent with the transient impairment in retinal primary plexus development observed here in *Elk3(−/−)* mice, which also displayed reduced Tie1 expression. We thus hypothesize that impairment in the functionality of the Tie1/Ang-2 signaling system accounts – in part - for both phenotypic irregularities of *Elk3(−/−)* mice, namely transient inhibition of retinal primary plexus formation

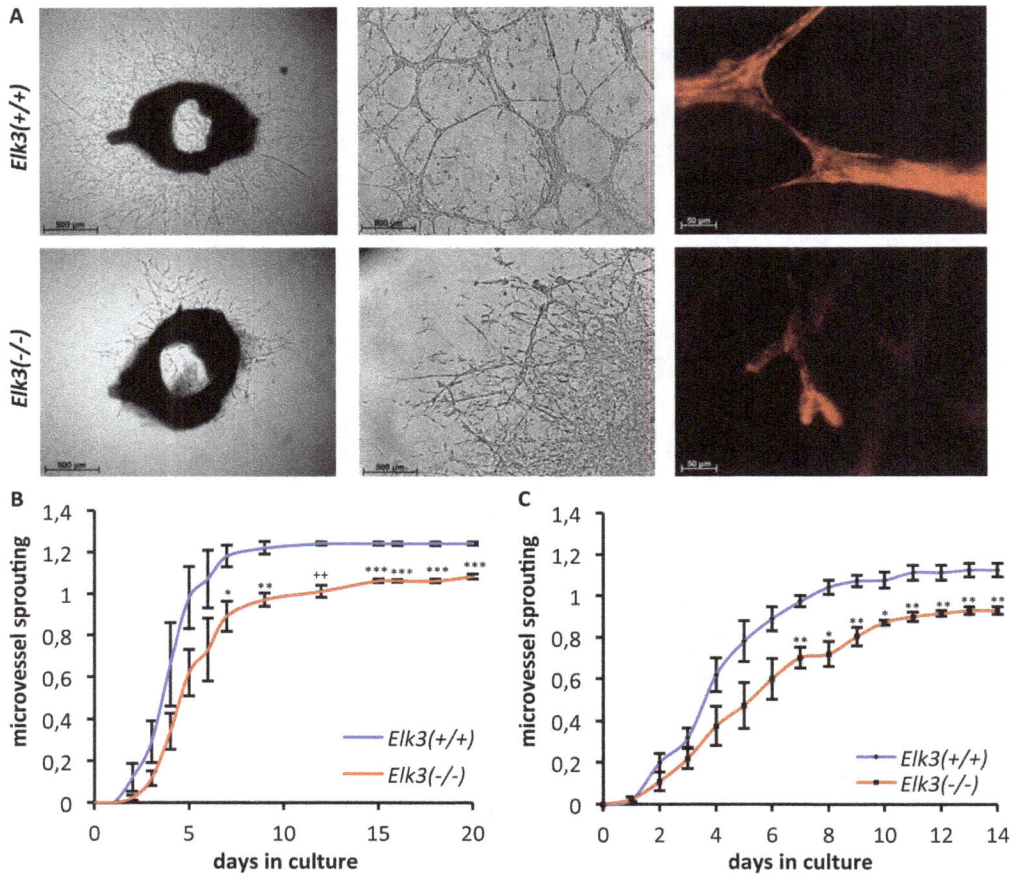

Figure 6. Microvessel sprouting and microtube formation is impaired in P10 and adult *Elk3(−/−)* knockout aortic ring explants. (A left) Aortic rings from *Elk3(+/+)* control animals show robust microvessel sprouting on day 5 of culture. In contrast, aortic rings from *Elk3(−/−)* knockout animals show drastically reduced microvessel sprouting. (A middle) Control *Elk3(+/+)*, but not *Elk3(−/−)* knockout aortic ring endothelial cells form microtubes in Matrigel after three weeks of culture. (A right) Phalloidin staining of aortic ring endothelial cells cultivated in Matrigel shows interconnected ECs and tip cells with filopodia in control explants, whereas *Elk3(−/−)* knockout aortic ring endothelial cells lack connections and instead have degenerated bulbs. (B, C) Kinetics of aortic ring microvessel sprouting for four pairs of adult (B) and four pairs of P10 (C) *Elk3(+/+)* control and *Elk3(−/−)* knockout animals observed during *in vitro* growth (for each time point mean +/− s.e.m. presented). Scale bar in (A left and middle) 500 μm, in (A right) 50 μm.

and adult retinal arterial tortuousity. We do not exclude potential contributions of the Tie2 co-receptor. We further hypothesize that Elk3, but not Elk1 or Elk4, is involved in transcriptional regulation of *Tie1* expression. *Tie1* may represent a direct or indirect Elk3 target gene. We note that approximately 1.6 kb upstream of the murine *Tie1* promoter, there is a canonical SRF-binding CArG-box with the sequence CCTTAATTGG. This element, however, is not conserved at this position in the human genome. Future

Table 3. Comparison of retinal phenotypes in the different knockout mouse models.

Knockout mouse model	*Srf* [IECKO]	*Mrtf-a*[(−/−)] *Mrtf-b* [IECKO]	*Elk1/Elk4* [dKO]	*Elk3 KO*
	Post-natal analysis			
Radial outgrowth	drastically reduced[#]	drastically reduced[#]	unaffected[#]	transiently reduced at early stages[*]
Tip cell morphology	drastically altered[#]	drastically altered[#]	unaffected[#]	unaffected[*]
Distal microaneurysms	present[#]	present[#]	absent[#]	absent[*]
Deep plexi	absent[#]	absent[#]	present[#]	present[*]
	Adult analysis			
Neovascular lesions	present[#]	present[§]	absent[*]	absent[*]
Tortuous arteries	absent[#]	absent[§]	absent[*]	present[*]

([*] this study, [#] published in Weinl et al., 2013, [§] unpublished observations).

studies will investigate whether a functionally relevant ternary complex of SRF and Elk3 is formed with this CArG-box *in vivo* and wether the postulated complex shows preference for Elk3 over Elk1 or Elk4. In light of the findings by D'Amico et al. [36], our data suggest that Elk3 represents a potential target for tumor therapy.

Alternatively, or in addition, reduced retinal expression at P6 and P10 of the immediate-early and proliferation-associated genes *Egr-1*, *Egr-2* and c-*fos* might have contributed to the transient delay in retinal angiogenesis of *Elk3(−/−)* mice. However, our measurements (Ki67 marker quantitation for proliferating cells at P6, vessel width at P6, P8 and adult animals) did not reveal any differences in proliferation of retinal endothelial cells at any of the investigated time points. We have therefore no direct experimental evidence for Elk3 impairment affecting proliferation of retinal endothelial cells.

In a separate study, human ELK3 was argued to inhibit angiogenic functions of HUVEC cells *in vitro* [37]. While this finding appears to differ with our report, the specific conditions and cells studied by Heo and Cho (2014) may have evoked the inhibitory role of Elk3, and could have involved Elk3-dependent changes in Tie1 expression in combination with inhibitory Ang-2 signaling, as suggested by this study.

The *Elk3(−/−)* mice differ from other mouse and rat models for tortuousity. In the rat ROP model, tortuousity is prevalent at young age and then decreases [38]. In contrast, *Elk3(−/−)* retinal arteries are completely normal in young animals, tortuousity is first obvious at four weeks of age and persists into later ages (2–8 months). The rat model of type-2 diabetic retinopathy displays tortuous retinal vessels that almost completely lack pericytes, microaneurysms and higher vessel diameters, and irregular retinal layering [39]. In contrast, *Elk3(−/−)* knockout retinal vessels have a normal smooth muscle coverage. Mutations in the *Col4a1* gene encoding procollagen type IVα1 result in tortuous arteries in mice with the C57BL/6J background [31]. We did not detect any significant changes in collagenIV levels between control and *Elk3(−/−)* knockout retinae as judged by antibody staining on adult retinal flat-mounts and qRT-PCR using whole retinal adult tissue. Tortuous vessels are commonly seen after injection of TNFα in mice [40], in a rat model of Oxygen Induced Retinopathy (OIR) [38] and in patients with cyanotic congenital heart disease [41]. Tortuousity might increase perfusion of avascular regions of the retina by reducing blood flow. All of these conditions are associated with increased VEGF expression. In contrast, *Vegf* RNA levels are normal in adult *Elk3(−/−)* knockout retinae displaying tortuousity. Furthermore, retinal layering and layer thickness are normal in *Elk3(−/−)* knockout mice, in contrast to the TNFα-injection mouse model [40].

Vessel tortuousity is observed in a number of human pathologies, for example in an aggressive form of ROP that additionally displays rapid retinal detachment, leakage of blood vessels and severe dilations [19]. In *Elk3(−/−)* knockout mice leakage of affected blood vessels was not detected by *in vivo* SLO angiography, which is consistent with unchanged VEGF levels. In some other human patients, changes in thickness of vessels are correlated with occurrence of abnormally shaped vessels. In patients with aortic isthmic coarctation, retinal arteriolar, but not venular diameter, was reduced [42,43]. In the Elk3 deficient arteries, proliferation was unchanged, as we did not detect any change in diameter of abnormally shaped adult arteries. Venular tortuousity has been observed in some human patients diagnosed with aortic isthmic coarctation [42,43] and in a screen for abnormalities of ocular fundi in monkeys [44]. Interestingly, only arteries are affected in the *Elk3(−/−)* eyes, as in the rat model of

OIR [38], in humans with ATS (arterial tortuousity syndrome) [45], and in the mouse TNFα injection model [40]. Abnormally shaped vessels are sometimes correlated with vision loss. ERGs are altered in ROP eyes [38], TNFα injected mice [40], and monocular vision loss during an exercise marathon run [46]. However, some patients with tortuous blood vessels and elevated VEGF levels have no ocular complaints [41]. As revealed by ERG measurements, vision was not impaired in adult *Elk3(−/−)* knockout mice. Blood pressure or hypertension could be expected to affect arterial shape. However, human patients with aortic isthmic coarctation after operative repair had retinal arteriolar tortuousity, but no hypertension, and blood pressure was normal [42,43], suggesting that vessel tortuousity is not necessarily correlated with hypertension. In agreement, we did not detect any abnormalities in blood pressure of *Elk3(−/−)* knockout animals.

Interestingly, a recent clinical characterization of FEVR patients (familial exudative vitreoretinopathy), using wide-field fluorescein angiography, revealed hitherto unrecognized, frequent vessel tortuousity among these patients [20]. We therefore note that post-natal impairments in retinal plexus formation and vessel tortuousity are shared pathological features of some human FEVR patients and murine knockout models of the SRF transcriptional system. The latter is evidenced by endothelial depletion of SRF itself [8], endothelial depletion of the SRF cofactors MRTF-A and −B [8], and constitutive depletion of the SRF cofactor Elk3 (this study). It remains an intriguing, but testable possibility that mutations in Elk3 alleles might contribute to FEVR pathology.

Using the aortic ring assay [33], we tested if endothelial cells of an origin other than the retinal blood vessel system were affected by the absence of Elk3. This turned out to be the case. Aortic rings explanted from P10 or adult *Elk3(−/−)* animals showed impairments in microvessel sprouting and tube formation. While this defect mirrors the post-natal delay in retinal angiogenesis of *Elk3(−/−)* mice, it does not reflect the transient nature of this effect. The observed impairment in *Elk3(−/−)* aortic ring adherence functions, leading to the formation of retraction bulbs, might however reflect specific functions of Elk3 in regulating adhesion-mediated cell behaviours [35].

In conclusion, this study shows that Elk3 has a distinct role in determining retinal RNA levels of immediate-early genes and genes encoding the angiogenic receptors Tie1 and Tie2. Elk3 is involved in ensuring proper radial outgrowth and arterial length in the mouse retina, which is consistent with previous *in vivo* and *in vitro* studies [21,34]. Interestingly, the new *Elk3(−/−)* mouse model described in our study has a highly penetrant phenotype of tortuous vessels with distinct features that could be used to study mechanisms of angiogenesis and vessel formation and could thus lead to a better understanding of human pathologies displaying tortuous vessels, including ROP and FEVR.

Supporting Information

Figure S1 The targeting vector was made as follows. The 5′ (4.3 kb), 3′ (3 kb) and inter-loxP (2.37 kb) fragments were PCR amplified on 129sv genomic DNA and sequentially subcloned in an ICS proprietary vector containing the LoxP sites and a Neo cassette flanked by FRT sites (Figure S1). The linearized construct was electroporated in 129S2/SvPas mouse embryonic stem (ES) cells. After selection, targeted clones were identified by PCR using external primers and further confirmed by Southern blotting with 5′ external probe. Two positive ES clones were injected into C57BL/6J blastocysts, and derived male chimeras gave germline transmission. The excision of the neomycin-resistance cassette was performed *in vivo* by breeding the chimeras with a Flp deleter line (C57BL/6J genetic background). The Flp transgene was segregated by breeding the first germ line mice with a wild type C57BL/6J animal. Constitutive KO mice were generated by breeding floxed-allele heterozygotes with a Cre deleter line followed by segregation in a further breeding step. The initial targeting vector contained a deletion of 104 bp (indicated by a red triangle), which was inconsequential regarding generation of the KO locus. Subseqent to Cre activation, deletion of genomic sequences extends from − 1720 to +650 relative the major transcription start site (TSS, +1), which corresponds to the first nucleotide of Elk3-001 EN-SMUST00000008542 (mouse GRCm38, Ensembl). The location of primers used for genotyping is indicated by P1, P3 and P4. Use of primers P1 and P3 detect the WT allele (PCR product size 363 bp), use of primers P3 and P4 amplify sequences surrounding the region that is deleted in the KO, and therefore detect a shorter fragment in Elk3 KO mice (PCR product size 230 bp, the 2480 bp product is not amplified under the PCR conditions used). Features are not drawn to scale. Primer sequences: primer P1: 5′-GGTTCCTCCTAGAAATCTCCCCAAG-3′; primer P3: 5′-TTTGCACTCAGGGTGTCTCCTCC-3′; primer P4: 5′-CA-CAGTTCACCTGATGGCTCACTC-3′. PCR conditions: 1×: 94°C 3 min. 2×: 94°C 1 min., 62°C 1 min., 72°C 1 min. 30×: 94°C 30 sec., 62°C 30 sec., 72°C 30 sec. 1×: 72°C 3 min. and cooling to 4°C.

Figure S2 Measurement of arterial length on adult *Elk3(+/+)* wildtype and *Elk3(−/−)* knockout retinal flat-mount preparations. For quantitative analysis, tortuous length (red line) and idealized length (yellow line) are measured in µm in both wildtype and knockout retinal flat-mounts stained with ILB4, and subsequently a tortuosity factor as defined as the ratio red line/yellow line is calculated and used to characterize tortuosity: a value close to 1 states no tortuosity (as shown for wildtype arteries), whereas a value > 1 is a hallmark of vessel tortuosity (as shown for knockout arteries). Values for WT retinae are normalized to 1. The value for knockout arteries with 1.06 (knockout arteries are on average 6% longer than wildtype arteries) is significantly different compared to WT as tested by Student's t-test statistics (p<0.001 *** as stated in Table 2). The measurements were performed on n = 9 WT retinae and n = 9 knockout retinae from different animals including 36 WT arteries and 30 knockout arteries in total.

Figure S3 Blood pressure measurements in female and male *Elk3(+/+)* control and *Elk3(−/−)* knockout mice (n = number of animals analysed). The data shown are means +/− s.e.m., ns not significant.

Figure S4 Retinal function is not impaired in adult *Elk3*-deficient mice. Electroretinographic data of adult *Elk3*(+/+) (black) and *Elk3*(−/−) mice (red). (A) Representative scotopic reponses at -2 (top) and 1.5 (middle) log cd*s/m², as well as a photopic response at 1.5 log cd*s/m² (bottom) flash intensity. Scotopic (B) and photopic (C) b-wave amplitudes from *Elk3* control mice and *Elk3*-deficient mice are plotted as a function of the logarithm of the flash intensity. In the box-and whisker-plot, boxes indicate the 25% and 75% quantile range, whiskers indicate the 5% and 95% quantiles, and the asterisks indicate the median of the data.

Figure S5 Analysis of astrocyte migration visualized by GFAP and ILB4 co-staining on *Elk3(+/+)* wildtype and *Elk3(−/−)* knockout retinal flat-mount preparations of different post-natal ages. No difference was observed in astrocyte migration towards the retinal periphery between *Elk3*(+/+) and *Elk3*(−/−) mice at all ages analysed (P4, 6 and 8). Number of analysed retinae of (WT/KO) genotype: P4 (10/6 retinae), P6 (8/8 retinae), P8 (12/8 retinae). ILB4 co-staining (not shown in this figure) was used to evaluate radial outgrowth of retinal blood vessels. Scale bars 100 µm.

Figure S6 P6 retinal flat-mounts of *Elk3(+/+)* and *Elk3(−/−)* mice were co-stained with ILB4 (green) and collagenIV (red). Overlay of both images results in the merge image (yellow). To quantify for vessel regression, number of vessels exclusively stained for collagenIV (as highlighted by white arrows), but not for ILB4, were counted per vascularized area. No difference was observed between both genotypes (ns not significant). Scale bars ILB4, CollagenIV and merge images 100 µm, zoom 50 µm.

Figure S7 (A) Western Blot analysis for P-Cofilin levels of two representative pairs of *Elk3(+/+)* control and *Elk3(−/−)* knockout adult whole retinal tissue, GAPDH was used as a loading control. (B) Quantitative Western Blot analysis of five pairs of *Elk3*(+/+) control and *Elk3*(−/−) knockout adult whole retinal tissue. P-Cofilin protein levels were calculated in relation to GAPDH (n = 5 independent experiments), ns not significant.

Table S1 Primer sequences for qRT-PCR of mouse tissue. Shown are forward (fw) and reverse (rev) sequences for analysed target genes. Gapdh was used as a housekeeping gene for normalization in all experiments.

Table S2 Measurement of proliferation by Ki67 and ILB4 co-staining of P6 and measurement of blood vessel width on ILB4 stained P6 and P8 *Elk3(+/+)* wildtype and *Elk3(−/−)* knockout retinal flat-mount preparations. Retinal flat-mounts of *Elk3*(+/+) WT and *Elk3*(−/−) KO P6 animals were co-stained with ILB4 and Ki67 and photographed at 20× magnification. On these images, Ki67 positive endothelial cells per vessel length were measured. Subsequently, Ki67 positive endothelial cells per 100 µm were calculated and all values of the WT were normalized to 100%. ns = not significant as tested by Student's t-test (p>0.05). For measurement of width, P6 and P8 ILB4-stained retinal flat-mounts were analysed. For width measurement, arteries and veins were analysed separately by outlining blood vessel Area (A) and blood vessel Length (L) and calculating mean width by Length/Area (L/A), followed by normalization of WT values to 100% (ns = not significant).

Acknowledgments

The *Elk3*(−/−) mouse mutant line was established and phenotyped in collaboration with the Genetic Engineering and Model Validation Department of the Mouse Clinical Institute (Institut Clinique de la Souris, MCI/ICS). We acknowledge the contribution of the Treisman laboratory (London) in the initial breeding of *Elk1/Elk4^dKO* mice.

Author Contributions

Conceived and designed the experiments: C. Wasylyk C. Weinl MJR BW AN. Performed the experiments: C. Wasylyk C. Weinl MGG SB HR CS MJR VS. Analyzed the data: C. Weinl MGG SB CS MJR MS VS. Contributed reagents/materials/analysis tools: C. Wasylyk MJR MS BW AN. Contributed to the writing of the manuscript: C. Weinl BW AN.

References

1. Carmeliet P, Jain RK (2000) Angiogenesis in cancer and other diseases. Nature 407: 249–257.
2. Adams RH, Alitalo K (2007) Molecular regulation of angiogenesis and lymphangiogenesis. Nature reviews Molecular cell biology 8: 464–478.
3. Gerhardt H, Golding M, Fruttiger M, Ruhrberg C, Lundkvist A, et al. (2003) VEGF guides angiogenic sprouting utilizing endothelial tip cell filopodia. The Journal of cell biology 161: 1163–1177.
4. Pitulescu ME, Schmidt I, Benedito R, Adams RH (2010) Inducible gene targeting in the neonatal vasculature and analysis of retinal angiogenesis in mice. Nature protocols 5: 1518–1534.
5. Fruttiger M (2002) Development of the mouse retinal vasculature: angiogenesis versus vasculogenesis. Investigative ophthalmology & visual science 43: 522–527.
6. Norman C, Runswick M, Pollock R, Treisman R (1988) Isolation and properties of cDNA clones encoding SRF, a transcription factor that binds to the c-fos serum response element. Cell 55: 989–1003.
7. Franco CA, Blanc J, Parlakian A, Blanco R, Aspalter IM, et al. (2013) SRF selectively controls tip cell invasive behavior in angiogenesis. Development 140: 2321–2333.
8. Weinl C, Riehle H, Park D, Stritt C, Beck S, et al. (2013) Endothelial SRF/MRTF ablation causes vascular disease phenotypes in murine retinae. The Journal of clinical investigation 123: 2193–2206.
9. Miano JM (2010) Role of serum response factor in the pathogenesis of disease. Laboratory investigation; a journal of technical methods and pathology 90: 1274–1284.
10. Arsenian S, Weinhold B, Oelgeschlager M, Ruther U, Nordheim A (1998) Serum response factor is essential for mesoderm formation during mouse embryogenesis. The EMBO journal 17: 6289–6299.
11. Posern G, Treisman R (2006) Actin' together: serum response factor, its cofactors and the link to signal transduction. Trends in cell biology 16: 588–596.
12. Esnault C, Stewart A, Gualdrini F, East P, Horswell S, et al. (2014) Rho-actin signaling to the MRTF coactivators dominates the immediate transcriptional response to serum in fibroblasts. Genes & development 28: 943–958.
13. Shaw PE, Schroter H, Nordheim A (1989) The ability of a ternary complex to form over the serum response element correlates with serum inducibility of the human c-fos promoter. Cell 56: 563–572.
14. Buchwalter G, Gross C, Wasylyk B (2004) Ets ternary complex transcription factors. Gene 324: 1–14.
15. Wang DZ, Li S, Hockemeyer D, Sutherland L, Wang Z, et al. (2002) Potentiation of serum response factor activity by a family of myocardin-related transcription factors. Proceedings of the National Academy of Sciences of the United States of America 99: 14855–14860.
16. Cen B, Selvaraj A, Burgess RC, Hitzler JK, Ma Z, et al. (2003) Megakaryoblastic leukemia 1, a potent transcriptional coactivator for serum response factor (SRF), is required for serum induction of SRF target genes. Molecular and cellular biology 23: 6597–6608.
17. Sasazuki T, Sawada T, Sakon S, Kitamura T, Kishi T, et al. (2002) Identification of a novel transcriptional activator, BSAC, by a functional cloning to inhibit tumor necrosis factor-induced cell death. The Journal of biological chemistry 277: 28853–28860.
18. Olson EN, Nordheim A (2010) Linking actin dynamics and gene transcription to drive cellular motile functions. Nature reviews Molecular cell biology 11: 353–365.
19. Nishina S, Yokoi T, Kobayashi Y, Hiraoka M, Azuma N (2009) Effect of early vitreous surgery for aggressive posterior retinopathy of prematurity detected by fundus fluorescein angiography. Ophthalmology 116: 2442–2447.
20. Kashani AH, Brown KT, Chang E, Drenser KA, Capone A, et al. (2014) Diversity of Retinal Vascular Anomalies in Patients with Familial Exudative Vitreoretinopathy. Ophthalmology.
21. Ayadi A, Zheng H, Sobieszczuk P, Buchwalter G, Moerman P, et al. (2001) Net-targeted mutant mice develop a vascular phenotype and up-regulate egr-1. The EMBO journal 20: 5139–5152.
22. Cesari F, Brecht S, Vintersten K, Vuong LG, Hofmann M, et al. (2004) Mice deficient for the ets transcription factor elk-1 show normal immune responses and mildly impaired neuronal gene activation. Molecular and cellular biology 24: 294–305.
23. Costello PS, Nicolas RH, Watanabe Y, Rosewell I, Treisman R (2004) Ternary complex factor SAP-1 is required for Erk-mediated thymocyte positive selection. Nature immunology 5: 289–298.
24. Costello P, Nicolas R, Willoughby J, Wasylyk B, Nordheim A, et al. (2010) Ternary complex factors SAP-1 and Elk-1, but not net, are functionally equivalent in thymocyte development. Journal of immunology 185: 1082–1092.
25. Weinhold B, Schratt G, Arsenian S, Berger J, Kamino K, et al. (2000) Srf(−/−) ES cells display non-cell-autonomous impairment in mesodermal differentiation. The EMBO journal 19: 5835–5844.
26. Iyer NV, Kotch LE, Agani F, Leung SW, Laughner E, et al. (1998) Cellular and developmental control of O2 homeostasis by hypoxia-inducible factor 1 alpha. Genes & development 12: 149–162.
27. Seeliger MW, Beck SC, Pereyra-Munoz N, Dangel S, Tsai JY, et al. (2005) In vivo confocal imaging of the retina in animal models using scanning laser ophthalmoscopy. Vision research 45: 3512–3519.
28. Tanimoto N, Muehlfriedel RL, Fischer MD, Fahl E, Humphries P, et al. (2009) Vision tests in the mouse: Functional phenotyping with electroretinography. Frontiers in bioscience 14: 2730–2737.
29. Alberti S, Krause SM, Kretz O, Philippar U, Lemberger T, et al. (2005) Neuronal migration in the murine rostral migratory stream requires serum response factor. Proceedings of the National Academy of Sciences of the United States of America 102: 6148–6153.
30. Feng Y, Vom Hagen F, Wang Y, Beck S, Schreiter K, et al. (2009) The absence of angiopoietin-2 leads to abnormal vascular maturation and persistent proliferative retinopathy. Thrombosis and haemostasis 102: 120–130.
31. Gould DB, Phalan FC, van Mil SE, Sundberg JP, Vahedi K, et al. (2006) Role of COL4A1 in small-vessel disease and hemorrhagic stroke. The New England journal of medicine 354: 1489–1496.
32. Behr M, Riedel D, Schuh R (2003) The claudin-like megatrachea is essential in septate junctions for the epithelial barrier function in Drosophila. Developmental cell 5: 611–620.
33. Nicosia RF (2009) The aortic ring model of angiogenesis: a quarter century of search and discovery. Journal of cellular and molecular medicine 13: 4113–4136.
34. Zheng H, Wasylyk C, Ayadi A, Abecassis J, Schalken JA, et al. (2003) The transcription factor Net regulates the angiogenic switch. Genes & development 17: 2283–2297.
35. Wozniak MA, Cheng CQ, Shen CJ, Gao L, Olarerin-George AO, et al. (2012) Adhesion regulates MAP kinase/ternary complex factor exchange to control a proliferative transcriptional switch. Current biology: CB 22: 2017–2026.
36. D'Amico G, Korhonen EA, Anisimov A, Zarkada G, Holopainen T, et al. (2014) Tie1 deletion inhibits tumor growth and improves angiopoietin antagonist therapy. The Journal of clinical investigation 124: 824–834.
37. Heo SH, Cho JY (2014) ELK3 suppresses angiogenesis by inhibiting the transcriptional activity of ETS-1 on MT1-MMP. International journal of biological sciences 10: 438–447.
38. Favazza TL, Tanimoto N, Munro RJ, Beck SC, Garcia Garrido M, et al. (2013) Alterations of the tunica vasculosa lentis in the rat model of retinopathy of prematurity. Documenta ophthalmologica Advances in ophthalmology 127: 3–11.
39. Saidi T, Mbarek S, Omri S, Behar-Cohen F, Chaouacha-Chekir RB, et al. (2011) The sand rat, Psammomys obesus, develops type 2 diabetic retinopathy similar to humans. Investigative ophthalmology & visual science 52: 8993–9004.
40. Robinson R, Ho CE, Tan QS, Luu CD, Moe KT, et al. (2011) Fluvastatin downregulates VEGF-A expression in TNF-alpha-induced retinal vessel tortuosity. Investigative ophthalmology & visual science 52: 7423–7431.
41. Tsui I, Shamsa K, Perloff JK, Lee E, Wirthlin RS, et al. (2009) Retinal vascular patterns in adults with cyanotic congenital heart disease. Seminars in ophthalmology 24: 262–265.
42. Shamsa K, Perloff JK, Lee E, Wirthlin RS, Tsui I, et al. (2010) Retinal vascular patterns after operative repair of aortic isthmic coarctation. The American journal of cardiology 105: 408–410.
43. Pressler A, Esefeld K, Scherr J, Ali M, Hanssen H, et al. (2010) Structural alterations of retinal arterioles in adults late after repair of aortic isthmic coarctation. The American journal of cardiology 105: 740–744.
44. Suzuki MT, Narita H, Cho F, Fukui M, Honjo S (1985) [Abnormal findings in the ocular fundi of colony-born cynomolgus monkeys]. Jikken dobutsu Experimental animals 34: 131–140.
45. Meyer S, Faiyaz-Ul-Haque M, Zankl M, Sailer NL, Marx N, et al. (2005) [Arterial tortuosity syndrome]. Klinische Padiatrie 217: 36–40.
46. Labriola LT, Friberg TR, Hein A (2009) Marathon runner's retinopathy. Seminars in ophthalmology 24: 247–250.

14

Zebrafish *WNK Lysine Deficient Protein Kinase 1 (wnk1)* Affects Angiogenesis Associated with VEGF Signaling

Ju-Geng Lai[1⦿], **Su-Mei Tsai**[1⦿], **Hsiao-Chen Tu**[1,2⦿], **Wen-Chuan Chen**[1], **Fong-Ji Kou**[1], **Jeng-Wei Lu**[1], **Horng-Dar Wang**[2], **Chou-Long Huang**[3]*, **Chiou-Hwa Yuh**[1,4,5,6]*

1 Institute of Molecular and Genomic Medicine, National Health Research Institutes, Zhunan Town, Miaoli, Taiwan, ROC, 2 Institute of Biotechnology, National Tsing Hua University, Hsinchu, Taiwan, ROC, 3 Departments of Medicine, University of Texas Southwestern Medical Center, Dallas, Texas, United States of America, 4 College of Life Science and Institute of Bioinformatics and Structural Biology, National Tsing-Hua University, Hsinchu, Taiwan, ROC, 5 Department of Biological Science and Technology, National Chiao Tung University, Hsinchu, Taiwan, ROC, 6 College of Medicine, Kaohsiung Medical University, Kaohsiung, Taiwan, ROC

Abstract

The WNK1 (WNK lysine deficient protein kinase 1) protein is a serine/threonine protein kinase with emerging roles in cancer. WNK1 causes hypertension and hyperkalemia when overexpressed and cardiovascular defects when ablated in mice. In this study, the role of Wnk1 in angiogenesis was explored using the zebrafish model. There are two zebrafish *wnk1* isoforms, *wnk1a* and *wnk1b*, and both contain all the functional domains found in the human WNK1 protein. Both isoforms are expressed in the embryo at the initiation of angiogenesis and in the posterior cardinal vein (PCV), similar to fms-related tyrosine kinase 4 (*flt4*). Using morpholino antisense oligonucleotides against *wnk1a* and *wnk1b*, we observed that *wnk1* morphants have defects in angiogenesis in the head and trunk, similar to *flk1/vegfr2* morphants. Furthermore, both *wnk1a* and *wnk1b* mRNA can partially rescue the defects in vascular formation caused by *flk1/vegfr2* knockdown. Mutation of the kinase domain or the Akt/PI3K phosphorylation site within *wnk1* destroys this rescue capability. The rescue experiments provide evidence that *wnk1* is a downstream target for Vegfr2 (vascular endothelial growth factor receptor-2) and Akt/PI3K signaling and thereby affects angiogenesis in zebrafish embryos. Furthermore, we found that knockdown of vascular endothelial growth factor receptor-2 (*flk1/vegfr2*) or vascular endothelial growth factor receptor-3 (*flt4/vegfr3*) results in a decrease in *wnk1a* expression, as assessed by *in situ* hybridization and q-RT-PCR analysis. Thus, the Vegf/Vegfr signaling pathway controls angiogenesis in zebrafish via Akt kinase-mediated phosphorylation and activation of Wnk1 as well as transcriptional regulation of *wnk1* expression.

Editor: Ramani Ramchandran, Medical College of Wisconsin, United States of America

Funding: This research was supported by grants from the NSC grant from Taiwan (99-3112-B-400-010, 101-2321-B-400-017 and 102-2321-B-400-016) to C.H.Y., and the NIH grant from USA (RO1DK59530) to C.L.H. The funders had no role in study design, data collection and analysis, decision to publish, or preparation of the manuscript.

Competing Interests: The authors have declared that no competing interests exist.

* Email: chyuh@nhri.org.tw (CHY); Chou-Long.Huang@UTSouthwestern.edu (CLH)

⦿ These authors contributed equally to this work.

Introduction

The development of the vascular system occurs via vasculogenesis and angiogenesis. Vasculogenesis refers to the de novo formation of vessels [1]; in angiogenesis, new blood vessels form by remodeling and extending old ones [2]. The most important molecules governing angiogenesis are the VEGF (vascular endothelial growth factor) family members and their receptors [3]. There are three different VEGF receptors, VEGFR1 (FLT1), VEGFR2 (KDR/FLK1) and VEGFR3 (FLT4). VEGFR2 mediates the majority of the downstream angiogenic effects of VEGF. These angiogenic effects include changes in microvascular permeability and endothelial cell proliferation, invasion, migration and survival. Upon activation by the binding of VEGF, the VEGFR2 tyrosine kinase phosphorylates downstream kinases, such as the phosphoinositide-dependent protein kinase (PI3 kinase), which then phosphorylates and activates the protein kinase Akt/PKB1. Multiple Akt/PKB substrates have been discovered, and WNK1 is a novel Akt/PKB substrate in insulin-stimulated 3T3-L1 adipocytes [4].

WNK1 (WNK lysine deficient protein kinase 1) protein is a novel mammalian serine/threonine protein kinase that lacks the invariant catalytic lysine found in subdomain II of all MAPKs, which is crucial for binding ATP and instead contains a catalytic lysine at position 233 in subdomain I [5]. Wnk1 cDNA was identified in a screen for MAPK family members in the mouse brain [5]. *WNK1* was found to be overexpressed in invasive colorectal cell lines [6]. WNK1 activates ERK5 by phosphorylating MEKK2/3, which is upstream of ERK5 in human embryonic kidney 293 (HEK293) cells [7]. Knocking down Wnk1 in the C17.2 mouse neural progenitor cell line resulted in decreased Erk5 activity, which reduced cell proliferation, migration and differentiation [8]. Other reports indicate that the WNK1 protein has a protein kinase AKT/protein kinase B (PKB) phosphorylation consensus sequence, and it has been shown that AKT kinase phosphorylates threonine 60 (Thr60) of WNK1 [9]. It is possible that during angiogenesis, VEGF/VEGFR2 phosphorylates and activates PI3 kinase, which then phosphorylates and activates AKT kinase, which might then phosphorylate WNK1.

WNK kinases contain an autophosphorylation domain, and serine 382 in the activation loop was shown to be required for autophosphorylation. The autoinhibitory domain, which is conserved in all four WNKs, suppresses the activity of the WNK1 kinase domain, and the two key residues required for the function of the autoinhibitory domain have been identified [10].

Overexpression of WNK1 causes hypertension and hyperkalemia in humans by altering renal Na^+ and K^+ transport [11]. WNK1 activates the downstream protein kinases STE20/SPS1-related proline-alanine-rich protein kinase (SPAK) and oxidative stress responsive 1 (OSR1) through phosphorylation of the t-loop in the catalytic domain [12,13,14,15]. Activated SPAK and OSR1 associate and then phosphorylate and activate other ion co-transporters, including $Na^+/K^+/2Cl^-$ co-transporter 1 (NKCC1) [16,17]. NKCC1 is a ubiquitous ion transporter [18] that controls cell volume and maintains osmostasis through absorption of Na^+, K^+ and Cl^- ions [19,20], suggesting that under hyperosmotic conditions, WNK1 can regulate the activity of NKCC1 through SPAK and OSR1 [21].

In the past, all research on WNK1 has focused on its function in cancer cell proliferation, differentiation, migration and apoptosis. In studies of somatic cells, WNK1 involvement in renal Na^+ and K^+ transport is also well known. However, the physiological function of WNK1 outside the kidney remains unclear. Using gene disruption and rescue in mice, Xie et al. found that Wnk1 function is required for embryonic angiogenesis and cardiac development, with *Wnk1* deletion affecting artery-vein specification [22]. The mechanism by which Wnk1 affects angiogenesis, however, remains largely unknown.

The zebrafish has emerged as a powerful vertebrate model system for development [23,24], organogenesis [25,26,27], vasculogenesis [1], neurogenesis [28,29] and carcinogenesis [30,31]. Zebrafish and other vertebrates have highly conserved genomic sequences; thus, zebrafish can be used to analyze the developmental process of embryo formation as well as human disease pathology [1,32]. Moreover, a range of forward and reverse genetic methods, including antisense morpholino oligonucleotide (MO)-based knockdown and Tol2 transgenesis, have been developed for functional analysis of genes in zebrafish [33,34]. Green fluorescent protein (GFP) under the control of the *fli1* or *flk1* regulatory region is specifically expressed in angioblasts [35,36]. The existence of transgenic lines expressing vessel-specific GFP also facilitates the study of vasculogenesis and angiogenesis in zebrafish.

Previous studies have shown that Wnk1 homozygous mutant mice die at E13 and have significant defects in angiogenesis, whereas Wnk1 heterozygous mice and wild-type mice do not differ significantly in hypotension, embryogenesis or angiogenesis [22,37]. To further understand the role of Wnk1 in angiogenesis, we used the vessel-specific transgenic zebrafish line *Tg(fli1:EGFP)*. We found that knockdown of *wnk1* by MOs led to defects in the angiogenic sprouting of intersegmental vessels (ISVs). Unlike Wnk1 mutant mice, *wnk1* zebrafish morphants survive. Analysis of these morphants has furthered our understanding of the role Wnk1 plays during angiogenesis and helped to identify the signaling pathway through which Wnk1 functions.

Materials and Methods

Zebrafish husbandry

Zebrafish embryos, larvae, and adult fish were maintained in the Zebrafish Core Facility at NTHU-NHRI (ZeTH) according to established protocols and methods [38]. Animal use protocols for zebrafish were approved by the Institutional Animal Care Use Committee (IACUC) of the National Health Research Institutes. The animal protocol number is NHRI-IACUC-096037-A.

Resources for sequence information

The zebrafish genomic sequence of WNK1 (NW_001878589) was obtained from the National Center for Biotechnology Information (NCBI). The human WNK1 protein sequence (gi|2711660|NP_061852.1) was obtained from the NCBI databank and used in a tBlastn search of the zebrafish RefSeq RNA database to identify zebrafish Wnk1 homologs.

RNA extraction, RT-PCR and quantitative polymerase chain reaction (q-RT-PCR)

Total RNA was extracted from twenty embryos at different embryonic stages with a NucleoSpin RNA II kit (MACHEREY-NAGEL). Complement DNA was synthesized from 900 ng of RNA using MutiScribe Reverse Transcriptase with the following program: 25°C-10 min → 48°C-30 min → 95°C-5 min → 12°C-indefinite. After the RT reaction, we diluted the cDNA 20-fold and performed the q-RT-PCR as described below.

Quantitative PCR studies were performed on selected clones using gene-specific primers. The rate of PCR amplification in one population vs. another (after normalizing against housekeeping genes) reflects differences in the expression of the gene in the two populations. We used GFP DNA as our standard to calculate the number of molecules after a given cycle number. Each q-RT-PCR Ct (cycle number) can be converted into number of molecules according to the standard curve and then converted into molecules per embryo by dividing by the number of embryos used.

DNA constructs: cloning and vectors

The *wnk1a* and *wnk1b* cDNA was generated by PCR amplification. The primers used to amplify the *wnk1a* and *wnk1b* cDNA are listed below.

wnk1a -F-*NotI*: 5′-ATAT**GCGGCCGC***ATG*GT-CAAGTTCCTTTCCCC-3′ (bold letters indicate a *NotI* site, and *italic letters* denote the translation initiation site).

wnk1a-OUT-R: 5′-ACCCATTCGTGCCTCTATCA-3′.

wnk1b- F-*NotI*: 5′-ATAT**GCGGCCGC**CTGGAAAG*ATG*T-CATCGGAAA-3′ (bold letters indicate a *NotI* site, and *italic letters* denote the translation initiation site).

wnk1b- OUT-R: 5′-CGTGGCATATTTGTGAGCAT-3′.

The PCR product was cloned into a cloning vector using the T&A cloning kit (Yeastern Biotech, catalog # YC001) and TaKaRa DNA ligation kit (TAKARA BIO INC, catalog #6024).

Rat Wnk1(1–449) was generated by PCR amplification from rat Wnk1(1–491)/pCMV5-Myc (kindly provided by Dr. Huang C. L., who obtained from Dr. Cobb's lab). The primers used to amplify the rat Wnk1(1–449) are listed below.

Rat-*EcoRI*-Wnk1(1–449)-F: 5′-ATCG**GAATTC***A*TGTCT-GACGGCACCGCAGA-3′.(bold letters indicate an *EcoRI* site, and *italic letters* denote the translation initiation site).

Rat-*XbaI*-Wnk1(1–449)-R: 5′- ATCG**TCTAGA**AATTGC-TACTTTGTCAAAAC-3′ (bold letters indicate an *XbaI* site).

Rat-Wnk1-seq-F: 5′-CCTAGTGTACCCGCAGTGGT-3′.

Rat-Wnk1-seq-R1: 5′-ACCACTGCGGGTACACTAGG-3′.

Rat-Wnk1-seq-R2: 5′-TAGCCATCTCAAGCATGCAC-3′.

The PCR product was digested with *EcoRI* and *XbaI* (NEW ENGLAND Biolabs Inc., catalog #R0101L and #R0145L), purified with a MinElute PCR Purification Kit (QIAGEN, catalog #28006), and subsequently cloned into an *EcoRI*- and *XbaI*-linearized pCS2+ vector using the T&A cloning kit (Yeastern

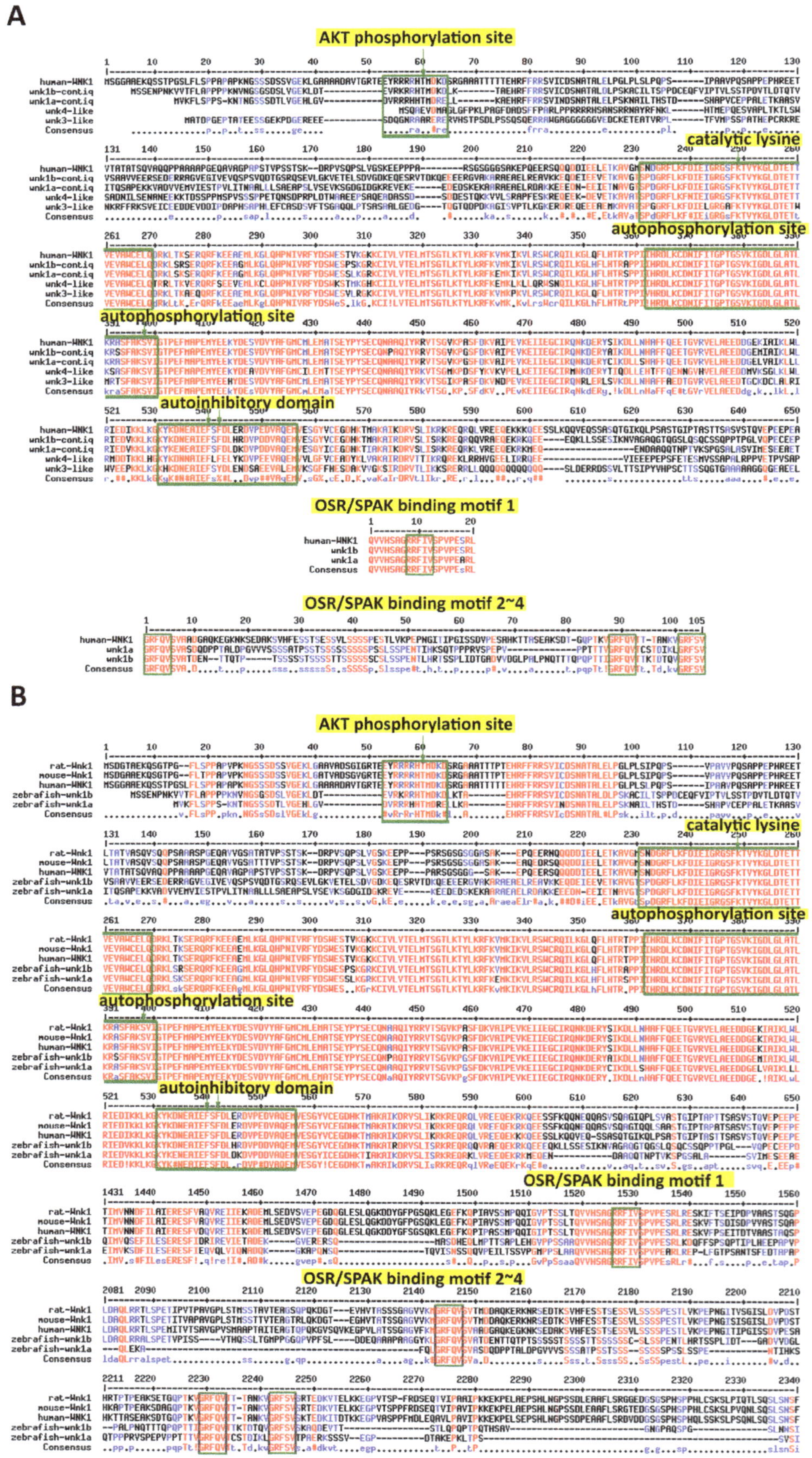
A
AKT phosphorylation site
catalytic lysine
autophosphorylation site
autophosphorylation site
autoinhibitory domain
OSR/SPAK binding motif 1
OSR/SPAK binding motif 2~4
B
AKT phosphorylation site
catalytic lysine
autophosphorylation site
autophosphorylation site
autoinhibitory domain
OSR/SPAK binding motif 1
OSR/SPAK binding motif 2~4

Figure 1. Sequence comparison between human WNK1 and zebrafish Wnk proteins. (A) Alignment of four zebrafish Wnks with the human WNK1 protein sequence. The WNK1 signature domain is highlighted. The AKT phosphorylation site at threonine 60 (arrow) in WNK1 is specific to Wnk1a and Wnk1b. The catalytic lysine (arrow) is located in a highly conserved region among all Wnk1s. The autophosphorylation site and the autoinhibitory domain are conserved between all four Wnk1s. The four OSR/SPAK binding motifs found in human WNK1 are specific to Wnk1a and Wnk1b. (B) Alignment of WNK1 protein sequences from mouse, rat, human and zebrafish.

Biotech, catalog # YC001) and TaKaRa DNA ligation kit (TAKARA BIO INC, catalog #6024).

Microinjection

Microinjections were carried out as previously described [38]. For the MO experiments, we injected 2.5–15 ng of MO were microinjected into each one-cell-stage embryo. For the RNA injections, 150–600 pg of mRNA was microinjected into each one cell-stage embryo.

Site-directed mutagenesis

We utilized the QuikChange II Site-Directed Mutagenesis Kit from Stratagene to generate the kinase dead and Akt phosphorylation site mutations in *wnk1*. *wnk1* cDNA in the yT&A vector (50 ng) was used as the template DNA in each reaction. Following amplification (95°C for 5 minutes, 18 cycles of 95°C for 30 seconds, 70°C for 30 seconds, and 68°C for 7 minutes 30 seconds), the product was treated with 1 µl of the *Dpn*I (10 U/µl) restriction enzyme to digest the parental methylated and hemimethylated dsDNA. The nicked vector DNA containing the desired mutations was then transformed into XL-1Blue super competent cells for nick repair and amplification.

The oligonucleotide sequences used to generate the mutations are given below. The underlined bases denote the mutation sites for site-directed mutagenesis.

Akt phosphorylation site mutant:

wnk1a 35 point mutation-F: 5′-CCGTCGTCGCCAC-CACGCCATGGATCGAGAACTGC-3′.

wnk1a 35 point mutation-R: 5′-GCAGTTCTCGATC-CATGGCGTGGTGGCGACGACGG-3′.

Kinase-dead mutant:

wnk1a 206 point mutation-F: 5′-TAGGACGTGGC-TCTTTTTGTACGGTCTACAAGGGACTG-3′.

wnk1a 206 point mutation-R: 5′-CAGTCCCTTGTA-GACCGTACAAAAAGAGCCACGTCCTA-3′.

Morpholinos used to knockdown gene expression

Morpholino oligonucleotides (MOs) were custom-made by Gene Tools (Philomath, OR, USA) and injected at doses that generated distinct gene knockdown effects while yielding the highest proportion of living embryos with the knockdown phenotype. The MO sequences and target sites are given below.

wnk1a ATG MO: 5′-ACTTGACCATCTTGTCGTTGA-GATT-3′

(Against *wnk1a* translation start codon, −15 to +10.)

wnk1a 5MM MO: 5′-ACTTCACGATCTTCTCCTTGA-CATT-3′

(Against *wnk1a* translation start codon, −15 to +10, but containing the five underlined mismatches.)

wnk1a Up MO: 5′-TCCACCAAGTGGAGCGTGAAGT-TAG-3′

(Against *wnk1a* upstream of translation start codon, −52 to −28.)

wnk1b Up MO: 5′-TGCGTAAATTTCCTGCTCTTGCTT-3′

(Against *wnk1b* upstream of translation start codon, −100 to −77.)

wnk1b ATG MO: 5′-TGGGATTTTCCGATGACATC-TTTCC-3′

(Against *wnk1b* translation start codon, −6 to +19.)

flk1 MO: 5′-GTCTGTTAAAATAACGTCCCGAATG-3′

(Against *flk1* upstream of translation start codon, −28 to −4.)

flt4 MO: 5′-CTCTTCATTTCCAGGTTTCAAGTCC-3′

(Against *flt4* translation start codon, −17 to +8.)

pi3kc2α: 5′-TATGTGGGCCATGGTGTCAGCTCT-3′

(Against *pi3kc2α* translation start codon, −12 to +12.)

Lyophilized MOs were resuspended to a final concentration of 10 mM in sterilized ddH₂O, and the solution was heated for 5 minutes at 65°C to dissociate aggregates of the powder. The MO solution was divided into 10-µl aliquots. Before use, each aliquot was heated to 65°C for 5 to 10 minutes and then cooled to room temperature.

In vitro transcription of mRNA

We used the mMESSAGE mMACHINE T7 Ultra kit (Applied Biosystems, catalog # AM1345) for *in vitro* transcription of wild-type *wnk1a* and *wnk1b* and the two *wnk1a* mutants. The synthesized mRNAs were checked by agarose gel electrophoresis with RNA Millennium Markers (Applied Biosystems catalog # AM7150) for integrity. The concentration of *in vitro* transcribed mRNA was determined using a NanoDrop ND-1000 UV-Vis Spectrophotometer. Rat Wnk1(1–449) mRNA was generated from a pCS2+ vector construct by *in vitro* transcription using the mMESSAGE mMACHINE SP6 kit (Applied Biosystems, catalog # AM1340).

Whole-mount *in situ* hybridization (WMISH)

Whole-mount *in situ* hybridization was carried out as previously described [38].

To generate probes for *in situ* hybridization, we first amplified *wnk1a*, *wnk1b*, *flt4*, *vegfc*, and *etv2* cDNA by PCR. The primers used to generate the DNA templates are listed in the supporting data (Data S1). We used the MEGAscript T7 kit (Ambion, catalog # AM1333) for *in vitro* transcription of digoxigenin (DIG)-labeled and fluorescein-labeled probes. Zebrafish embryos were collected and fixed in 4% paraformaldehyde at the indicated time points. To optimize hybridization, 5% dextran sulfate was added to the hybridization buffer for the DIG-labeled probes [39]. After post-hybridization washes to remove excess probe, the embryos were blocked with 1% blocking reagent (Roche Molecular Biochemicals, Mannheim, Germany) for 1 hour and then incubated overnight with pre-absorbed alkaline phosphatase (AP)-conjugated anti-DIG antibody (Roche Molecular Biochemical; 1:2000 dilution) at 4 °C. Transcripts were visualized by AP-based NBT/BCIP staining under identical conditions and staining times.

To confirm the localization of *wnk1a* and *wnk1b* in the PCV of zebrafish embryo, double *in situ* hybridization was performed using fluorescein-labeled *wnk1a* or *wnk1b* probe mixed with DIG-labeled *flt4* probe and detected with an AP-conjugated anti-fluorescein antibody followed by an AP-conjugated anti-DIG antibody. The *wnk1a* and *wnk1b* transcripts were visualized by AP-based NBT/BCIP, and the *flt4* and *vegfc* transcripts were visualized by AP-based fast red (Roche Molecular Biochemicals, Mannheim, Germany) staining. Therefore, *wnk1a* and *wnk1b*

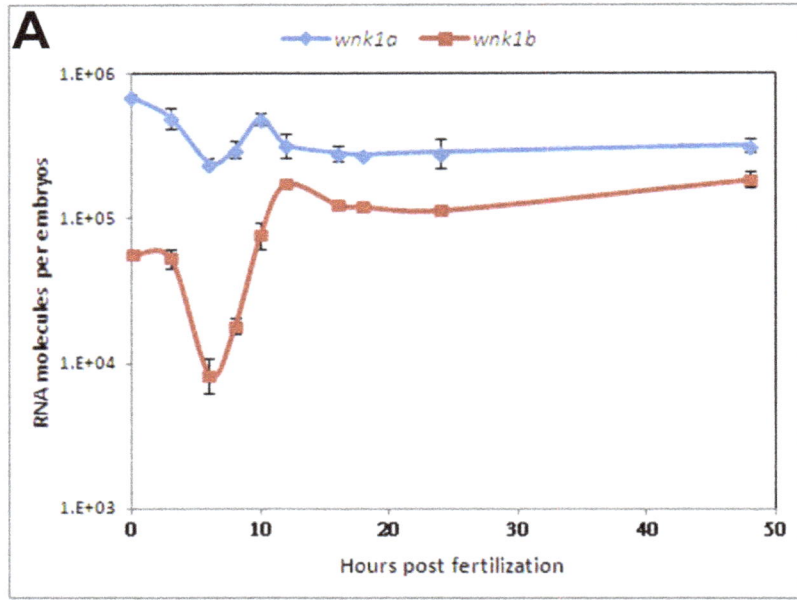

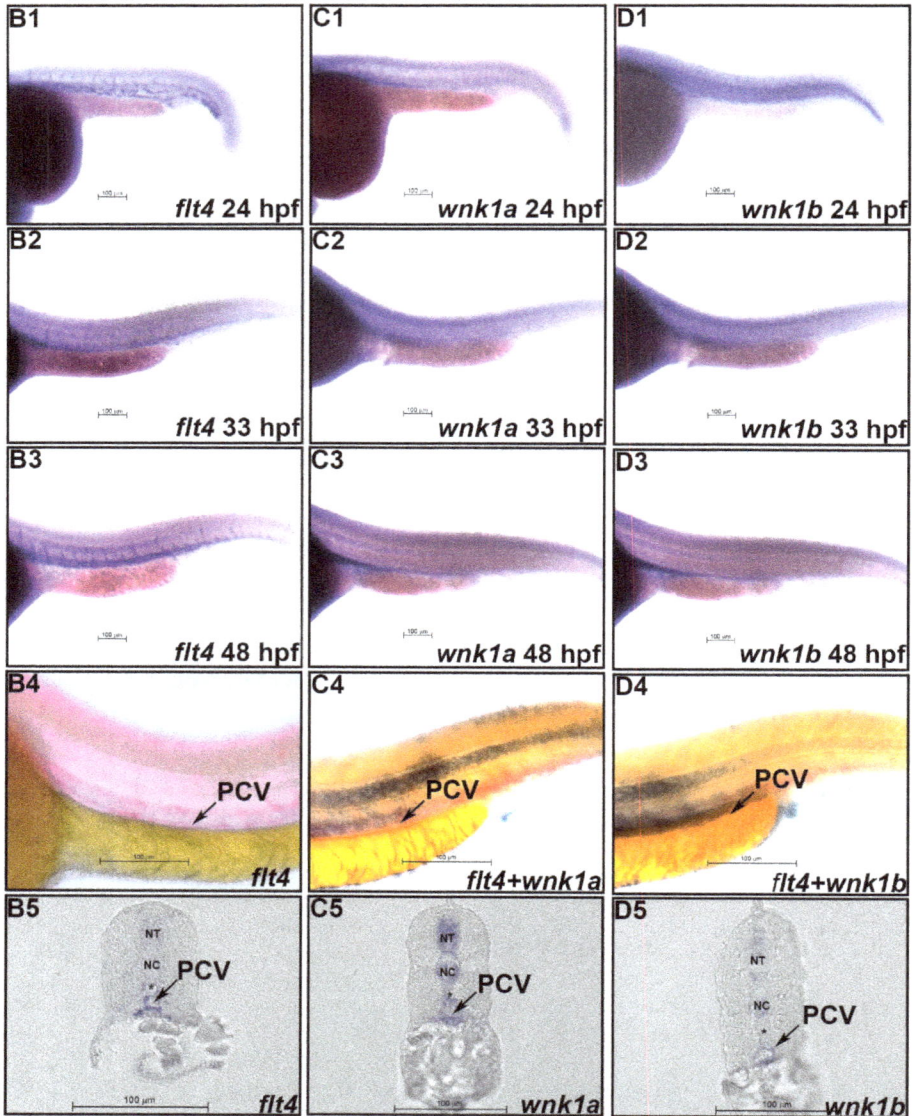

Figure 2. Spatial and temporal expression patterns of *wnk1a* **and** *wnk1b.* (A) *wnk1a* and *wnk1b* mRNA expression profiles as determined by q-RT-PCR. At least three replicates were performed, and the average number of molecules was calculated using a standard curve from a q-RT-PCR assay. The standard deviations are shown in the graph. The red and blue lines indicate the *wnk1a* and *wnk1b* expression profiles, respectively. (B~D) Whole-mount *in situ* hybridization for *flt4* (B) *wnk1a* (C), and *wnk1b* (D) was performed at the indicated time points. *flt4* (B1~B3), *wnk1a* (C1~C3), and *wnk1b* (D1~D3) mRNA expression in the tail is shown at 24, 33 and 48 hpf. Double *in situ* hybridization for *flt4* alone (B4), *wnk1a*+*flt4* (C4), and *wnk1b*+*flt4* (D4) shows the co-localization of *wnk1a* and *wnk1b* with *flt4* in the PCV. Expression of *flt4* (B5), *wnk1a* (C5) and *wnk1b* (D5) is seen in the PCV (arrow) in sections from stained embryos. *wnk1a* and *wnk1b* are also expressed in the neural tube (NT) and notochord (NC). The dorsal aorta (*) is negative for *wnk1a* and *wnk1b* expression. Scale bar: 100 μm.

expression appears blue while *flt4* expression is labeled in red. In between visualization of the fluorescein- and DIG-labeled probes, the AP enzymatic reaction was inactivated by incubating embryos in 100 mM glycine-hydrochloride (pH2.2) for 30 minutes.

Construction of *wnk1a-GFP* and *wnk1b-GFP* for testing morpholino knockdown efficiency and specificity

To test the knockdown efficiency of *wnk1a* and *wnk1b* MOs, 263-bp and 286-bp fragments of *wnk1a* and *wnk1b* mRNA containing the MO targeting sites were amplified from zebrafish cDNA by PCR. For the *wnk1a-GFP* construct, the primers used were *wnk1a*-EcoRI (5′-AATA**GAATTC**TTCCACTTGGTT-TAAAGCGG-3′, bold letters indicate an *EcoRI* site) and *wnk1a*-BamHI (5′-AATA**GGATCC**GCCTTCAGCAGTTCTC-GATC-3′, bold letters indicate a *BamHI* site). For the *wnk1b-GFP* construct, the primers used were *wnk1b*-EcoRI (5′-AATA-**GAATTC**AACTCTGTGGTTCACGTGAG-3′, bold letters indicate an *EcoRI* site) and *wnk1b*-BamHI (5′- AATA**G-GATCC**TGGCGTCGCTTTCTGAC-3′, bold letters indicate a *BamHI* site). The PCR products were cloned into the pEGFP-N1 plasmid. Linearized *wnk1a-GFP* and *wnk1b-GFP* plasmids (200 pg) were microinjected into one-cell-stage embryos along with 10 ng of various *wnk1a* and *wnk1b* MOs as shown in Fig. S1.

Fluorescent microscopy

Embryos were removed from their chorions with watchmaker forceps. For live imaging, the embryos were anesthetized with 0.168 mg/ml tricaine (Sigma, catalog # A-5040) and placed on a 1% agarose plate. For imaging of fixed tissues, the embryos were incubated in a 4% formaldehyde-PBS (1x PBS) solution overnight at 4°C, washed with PBST (1x PBS, 0.1% Tween 20) and then mounted in 1% PBS-low melt agarose (Zymeset). Embryos of different stages were collected for GFP visualization and photography. All imaging was performed on a Zeiss SteREO Discovery.V8 fluorescent microscope equipped with a Zeiss AxioCam MRc CCD camera.

Results

Identification of zebrafish *wnk1* and cloning of full-length *wnk1* cDNA

To identify the zebrafish *wnk1* orthologue, the human WNK1 protein sequence was used to search the translated zebrafish RefSeq RNA database using tBLASTn. Four sequences, XM_684564.5 (*wnk1*), XM_002666846.2 (*wnk1*), XM_003201205.1 (*wnk3*-like), and XM_680072.5 (*wnk4*-like), were found to be homologous to human WNK1.

We designed primers based on the first two homologs and cloned *wnk1* from zebrafish using RT-PCR. The zebrafish *wnk1a* cDNA is 4794 bp long, which is slightly different from the previously reported NCBI GenBank sequence XM_678215.3 and very similar to XM_002666846.2. The zebrafish *wnk1b* cDNA is 5730 bp long and similar to XM_684564.5 with large internal deletions.

The translated amino acid sequences of the four zebrafish *wnks* were compared with the human WNK1 protein sequence (Fig. 1A). As in human WNK1, a glycine in the glycine string of the MAPK motif is replaced by lysine in all four Wnk1 homologs in zebrafish. Additionally, all four zebrafish Wnk proteins contain an auto-inhibitory domain and a serine residue that is susceptible to auto-phosphorylation (Fig. 1A).

Among the four mammalian WNK family members, only WNK1 has an Akt phosphorylation site and the four RFXV (arginine-phenylalanine-any amino acid-valine) motifs required for binding to oxidative stress responsive 1 (OSR1) and STE20/SPS1-related proline-alanine-rich protein kinase (SPAK). Akt can phosphorylate WNK1, and OSR1 and SPAK are endogenous substrates for WNK1. Of the four zebrafish Wnks, only Wnk1a and Wnk1b have the Akt phosphorylation site and four OSR1/SPAK binding motifs (Fig. 1A). Based on these unique signatures, we confirmed that zebrafish *wnk1a* and *wnk1b* are mammalian *WNK1* homologs.

The WNK1 amino acid sequences from rat, mouse, human and zebrafish were also compared (Fig. 1B). In all examined species, the Wnk1 protein exhibited strong similarity in the AKT phosphorylation site, the catalytic domain, the autophosphorylation domain, the autoinhibitory domain and four OSR/SPAK binding domains. Previous work on Wnk1 has identified important residues for each of the domains [10]; these residues are also conserved between species. The rat Wnk1(1–449) truncation has been proven to be constitutively active using an *in vitro* kinase assay [10].

Spatial and temporal expression of *wnk1* in zebrafish development

To understand the role of *wnk1* in embryogenesis, we examined the temporal expression profile of *wnk1* by quantitative *reverse transcription polymerase chain reaction* (q-RT-PCR) (Fig. 2A). *wnk1a* and *wnk1b* mRNAs are maternally deposited, and zygotic expression of both begins as early as 10 hpf (hours post fertilization) and remains high at all stages examined. The expression of *flk1/vegfr2* begins as early as the 5 to 9 somite stage (12 to 15 hpf) in the intermediate cell mass of the mesoderm [40] and the 14 to 19 somite stage (16 to 19 hpf) in the head and vessel endothelial cells [41]. Additional studies have reported that *flk1/vegfr2* is expressed in the intersegmental vessels at 24 hpf [42] when the single circulatory loop in zebrafish is established [43,44]. Overall, the temporal expression of *wnk1* is consistent with its role in angiogenesis. We did not detect significant expression of *wnk3* or *wnk4* in the zebrafish embryo prior to 48 hpf (data not shown).

q-RT-PCR was performed using cDNA from whole embryos, including non-vascular tissues. We next examined *wnk1a* and *wnk1b* expression in blood vessels by whole-mount *in situ* hybridization. At 3 hpf, maternal *wnk1a* and *wnk1b* mRNA are ubiquitously expressed in embryos (Fig. S2-A1, B1). At 6 and 8 hpf, expression of both *wnk1a* and *wnk1b* transcripts is decreased (Fig. S2-A2, A3, B2, B3). At 10 and 12 hpf, zygotic *wnk1a* and *wnk1b* are expressed ubiquitously (Fig. S2-A4, A5, B4, B5). At 18

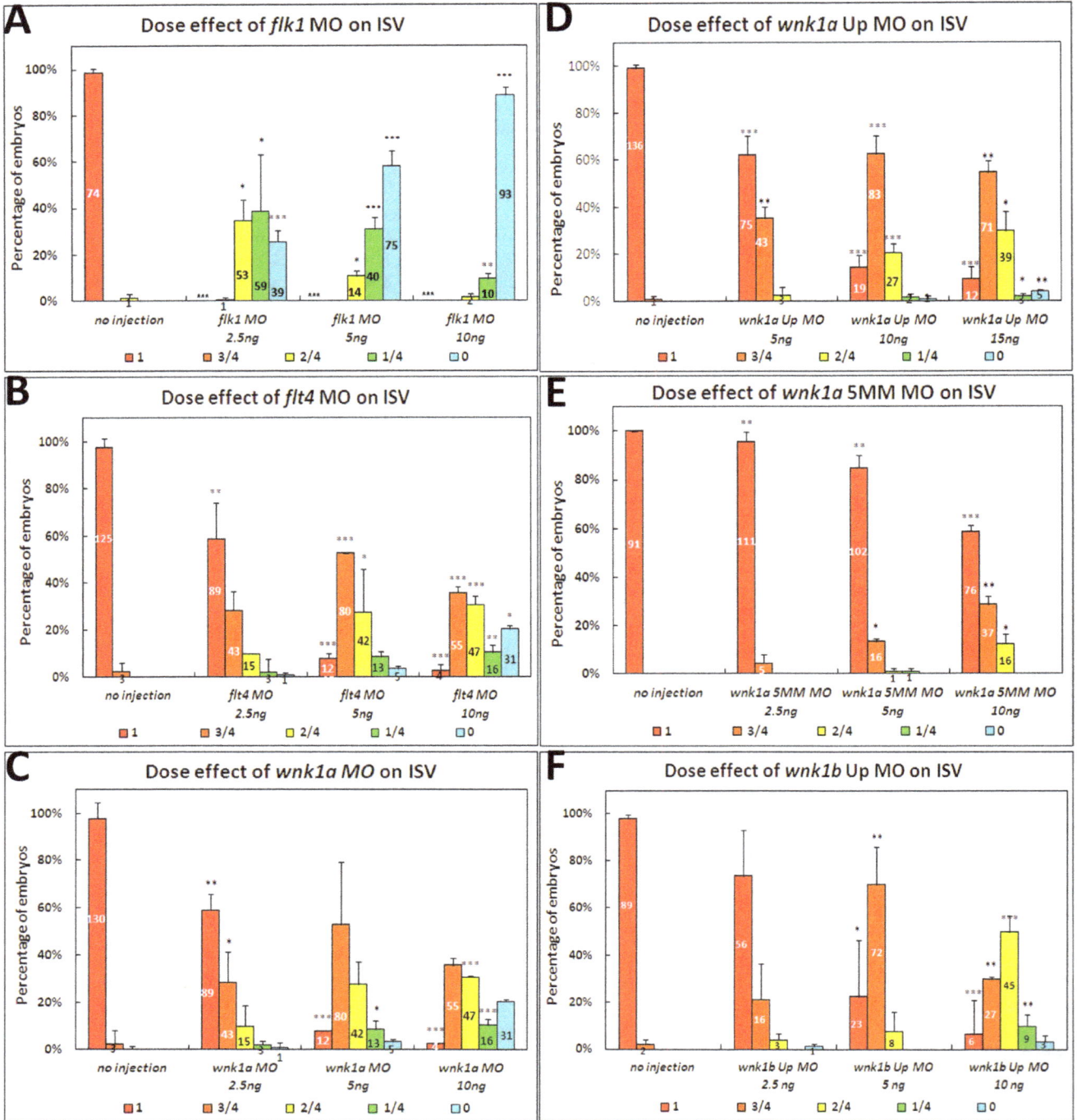

Figure 3. Statistical analysis of the length of intersegmental vessels in *flk1*, *flt4*, *wnk1a*, *wnk1a* 5MM, *wnk1a* upstream and *wnk1b* upstream morpholino-injected embryos. The effects of (A) *flk1* MO, (B) *flt4* MO, (C) *wnk1a* MO, (D) *wnk1a* 5 base mismatch MO, (E) *wnk1a* upstream MO, and (F) *wnk1b* upstream MO on the length of intersegmental vessels. Morpholino injection has a dose-dependent effect on intersegmental vessel formation and growth. All experiments were performed at least three times, and the average ISV length was calculated along with the standard deviation, which is labeled on each bar. Red indicates that the ISVs grew to full length, orange indicates that the ISVs were 75% of the normal length, yellow indicates 50%, green indicates 25%, and light blue indicates that no ISVs were observed in the embryos. The differences between treatments were assessed using a two-tailed Student's *t*-test. Significant differences between the morphants and controls are indicated (∗, $P<0.05$; ∗∗, $P<0.01$; and ∗∗∗, $P<0.001$).

hpf, *wnk1a* is strongly expressed in head and somite tissues (Fig. S2-A6), whereas *wnk1b* is also expressed in the notochord (Fig. S2-B6). Similarly, from 24 to 48 hpf, *wnk1a* is detected in the head,

neural tube, somite, and PCV (Fig. S2-A7∼A12), whereas *wnk1b* is detected in all those tissues plus the notochord. Similar to *wnk1a*, *wnk1b* is expressed in the PCV after 33 hpf (Fig. S2-

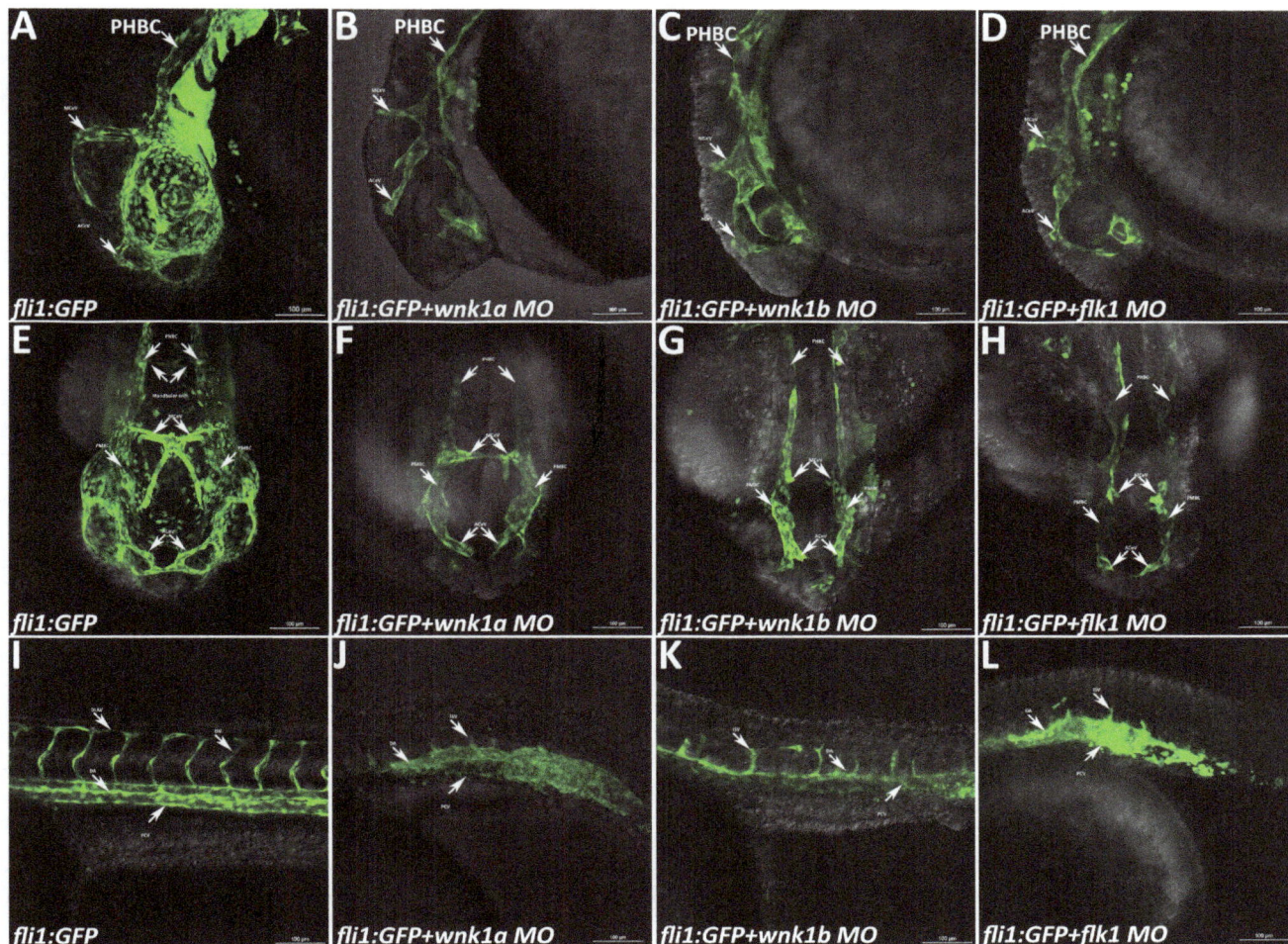

Figure 4. Phenotype of *Tg(fli1:GFP)* embryos injected with various morpholinos and imaged with a confocal microscope. (A–D) Lateral views of the heads of uninjected control embryos and *wnk1a*, *wnk1b* and *flk1* morphants at 33 hpf. (E–H) Frontal views of the heads of uninjected control embryos and *wnk1a*, *wnk1b* and *flk1* morphants at 33 hpf. (I–L) Lateral views of the trunk in uninjected control embryos and *wnk1a*, *wnk1b* and *flk1* morphants at 33 hpf. Important vessels are indicated with arrows and labeled, with the full name given in the text. Scale bar: 100 μm.

B7~B12). We used *flt4*, which is known to be expressed in the posterior cardinal vein (PCV), as a marker and found that both *wnk1a* and *wnk1b* are expressed in the PCV from 24 to 48 hpf (Fig. 2A1~A3, B1~B3 and C1~C3).

To confirm the localization of *wnk1a* and *wnk1b* in the PCV of zebrafish embryos, double *in situ* hybridization with antisense *wnk1a* or *wnklb* riboprobes and a *flt4* riboprobe was performed. The *flt4* transcript was detected with an AP-conjugated anti-DIG antibody and visualized with AP-Fast Red (Fig. 2A4) while *wnk1a* and *wnk1b* were detected with an AP-conjugated anti-fluorescein antibody. Our data showed that *wnk1a* and *wnk1b* colocalized with *flt4* in the PCV. We also observed *wnk1a* and *wnk1b* expression in the notochord (Fig. 2B4, C4). Embryos hybridized with the sense probes for *wnk1a* and *wnk1b* have no staining, indicating that the staining observed with the antisense probe is specific (Fig. S2-A13 and B13). Thus, colocalization studies using double *in situ* hybridization to detect both *wnk1a* or *wnk1b* and the PCV marker *flt4* in the same embryo indicate that *wnk1a* and *wnk1b* are expressed in vascular structures specific to the PCV.

We also examined sections of embryos following whole-mount *in situ* hybridization for *flt4*, *wnk1a* or *wnk1b*. We found *flt4* expression in the PCV whereas *wnk1a* and *wnk1b* expression was

observed in the PCV, the neural tube (NT) and the notochord (NC) (Fig. 2A5, B5 and C5). All of these results suggest that *wnk1a* and *wnk1b* are indeed expressed in the vascular structures of the PCV.

Quantitative analysis of the effect of *wnk1* knockdown on angiogenesis

To investigate the functional role of *wnk1* in zebrafish embryos, we used the *Tg(fli1:EGFP)* strain, which allows immediate and direct *in situ* monitoring of vessel formation. Translation of endogenous *wnk1* was suppressed in *Tg(fli1:EGFP)* by targeting *wnk1a* and *wnk1b* with specific antisense morpholino oligonucleotides (MOs). Morpholino specificity was verified by testing their ability to suppress the expression of a fusion protein that contained the targeted *wnk1* sequence (Fig. S1). The primer and nucleotide sequence for the *wnk1a-GFP* and *wnk1b-GFP* constructs are provided in the supporting data (Data S1). Figure S1 shows the target sites for the MOs, the number of injected embryos, and the quantification of GFP expression in the morphants. Morpholinos that target the 5'UTRs of *wnk1a* and *wnk1b* also efficiently inhibit the expression of the corresponding GFP fusion construct (Fig. S1-

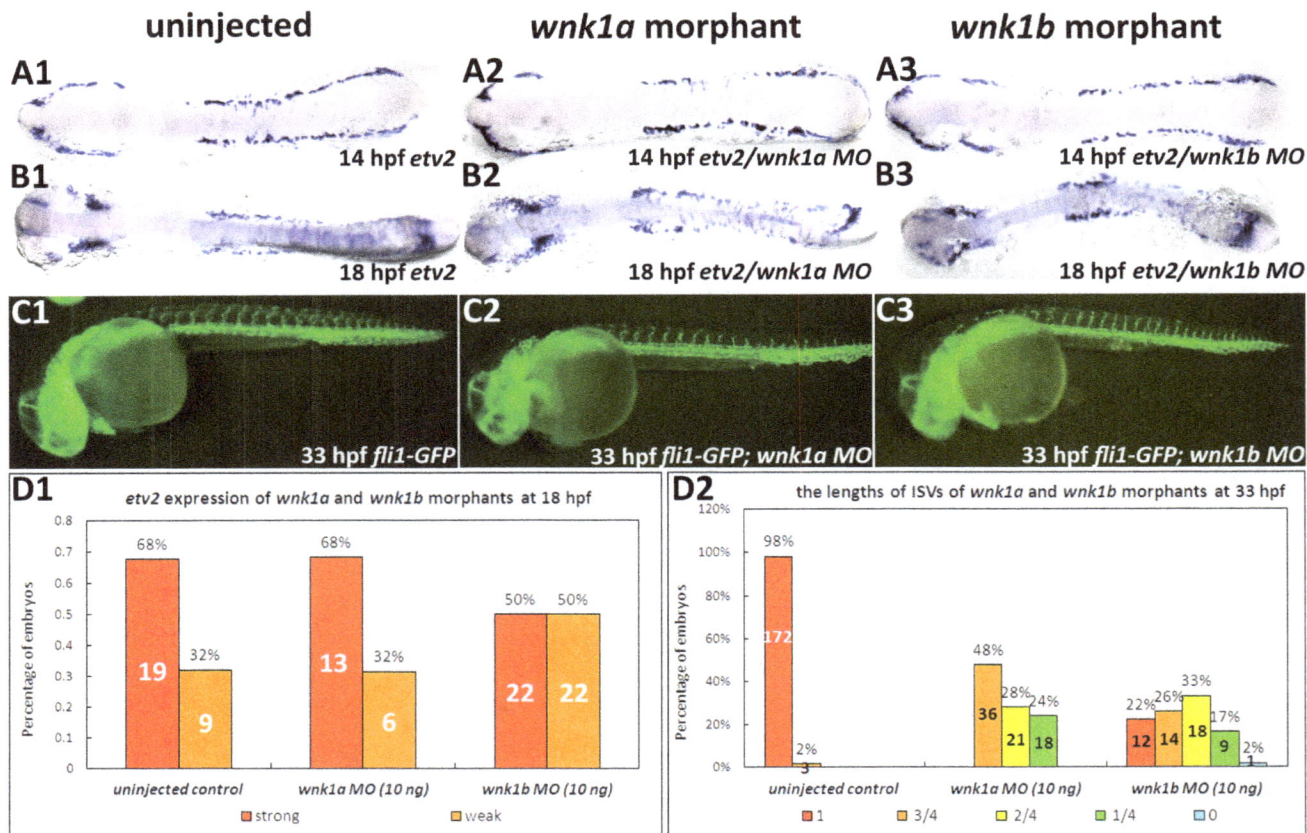

Figure 5. Effect of *wnk1a* or *wnk1b* knockdown on vasculogenesis and angiogenesis in *Tg(fli1:GFP)* embryos. (A, B) Whole mount *in situ* hybridization for *etv2* at 14 and 18 hpf in uninjected control embryos (A1, B1), *wnk1a* morphants (A2, B2), and *wnk1b* morphants (A3, B3). Flat mounts of de-yolked embryos were prepared. (C) GFP fluorescence was used to assay ISV formation in uninjected control embryos (C1), *wnk1a* morphants (C2), and *wnk1b* morphants (C3) at 33 hpf. (D1) *etv2* expression in uninjected control, *wnk1a* and *wnk1b* morphants as a percentage of embryos exhibit strong or expression, (D2) ISV length in *wnk1a* and *wnk1b* morphants.

A4, B4). In contrast, the control MO does not suppress the expression of the GFP fusion protein (Fig. S1-A5, B5). Furthermore, *wnk1b* Up MOs do not inhibit *wnk1a-GFP* (Fig. S1-A6) and *wnk1a* MOs do not suppress *wnk1b-GFP* (Fig. S1-B6, B7). Our results demonstrate that *wnk1a* MOs specifically inhibit *wnk1a-GFP* expression and *wnk1b* MOs specifically inhibit *wnk1b-GFP* expression.

To determine the role that *wnk1* plays in angiogenesis, we designed and tested MOs against *wnk1a*, *wnk1b* and other genes required for angiogenesis. ISVs sprout and elongate dorsally from the DA and the PCV and connect to the DLAV between 29 and 36 hpf [45]. We analyzed embryos at 33 hpf, when the ISVs are forming. Because ISV development begins in the anterior trunk and proceeds posteriorly, we calculated the lengths of the ISVs from the middle of the yolk to the yolk extension. ISVs were observed in age-matched embryos and categorized as having extended over 100%, 75%, 50%, 25% or 0% of the distance from the DA (or PCV) to the DLAV (Fig. S3-A). Due to variations in the effects of morpholino injection from embryo to embryo, we examined many embryos in each group. The phenotype and motility of the embryos were classified as described in Fig. S3-B. The number of embryos analyzed (n) and the means, standard deviation and significance from three independent experiments are indicated in the figures.

In mice, VEGFR2 (KDR/FLK1) is the primary VEGFA receptor in the developing endothelial lineage and it is essential for endothelial differentiation during embryonic vasculogenesis as well as angiogenesis [46]. VEGFR2 also plays important roles in physiological as well as pathological postnatal angiogenesis [47]. In zebrafish, VEGFR2 is essential for angiogenesis only, and knockdown of *vegfr2/flk1* using morpholinos causes angiogenesis defects as shown by the shortening of ISVs (Fig. 3A). The inhibition of ISVs by *flk1* MO knockdown is dose-dependent.

VEGFR3 (Flt4) is predominantly expressed in embryonic blood endothelium, lymphatic endothelial cells, monocytes and macrophages [48]. VEGFR3 is important in lymphangiogenesis, but recent studies have shown that VEGFR3 also functions during sprouting angiogenesis [49]. In mouse, blocking VEGFR3 suppresses angiogenic sprouting and reduces the retina vessel density [50]. We found that *flt4* MOs inhibit the formation of ISVs, although to a lesser extent than *flk1* MOs (Fig. 3B).

Compared with *vegfr2* and *vegfr3* morphants, *wnk1a* morphants display a similar inhibition of ISV growth (Fig. 3C), suggesting that *wnk1a* is involved in angiogenesis in the vessel during sprouting or elongation. A 5-base mismatch (5MM) control morpholino has no inhibitory activity, with ISV lengths in the morphants comparable to those in wild-type embryos (Fig. 3D). A second morpholino targeted to the 5′-untranslated region of *wnk1a* causes similar inhibition (Fig. 3E). We also designed a

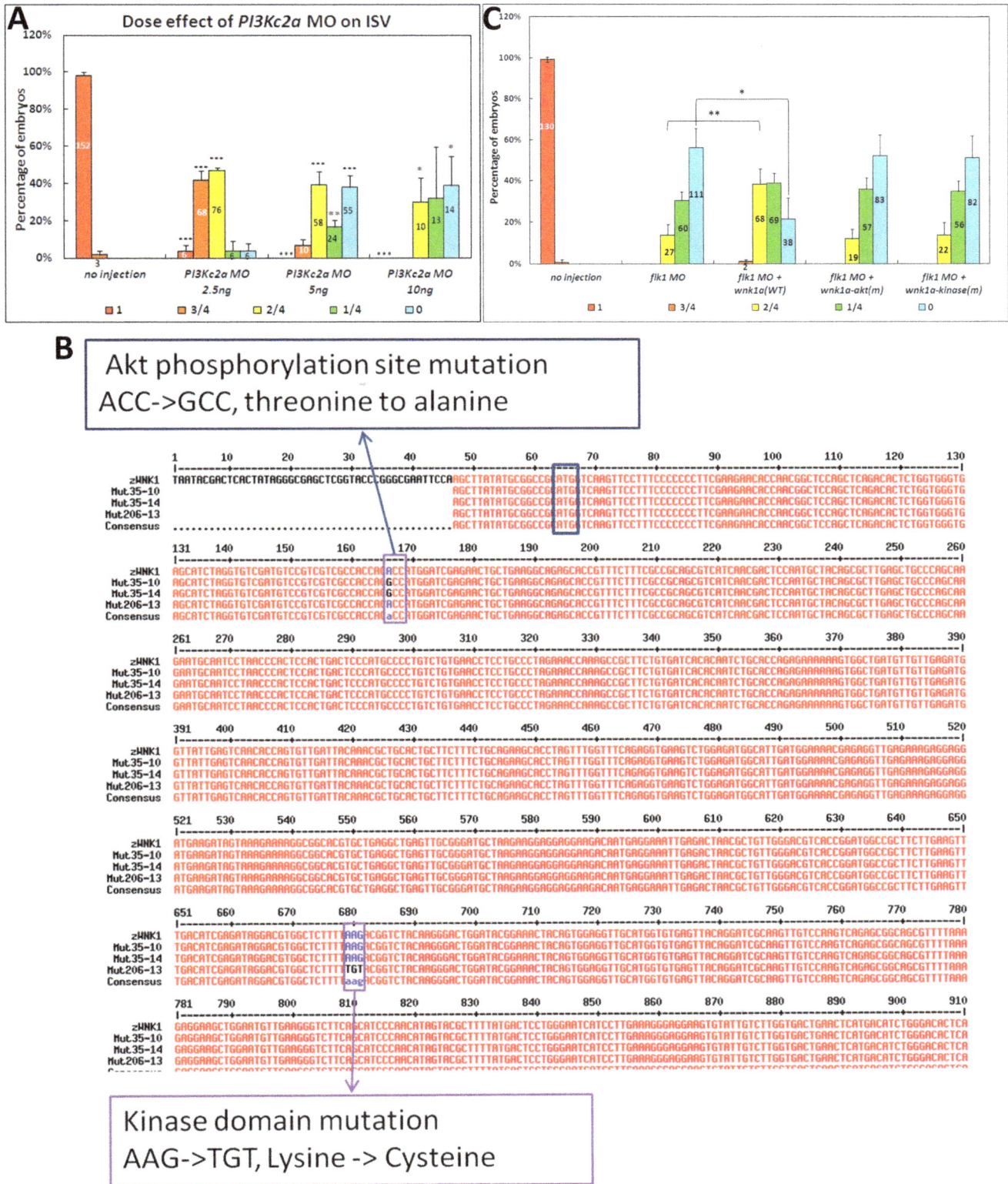

Figure 6. Effect of knockdown of the PI3K ortholog on ISVs and the rescue effects of wild-type wnk1a, wnk1a containing an Akt phosphorylation site mutation and kinase-deficient wnk1a on flk1 morphants. (A) The effects of pi3kc2α MO on the length of intersegmental vessels. (B) Two Thr35 mutations and one Lys206 mutation were generated using site-directed mutagenesis. The sequence of wild-type wnk1a aligned with Thr35 and Lys206 mutants, which are Akt phosphorylation site and kinase domain mutants, respectively. (C) Co-injection of wnk1a mRNA rescues flk1 morphants. Quantitative analysis of the length of the ISVs in flk1 morphants co-injected with various wnk1a mRNAs. Experiments were performed at least three times, and the number of embryos analyzed is shown in the bar graph. Red indicates that the ISVs grew to full length, orange indicates that the ISVs were 75% of the normal length, yellow indicates 50%, green indicates 25%, and light blue indicates no ISVs

were observed in the embryos. The differences between treatments were assessed using a two-tailed Student's t-test. Significant differences between the morphants and controls are indicated (*, $P<0.05$; **, $P<0.01$; and ***, $P<0.001$).

translation-inhibiting MO and an upstream MO for *wnk1b* knockdown and found that the *wnk1b* upstream MO significantly inhibits ISV growth (Fig. 3F).

Zebrafish *wnk1* knockdown results in defective angiogenesis but not vasculogenesis

Representative age/somite matched images of uninjected *Tg(fli1:EGFP)* embryos as well as *wnk1a*, *wnk1b*, and *flk1* morphants are shown in Figure 4. Since *wnk1a* and *wnk1b* are expressed strongly in the head as well as the trunk, we examined the embryos from a lateral head view (Fig. 4A–D), a frontal head view (Fig. 4E–H), and a lateral trunk view (Fig. 4I–L). Knockdown of either *wnk1a* or *wnk1b* causes significant defects in angiogenesis in both the head and trunk vessels. The vessel formation defects caused by knockdown of *wnk1a* or *wnk1b* in zebrafish are similar

to the defects observed in *Wnk1* mutant mice, which include atresic branches of the internal carotid artery and primary head veins and disorganization of the intersomitic vessels and their branches [22]. Knockdown of either *wnk1a* or *wnk1b* in zebrafish inhibits the density and formation of vessels in the head region and body (Fig. 4). Notably, only the formation of small vessels in the head, such as the caudal division of the internal carotid artery (CaDI), the primitive mesencephalic artery (PMsA) and the partial optic artery (OA), are inhibited. Major vessel structures, such as the vessels of the mandibular arch, the anterior (rostral) cerebral vein (ACeV), the cranial division of the internal carotid artery (CrDI), the middle cerebral vein (MCeV), the primordial hindbrain channel (PHBC), the primitive internal carotid artery (PICA), and the primordial midbrain channel (PMBC), are not affected by *wnk1a* MO (Fig. 4B, F, J) or *wnk1b* MO (Fig. 4C, G,

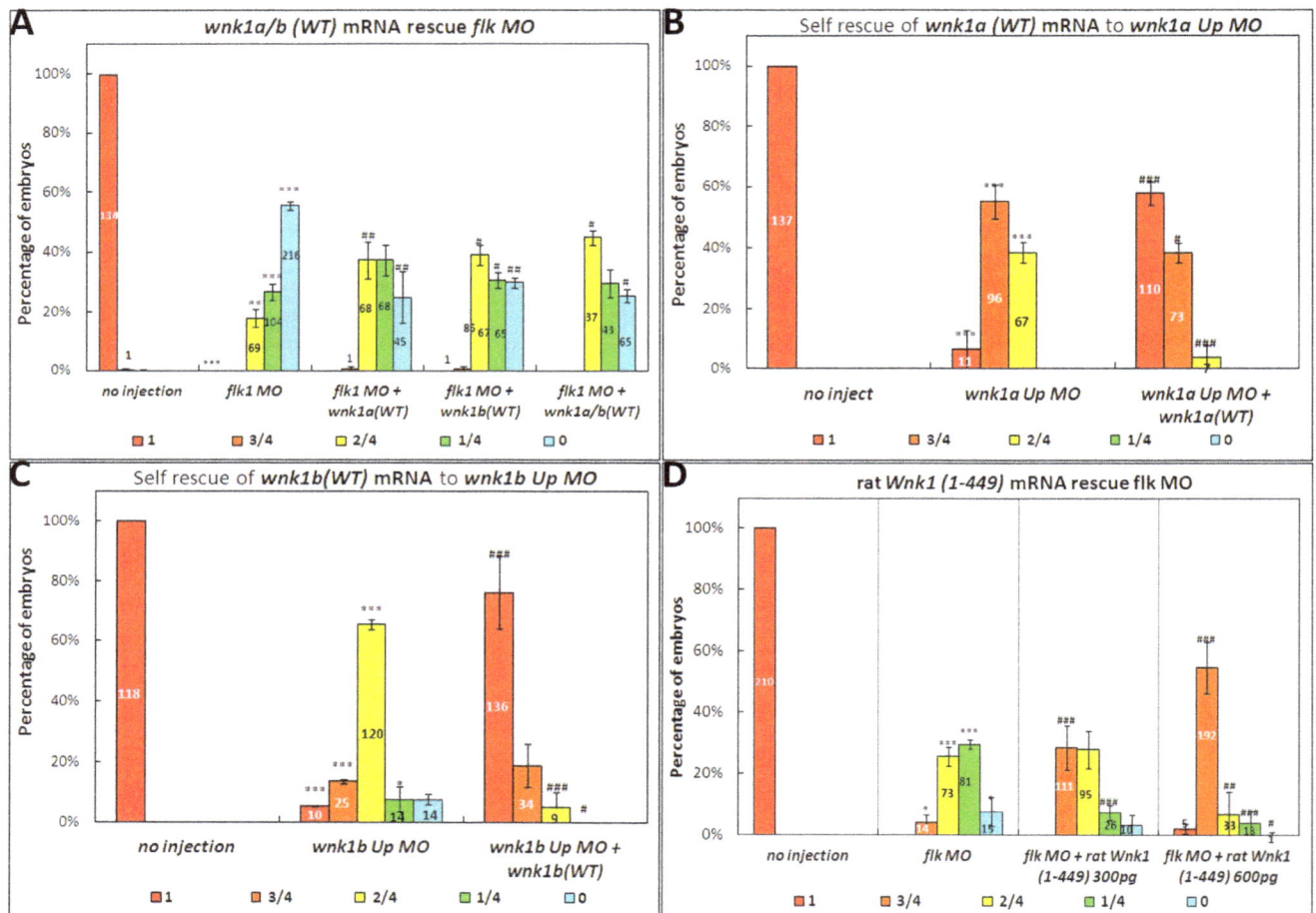

Figure 7. Effect of wild-type *wnk1a* and *wnk1b* mRNA injection on *flk1*, *wnk1a* and *wnk1b* morphants. (A) Co-injection of *wnk1a*, *wnk1b* or both *wnk1a* and *wnk1b* mRNA rescues *flk1* morphants. (B) Co-injection of *wnk1a* mRNA rescues the ISV defect caused by the *wnk1a* upstream MO. (C) Co-injection of *wnk1b* mRNA rescues the ISV defect caused by the *wnk1b* upstream MO. (D) Injection of rat *Wnk1(1–449)* rescues *flk1* morphants. Experiments were performed at least three times, and the number of embryos analyzed is shown in the bar graph. Red indicates that the ISVs grew to full length, orange indicates that the ISVs were 75% of the normal length, yellow indicates 50%, green indicates 25%, and light blue indicates no ISVs were observed in the embryos. The differences between treatments were assessed using a two-tailed Student's t-test. Significant differences between the morphants and controls are indicated (*, $P<0.05$; **, $P<0.01$; and ***, $P<0.001$); significant differences between co-injection of RNA with morpholino and morpholino alone are also indicated (#, $P<0.05$; ##, $P<0.01$; and ###, $P<0.001$).

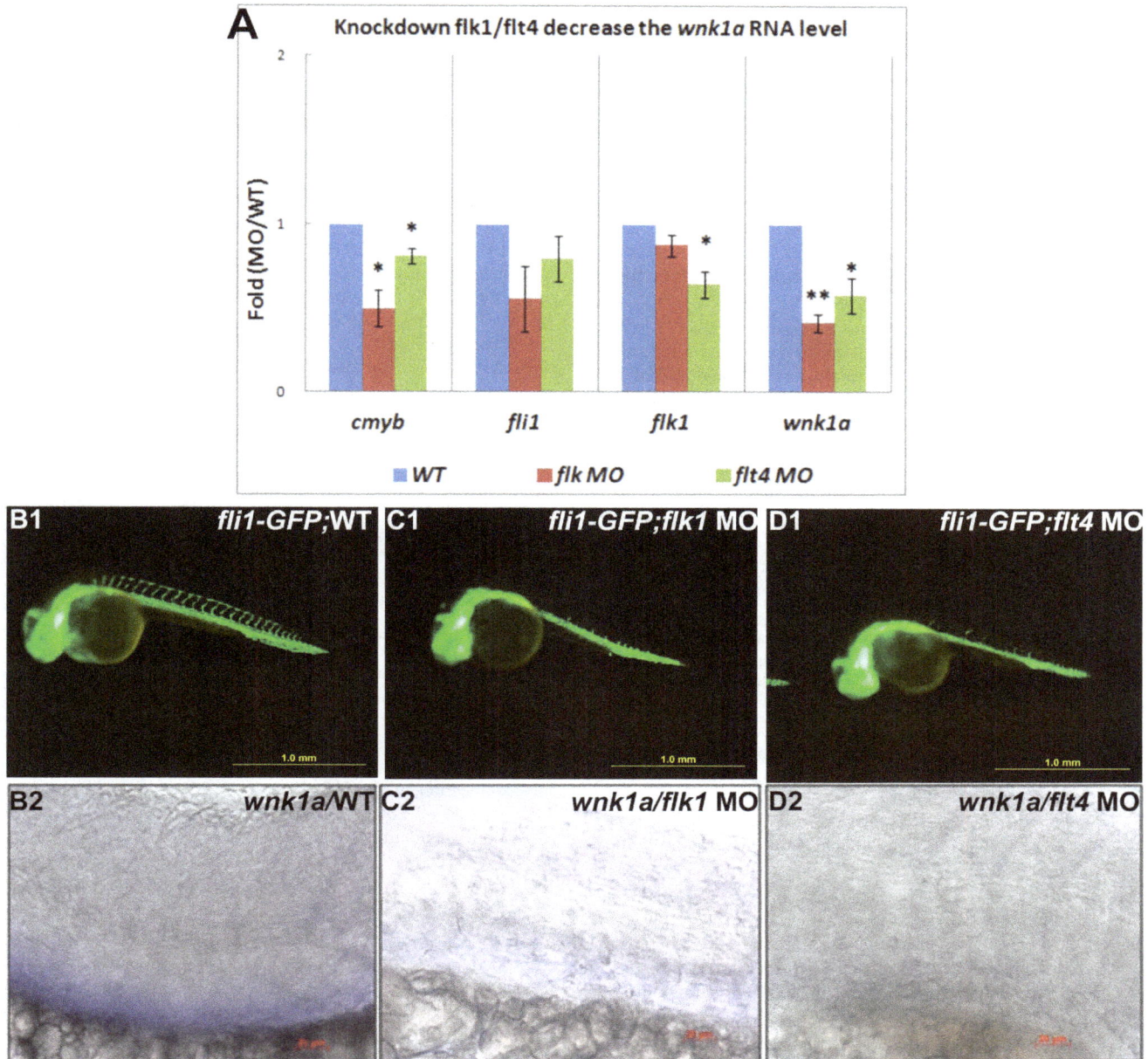

Figure 8. Injections of *flk1* MO and *flt4* MO decrease *wnk1* mRNA expression. (A) Relative fold-change comparisons between *flk1* and *flt4* morphants and uninjected controls. Comparison of mRNA expression levels at 33 hpf for important transcription factors, receptors, and *wnk1*. Blue, red, and green bars denote mRNA expression in wild-type embryos, *flk1* morphants and *flt4* morphants, respectively. The x-axis indicates the expressed genes, and the y-axis shows the fold differences between the morphants and the control. The differences between treatments were assessed using a two-tailed Student's *t*-test. Significant differences between the morphants and the controls are indicated (*, $P<0.05$ and**, $P<0.01$). (B1, C1, D1) The ISVs are affected in morphants compared with wild-type embryos. (B2, C2 and D2) The expression of *wnk1a* is reduced in the PCV in *flk1* and *flt4* morphants. *wnk1a* mRNA was detected with *in situ* hybridization in wild-type embryos (B2), *flk1* morphants (C2) and *flt4* morphants (D2).

K); this result is similar to that seen in *flk1* morphants (Fig. 4D, H, L).

In the trunk, we found that growth of the intersegmental vessels (ISVs) is inhibited in *wnk1* morphants and that formation of the dorsal longitudinal anastomotic vessel (DLAV) is also affected. However, blood vessels formed by the vasculogenesis process, including the dorsal aorta (DA), the caudal artery (CA), the caudal vein (CV) and the posterior cardinal vein (PCV), are not affected (Fig. 4I–L). The phenotype of zebrafish *wnk1* morphants is consistent with that of *wnk1* knockout mice, with effects on angiogenesis but not vasculogenesis [22].

Expression of the vasculogenesis marker *etv2* is unaffected in *wnk1* morphants

To further verify that *wnk1* functions in angiogenesis rather than vasculogenesis, we examined the expression of the vasculogenesis marker *etv2* in somite matched control, *wnk1a and wnk1b* morphants. The embryonic expression of *etv2* is restricted to the earliest precursors of vascular endothelial cells. Morpholino knockdown of *etv2* results in the absence of vasculogenesis [51]. *wnk1a* and *wnk1b* morpholinos were injected into *fli1:GFP* embryos, and the effect on ISVs was assayed. We found that there is no difference in *etv2* expression between the *wnk1a* or *wnk1b* morphants and control embryos at 14 hpf (Fig. 5A1– A3) and 18 hpf (Fig. 5B1– B3), whereas the development of ISVs is significantly affected (Fig. 5C1–C3). The quantified results for *etv2* expression at 18 hpf and the length of ISVs at 33 hpf were shown in Figure 5D1 and D2 respectively.

Knockdown of endothelial-specific *pi3kc2α* inhibits the growth of intersegmental vessels

Previous studies have demonstrated that VEGF/VEGFR signaling regulates endothelial cell survival and growth through the activation of the PI3K/Akt pathway, and endothelial cell permeability through the activation of endothelial NO synthase (eNOS) [52,53,54]. The WNK1 protein contains an Akt phosphorylation motif; therefore, we suspect that Wnk1 participates in angiogenesis after being phosphorylated and activated by Akt kinase downstream of Vegf/Vegfr signaling.

To further analyze whether Wnk1 acts through the Vegf/Vegfr2-PI3K/Akt pathway in endothelial cell activation, we wanted to inhibit PI3K, which falls between Vegfr2 and Wnk1 in the proposed signaling cascade, to check the integrity of this pathway in angiogenesis. To date, there are eight known PI3K isoforms with varying structural features and lipid substrate preferences; they are divided into three classes (class I, class II and class III), and these isoforms are involved in metabolic control, immunity, angiogenesis and cardiovascular homeostasis [55]. From the literature, we know that endothelial cells only express PI3KC2α [56]. From an NCBI GenBank search, we found that the zebrafish gene phosphoinositide-3-kinase, class 2, alpha polypeptide (*pik3c2a*) is similar to the human *PI3KC2α* homologs. The *pi3kc2α* mRNA expression pattern from ZFIN (Bernard Thisse's group, Expression of the zebrafish genome during embryogenesis. ZFIN Direct Data Submission (http://zfin.org/cgi-bin/webdriver?MIval = aa-ZDB_home.apg)) showed that *pi3kc2α* is expressed in axial vasculature at 24 hpf (Fig. S4), providing support for a role for *pi3kc2α* in angiogenesis.

We then designed a MO to knockdown *pik3c2a*. The *pi3kc2α* morphant exhibits growth inhibition in the ISVs similar to that observed in the *vegfr2, wnk1a* and *wnk1b* morphants (Fig. 6A), suggesting that Pi3kc2α and Wnk1 may be part of the same pathway. We hypothesized that upon Vegf binding to Vegfr, Pi3kc2α is activated, which phosphorylates and activates Wnk1, which in turn activates downstream targets. Additionally, we found that injection of 10 ng of *pi3kc2α* MO into embryos significantly increases mortality relative to controls, suggesting that Pi3kc2α might participate in other physiological functions, possibly through other signaling pathways. The number of embryos examined and the phenotypic and mortality analyses of *pi3kc2a* morphants versus other morphants are provided in Fig. S5.

Partial Rescue of the angiogenesis defect in *vegfr2* morphants by wild-type, but not Akt-phosphorylation site mutant or kinase-dead mutant, *wnk1a* mRNA

Based on the results presented in Figure 3 and 6A, we hypothesized that the binding of Vegf to Vegfr2 activates Wnk1a through phosphorylation by the PI3K-Akt kinase cascade. To test this theory, we used site-directed mutagenesis to generate two mutants of Wnk1a, one missing the Akt phosphorylation site and the other lacking kinase activity (Fig. 6B). We transcribed mRNA for wild-type *wnk1a* and the two mutants *in vitro* and then co-injected these with the *vegfr2* MO for rescue experiments.

Figure 6C illustrates the result of the rescue experiments. Co-injection of *vegfr2* MO with wild-type *wnk1a* RNA, but not *wnk1a-akt(m)* or *wnk1a-kinase(m)*, leads to a statistically significant increase in angiogenesis compared with vegfr2 MO injection alone. Representative images of rescued morphants are provided in Figure S6. Notably, the rescue is incomplete: ISVs in the *vegfr2* morphants rescued with *wnk1a* RNA are only half as long as in wildtype. It is possible that some Vegfr2 activity remains in morphant embryos, and hence wild-type Wnk1 can be activated and subsequently phosphorylate downstream targets to achieve rescue. Therefore, the rescue is partially due to the morpholino knockdown the Vegfr2.

Because there are two Wnk1 isoforms in zebrafish, we wondered if the ISVs could be completely rescued by providing both isoforms. Co-injection of both *wnk1a* and *wnk1b* mRNA with *flk1* MO, however, is comparable to co-injection with *wnk1a* or *wnk1b* RNA alone (Fig. 7A). Wild-type *wnk1a* and *wnk1b* mRNA fully rescue the angiogenesis defects in *wnk1a* and *wnk1b* morphants, respectively (Fig. 7B and 7C). Thus, the partial rescue is not due to poor quality or low abundance of the mRNA.

Because no biochemical assays have been performed to confirm the expected effects of truncation on zebrafish *wnk1a* and *wnk1b*, we used a constitutively active rat Wnk1 truncation, for which biochemical data are available, in rescue assays. Previous biochemical studies on rat Wnk1 have demonstrated that the Wnk1(1–449) truncation is constitutively active due to the lack of an autoinhibitory domain [10]. The truncated form of Wnk1 was expected to be better able to rescue *flk1* morphants than wild-type Wnk1. We obtained rat Wnk1 cDNA from Dr. Cobb's lab, subcloned the Wnk1(1–449) fragment and then generated mRNA for co-injection with *flk1* MOs. We demonstrated that rat Wnk1(1–449) effectively rescues ISV formation in *flk1* morphants in a dose-dependent manner (Fig. 7D).

Knockdown of *flk1* or *flt4* decreases expression of *wnk1* mRNA

Another possible mechanism to explain how VEGF signal transduction affects angiogenesis through *wnk1* involves transcriptional regulation. VEGF signal transduction might also regulate *wnk1* gene expression. The co-localization of *flt4* (vegfr3) and *wnk1* in the PCV strengthens this possibility. Furthermore, we have analyzed *flk1* and *flt4* morphants for *wnk1* expression. q-RT-PCR analysis of *wnk1a* and other endothelial genes demonstrated a significant reduction in *wnk1a* RNA in *flk1* and *flt4* morphants relative to controls (Fig. 8A). Several genes for blood/vessel formation (*cmyb, fli1* and *flk1*) are also down regulated in *flk1* and *flt4* morphants. ISVs are inhibited by *flk1* and *flt4* MO injection (Fig. 8B1, C1 and D1) and expression of *wnk1a* in the PCV is decreased in *flk1* and *flt4* morphants compared with uninjected controls (Fig. 8 B2, C2 and D2).

Discussion

In this study, we found that knockdown of *vegfr2, vegfr3, wnk1* or *pi3kc2a* causes angiogenesis defects. From published works, we also know that Wnk1 can be phosphorylated by Akt kinase, and our zebrafish Wnk1a protein sequence contains an Akt phosphorylation site. Therefore, we propose that Wnk1a is downstream of the Vegfr2/Fkl1-PI3K-Akt signaling pathway in zebrafish. In *wnk1a* mRNA rescue experiments, we found that wild-type *wnk1a*, but not *wnk1a* with an Akt phosphorylation site mutation, partially rescues the angiogenesis defect of *vegfr2* knockdown. The finding that the Akt site mutant fails to rescue the angiogenesis defect of *flk1* morphants supports the hypothesis that binding of Vegf to Vegfr2 activates PI3K and Akt kinase, which then phosphorylate Wnk1 to regulate angiogenesis. In addition, we found that rat Wnk1(1–449), a constitutively active form that lacks the autoinhibitory domain, effectively rescues the *flk1* morphant. One important question arising from these results, though, is why wild-type *wnk1a* RNA rescues *flk1* morphants if the function of Vegfr2/Flk1 pathway is to phosphorylate and activate Wnk1.

To address this issue, we postulated that the Vegfr2 pathway might also regulate the expression of *wnk1a*. We performed real-time q-RT-PCR and *in situ* hybridization to investigate this possibility. Our q-RT-PCR results reveal that knockdown of either *flk1* or *flt4* causes a decrease in the *wnk1a* mRNA level. The reduction in *wnk1a* expression is modest, perhaps because *wnk1a* is broadly expressed in a variety of tissues, including some not affected by the relatively vascular-specific knockdown of *flk1* or *flt4*. The *in situ* hybridization results also suggest that the expression of *wnk1a* in the PCV is decreased in *flk1* and *flt4* morphants. Together, the q-RT-PCR and *in situ* results support the notion that the expression of *wnk1a* is down regulated by knockdown of *flk1* and *flt4*. This downregulation of *wnk1a* would explain why co-injection of wild-type *wnk1a* RNA rescues the angiogenesis defect of *fkl1* morphants. Because morpholino knockdown is incomplete, residual Flk1 protein must remain in *flk1* morphants. It is conceivable that overexpression of Wnk1a proteins (by mRNA injection) can partially overcome decreased phosphorylation of Wnk1a by the Flk1-PI3K-Akt cascade. How Vegfr2/Flk1 regulates *wnk1a* expression remains unknown and awaits future investigation.

Angiogenesis comprises four main steps: selection of sprouting endothelial cells, sprout outgrowth and guidance, sprout fusion, and perfusion/maturation [49]. These processes are regulated by different growth factors, receptors and downstream signal molecules. In the *wnk1a* morphants, we observed that the number of endothelial cells participating in the ISVs and the intervals between ISVs are similar to those in wild-type embryos. Knockdown of *wnk1* suppresses the growth of the ISV toward the DLAV. We also found that ISVs become straighter and finer in embryos overexpressing *wnk1a* mRNA than in wild-type embryos (Fig. S5). Therefore, we speculate that Wnk1a may be involved in sprout outgrowth, migration and elongation of the selected tip cells, rather than in the selection of sprouting endothelial cells or lateral inhibition among endothelial cells. We speculate that Wnk1a has no interaction with the Notch signaling pathway, which is involved in lateral inhibition.

The expression pattern of *WNK1* is ubiquitous in human, mouse and zebrafish. In a previous study [22], it was found that *Wnk1* mRNA is expressed in endothelial tissue such as the heart, the brachial arches, the dorsal aorta, pericytes and other manifestations of the cardiovascular system. *Wnk1* is also expressed in the neural tube and the gut. From our *in situ* data, we found the zebrafish *wnk1* is expressed in the neural tube, notochord, and the vascular structure-posterior cardinal vein (PCV). In *Wnk1*-null mice, *Wnk1* mRNA was absent in all these tissues. Using a Cre recombinase system, endothelial-specific Wnk1 expression rescues angiogenesis in *Wnk1*-null mice. This result suggests that *Wnk1* expression in tissues beyond the vascular endothelial cells is not necessary for angiogenesis. Although we have not shown that endothelial-specific *wnk1* can rescue angiogenesis in zebrafish *wnk1* null mutants, we believe the function of *wnk1* in angiogenesis is highly conserved among

vertebrates. Only endothelial-specific expression of *wnk1* can rescue angiogenesis in the *Wnk1*$^{-/-}$ background [22].

VEGF is an important factor in promoting angiogenesis. Compared with normal tissues, most tumors grow faster *in vivo* and often require additional blood to supply the necessary nutrients and oxygen; thus, many tumors secrete various angiogenic factors and induce vascular endothelial cells to promote proliferation and tumor expansion. In the healthy body, the role of VEGF is limited mainly to wound healing and menstruation. However, in the process of tumor growth and metastasis, VEGF and downstream genes play an indispensable role. Therefore, VEGF therapies that inhibit the formation of new blood vessels have become very important in cancer treatment. In future work, we will xenotransplant cancer cells into *Tg(fli1:EGFP)* zebrafish to observe angiogenesis occurring near the cancer cells in live animals. Using drugs that inhibit VEGF as well as the *wnk1* morpholino antisense oligonucleotides, we will test the feasibility of using anti-*wnk1* MOs to inhibit angiogenesis, tumor growth and metastasis.

Supporting Information

Figure S1   Morpholino specificity revealed by co-injections of *wnk1a-GFP* or *wnk1b-GFP* with various morpholinos. (A1, B1) Schematic of *wnk1a-GFP* and *wnk1b-GFP* constructs and the location of morpholino target sites. (A2, B2) Injection of *wnk1a-GFP* or *wnk1b-GFP* only. Co-injection of *wnk1a-GFP* or *wnk1b-GFP* with (A3, B3) *wnk1a* or *wnk1b* MOs targeted to the ATG, (A4, B4) *wnk1a* or *wnk1b* MOs that bind upstream of the translation start site, (A5, B5) scrambled control MOs, (B6) MOs targeted to the other isoform's ATG, and (A6, A7) MOs targeted to the 5′ untranslated region of the other isoform.

Figure S2   Temporal expression patterns of *wnk1a* and *wnk1b*. Whole mount *in situ* hybridization to detect *wnk1a* (A1~A12) and *wnk1b* (B1~B12) mRNA expression was performed at the indicated time points. Whole mount *in situ* hybridization of sense probes for *wnk1a* (A13) and *wnk1b* (B13) at 48 hpf showed no signal. All pictures are lateral views. Scale bar: 100 μm.

Figure S3   Measurement of the length of ISVs and representative images of phenotypic classification. (A1) Illustration of the region used to measure the ISVs. (A2~A6) ISVs categorized as having extended over 100%, 75%, 50%, 25% or 0% of the distance from the DA (or PCV) to the DLAV at 33 hpf. (B1~B4) Phenotypes were characterized as normal, class 1, class 2 or class 3 at 24 hpf.

Figure S4   Whole mount *in situ* hybridization for *pi3kc2a* mRNA at the indicated time points. Images were obtained from ZFIN.

Figure S5   Phenotypic classification of 24 hpf *flk1* morphants. *flt4* morphant (A), *pi3kc2a* morphant (B), *wnk1a* morphant (C), *wnk1a* UP morphant (D) and *wnk1a* 5 MM morphant (F). For each morphant, there are two figures. The first figure shows the number of embryos analyzed, and the second figure shows the percentage of morphants displaying a phenotype.

Figure S6   Phenotype of *Tg(fli1:GFP)* embryos injected with various morpholinos and imaged with a florescence

microscope. (A–E) Uninjected control embryos (A), *flk1* morphants (B) and *flk1* morphants co-injected with wnk1a (WT) mRNA (C), *wnk1a*-akt(m) mRNA (D), or *wnk1a*-kinase(m) mRNA (E) at 33 hpf. (F–H) Frontal views of the heads of uninjected control embryos (F), *wnk1b* morphants (G) or *wnk1b* morphants co-injected with *wnk1b* mRNA at 33 hpf. (I and J) *wnk1a* mRNA injected embryo (I) compared to wild-type control (J) at 29 hpf.

Data S1 Detailed information regarding q-RT-PCR primers, *in situ* probe location, morpholino design, and *wnk1*-GFP constructs.

References

1. Baldessari D, Mione M (2008) How to create the vascular tree? (Latest) help from the zebrafish. Pharmacol Ther 118: 206–230.
2. Risau W (1997) Mechanisms of angiogenesis. Nature 386: 671–674.
3. Shibuya M (2008) Vascular endothelial growth factor-dependent and -independent regulation of angiogenesis. BMB Rep 41: 278–286.
4. Jiang ZY, Zhou QL, Holik J, Patel S, Leszyk J, et al. (2005) Identification of WNK1 as a substrate of Akt/protein kinase B and a negative regulator of insulin-stimulated mitogenesis in 3T3-L1 cells. J Biol Chem 280: 21622–21628.
5. Xu B, English JM, Wilsbacher JL, Stippec S, Goldsmith EJ, et al. (2000) WNK1, a novel mammalian serine/threonine protein kinase lacking the catalytic lysine in subdomain II. J Biol Chem 275: 16795–16801.
6. Verissimo F, Jordan P (2001) WNK kinases, a novel protein kinase subfamily in multi-cellular organisms. Oncogene 20: 5562–5569.
7. Xu BE, Stippec S, Lenertz L, Lee BH, Zhang W, et al. (2004) WNK1 activates ERK5 by an MEKK2/3-dependent mechanism. J Biol Chem 279: 7826–7831.
8. Sun X, Gao L, Yu RK, Zeng G (2006) Down-regulation of WNK1 protein kinase in neural progenitor cells suppresses cell proliferation and migration. J Neurochem 99: 1114–1121.
9. Vitari AC, Deak M, Collins BJ, Morrice N, Prescott AR, et al. (2004) WNK1, the kinase mutated in an inherited high-blood-pressure syndrome, is a novel PKB (protein kinase B)/Akt substrate. Biochem J 378: 257–268.
10. Xu BE, Min X, Stippec S, Lee BH, Goldsmith EJ, et al. (2002) Regulation of WNK1 by an autoinhibitory domain and autophosphorylation. J Biol Chem 277: 48456–48462.
11. Wilson FH, Disse-Nicodeme S, Choate KA, Ishikawa K, Nelson-Williams C, et al. (2001) Human hypertension caused by mutations in WNK kinases. Science 293: 1107–1112.
12. Richardson C, Rafiqi FH, Karlsson HK, Moleleki N, Vandewalle A, et al. (2008) Activation of the thiazide-sensitive Na+-Cl− cotransporter by the WNK-regulated kinases SPAK and OSR1. J Cell Sci 121: 675–684.
13. Zagorska A, Pozo-Guisado E, Boudeau J, Vitari AC, Rafiqi FH, et al. (2007) Regulation of activity and localization of the WNK1 protein kinase by hyperosmotic stress. J Cell Biol 176: 89–100.
14. Anselmo AN, Earnest S, Chen W, Juang YC, Kim SC, et al. (2006) WNK1 and OSR1 regulate the Na+, K+, 2Cl- cotransporter in HeLa cells. Proc Natl Acad Sci U S A 103: 10883–10888.
15. Moriguchi T, Urushiyama S, Hisamoto N, Iemura S, Uchida S, et al. (2005) WNK1 regulates phosphorylation of cation-chloride-coupled cotransporters via the STE20-related kinases, SPAK and OSR1. J Biol Chem 280: 42685–42693.
16. Gagnon KB, England R, Delpire E (2006) Characterization of SPAK and OSR1, regulatory kinases of the Na-K-2Cl cotransporter. Mol Cell Biol 26: 689–698.
17. Richardson C, Alessi DR (2008) The regulation of salt transport and blood pressure by the WNK-SPAK/OSR1 signalling pathway. J Cell Sci 121: 3293–3304.
18. Orlov SN, Gossard F, Pausova Z, Akimova OA, Tremblay J, et al. (2010) Decreased NKCC1 activity in erythrocytes from African Americans with hypertension and dyslipidemia. Am J Hypertens 23: 321–326.
19. Flatman PW (2007) Cotransporters, WNKs and hypertension: important leads from the study of monogenetic disorders of blood pressure regulation. Clin Sci (Lond) 112: 203–216.
20. Gamba G (2005) Molecular physiology and pathophysiology of electroneutral cation-chloride cotransporters. Physiol Rev 85: 423–493.
21. Vitari AC, Deak M, Morrice NA, Alessi DR (2005) The WNK1 and WNK4 protein kinases that are mutated in Gordon's hypertension syndrome phosphorylate and activate SPAK and OSR1 protein kinases. Biochem J 391: 17–24.
22. Xie J, Wu T, Xu K, Huang I, Cleaver O, et al. (2009) Endothelial-specific expression of WNK1 kinase is essential for angiogenesis and heart development in mice. Am J Pathol: 1315–1321.
23. Driever W, Stemple D, Schier A, Solnica-Krezel L (1994) Zebrafish: genetic tools for studying vertebrate development. Trends Genet 10: 152–159.
24. Lele Z, Krone PH (1996) The zebrafish as a model system in developmental, toxicological and transgenic research. Biotechnol Adv 14: 57–72.
25. Drummond IA (2000) The zebrafish pronephros: a genetic system for studies of kidney development. Pediatr Nephrol 14: 428–435.
26. Langenberg T, Brand M, Cooper MS (2003) Imaging brain development and organogenesis in zebrafish using immobilized embryonic explants. Dev Dyn 228: 464–474.
27. Glickman NS, Yelon D (2002) Cardiac development in zebrafish: coordination of form and function. Semin Cell Dev Biol 13: 507–513.
28. Avanesov A, Malicki J (2004) Approaches to study neurogenesis in the zebrafish retina. Methods Cell Biol 76: 333–384.
29. Lam CS, Marz M, Strahle U (2009) gfap and nestin reporter lines reveal characteristics of neural progenitors in the adult zebrafish brain. Dev Dyn 238: 475–486.
30. Goessling W, North TE, Zon LI (2007) Ultrasound biomicroscopy permits in vivo characterization of zebrafish liver tumors. Nat Methods 4: 551–553.
31. Peterson SM, Freeman JL (2009) Cancer cytogenetics in the zebrafish. Zebrafish 6: 355–360.
32. Amsterdam A, Hopkins N (2006) Mutagenesis strategies in zebrafish for identifying genes involved in development and disease. Trends Genet 22: 473–478.
33. Malicki JJ, Pujic Z, Thisse C, Thisse B, Wei X (2002) Forward and reverse genetic approaches to the analysis of eye development in zebrafish. Vision Res 42: 527–533.
34. Malicki J (2000) Harnessing the power of forward genetics–analysis of neuronal diversity and patterning in the zebrafish retina. Trends Neurosci 23: 531–541.
35. Lawson ND, Weinstein BM (2002) In vivo imaging of embryonic vascular development using transgenic zebrafish. Dev Biol 248: 307–318.
36. Jin SW, Beis D, Mitchell T, Chen JN, Stainier DY (2005) Cellular and molecular analyses of vascular tube and lumen formation in zebrafish. Development 132: 5199–5209.
37. Zambrowicz BP, Abuin A, Ramirez-Solis R, Richter LJ, Piggott J, et al. (2003) Wnk1 kinase deficiency lowers blood pressure in mice: a gene-trap screen to identify potential targets for therapeutic intervention. Proc Natl Acad Sci U S A 100: 14109–14114.
38. Tseng WF, Jang TH, Huang CB, Yuh CH (2011) An evolutionarily conserved kernel of gata5, gata6, otx2 and prdm1a operates in the formation of endoderm in zebrafish. Dev Biol 357: 541–557.
39. Lauter G, Soll I, Hauptmann G (2011) Two-color fluorescent in situ hybridization in the embryonic zebrafish brain using differential detection systems. BMC Dev Biol 11: 43.
40. Tao S, Cai Y, Sampath K (2009) The Integrator subunits function in hematopoiesis by modulating Smad/BMP signaling. Development 136: 2757–2765.
41. Siekmann AF, Standley C, Fogarty KE, Wolfe SA, Lawson ND (2009) Chemokine signaling guides regional patterning of the first embryonic artery. Genes Dev 23: 2272–2277.
42. Zeng XXI, Zheng XJ, Xiang Y, Cho HP, Jessen JR, et al. (2009) Phospholipase D1 is required for angiogenesis of intersegmental blood vessels in zebrafish. Developmental Biology 328: 363–376.
43. Nicoli S, De Sena G, Presta M (2009) Fibroblast growth factor 2-induced angiogenesis in zebrafish: the zebrafish yolk membrane (ZFYM) angiogenesis assay. J Cell Mol Med 13: 2061–2068.
44. Habeck H, Odenthal J, Walderich B, Maischein H, Schulte-Merker S (2002) Analysis of a zebrafish VEGF receptor mutant reveals specific disruption of angiogenesis. Curr Biol 12: 1405–1412.
45. Isogai S, Horiguchi M, Weinstein BM (2001) The vascular anatomy of the developing zebrafish: an atlas of embryonic and early larval development. Dev Biol 230: 278–301.

Acknowledgments

We would like to thank the Taiwan Zebrafish Core Facility at NTHU-NHRI for providing fish lines and resources; TZeTH is supported by a grant from the NSC (102-2321-B-400-018). We are thankful to B. Thisse for providing the *in situ* data for phosphoinositide-3-kinase, class 2, alpha polypeptide. Additional funding provided to C.H.Y. by the National Health Research Institute is gratefully acknowledged.

Author Contributions

Conceived and designed the experiments: CHY SMT HCT JGL WCC FJK JWL. Performed the experiments: SMT HCT JGL WCC FJK JWL. Analyzed the data: SMT HCT JGL WCC FJK CHY. Contributed reagents/materials/analysis tools: CLH. Wrote the paper: CHY. Contributed to the intellectual discussion: CLH HDW. Helped the project all the way through: CLH.

46. Hirashima M (2009) Regulation of endothelial cell differentiation and arterial specification by VEGF and Notch signaling. Anat Sci Int 84: 95–101.

47. Shibuya M (2006) Differential roles of vascular endothelial growth factor receptor-1 and receptor-2 in angiogenesis. J Biochem Mol Biol 39: 469–478.

48. Jakobsson L, Bentley K, Gerhardt H (2009) VEGFRs and Notch: a dynamic collaboration in vascular patterning. Biochem Soc Trans 37: 1233–1236.

49. Adams RH, Alitalo K (2007) Molecular regulation of angiogenesis and lymphangiogenesis. Nat Rev Mol Cell Biol 8: 464–478.

50. Tammela T, Zarkada G, Wallgard E, Murtomaki A, Suchting S, et al. (2008) Blocking VEGFR-3 suppresses angiogenic sprouting and vascular network formation. Nature 454: 656–660.

51. Sumanas S, Lin S (2006) Ets1-related protein is a key regulator of vasculogenesis in zebrafish. PLoS Biol 4: e10.

52. Dayanir V, Meyer RD, Lashkari K, Rahimi N (2001) Identification of tyrosine residues in vascular endothelial growth factor receptor-2/FLK-1 involved in activation of phosphatidylinositol 3-kinase and cell proliferation. J Biol Chem 276: 17686–17692.

53. Fujio Y, Walsh K (1999) Akt mediates cytoprotection of endothelial cells by vascular endothelial growth factor in an anchorage-dependent manner. J Biol Chem 274: 16349–16354.

54. Makinen T, Veikkola T, Mustjoki S, Karpanen T, Catimel B, et al. (2001) Isolated lymphatic endothelial cells transduce growth, survival and migratory signals via the VEGF-C/D receptor VEGFR-3. EMBO J 20: 4762–4773.

55. Vanhaesebroeck B, Guillermet-Guibert J, Graupera M, Bilanges B (2010) The emerging mechanisms of isoform-specific PI3K signalling. Nat Rev Mol Cell Biol 11: 329–341.

56. El Sheikh SS, Domin J, Tomtitchong P, Abel P, Stamp G, et al. (2003) Topographical expression of class IA and class II phosphoinositide 3-kinase enzymes in normal human tissues is consistent with a role in differentiation. BMC Clin Pathol 3: 4.

15

The Hemodynamically-Regulated Vascular Microenvironment Promotes Migration of the Steroidogenic Tissue during Its Interaction with Chromaffin Cells in the Zebrafish Embryo

Chih-Wei Chou, You-Lin Zhuo, Zhe-Yu Jiang, Yi-Wen Liu*

Department of Life Science, Tunghai University, Taichung, Taiwan

Abstract

Background: While the endothelium-organ interaction is critical for regulating cellular behaviors during development and disease, the role of blood flow in these processes is only partially understood. The dorsal aorta performs paracrine functions for the timely migration and differentiation of the sympatho-adrenal system. However, it is unclear how the adrenal cortex and medulla achieve and maintain specific integration and whether hemodynamic forces play a role.

Methodology and Principal Findings: In this study, the possible modulation of steroidogenic and chromaffin cell integration by blood flow was investigated in the teleostean counterpart of the adrenal gland, the interrenal gland, in the zebrafish (*Danio rerio*). Steroidogenic tissue migration and angiogenesis were suppressed by genetic or pharmacologic inhibition of blood flow, and enhanced by acceleration of blood flow upon norepinephrine treatment. Repressed steroidogenic tissue migration and angiogenesis due to flow deficiency were recoverable following restoration of flow. The regulation of interrenal morphogenesis by blood flow was found to be mediated through the vascular microenvironment and the Fibronectin-phosphorylated Focal Adhesion Kinase (Fn-pFak) signaling. Moreover, the knockdown of *krüppel-like factor 2a* (*klf2a*) or *matrix metalloproteinase 2* (*mmp2*), two genes regulated by the hemodynamic force, phenocopied the defects in migration, angiogenesis, the vascular microenvironment, and pFak signaling of the steroidogenic tissue observed in flow-deficient embryos, indicating a direct requirement of mechanotransduction in these processes. Interestingly, epithelial-type steroidogenic cells assumed a mesenchymal-like character and downregulated β-Catenin at cell-cell junctions during interaction with chromaffin cells, which was reversed by inhibiting blood flow or Fn-pFak signaling. Blood flow obstruction also affected the migration of chromaffin cells, but not through mechanosensitive or Fn-pFak dependent mechanisms.

Conclusions and Significance: These results demonstrate that hemodynamically regulated Fn-pFak signaling promotes the migration of steroidogenic cells, ensuring their interaction with chromaffin cells along both sides of the midline during interrenal gland development.

Editor: Sheng-Ping Lucinda Hwang, Institute of Cellular and Organismic Biology, Taiwan

Funding: CWC, YLZ, ZYJ, and YWL were supported by Ministry of Science and Technology (http://web1.most.gov.tw/) grants (101-2313-B-029-001, 102-2628-B-029-002-MY3 and 102-2321-B-400-018). The funder had no role in study design, data collection and analysis, decision to publish, or preparation of the manuscript.

Competing Interests: The authors have declared that no competing interests exist.

* Email: dlslys@thu.edu.tw

Introduction

Although blood vessels have long been known to respond to hemodynamic forces through mechanotransduction, only recently have researchers begun to understand the influence of hemodynamics on organogenesis through modulation of cellular behaviors, the extracellular matrix (ECM) microenvironment, as well as cell signaling events [1]. The early zebrafish embryo does not rely on blood circulation to transport oxygen [2], making it an excellent *in vivo* model for studying the effect of blood flow on development. Various genetic and pharmacological approaches have been developed in the zebrafish model, which have revealed

the crucial role of hemodynamics in the morphogenesis of heart, kidney, and brain vasculature [3,4,5,6]. Moreover, it is possible to study the role of hemodynamics in establishing the architecture of endocrine tissues in the zebrafish embryo, since the specification and differentiation of a variety of endocrine cells proceed even in the complete absence of vasculature [7,8,9,10,11].

How the adrenal cortex and medulla—arising because of distinct cell fate decisions in physically separated precursor cells—assemble to form the adrenal gland remains incompletely understood. The adrenal cortex is comprised of steroidogenic cells differentiated from the intermediate mesoderm, while the medulla contains chromaffin cells that originate from the neural crest and are subsequently segregated from the sympatho-adrenal lineage [12]. Mice deficient in the transcription factor steroidogenic factor-1 (SF-1, NR5A1) lack an adrenal cortex, but exhibit normal differentiation of chromaffin cells, half of which are present in the suprarenal region, arguing against a role for the adrenal cortex in attracting chromaffin cells [13]. However, ectopic adrenocortical cells in the mouse thorax, induced through the transgenic overexpression of SF-1, are capable of recruiting sympatho-adrenal progenitors [14]. These findings suggestive of an undefined role of the adrenal cortex have been clarified by the recent demonstration of the dorsal aorta (DA) as a morphogenetic center that instructs the specification and segregation of the sympatho-adrenal lineage in the chick embryo [15]. The DA and the adrenal cortex both secrete Neuregulin 1, which attracts chromaffin cells to the suprarenal region. However, the existence of shared paracrine factors does not explain why chromaffin cells colonize the adrenal cortex rather than non-adrenal regions surrounding the DA, and additional molecular and cellular factors could participate in the integration of steroidogenic and chromaffin cells. It was hypothesized that in addition to instructing the migration and differentiation of chromaffin cells, the vasculature near the adrenal gland also specifies the behavior of adrenocortical cells, thereby promoting cortex-medulla amalgamation. This possibility was investigated in the present study in zebrafish, an established model for exploring the development and diseases of the cardiovascular and endocrine systems.

The teleostean interrenal gland is functionally equivalent to the adrenal gland in mammals, with steroidogenic and chromaffin cell populations arising from conserved molecular programs [16,17,18]. The integration of these two cell types occurs between 1.5 and 3 days post-fertilization (dpf), which is immediately followed by de novo cortisol synthesis in response to stress [18,19,20]. Within the same temporal window, the interrenal vessel (IRV) is patterned along with a vessel-derived, Fibronectin (Fn)-enriched microenvironment [21], which is essential for IRV growth, steroidogenic tissue morphogenesis, and positioning the interrenal organ. Nevertheless, little is known about how the Fn-enriched interrenal microenvironment is regulated and the cellular mechanisms governing morphogenetic movements during integration.

Previous studies have shown that Klf2a and MMP2 are hemodynamically regulated: KLF2 is a transcription factor activated in cultured endothelial cells by fluid shear stress from laminar flow [22,23], and the endothelial expression of mouse Klf2 and its ortholog klf2a in zebrafish reflects an increase in fluid-generated forces, while a loss of function leads to defective smooth muscle tone [24]. MMPs are known to mediate ECM remodeling and enable reshaping of tissues through peptidase activity [25]. In the zebrafish embryo, mmp2 is expressed in the endothelium of developing axial vasculature in a flow-dependent manner [5]; and in rats and cultured cells, MMP2 activity in glomerular mesangial cells is induced by stretch [26,27] and regulated by cyclic strains in the endothelium resulting from turbulent flow, which modulates the migration of vascular smooth muscle cells [28,29]. Moreover, MMP2 cleaves a variety of ECM molecules, including type IV collagen, vitronectin, and fibronectin [30,31]. Abundant RNA transcripts of both klf2a and mmp2 are restrictively localized at the axial vasculature at around Prim-25 stage (36 hpf) during zebrafish development [5,32], which is temporally correlated with the initiation of interrenal medial extension and angiogenesis. Furthermore, the nascent DA in the zebrafish does not recruit mural cells until 3 dpf [33], and differentiated vascular smooth muscle cells appear only after 7 dpf [34]; it was therefore hypothesized that hemodynamic forces could be transduced

through the endothelium to influence closely associated interrenal cells.

In this study, the possible role of blood flow for the integration of steroidogenic and chromaffin cells was examined in the zebrafish interrenal gland, by using genetic and pharmacological approaches to abolish blood flow in the embryo. The vascular structure and associated ECM microenvironment in the interrenal region were examined for changes in the architecture of the developing interrenal tissue. The modulation of interrenal morphogenesis by blood flow through mechanotransduction was investigated by knocking down the mechanosensitive proteins Krüppel-like factor 2a (Klf2a) and Matrix metalloproteinase (Mmp)2. In addition, we demonstrated that steroidogenic cells undergo an epithelial-to-mesenchymal transition (EMT)-like change during organ assembly, which was correlated with a reduction in epithelial and a rise in mesenchymal markers. During EMT, which occurs at many critical steps during embryonic development, cell-cell contacts and polarity are lost and the cytoskeleton is extensively remodeled [35]. The present findings underscore the role of hemodynamics in regulating Fn-phosphorylated Focal adhesion kinase (pFak) signaling in the developing interrenal tissue, which in turn induces an EMT-like transformation in steroidogenic cells. Thus, in addition to the known chemoattractive function for chromaffin cells, the axial vasculature regulates the migration of steroidogenic cells through hemodynamically regulated signaling.

Methods

Ethics Statement

All of the zebrafish-use protocols in this research were reviewed and approved by the Institutional Animal Care and Use Committee of Tunghai University (IRB Approval NO. 101–12).

Zebrafish Husbandry

Zebrafish (Danio rerio) were reared according to standard protocols [36]. Embryos were obtained from natural crosses of wild-type or transgenic fish, and staged as previously described [37]. The following lines were used: Tg(wt1b: GFP)(line 1) [38] (a gift from Christoph Englert, Fritz-Lipmann Institute, Jena, Germany); Tg(ff1bEx2: GFP) [39] (a gift from Dr. Woon-Khiong Chan, National University of Singapore); and Tg(kdrl: EGFP)^{s843} [40] (a gift of Didier Stainier, University of California, San Francisco, CA, USA).

3β-Hydroxysteroid Dehydrogenase (3β-Hsd) Staining, In Situ Hybridization (ISH), Immunohistochemistry (IHC), Densitometry and Imaging

Embryos used for histological analysis were treated with 0.03% phenylthiourea (Sigma) from 12 h post-fertilization (hpf) onwards to inhibit pigmentation. The 3β-Hsd activity staining, ISH [9], and IHC [41] were performed with modifications according to previously published methods.

To delineate the morphology of steroidogenic interrenal tissue, histochemical staining for 3β-Hsd enzymatic activity was performed on whole embryos, and Nomarski images were captured using a BX51 microscope (Olympus).

For whole-mount ISH, digoxigenin (DIG)- and fluorescein-labeled antisense riboprobes were synthesized from linearized plasmids of dopamine β hydroxylase (dβh) and ff1b (nr5a1a) genes, respectively; the probes were detected with alkaline phosphatase-conjugated anti-DIG or -fluorescein antibody (Roche), and visualized with 5-bromo-4-chloro-3-indolyl-phosphate/nitro blue tetrazolium (Promega) or Fast Red (Roche). Stained embryos were flat-mounted and photographed under an Axioplan II microscope (Zeiss).

For IHC experiments, *Tg(fflbEx2: GFP)* and *Tg(kdrl: EGFP)*[s843] embryos were fixed and embedded in 4% NuSieve GTG low-melting agarose (Lonza), cut into 100- μm sections with a VT1000M vibratome (Leica), and permeabilized with phosphate-buffered saline (PBS) containing 1% Triton X-100 before incubation with rabbit anti-human Fn (Sigma), mouse anti-human pFak (pY397) (BD Transduction Laboratories), mouse anti-chicken β-Catenin (Sigma), mouse anti-pig Vimentin (V9) (Abcam), and rabbit anti-zebrafish E-cadherin (Cdh1) (GeneTex) antibodies at 1:200, 1:100, 1:50, 1:200 and 1:200 dilutions, respectively. Dylight 594- and 650-conjugated anti-rabbit or anti-mouse IgG (abcam) were used as secondary antibodies at 1:200 dilution. Images were captured with an LSM510 confocal microscope with version 3.5 software (Zeiss).

For the quantification of 3β-Hsd activity, images of deyolked embryos in each group were taken with identical illumination and magnification using Axioskop 2 Plus microscope equipped with AxioVision 3.0 software (Carl Zeiss). Signal area and density were measured using Image Gauge Program, version 4.0 (Fuji Photo Film). Videos of embryos oriented with the anterior toward the left were taken by using an SMZ1500 microscope equipped with an AM4023X Dino-Eye eyepiece camera (Nikon).

Microinjection of Antisense Morpholino Oligonucleotides (MOs)

The MO for *cardiac troponin T2a* (*tnnt2a*MO) (5'-CAT GTT TGC TCT GAT CTG ACA CGC A-3') [42], along with *klf2a*MO (5'-GGA CCT GTC CAG TTC ATC CTT CCA C-3') [43], and *mmp2*MO (5'-GGG AGC TTA GTA AAC ACA AAC CTG T-3') [44] were synthesized by Genetools LLC and diluted in 1× Danieau solution, before injection into one- to two-cell stage embryos using a Nanoject (Drummond Scientific Company) at dosages of 1.0, 1.2, and 1.2 pmole per embryo, respectively.

Pharmacological Treatment

Camptothecin (Sigma # C9911) treatment was performed according to a previously described method [45] with modifications. The compound (60 μM in 0.1% dimethyl sulfoxide [DMSO]) was applied to 48 hpf embryos, which were harvested at 57 hpf for the 3β-Hsd activity assay. The treatment of embryos with 2,3-butanedione 2-monoxime (2,3-BDM; Sigma #B0753) was as described in an earlier report [46], except that dechorionated embryos were immersed in various concentrations of 2,3-BDM starting from 1.5 dpf. Norepinephrine treatment was performed by treating dechorionated embryos with 0.01, 0.1 or 1 mM norepinephrine (Sigma A7257) freshly prepared in egg water. L-NAME treatment was performed by treating dechorionated embryos with freshly prepared 100 μM Nω-nitro-L-arginine methyl ester (L-NAME) (#N5751, Sigma) in egg water with 0.1% DMSO at 36 hpf. For L-arginyl-L-glycyl-L-aspartic acid (RGD; #G1269, Sigma) treatment, the peptide was reconstituted to 1 mM in filter-sterilized egg water and applied to dechorionated embryos at a final concentration of 100 μM at 26 hpf; embryos were collected at 2.5 dpf and fixed for histological assays.

Statistical Analysis

All quantitative data are expressed as the mean ± standard error of the mean. Data were evaluated by analysis of variance (ANOVA), followed by Duncan's new multiple range test (Duncan's multiple test) or Student's t test. $P < 0.05$ was considered statistically significant.

Results

Blood Flow is Required for the Morphogenesis of Kidney Glomerulus and Interrenal Tissue

The hemodynamic force drives the assembly of zebrafish kidney glomeruli at the midline [5]. Since the kidney and interrenal gland develop in parallel [16], with the DA acting as the source of angiogenesis in both organs [21,47], the role of blood flow in the morphogenesis of the interrenal gland was assessed. Kidney and interrenal tissue morphology was visualized by staining for 3β-Hsd enzymatic activity in *Tg(wt1b: GFP)* embryos, in which GFP is expressed in the glomerular podocytes, pronephric tubules, and proximal pronephric ducts [38,48], as well as in the exocrine pancreas due to a possible position effect of transgene insertion. The MO against *tnnt2a*, a gene essential for sarcomere assembly and heart contractility [42], was injected into *Tg(wt1b: GFP)* embryos, and 100% of the *tnnt2a* morphants (n = 56) displayed completely abolished heartbeat and blood flow. Consistent with the previous study [5], bilateral kidney glomeruli in control embryos assembled at the midline by 54 hpf, but failed to fuse in *tnnt2a* morphants (Figure 1A). The steroidogenic tissue in blood flow-deficient embryos grew as a round, tightly packed cell aggregate, without extending protrusions as in the case of controls. The extent of migration was quantified by measuring the distance between the tip of medially extending steroidogenic tissue and the midline, and although there was no difference at 54 hpf, the distance was decreased in morphants relative to control embryos at 77 hpf (Figure 1B). The inhibition of medial extension was not due to growth arrest of interrenal tissue, since organ size—as assessed by densitometric analysis of 3β-Hsd activity staining—was similar in *tnnt2a*MO-injected and control embryos at all stages examined (Figure 1C). To further evaluate the effect of tissue growth on interrenal morphogenetic movement, embryos were treated with camptothecin, which blocks cell proliferation in zebrafish embryos [45], from 48 to 57 hpf. Camptothecin-treated embryos showed an 18% reduction in interrenal tissue size compared to controls. Notably, the formation of protrusions was unaffected by camptothecin treatment (Figure 1D), suggesting that cell growth is not the major determinant for interrenal medial extension. Taken together, these results indicate that blood flow is required for the morphogenetic movement of both kidney and interrenal tissues. Based on the early defects in the ventral DA caused by *tnnt2a* knockdown [49,50], experiments were performed to establish whether interrenal morphogenetic movement during the temporal window of organ assembly is specifically subject to regulation by blood flow.

Medial Extension of Steroidogenic Tissue during Interrenal Organ Assembly is Regulated by Blood Flow

The pharmacological agent 2,3-BDM, which affects heart rate without affecting cell viability, has previously been used to evaluate the role of blood flow in zebrafish organogenesis [5,6,51]. To rule out the possibility that defective medial extension of the interrenal tissue in *tnnt2a* morphants was due to an early effect on blood vessel morphogenesis, blood flow was inhibited in embryos by application of 2,3-BDM from 1.5 dpf, by which interrenal medial extension and organ assembly are initiated (Figure 2). The 2,3-BDM treatment on zebrafish embryos leads to decreased myofibrillar ATPase and myocardial force in a dose-dependent manner, which affects heart rate at a concentration as low as 2 mM and is sufficient to eliminate blood flow at 6 mM [46]. Consistent with the previous study, a concentration of 6 mM produced a 53% reduction in heart rate and a cessation of blood flow (Video S1) compared to control embryos (Video S2). A lower

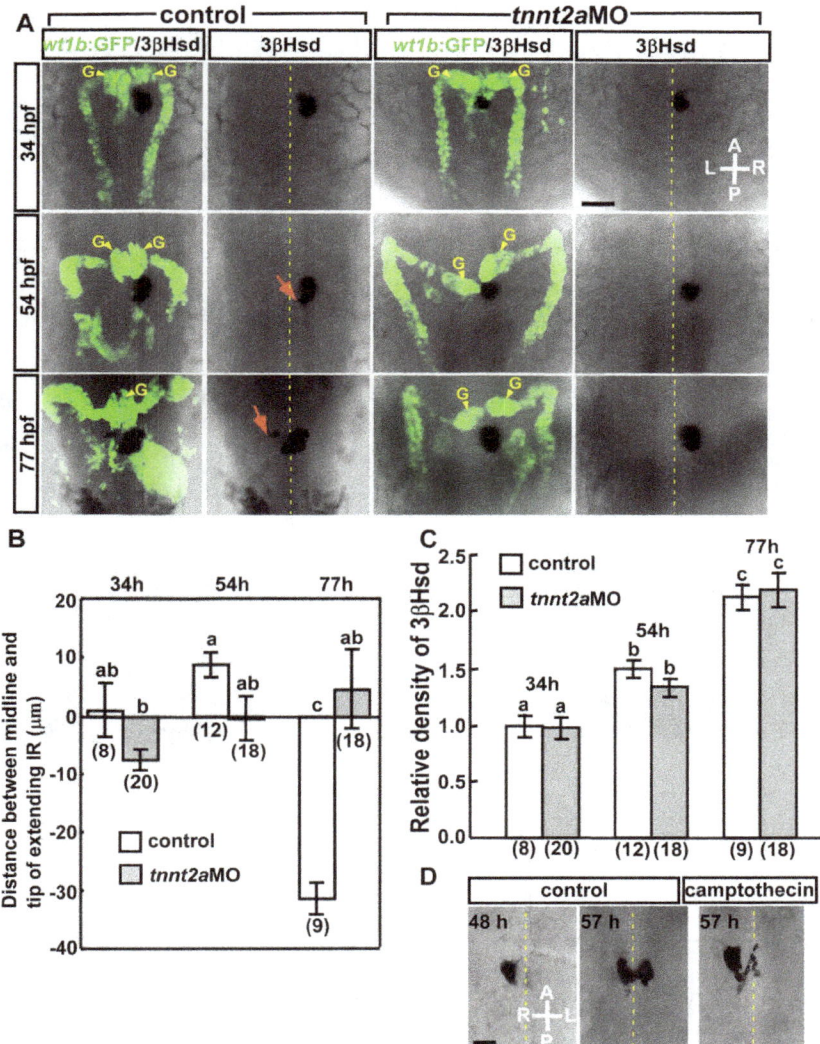

Figure 1. Morphology of pronephros and interrenal tissue in the absence of blood flow. (A) The interrenal steroidogenic tissue positive for 3β-Hsd activity forms an extension that protrudes toward the midline by 54 hpf (cell protrusions marked by red arrows), while kidney glomeruli delineated by *wt1b*: GFP expression (G, yellow arrowheads) assemble at the midline. Morphogenetic movements of kidney glomeruli and steroidogenic tissues are defective in the *tnnt2a* morphant. All panels show dorsal views of representative embryos. (B) Quantification of effects of *tnnt2a*MO injection on interrenal migration. The distance between the midline and the migrating tip of steroidogenic tissue was designated as positive if the migrating tip had not reached the midline, and negative if the tip had migrated across the midline. (C) Relative density of steroidogenic tissue, as assessed by 3β-Hsd activity staining in the ventral surface, in *tnnt2a* morphants compared to wild-type controls. The number of embryos in each group is indicated in parentheses in (B) and (C). Histograms with different letters above them are significantly different (ANOVA and Duncan's multiple test, $P<0.05$). (D) Effect of camptothecin treatment from 48 to 57 hpf on 3β-Hsd activity in steroidogenic cells. A, anterior; P, posterior; L, left; R, right. Broken yellow lines indicate position of the midline. Abbreviations: glomerulus (G). Scale bar, 50 μm.

concentration of 2,3-BDM (2 mM) caused a 26% decrease in heart rate and a visibly weakened blood flow (Video S3). To examine the morphology of the DA adjacent to the kidney and interrenal regions, 2,3-BDM was applied to *Tg(kdrl: EGFP)*[s843] embryos that express GFP in the developing blood vascular structure [40], which were then harvested at 2.5 dpf, when the migration of interrenal cells can be clearly observed [19]. Treatment with 2 or 6 mM 2,3-BDM suppressed interrenal medial extension across the midline (Figure 2B, B'', C, C''), with similar effects observed at both concentrations (Figure 2D). However, the interrenal tissue had more protrusions at 2 than at 6 mM 2,3-BDM (Figure 2B, C), suggesting that the effect of 2,3-BDM was dose-dependent. In contrast, the morphology of the DA

and the pronephric glomerulus was unperturbed by 2,3-BDM treatment. Thus, the inhibition of medial extension of the interrenal tissue caused by loss of blood flow was not due to a general defect in the DA.

Conversely, as the heart rate was accelerated by norepinephrine treatment from 33 hpf, a significant enhancement of interrenal tissue extension was detected at 2 dpf (Figure 2E-E'', F-F'', G-G'', H). Norepinephrine accelerated the heart rate of developing embryos in a dose-dependent manner (Figure S1). 0.01, 0.1 and 1 mM of norepinephrine treatments on embryos at 33 hpf led to a 23%, 29% and 41% increase of heart rate, respectively. Compared to the control embryo (Figure 2E), both 0.1 and 1 mM of norepinephrine treatements led to a more evident migratory

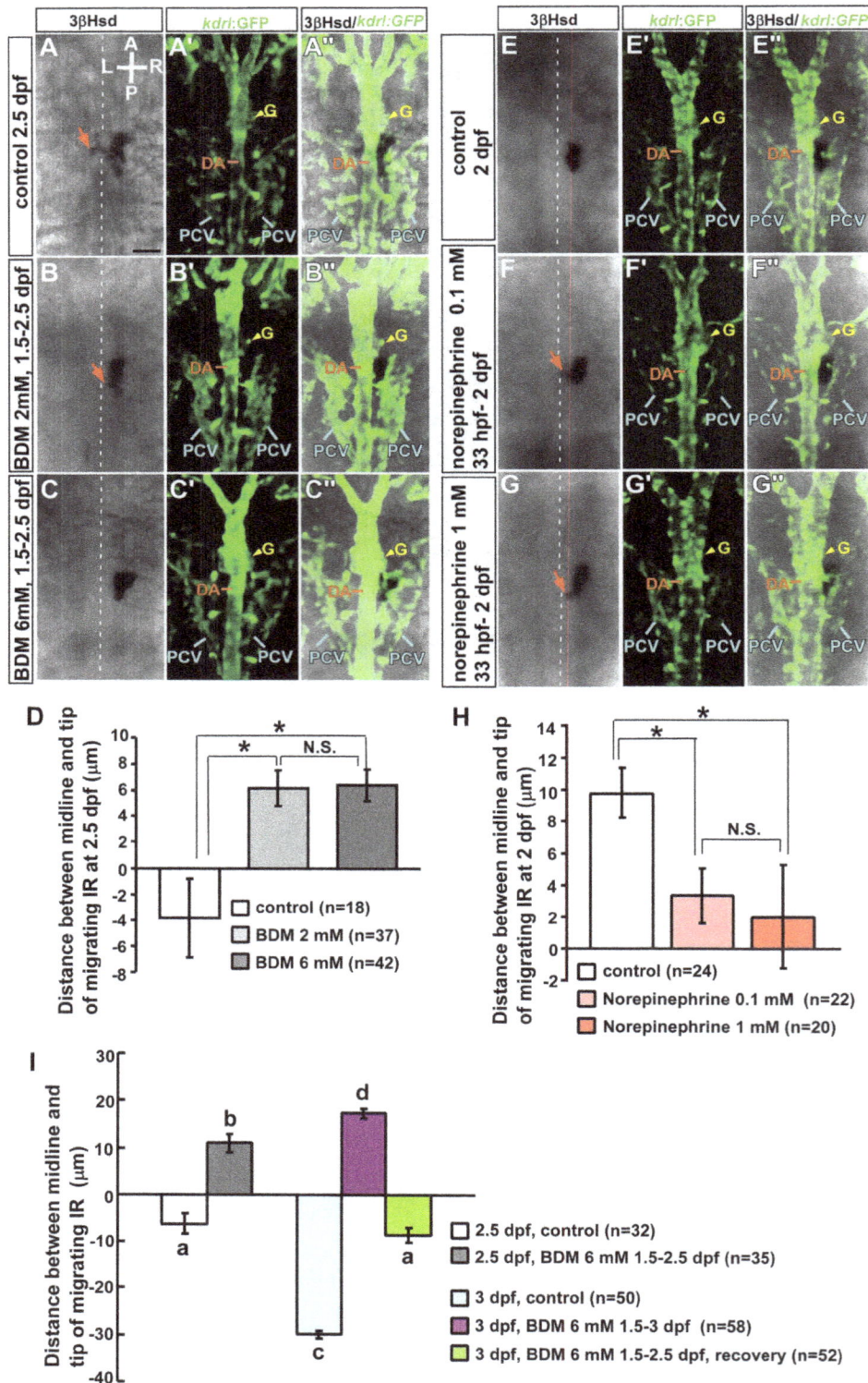

Figure 2. Effects of 2,3-BDM and norepinephrine on morphogenetic movements of interrenal tissue. For repression of blood flow, *Tg(kdrl: GFP)^{s843}* embryos were treated with (A–A″) vehicle (control), or 2,3-BDM at a concentration of (B–B″) 2 mM or (C–C″) 6 mM from 1.5 dpf. A suppression of the medial extension of steroidogenic cells was observed in 2,3-BDM-treated embryos at 2.5 dpf, while the morphology of the DA and the pronephric glomerulus (yellow arrowheads) appeared unperturbed. Protrusions (red arrow) formed at the lower concentration; the phenotype was more severe at the higher concentration. For acceleration of blood flow, *Tg(kdrl: GFP)^{s843}* embryos were treated with (E–E″) vehicle (control), or norepinephrine at a concentration of (F–F″) 0.1 mM or (G-G″) 1 mM from 33 hpf. An enhancement of interrenal medial extension, as evidenced by the formation of protrusions, was observed in norepinephrine-treated embryos at 2 dpf. The effects of 2,3-BDM and norepinephrine treatments on interrenal migration were quantified in (D) and (H), respectively. The distance between the midline and migrating tip of steroidogenic tissue was

designated as positive if the migrating tip had not reached the midline, and negative if the tip had migrated across the midline. *P<0.05; N.S., not significant (Student's t-test). (I) Suppressing effect of interrenal cell migration by 2,3-BDM at 6 mM from 1.5 dpf was reversible at 3 dpf, as the 2,3-BDM applied from 1.5 dpf was washed out at 2.5 dpf for restoring blood flow. The interrenal tissue in recovered embryos extended across the midline at 3 dpf and displayed a migration distance not significantly different from that in control embryos at 2.5 dpf. Histograms with different letters above them are significantly different (ANOVA and Duncan's multiple test, P<0.05). A, anterior; P, posterior; L, left; R, right. Broken white lines indicate position of the midline. Abbreviations: glomerulus (G), posterior cardinal vein (PCV). Scale bar, 50 µm.

phenotype of interrenal tissue, as verified from the extending protrusions (red arrows in Figure 2F, G), which was consistent with the results of the quantification of interrenal tissue extension (Figure 2H). However, no significant difference in steroidogenic tissue extension could be detected between embryos treated with 0.1 or 1 mM of norepinephrine. Norepinephrine at 0.01 mM also enhanced steroidogenic tissue extension (4.3±2.0 µm, n = 24) compared to control embryos, while no significant statistical difference was found among norepinephrine treatments at 0.01, 0.1 and 1 mM. Our results thus indicated that a moderate elevation of heart rate by 23% was sufficient to promote migration of steroidogenic interrenal cells, although further increase of heart rate by treating with higher concentrations of norepinephrine did not lead to a dose-dependent enhancing effect on interrenal medial extension.

To confirm the relationship between blood flow and steroidogenic cell migration, we further tested whether interrenal medial extension repressed by 2,3-BDM treatment could be recovered by restoring the blood flow (Figure 2I, Figure S2). Steroidogenic tissue migrated across the midline by 2.5 dpf (Figure S2A, A'') and continued to extend and form a bilobed organ structure by 3 dpf (Figure S2C, C''). Extension of steroidogenic tissue was arrested as 2,3-BDM at 6 mM was applied to embryos from 1.5 dpf onwards (Figure S2B, B'', D, D''). The steroidogenic tissue extension in 2,3-BDM-treated embryos was recovered at 3 dpf as 2,3-BDM was washed out at 2.5 dpf (Figure S2E, E''). The interrenal tissue in 2,3-BDM-treated embryos appeared to be located further away from the midline at 3 dpf than at 2.5 dpf (Figure 2I), possibly due to continuous growth of peri-interrenal structures from 2.5 to 3 dpf. It is interesting to note that there was no significant difference of migration distance between control embryos at 2.5 dpf and recovered embryos at 3 dpf (Figure 2I), implying that the inhibited interrenal medial extension by 2,3-BDM treatment from 1.5 to 2.5 dpf could be rescued by resuming blood flow for 12 hours. Taken together, results in Figure 2 demonstrated that pharmacologic repression and acceleration of heart rates are well correlated with the extent of interrenal medial extension. Furthermore, the inhibited steroidogenic tissue extension caused by arrested blood flow was recoverable following restoration of blood flow, providing strong evidence that migratory activity of interrenal steroidogenic cells is indeed modulated by blood flow.

Blood Flow Regulates IRV Extension during Interrenal Organ Assembly

Interrenal medial extension temporally coincides with IRV angiogenesis, which is promoted by the IRV-associated vascular microenvironment [21], and therefore the effect of reduced blood flow on IRV angiogenesis was examined from 1.5 to 2.5 dpf (Figure 3). IRV growth was initiated normally when blood flow was inhibited starting at 1.5 dpf. However, in embryos treated with 2 or 6 mM 2,3-BDM, IRV lengths were reduced and the vessels reached but did not extend ventrally through the interrenal tissue, with a more severe phenotype observed at the higher concentration (Figure 3B'–C', D), indicating a dose-dependent effect of 2,3-BDM on IRV extension. Our previous study showed that IRV directionality, but not initiation of angiogenesis, is perturbed in the

tnnt2a morphant [21]; accordingly, the present results indicated that the blood flow was not required for the sprouting of the IRV from the DA, but may play a role in its extension. Furthermore, the interrenal tissue in 2,3-BDM-treated embryos (Figure 3B–B', C–C') and tnnt2a morphants [21] only interacted with the tip of the IRV but not the DA, while the extending interrenal tissue in the control embryo remained closely associated with both the ventral DA and the IRV (Figure 3A–A').

To test whether accelerated blood flow could promote extension of the IRV, embryos were treated with norepinephrine at 0.1 or 1 mM at 33 hpf and harvested at 2 dpf for analysis (Figure 3E-G, E'-G'). It was found that norepinephrine at both concentrations significantly increased length of the IRV (Figure 3H), yet no difference in the IRV growth was observed between 0.1 and 1 mM of norepinephrine treatments. The promoting effects of norepinephrine treatments on extension of the IRV were therefore highly correlated with those on interrenal medial extension (Figure 2H). Similar to the case of interrenal medial extension in Figure 2I, restoring blood flow by 2,3-BDM washout after the treatment from 1.5 to 2.5 dpf led to a recovery of IRV growth at 3 dpf, with the IRV length in 3-dpf recovered embryos not significantly different from that in 2.5-dpf control embryos (Figure 3I, S3).

Our results from pharmacologic inhibition and acceleration of blood flow therefore strongly support that blood flow regulates both interrenal medial extension and IRV growth during interrenal organ assembly. While the processes of interrenal medial extension and IRV growth occur synchronously during development [21], they are both influenced by blood flow in a highly correlated manner. Therefore, it leads to the hypothesis that there might be a common flow-regulated molecular and cellular mechanism by which both interrenal medial extension and IRV angiogenesis are regulated. The initiation of IRV angiogenesis requires deposition of Fn at the ventral DA near the interrenal tissue, and the accumulation of this protein in the local microenvironment supports IRV extension [21]. While the interrenal tissue is closely associated with both the DA and the IRV, vessel-derived Fn functions at the tissue-vessel interface and thus modulates the migration of steroidogenic cells [19]. Therefore, it is possible that the vascular microenvironment established during IRV angiogenesis is regulated by blood flow, which in turn modulates the migration of steroidogenic cells.

Blood Flow is Required for Patterning the Fn-rich Microenvironment and pFak Distribution in the Interrenal Region

Possible perturbations in the interrenal microenvironment of blood flow-deficient embryos were assessed using the Tg(ff1bEx2: GFP) line, in which the GFP expression recapitulates the endogenous expression of ff1b [52]—the teleostean ortholog of mammalian SF-1—and marks the ontogeny of steroidogenic interrenal tissue [16,17]. Embryos were examined for expression of Fn and pFak (Figure 4). The elimination of blood flow by tnnt2aMO injection (Figure 4B–B') or 6 mM 2,3-BDM treatment (Figure 4C–C'') did not diminish Fn accumulation in the interrenal microenvironment (Figure 4D). However, Fn was

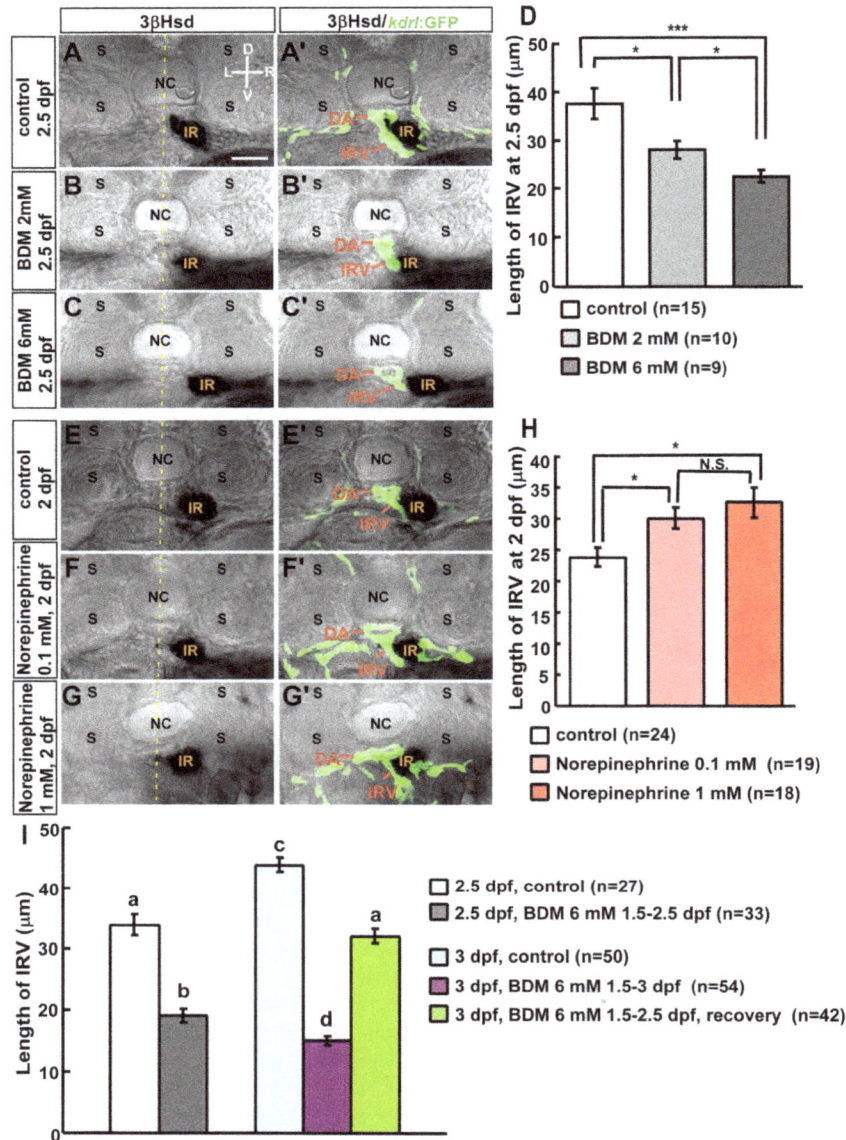

Figure 3. Effects of 2,3-BDM and norepinephrine on IRV formation. For repression of blood flow, Tg(kdrl: GFP)^s843 embryos were treated with (A–A') vehicle (control), or 2,3-BDM at a concentration of (B–B') 2 mM or (C–C') 6 mM from 1.5 dpf, and harvested at 2.5 dpf. For acceleration of blood flow, Tg(kdrl: GFP)^s843 embryos were treated with (E-E') vehicle (control), or norepinephrine at a concentration of (F–F') 0.1 mM or (G-G') 1 mM from 33 hpf, and harvested at 2 dpf. Transverse sections of harvested embryos were subject to analysis of 3β-Hsd activity (black) and GFP expression (green). IRV lengths of 2,3-BDM- or norepinephrine-treated embryos were quantified in (D) and (H), respectively; which were verified from confocal Z-stacks covering the full range of IRV growth, and measurements were made from single focal planes displaying the maximal range of ventrally extending IRV. *$P < 0.05$, ***$P < 0.0005$, N.S., not significant (Student's t-test). (I) Repressing effect of 2,3-BDM (6 mM) on IRV growth was reversible at 3 dpf, as the 2,3-BDM applied from 1.5 dpf was washed out at 2.5 dpf. The IRV length in recovered embryos at 3 dpf was not significantly different from that in control embryos at 2.5 dpf. Histograms with different letters above them are significantly different (ANOVA and Duncan's multiple test, $P < 0.05$). D, dorsal; V, ventral; L, left; R, right. Abbreviations: interrenal tissue (IR), notochord (NC), somite (S). Scale bar, 25 μm.

abnormally distributed, raising the possibility that in the absence of blood flow, the polymerization of Fn into fibrils was disrupted. To verify whether aberrant Fn deposition perturbed signaling events within the interrenal tissue, the localization of pFak—a downstream effector of Fn-Integrin signaling and an indicator of the dynamic reorganization of focal adhesions during cell migration—was examined (Figure 4A–C"). Indeed, pFak level within the interrenal tissue was significantly reduced compared to control embryos (Figure 4E), suggesting a disruption of Integrin-

mediated signaling. In contrast, pFak distribution was readily detected at the somites, gut tube, and swim bladder in tnnt2a morphants (Figure 4B, B') and 2,3-BDM-treated embryos (Figure 4C, C'). These results indicate that the interrenal microenvironment established during IRV angiogenesis is perturbed by reduced blood flow, resulting in the suppression of Fn-pFak signaling and steroidogenic cell migration.

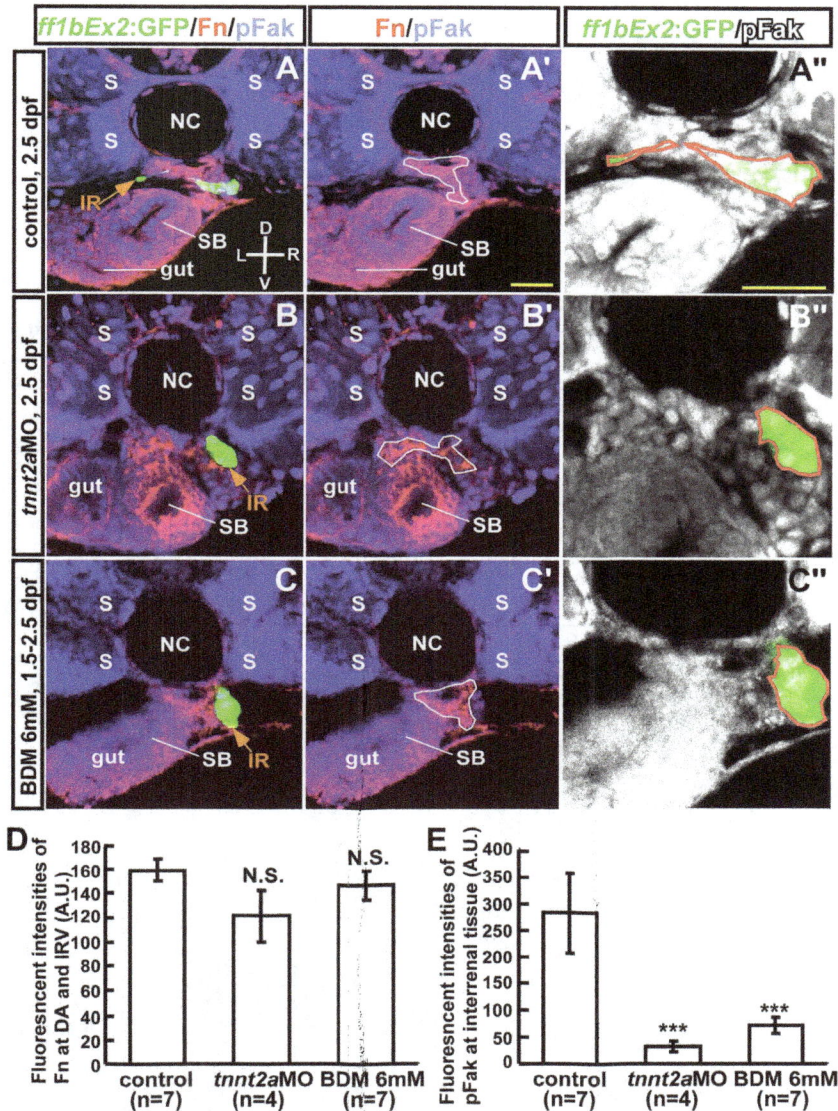

Figure 4. Effect of blood flow inhibition on the ECM microenvironment and pFak distribution in interrenal steroidogenic tissue. Transverse sections of *Tg(ff1bEx2: GFP)* embryos were (A–A″) uninjected (control), (B–B″) injected with *tnnt2a*MO, or (C–C″) treated with 6 mM 2,3-BDM from 1.5 dpf. Embryos were harvested at 2.5 dpf and assayed for expression of GFP (green), Fn (red), and pFak (blue in A–C and A′–C′; white in A″–C″). Images are single confocal planes showing the maximal transverse dimension of *ff1b*GFP-expressing steroidogenic tissue of a representative embryo, with magnified views shown in (A″–C″). (D) Fluorescence intensity of Fn in the DA and IRV selected as regions of interest (ROI; white lines in A′–C′) normalized to the size of the ROI. (E) Total fluorescence intensities of pFak within the steroidogenic tissue (ROI marked by orange lines in A″–C″) were normalized to the size of the cluster. The difference between the treatment and the control groups was analyzed by Student's t-test. ***$P <$ 0.001, N.S., not significant. D, dorsal; V, ventral; L, left; R, right. Abbreviations: arbitrary units (A.U.), interrenal tissue (IR), notochord (NC), somite (S), swim bladder (SB). Scale bar, 25 μm.

Klf2a and MMP2 are Required for Migration, Angiogenesis, and Fn-pFak signaling in the interrenal tissue

To confirm whether hemodynamics, and not circulating factors, account for the effect of blood flow on steroidogenic tissue migration and angiogenesis, the role of Klf2a and MMP2 in interrenal morphogenesis was evaluated (Figure 5). While *Klf2a* deficiency leads to heart failure at 3 dpf [24], as evidenced by pericardial edema and venous pooling of blood around the yolk sac, a heart rate similar to that of control embryos is observed at 2 dpf [3]. In the present study, only mild cardiac edema was observed at 2.5 dpf, and circulation was unaffected, making it possible to evaluate the specific effect of hemodynamic forces on interrenal development at this stage. Consistent with the previous finding that primary vascular structures are not perturbed in the *klf2a* morphant [24], the axial vasculature was grossly normal in the peri-interrenal region at 2.5 dpf (Figure 5B′). However, the migration of steroidogenic cells was inhibited (Figure 5B, D), and IRV growth and directionality were perturbed (Figure 5F, H). In contrast to the *tnnt2a* morphant and 2,3-BDM-treated embryos in which the steroidogenic tissue and DA were not closely associated (Figure 3) [21], the interrenal tissue was proximal to the DA in the

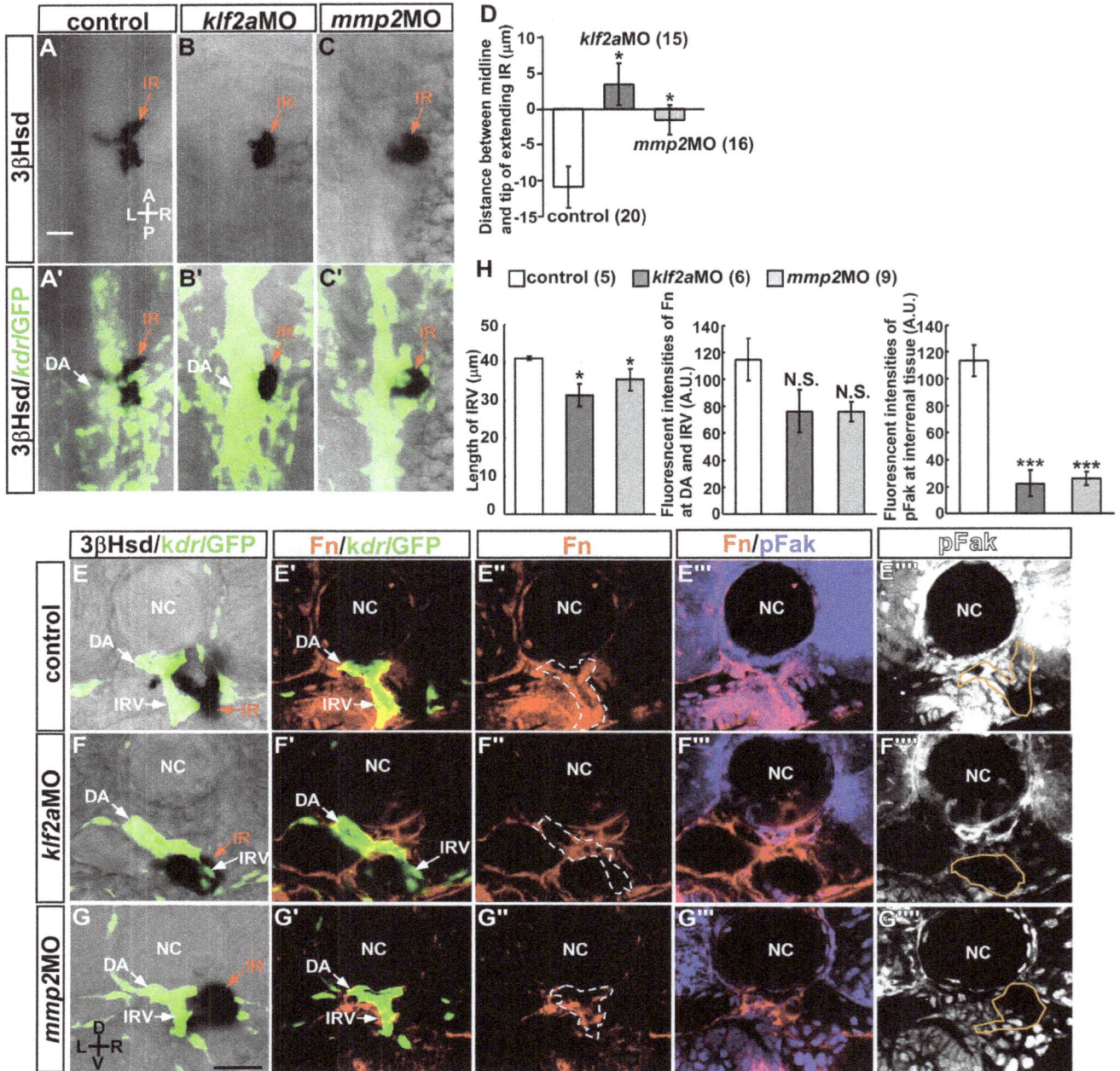

Figure 5. Suppression of interrenal tissue migration in *klf2a* and *mmp2* morphants. Dorsal view of interrenal steroidogenic tissue (IR, red arrows) as detected by 3β-Hsd activity staining, with adjacent vasculature marked by GFP expression. Tg(kdrl: GFP)^s843 embryos were (A, A') uninjected (control), or injected with (B, B') *klf2a*MO or (C, C') *mmp2*MO. (D) Quantification of the effects of MO-mediated gene knockdown on interrenal migration. The distance between the midline and the migrating tip of steroidogenic tissue was designated as positive if the migrating tip had not reached the midline and negative if it had crossed the midline. The number of embryos in each group is indicated in parentheses. The extent of interrenal medial extension of control 2.5-dpf embryos in panel 5D was not statistically different from those in Figure 2D and 2I. Fn and pFak expression in the interrenal region was examined in (E–E'''') uninjected (control), and (F–F'''') *klf2a*MO- and (G–G'''') *mmp2*MO-injected embryos by IHC. Images show transverse sections of a representative embryo from each treatment group. (H) Quantification of the effects of *klf2a*MO and *mmp2*MO on IRV growth, Fn level in the vicinity of the DA and IRV (ROI marked by broken lines in E''–G''), and pFak level in the steroidogenic tissue (ROI marked by orange lines in E''''–G''''). The number of embryos in each group is indicated in parentheses. Fluorescence intensities of Fn and pFak were normalized to their respective ROI sizes. The difference between the treatment and the control groups was analyzed by Student's t-test. *P< 0.05, ***P<0.001, N.S., not significant. A, anterior; P, posterior; L, left; R, right; D, dorsal; V, ventral. Abbreviations: notochord (NC). Scale bar, 25 μm.

klf2a morphant. Despite these phenotypic differences between blood flow-deficient and *klf2a* morphant embryos, both types of embryos showed abnormal Fn distribution and reduced pFak level in the interrenal area (Figure 5F–F'''', H).

Although blood flow regulates the generation of hematopoietic stem cells from the DA by a *klf2a*-nitric oxide (NO) pathway [49,50], steroidogenic interrenal tissue migration and angiogenesis were NO-independent (Figure S4). Treatment with the endothelial NO synthase inhibitor L-NAME from 1.5 to 2.5 dpf had no effect on interrenal tissue migration and angiogenesis, indicating that blood flow and Klf2a do not regulate interrenal morphogenesis through activation of NO signaling.

Embryos injected with 1.2 pmole *mmp2*MO had no major morphological abnormalities except for a kinked tail and mild (2%) reduction in heartbeat that did not cause any visible changes in blood flow. Nevertheless, morphants showed defects in migration, angiogenesis, and Fn-pFak signaling in the interrenal tissue (Figure 5C, D, G, H). This indicated that MMP2 activity may participate in the blood flow-regulated interrenal microenvironment. As observed upon *klf2a* knockdown, the steroidogenic tissue remained associated with both the DA and the IRV, suggesting that neither Klf2a nor MMP2 was essential for this association, which likely depends on other hemodynamically regulated molecules.

Medial Extension of the Interrenal Tissue Involves EMT-like Changes in Steroidogenic Cell Morphology that are Hemodynamically Regulated and pFak-Dependent

The interaction of cancerous epithelial cells with Fn *in vitro* promotes EMT [53,54]. The morphology of the interrenal steroidogenic tissue and the associated Fn-enriched microenvironment suggested that an EMT-like phenotypic change could occur during interrenal medial extension. An examination of interrenal tissue morphology by high resolution Nomarski microscopy revealed that while steroidogenic cells positive for 3β-Hsd activity formed a cluster to the right of the midline by 48 hpf (Figure 6A, B), protrusions were detected at 48 hpf that became more evident by 60 hpf (Figure 6C) and continuously spread across the midline until a bilobed structure was formed by 84 hpf (Figure 6E). During the morphogenetic movement, interrenal steroidogenic cells became more loosely associated with each other and demonstrated a mesenchymal-like phenotype with cell surface protrusions (Figure 6D, E). These morphological features likely reflected an EMT-like process during organ assembly.

To confirm whether interrenal steroidogenic cells undergo a transformation from epithelial to mesenchymal phenotypes, the expression of β-Catenin—a marker for adherent junctions in epithelial cells [55]—was examined. At 2 dpf, β-Catenin was clearly detected at cell-cell junctions of interrenal steroidogenic cells visible by GFP expression in *ff1bEx2: GFP* embryos (Figure 6F–F'), while at 2.5 dpf, β-Catenin was markedly reduced within the steroidogenic tissue cluster (Figure 6G–G'), reflecting the adoption of a mesenchymal-like character.

Since an EMT-like change occurred in steroidogenic cells during interrenal medial extension, the roles of hemodynamic forces and Fn-pFak signaling in this process was assessed. The accumulation of β-Catenin was observed in the interrenal tissue of blood flow-deficient embryos generated by *tnnt2a*MO microinjection (Figure 6H–H') or 6 mM 2,3-BDM treatment (Figure 6I–I'), providing evidence that blood flow induces an EMT-like change in steroidogenic cells. Since blood flow regulates interrenal medial migration via Fn-pFak signaling (Figure 4), Fn signaling was inhibited without perturbing blood flow to determine whether the EMT-like change in steroidogenic cells could be repressed.

The RGD peptide, an antagonist of Fn, was applied to *Tg(ff1bEx2: GFP)* embryos at a concentration of 100 μM starting from 26 hpf, when circulation is initiated; in these embryos, junctional β-Catenin distribution was significantly higher than in controls at 2.5 dpf (Figure 6J–J', M). RGD effectively reduced pFak level in the interrenal area (Figure S5), thus suggesting that the inhibition of pFak signaling was responsible for the observed suppression of EMT-like changes in steroidogenic cells. Moreover, β-Catenin accumulation at cell-cell junctions was evident in both *klf2a* and *mmp2* morphants at 2.5 dpf (Figure 6K–K', L–L', M) as compared to the control embryo.

Consistent with the results of β-Catenin expression, immunohistochemial analysis of E-cadherin, a central component of cell-cell adhesion junction which is required for the formation of epithelia [56,57], detected a clear epithelial phenotype of the interrenal tissue at 2 dpf (Figure S6A, A'). At 2.5 dpf, the E-cadherin expression was reduced at the interrenal tissue where a migratory phenotype was manifested (Figure S6B, B'). In contrast, junctional E-cadherin distribution at the interrenal tissue was not reduced in 2.5 dpf embryos where interrenal medial migration was suppressed by a disruption of either circulation (Figure S6C, C') or pFak-mediated signaling (Figure S6D, D'), or hemodynamics-regulated molecules (Figure S6E, E', F, F'). It was noted that RGD-treated embryos and *mmp2* morphants at 2.5 dpf displayed a higher expression level of junctional E-cadherin than control embryos at 2 dpf did (Figure S6G), with the underlying mechanism remaining unclear. Nevertheless, the immunohistochemistry results of β-Catenin and E-cadherin both indicated a clear reduction of epithelial nature at the interrenal tissue from 2 to 2.5 dpf. Moreover, mesenchymal phenotype of the interrenal tissue at 2.5 dpf correlated well with a rise of Vimentin expression in the *ff1b*-expressing steroidogenic cells (Figure S7A, A', B, B'). Vimentin, a type III intermediate filament protein and a widely used mesenchymal marker, plays a predominant role for inducing changes in cell shape, adhesion and motility during the EMT [58,59]. In contrast to the reduction of β-Catenin and E-cadherin during interrenal medial extension, the Vimentin expression is significantly increased from 2 to 2.5 dpf, and this accumulation of Vimentin was not detected in embryos deficient in either blood flow (Figure S7C, C') or pFak signaling (Figure S6D, D'), or hemodynamic transducers (Figure S7E, E', F, F'). Therefore, an inverse correlation between epithelial and mesenchymal markers was observed during interrenal medial expression. Taken together, these results indicate that blood flow, through mechanotransduction and Fn-pFak signaling, promotes EMT-like changes in steroidogenic cells during interrenal organ assembly.

Migration of Differentiated Chromaffin Cells Requires Blood Flow but is Independent of Mechanotransduction and Fn-Mediated Signaling

To determine whether blood flow also regulates the development of the chromaffin cell lineage, ISH was performed to detect transcript expression of *ff1b* and *dβh*, markers for steroidogenic and chromaffin cell lineages, respectively (Figure 7). Consistent with the findings of our earlier study [19], the integration of the two cell populations was detected as early as 36 hpf (Figure 7A–A'), and was not affected in *tnnt2a* morphants (Figure 7B–B'), while interrenal medial migration and organ assembly were observed at 56 hpf and 3 dpf (Figure 7C–C', E–E'), respectively. Since the medial extension of steroidogenic tissue was inhibited in *tnnt2a* morphants, chromaffin cells that reached the interrenal region remained closely associated with steroidogenic cells, and were located to the right of the midline (Figure 7D–D', F–F'). While the convergence of differentiated chromaffin cells colonizing

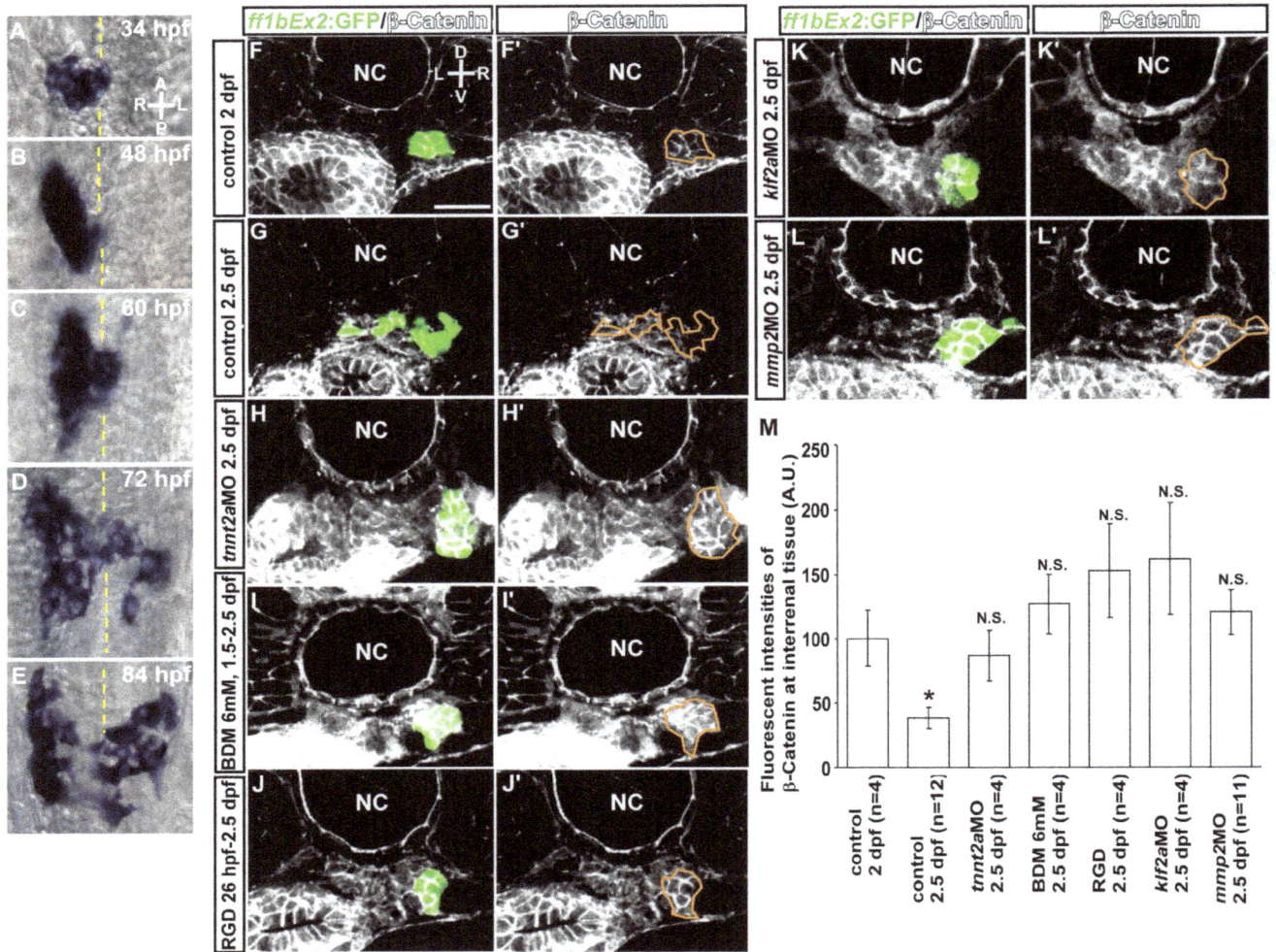

Figure 6. Steroidogenic cells are induced to undergo an EMT-like change by hemodynamic forces and pFak signaling. (A–E) Ventral view of the midtrunk from 34 to 84 hpf; steroidogenic cells become loosely associated and develop protrusions at the cell surface. The accumulation of β-Catenin at cell-cell junctions in the steroidogenic tissue can be seen in cross sections of Tg(ff1bEx2: GFP) embryos at (F, F') 2 dpf, but not at (G, G') 2.5 dpf. The decrease in junctional β-Catenin was not observed in (H, H') tnnt2a morphants, (I, I') 2,3-BDM- or (J, J') RGD-treated embryos, or (K, K') klf2a or (L, L') mmp2 morphants. Sections are shown of a representative embryo from each treatment group. (M) Fluorescence intensity of β-Catenin in ff1bGFP-expressing steroidogenic tissue (ROI marked by orange lines) is normalized to the size of the cluster, with the number of embryos indicated in parentheses. The difference between 2-dpf control group and any of the other groups was analyzed by Student's t-test. *P<0.05, N.S., not significant. A, anterior; P, posterior; L, left; R, right; D, dorsal; V, ventral. Broken yellow lines indicate position of the midline. Abbreviations: notochord (NC). Scale bar, 25 μm.

the interrenal organ was completed by 3 dpf in wild-type embryos (Figure 7E'), clusters of differentiated chromaffin cells were located outside the interrenal region in tnnt2a morphants (Figure 7F–F'), apparently due to the unsuccessful migration of chromaffin cells, indicating that although they are still capable of interacting with steroidogenic cells, their migration is defective in blood flow-deficient embryos, leading to an incomplete assembly of the interrenal organ.

Interestingly, while blood flow was required, mechanotransduction and Fn-pFak signaling were dispensable for chromaffin cell migration. Embryos injected with klf2aMO or mmp2MO, or treated with 100 μM RGD starting from 26 hpf, had defective medial migration of ff1b-expressing cells but normal convergence of chromaffin cells at the midline (Figure 7G–I, G'–I'), resulting in only partial integration of the two cell lineages. This implies that

the migration of steroidogenic and chromaffin cells are differentially modulated by blood flow.

Discussion

The results of this study indicate that in addition to supplying steroids and maintaining tissue homeostasis, blood flow ensures maximal interaction between steroidogenic and chromaffin cells in teleosts (Figure 8). During interrenal organ assembly, hemodynamic forces pattern the vascular microenvironment and regulate the morphology of steroidogenic cells and the associated angiogenic endothelium. The data presented here illustrate a mechanism by which an EMT-like process and tissue-tissue interactions can be modulated by blood flow. A disruption of the vascular microenvironment or mechanotransduction perturbs steroidogenic tissue morphogenesis but not chromaffin cell migration,

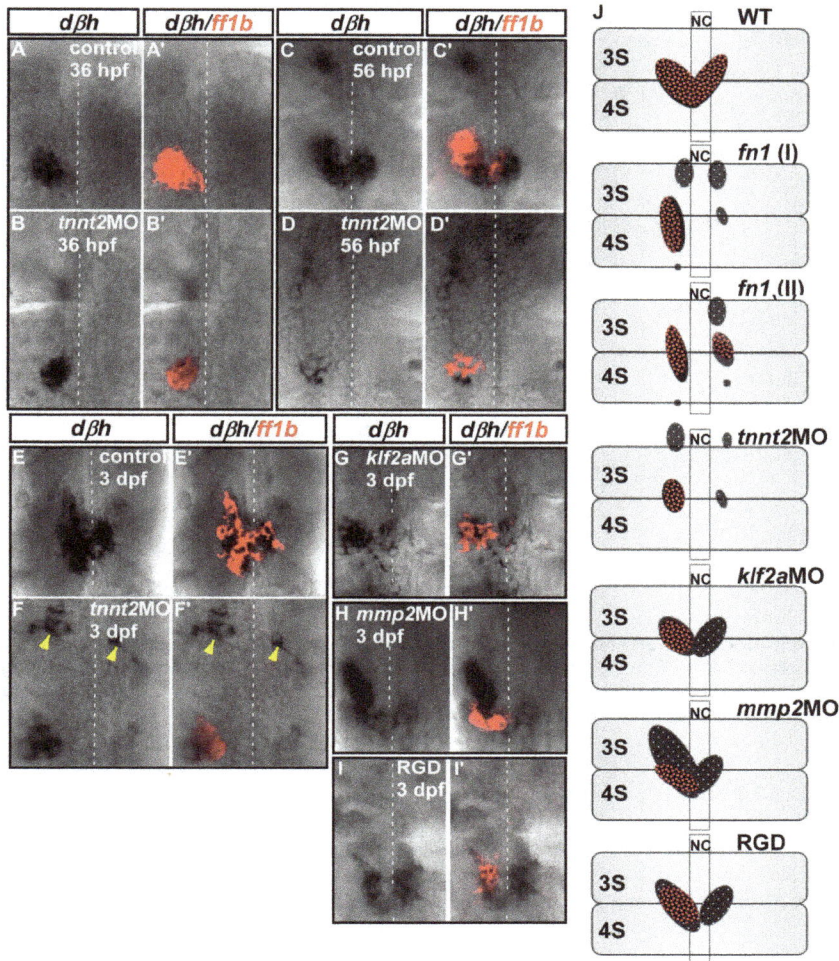

Figure 7. Interaction between interrenal steroidogenic and chromaffin cells in *tnnt2a*, *klf2a*, and *mmp2* morphants and RGD-treated embryos during interrenal gland assembly. Double ISH assays showing colocalization of *ff1b* (red) and *dbh* (black) transcripts in uninjected control embryos and *tnnt2a* morphants at (A, A'; B, B') 36 hpf (n = 3 and 6, respectively), (C, C'; D, D') 56 hpf (n = 3 and 5, respectively), and (E, E'; F, F') 3 dpf (n = 17 and 15, respectively), and in (G, G') *klf2a* (n = 9) and (H, H') *mmp2* (n = 8) morphants and (I, I') RGD-treated embryos (n = 18) at 3 dpf. Ventral flat mount views are shown for representative embryos in each group, oriented with anterior at the top. Yellow arrowheads indicate chromaffin cell clusters that failed to converge at the interrenal area in *tnnt2a* morphants. Broken white lines indicate position of the midline. (J) Schematic representation of various phenotypic defects associated with interrenal organ assembly. Panels show ventral views of wild-type, mutant, morphant, and drug-treated embryos at 3 dpf, oriented with anterior at the top. Phenotypes depicted for *cloche* (*clo*) and *fn1* mutants are based on previous reports [9,21]. Abbreviations: notochord (NC), the third somite (3S), the fourth somite (4S).

indicating that blood flow regulates these processes through different pathways.

The obstruction of blood flow in the zebrafish embryo produced a phenotype similar to that of the *fn1* mutant [19] (Figure 7), providing evidence that the interrenal Fn-enriched microenvironment is regulated by hemodynamic forces (Figure 4). However, while blood flow-deficient embryos have similar defects in steroidogenic and chromaffin cell migration, 20%–30% of *fn1* mutants exhibit a more severe phenotype, where the bilateral fusion of early interrenal tissues is unsuccessful (Figure 7). The variable expressivity of this phenotype in *fn1* mutants could be due to a more profound effect of Fn deficiency on early development prior to the onset of blood flow [41,60]. Indeed, early bilateral interrenal tissues arise in close association with pre-vascular angioblasts, and their fusion occurs in parallel with the assembly of axial vasculature independently of the initiation of blood flow [9,52].

The phenotype of the RGD-treated embryo—that is, defective migration of steroidogenic but not chromaffin cells—was different from that of the *fn1* mutant, in which the migration of both cell types was compromised (Figs. 7 and 8). Fn regulates the fusion of bilateral cardiac primordia, and is therefore essential for the development of myocardial epithelia [41]; thus, *fn1* mutants have impaired cardiac function and consequently, reduced blood flow, which may cause the aberrant migration of chromaffin cells. Nevertheless, these cell clusters in *fn1* mutants were more dispersed than in *tnnt2a* morphants (Figure 7J), suggesting that the presence of Fn ensures that the microenvironment stimulates chromaffin cell migration prior to the onset of circulation. Trunk neural crest cells, from which the sympathochromaffin lineage is derived, migrate along the medial surface of each somite but not the somite boundary where Fn accumulates [60,61]. However, disrupted somite formation in the *fn1* mutant leads to the uncoupling of slow- and fast-twitch muscle fibers, and hence a

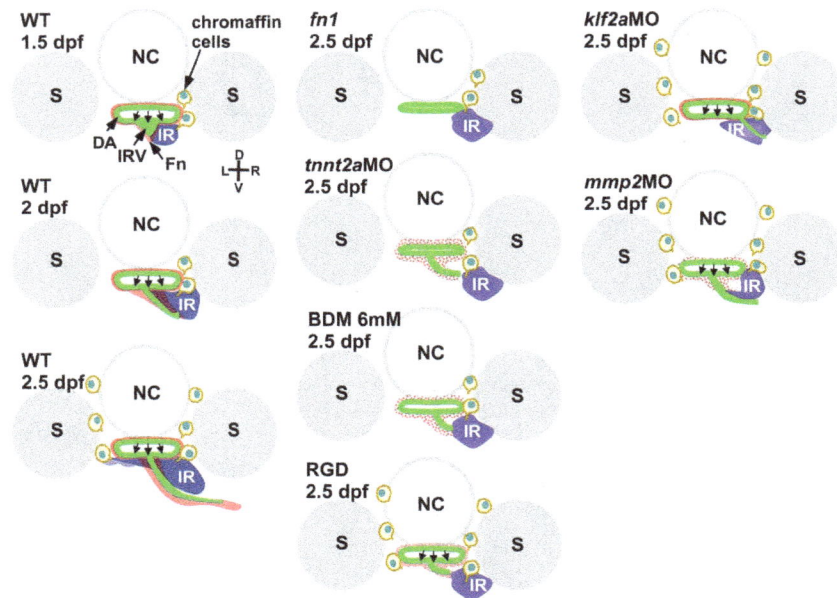

Figure 8. Schematic representation of interrenal steroidogenic tissue (IR) and chromaffin cell integration that takes place in the vicinity of the DA and extending IRV. An Fn-enriched microenvironment promotes medial extension of the steroidogenic tissue and culminates in steroidogenic-chromaffin interactions on both sides of the midline (left); various defects in extension lead to incomplete assembly of the interrenal organ (middle and right). D, dorsal; V, ventral; L, left; R, right. Abbreviations: notochord (NC). Somite (S).

disorganized myofibril pattern [62], which is another factor that could compromise chromaffin cell migration. In contrast, the RGD-treatment in this study was initiated at 26 hpf without evident perturbation of cardiac flow and somite morphology, which might explain why chomaffin cells migrate normally in RGD-treated embryos.

EMT is initiated by transforming, fibroblast, epithelial, and hepatocyte growth factors as well as the oncogene Harvey rat sarcoma. During this process, there is a downregulation of epithelial and concomitant upregulation of mesenchymal markers, while cells assume a proliferative and migratory character [35]. EMT is similar to the endothelial-to-mesenchymal transition (EnMT), a critical step in vertebrate heart development in which endothelial endocardial cells give rise to heart cushion cells that form the mesenchymal portion of septa and valves [63]. In various vertebrate models including zebrafish, alterations in hemodynamic forces during cardiogenesis have profound effects on cardiac septation and valvulogenesis [3,4,46,64], suggesting that EnMT is regulated by hemodynamics. The present study underscores a novel role for hemodynamics in the EMT-like behavior of vessel-associated endocrine cells via modulation of the vascular microenvironment and Fn-pFak signaling.

In addition to being an epithelial cell marker, β-Catenin also transduces canonical Wnt signals and is implicated in cell proliferation [65]. Cytoplasmic β-Catenin is stabilized upon activation of Wnt signaling, leading to its translocation to the nucleus, where it interacts with T-cell factors (TCFs) to stimulate the transcription of target genes. There was no obvious enrichment of nuclear β-Catenin detected in steroidogenic cells during interrenal organ assembly (Figure 6), and it is possible that canonical Wnt signaling is not involved in zebrafish interrenal development. Nevertheless, Wnt4 can inhibit β-Catenin/TCF signaling by redirecting nuclear β-Catenin to the membrane [66]. During mammalian sex differentiation, Wnt4 inhibits the migration of endothelial and steroidogenic cells into the female gonad

[67], and is also expressed in the outermost region of the adrenal cortex, where it may play a role in migration events that segregate adrenal and gonadal lineages during early development [68]. It therefore remains to be explored whether Wnt signals are directly or indirectly regulated by hemodynamic forces and thereby guide cell migration during interrenal organ assembly.

It will be of interest to explore whether other morphogens participate in the interrenal organogenesis. Pregnenolone, a steroid produced from cholesterol by the steroidogenic enzyme Cyp11a1, promotes cell migration by activating CLIP-170 and stabilizing microtubules [69,70]. The function of pregnenolone for cell movement has been well studied in the zebrafish gastrulation which is well before the onset of blood flow as well as interrenal organogenesis. While *cyp11a1* is expressed at the zebrafish interrenal tissue by 1 dpf [18], it remains unclear whether pregnelolone would also form a morphogen gradient during the interrenal morphogenetic movement. On the other hand, the molecular and cellular mechanisms by which blood flow regulates chromaffin cell migration remain to be explored. In the blood flow-deficient zebrafish embryo, the expression of endothelial CXCR4a is upregulated during collateral formation [71]. CXCR4a is the G protein-coupled receptor for the chemokine stromal cell-derived factor 1 (SDF-1). SDF-1, along with Bone Morphogenetic Proteins (BMPs) and Neuregulin 1 of the epidermal growth factor family, are the three groups of paracrine factors that participate in the generation of sympatho-adrenal progenitors from the neural crest [12,72,73,74]. BMPs are produced by the DA and are critical for the production of SDF-1 and Neuregulin 1 in the vicinity of the DA, while SDF-1 and Neuregulin 1 function as chemoattractants for the migration of neural crest cells [15]. It will therefore be intriguing to examine whether a loss of blood flow would influence the activity of SDF-1 through upregulating CXCR4a expression.

Supporting Information

Figure S1   Effect of norepinephrine on the heart beat of zebrafish. Norepinephrine treatments resulted in a dose-dependent increase of heart rate at 33 hpf. The difference between groups treated with various concentrations of norepinephrine was analyzed by Student's t-test. *$P<0.05$, ***$P<0.0005$.

Figure S2   Interrenal cell migration suppressed by 2,3-BDM was recovered following the removal of 2,3-BDM. The interrenl tissue stained by 3β-Hsd activity assay in the control *Tg(kdrl: GFP)*^{s843} embryo continued to extend across the midline from 2.5 dpf (A-A") to 3 dpf (C-C"), while migration of interrenal cells was repressed by 2,3-BDM treatment at 6 mM from 1.5 to 2.5 dpf (B-B") or 3 dpf (D-D"). Migration of interrenal cells was recovered at 3 dpf as 2,3-BDM was washed out at 2.5 dpf (E-E"). Protrusions of extending interrenal tissues (red arrows) were detected in control as well as recovered embryos. Broken white lines indicate position of the midline. Abbreviations: glomerulus (G), posterior cardinal vein (PCV). Scale bar, 50 μm.

Figure S3   Effects of blood flow inhibition on IRV growth was reversible following the removal of 2,3-BDM. The IRV in the control *Tg(kdrl: GFP)*^{s843} embryo continued to extend from 2.5 dpf (A, A') to 3 dpf (C, C'), while the IRV growth was repressed by 2,3-BDM treatment at 6 mM from 1.5 to 2.5 dpf (B, B') or 3 dpf (D, D'). Extension of IRV was recovered at 3 dpf as 2,3-BDM was washed out at 2.5 dpf (E, E'). The interrenal tissue (IR) was detected by 3β-Hsd acitivity assay. D, dorsal; V, ventral; L, left; R, right. Broken yellow lines indicate position of the midline. Abbreviations: notochord (NC), somite (S). Scale bar, 50 μm.

Figure S4   Effect of L-NAME on morphogenetic movements of interrenal steroidogenic tissue and IRV formation. (A–A") *Tg(kdrl: GFP)*^{s843} embryos treated with 100 μM L-NAME from 1.5 dpf onwards had interrenal steroidogenic tissue (IR) morphology (orange arrows) and (B–B") IRV length similar to control embryos (Figure 3A, A', D) at 2.5 dpf (n = 8). The activity of endothelial NO synthase was inhibited by L-NAME at concentrations higher than 10 μM [50]. D, dorsal; V, ventral; L, left; R, right. Abbreviations: posterior cardinal vein (PCV). Scale bar, 50 μm.

Figure S5   Effect of RGD treatment on pFAK distribution in the interrenal region. Transverse sections of *Tg(kdrl: GFP)*^{s843} embryos either untreated (control; n = 6) or treated with 100 μM RGD peptide (n = 10) from 26 hpf and harvested at 2.5 dpf for evaluation of 3β-Hsd activity and pFak level by IHC. Sections are shown of a representative embryo from each group, oriented with the dorsal side at the top. Abbreviations: interrenal tissue (IR), notochord (NC), somite (S).

Figure S6   Steroidogenic cells display a decrease of E-cadherin expression which is induced by hemodynamic forces and pFak signaling. E-cadherin in the fluorescent steroidogenic tissue of *Tg(ff1bEx2: GFP)* embryos was decreased from 2 dpf (A-A') to 2.5 dpf (B-B'). The decrease in E-cadherin was not observed in (C, C') *tnnt2a* morphants, (D, D') RGD-treated embryos, or (E, E') *klf2a* or (F, F') *mmp2* morphants. Sections are shown of a representative embryo from each treatment group. (F) Fluorescence intensity of E-cadherin in *ff1b*GFP-expressing steroidogenic tissue is normalized to the size of the cluster, with the number of embryos indicated in parenthesis. The difference between 2-dpf control group and any of the other groups was analyzed by Student's t-test. *$P<0.05$, **$P<0.005$, N.S., not significant. D, dorsal; V, ventral; L, left; R, right. Abbreviations: notochord (NC). Scale bar, 25 μm.

Figure S7   Steroidogenic cells display a rise of Vimentin expression which is induced by hemodynamic forces and pFak signaling. Vimentin in the steroidogenic tissue (marked by green fluorescence) of *Tg(ff1bEx2: GFP)* embryos was increased from 2 dpf (A-A') to 2.5 dpf (B-B'). The increase in Vimentin was not observed in (C, C') *tnnt2a* morphants, (D, D') RGD-treated embryos, or (E, E') *klf2a* or (F, F') *mmp2* morphants. Sections are shown of a representative embryo from each treatment group. (G) Fluorescence intensity of Vimentin in *ff1b*GFP-expressing steroidogenic tissue (ROI marked by orange lines) is normalized to the size of the cluster, with the number of embryos indicated in parenthesis. The difference between 2-dpf control group and any of the other groups was analyzed by Student's t-test. **$P<0.005$, N.S., not significant. D, dorsal; V, ventral; L, left; R, right. Abbreviations: notochord (NC). Scale bar, 25 μm.

Video S1   Complete blockage of blood flow in the posterior cardinal vein of a 36-hpf embryo treated with 6 mM 2,3-BDM.

Video S2   Normal blood flow in the posterior cardinal vein of a wild-type 36-hpf embryo.

Video S3   Partial reduction in blood flow in the posterior cardinal vein of a 36-hpf embryo treated with 2 mM 2,3-BDM.

Acknowledgments

The authors would like to thank Dr. Christoph Englert, Dr. Woon-Khiong Chan, and Prof. Didier Stainier for generously providing the zebrafish strains; Ru Shiangli, Jamie Lin, Yang Huang, Yusyuan Tian, Kuan-Chieh Wang and Hsin-Yu Hou for excellent technical assistance; Dr. Yi-Ching Lin for helpful advice on statistical analysis; and the Taiwan Zebrafish Core Facility, Zebrafish Core in Academia Sinica, and Zebrafish Core Facility at NTHU-NHRI (ZeTH) for assistance with fish culturing.

Author Contributions

Conceived and designed the experiments: YWL. Performed the experiments: CWC YLZ ZYJ YWL. Analyzed the data: CWC YLZ ZYJ YWL. Wrote the paper: YWL.

References

1. Culver JC, Dickinson ME (2010) The effects of hemodynamic force on embryonic development. Microcirculation 17: 164–178.
2. Pelster B, Burggren WW (1996) Disruption of hemoglobin oxygen transport does not impact oxygen-dependent physiological processes in developing embryos of zebra fish (Danio rerio). Circ Res 79: 358–362.
3. Vermot J, Forouhar AS, Liebling M, Wu D, Plummer D, et al. (2009) Reversing blood flows act through klf2a to ensure normal valvulogenesis in the developing heart. PLoS Biol 7: e1000246.

4. Hove JR, Koster RW, Forouhar AS, Acevedo-Bolton G, Fraser SE, et al. (2003) Intracardiac fluid forces are an essential epigenetic factor for embryonic cardiogenesis. Nature 421: 172–177.

5. Serluca FC, Drummond IA, Fishman MC (2002) Endothelial signaling in kidney morphogenesis: a role for hemodynamic forces. Curr Biol 12: 492–497.

6. Banjo T, Grajcarek J, Yoshino D, Osada H, Miyasaka KY, et al. (2013) Haemodynamically dependent valvulogenesis of zebrafish heart is mediated by flow-dependent expression of miR-21. Nat Commun 4: 1978.

7. Field HA, Dong PD, Beis D, Stainier DY (2003) Formation of the digestive system in zebrafish. II. Pancreas morphogenesis. Dev Biol 261: 197–208.

8. Field HA, Ober EA, Roeser T, Stainier DY (2003) Formation of the digestive system in zebrafish. I. Liver morphogenesis. Dev Biol 253: 279–290.

9. Liu YW, Guo L (2006) Endothelium is required for the promotion of interrenal morphogenetic movement during early zebrafish development. Dev Biol 297: 44–58.

10. Opitz R, Maquet E, Huisken J, Antonica F, Trubiroha A, et al. (2012) Transgenic zebrafish illuminate the dynamics of thyroid morphogenesis and its relationship to cardiovascular development. Dev Biol 372: 203–216.

11. Alt B, Elsalini OA, Schrumpf P, Haufs N, Lawson ND, et al. (2006) Arteries define the position of the thyroid gland during its developmental relocalisation. Development 133: 3797–3804.

12. Huber K (2006) The sympathoadrenal cell lineage: specification, diversification, and new perspectives. Dev Biol 298: 335–343.

13. Gut P, Huber K, Lohr J, Bruhl B, Oberle S, et al. (2005) Lack of an adrenal cortex in Sf1 mutant mice is compatible with the generation and differentiation of chromaffin cells. Development 132: 4611–4619.

14. Zubair M, Oka S, Parker KL, Morohashi K (2009) Transgenic expression of Ad4BP/SF-1 in fetal adrenal progenitor cells leads to ectopic adrenal formation. Mol Endocrinol 23: 1657–1667.

15. Saito D, Takase Y, Murai H, Takahashi Y (2012) The dorsal aorta initiates a molecular cascade that instructs sympatho-adrenal specification. Science 336: 1578–1581.

16. Hsu HJ, Lin G, Chung BC (2003) Parallel early development of zebrafish interrenal glands and pronephros: differential control by wt1 and ff1b. Development 130: 2107–2116.

17. Chai C, Liu YW, Chan WK (2003) Ff1b is required for the development of steroidogenic component of the zebrafish interrenal organ. Dev Biol 260: 226–244.

18. To TT, Hahner S, Nica G, Rohr KB, Hammerschmidt M, et al. (2007) Pituitary-interrenal interaction in zebrafish interrenal organ development. Mol Endocrinol 21: 472–485.

19. Chou CW, Chiu CH, Liu YW (2013) Fibronectin mediates correct positioning of the interrenal organ in zebrafish. Dev Dyn 242: 432–443.

20. Alsop D, Vijayan MM (2009) Molecular programming of the corticosteroid stress axis during zebrafish development. Comp Biochem Physiol A Mol Integr Physiol 153: 49–54.

21. Chiu CH, Chou CW, Takada S, Liu YW (2012) Development and fibronectin signaling requirements of the zebrafish interrenal vessel. PLoS One 7: e43040.

22. Parmar KM, Larman HB, Dai G, Zhang Y, Wang ET, et al. (2006) Integration of flow-dependent endothelial phenotypes by Kruppel-like factor 2. J Clin Invest 116: 49–58.

23. Dekker RJ, van Thienen JV, Rohlena J, de Jager SC, Elderkamp YW, et al. (2005) Endothelial KLF2 links local arterial shear stress levels to the expression of vascular tone-regulating genes. Am J Pathol 167: 609–618.

24. Lee JS, Yu Q, Shin JT, Sebzda E, Bertozzi C, et al. (2006) Klf2 is an essential regulator of vascular hemodynamic forces in vivo. Dev Cell 11: 845–857.

25. Page-McCaw A, Ewald AJ, Werb Z (2007) Matrix metalloproteinases and the regulation of tissue remodeling. Nat Rev Mol Cell Biol 8: 221–233.

26. Yasuda T, Kondo S, Homma T, Harris RC (1996) Regulation of extracellular matrix by mechanical stress in rat glomerular mesangial cells. J Clin Invest 98: 1991–2000.

27. Singhal PC, Sagar S, Garg P (1996) Simulated glomerular pressure modulates mesangial cell 72 kDa metalloproteinase activity. Connect Tissue Res 33: 257–263.

28. Cummins PM, von Offenberg Sweeney N, Killeen MT, Birney YA, Redmond EM, et al. (2007) Cyclic strain-mediated matrix metalloproteinase regulation within the vascular endothelium: a force to be reckoned with. Am J Physiol Heart Circ Physiol. pp. H28–42.

29. von Offenberg Sweeney N, Cummins PM, Birney YA, Cullen JP, Redmond EM, et al. (2004) Cyclic strain-mediated regulation of endothelial matrix metalloproteinase-2 expression and activity. Cardiovasc Res 63: 625–634.

30. Xu J, Rodriguez D, Petitclerc E, Kim JJ, Hangai M, et al. (2001) Proteolytic exposure of a cryptic site within collagen type IV is required for angiogenesis and tumor growth in vivo. J Cell Biol 154: 1069–1079.

31. Kenny HA, Kaur S, Coussens LM, Lengyel E (2008) The initial steps of ovarian cancer cell metastasis are mediated by MMP-2 cleavage of vitronectin and fibronectin. J Clin Invest 118: 1367–1379.

32. Corti P, Young S, Chen CY, Patrick MJ, Rochon ER, et al. (2011) Interaction between alk1 and blood flow in the development of arteriovenous malformations. Development 138: 1573–1582.

33. Santoro MM, Pesce G, Stainier DY (2009) Characterization of vascular mural cells during zebrafish development. Mech Dev 126: 638–649.

34. Miano JM, Georger MA, Rich A, De Mesy Bentley KL (2006) Ultrastructure of zebrafish dorsal aortic cells. Zebrafish 3: 455–463.

35. Acloque H, Adams MS, Fishwick K, Bronner-Fraser M, Nieto MA (2009) Epithelial-mesenchymal transitions: the importance of changing cell state in development and disease. J Clin Invest 119: 1438–1449.

36. Westerfield M (2000) The Zebrafish Book: Guide for the Laboratory Use of Zebrafish (Danio rerio). Eugene, OR.: Univ. of Oregon Press.

37. Kimmel CB, Ballard WW, Kimmel SR, Ullmann B, Schilling TF (1995) Stages of embryonic development of the zebrafish. Dev Dyn 203: 253–310.

38. Perner B, Englert C, Bollig F (2007) The Wilms tumor genes wt1a and wt1b control different steps during formation of the zebrafish pronephros. Dev Biol 309: 87–96.

39. Quek SI (2009) Molecular characterization of the zebrafish ff1b gene. Singapore: National University of Singapore.

40. Jin SW, Beis D, Mitchell T, Chen JN, Stainier DY (2005) Cellular and molecular analyses of vascular tube and lumen formation in zebrafish. Development 132: 5199–5209.

41. Trinh LA, Stainier DY (2004) Fibronectin regulates epithelial organization during myocardial migration in zebrafish. Dev Cell 6: 371–382.

42. Sehnert AJ, Huq A, Weinstein BM, Walker C, Fishman M, et al. (2002) Cardiac troponin T is essential in sarcomere assembly and cardiac contractility. Nat Genet 31: 106–110.

43. Nicoli S, Standley C, Walker P, Hurlstone A, Fogarty KE, et al. (2010) MicroRNA-mediated integration of haemodynamics and Vegf signalling during angiogenesis. Nature 464: 1196–1200.

44. Detry B, Erpicum C, Paupert J, Blacher S, Maillard C, et al. (2012) Matrix metalloproteinase-2 governs lymphatic vessel formation as an interstitial collagenase. Blood 119: 5048–5056.

45. Vasilyev A, Liu Y, Mudumana S, Mangos S, Lam PY, et al. (2009) Collective cell migration drives morphogenesis of the kidney nephron. PLoS Biol 7: e9.

46. Bartman T, Walsh EC, Wen KK, McKane M, Ren J, et al. (2004) Early myocardial function affects endocardial cushion development in zebrafish. PLoS Biol 2: E129.

47. Drummond IA, Majumdar A, Hentschel H, Elger M, Solnica-Krezel L, et al. (1998) Early development of the zebrafish pronephros and analysis of mutations affecting pronephric function. Development 125: 4655–4667.

48. Bollig F, Perner B, Besenbeck B, Kothe S, Ebert C, et al. (2009) A highly conserved retinoic acid responsive element controls wt1a expression in the zebrafish pronephros. Development 136: 2883–2892.

49. Wang L, Zhang P, Wei Y, Gao Y, Patient R, et al. (2011) A blood flow-dependent klf2a-NO signaling cascade is required for stabilization of hematopoietic stem cell programming in zebrafish embryos. Blood 118: 4102–4110.

50. North TE, Goessling W, Peeters M, Li P, Ceol C, et al. (2009) Hematopoietic stem cell development is dependent on blood flow. Cell 137: 736–748.

51. Watson O, Novodvorsky P, Gray C, Rothman AM, Lawrie A, et al. (2013) Blood flow suppresses vascular Notch signalling via dll4 and is required for angiogenesis in response to hypoxic signalling. Cardiovasc Res 100: 252–261.

52. Chou CW, Hsu HC, Quek SI, Chan WK, Liu YW (2010) Arterial and venous vessels are required for modulating developmental relocalization and laterality of the interrenal tissue in zebrafish. Dev Dyn 239: 1995–2004.

53. Park J, Schwarzbauer JE (2013) Mammary epithelial cell interactions with fibronectin stimulate epithelial-mesenchymal transition. Oncogene: doi: 10.1038/onc.2013.1118. [Epub ahead of print].

54. Sun XJ, Fa PP, Cui ZW, Xia Y, Sun L, et al. (2013) The EDA-containing cellular fibronectin induces epithelial mesenchymal transition in lung cancer cells through integrin alpha9beta1-mediated activation of PI3-K/Akt and Erk1/2. Carcinogenesis 35: 184–191.

55. Savagner P (2001) Leaving the neighborhood: molecular mechanisms involved during epithelial-mesenchymal transition. Bioessays 23: 912–923.

56. Cano A, Perez-Moreno MA, Rodrigo I, Locascio A, Blanco MJ, et al. (2000) The transcription factor snail controls epithelial-mesenchymal transitions by repressing E-cadherin expression. Nat Cell Biol 2: 76–83.

57. Moreno-Bueno G, Cubillo E, Sarrio D, Peinado H, Rodriguez-Pinilla SM, et al. (2006) Genetic profiling of epithelial cells expressing E-cadherin repressors reveals a distinct role for Snail, Slug, and E47 factors in epithelial-mesenchymal transition. Cancer Res 66: 9543–9556.

58. Mendez MG, Kojima S, Goldman RD (2010) Vimentin induces changes in cell shape, motility, and adhesion during the epithelial to mesenchymal transition. Faseb J 24: 1838–1851.

59. Vuoriluoto K, Haugen H, Kiviluoto S, Mpindi JP, Nevo J, et al. (2011) Vimentin regulates EMT induction by Slug and oncogenic H-Ras and migration by governing Axl expression in breast cancer. Oncogene 30: 1436–1448.

60. Koshida S, Kishimoto Y, Ustumi H, Shimizu T, Furutani-Seiki M, et al. (2005) Integrinalpha5-dependent fibronectin accumulation for maintenance of somite boundaries in zebrafish embryos. Dev Cell 8: 587–598.

61. Honjo Y, Eisen JS (2005) Slow muscle regulates the pattern of trunk neural crest migration in zebrafish. Development 132: 4461–4470.

62. Snow CJ, Peterson MT, Khalil A, Henry CA (2008) Muscle development is disrupted in zebrafish embryos deficient for fibronectin. Dev Dyn 237: 2542–2553.

63. Kovacic JC, Mercader N, Torres M, Boehm M, Fuster V (2012) Epithelial-to-mesenchymal and endothelial-to-mesenchymal transition: from cardiovascular development to disease. Circulation 125: 1795–1808.

64. Granados-Riveron JT, Brook JD (2012) The impact of mechanical forces in heart morphogenesis. Circ Cardiovasc Genet 5: 132–142.

65. Klaus A, Birchmeier W (2008) Wnt signalling and its impact on development and cancer. Nat Rev Cancer 8: 387–398.

66. Bernard P, Fleming A, Lacombe A, Harley VR, Vilain E (2008) Wnt4 inhibits beta-catenin/TCF signalling by redirecting beta-catenin to the cell membrane. Biol Cell 100: 167–177.

67. Jeays-Ward K, Hoyle C, Brennan J, Dandonneau M, Alldus G, et al. (2003) Endothelial and steroidogenic cell migration are regulated by WNT4 in the developing mammalian gonad. Development 130: 3663–3670.

68. Heikkila M, Peltoketo H, Leppaluoto J, Ilves M, Vuolteenaho O, et al. (2002) Wnt-4 deficiency alters mouse adrenal cortex function, reducing aldosterone production. Endocrinology 143: 4358–4365.

69. Weng JH, Liang MR, Chen CH, Tong SK, Huang TC, et al. (2013) Pregnenolone activates CLIP-170 to promote microtubule growth and cell migration. Nat Chem Biol 9: 636–642.

70. Hsu HJ, Liang MR, Chen CT, Chung BC (2006) Pregnenolone stabilizes microtubules and promotes zebrafish embryonic cell movement. Nature 439: 480–483.

71. Packham IM, Gray C, Heath PR, Hellewell PG, Ingham PW, et al. (2009) Microarray profiling reveals CXCR4a downregulated by blood flow in vivo and mediates collateral formation in zebrafish embryos. Physiol Genomics 38: 319–327.

72. Kasemeier-Kulesa JC, McLennan R, Romine MH, Kulesa PM, Lefcort F (2010) CXCR4 controls ventral migration of sympathetic precursor cells. J Neurosci 30: 13078–13088.

73. Britsch S, Li L, Kirchhoff S, Theuring F, Brinkmann V, et al. (1998) The ErbB2 and ErbB3 receptors and their ligand, neuregulin-1, are essential for development of the sympathetic nervous system. Genes Dev 12: 1825–1836.

74. Shah NM, Groves AK, Anderson DJ (1996) Alternative neural crest cell fates are instructively promoted by TGFbeta superfamily members. Cell 85: 331–343.

16

Lectin-Like Oxidized LDL Receptor-1 Is an Enhancer of Tumor Angiogenesis in Human Prostate Cancer Cells

Iván González-Chavarría[1], Rita P. Cerro[1], Natalie P. Parra[1], Felipe A. Sandoval[1], Felipe A. Zuñiga[2], Valeska A. Omazábal[3], Liliana I. Lamperti[2], Silvana P. Jiménez[1], Edelmira A. Fernandez[1], Nicolas A. Gutiérrez[1], Federico S. Rodriguez[1], Sergio A. Onate[4], Oliberto Sánchez[5], Juan C. Vera[1], Jorge R. Toledo[1]*

1 Biotechnology and Biopharmaceuticals Laboratory, Department of Pathophysiology, School of Biological Sciences, Universidad de Concepción, Concepción, Chile, 2 Department of Clinical Biochemistry and Immunology, School of Pharmacy, Universidad de Concepción, Concepción, Chile, 3 Department of Basic Sciences, Faculty of Medicine, Universidad Católica de la Santísima Concepción, Concepción, Chile, 4 Translational Research Unit, School of Medicine, Universidad de Concepción, Concepción, Chile, 5 Department of Pharmacology, School of Biological Sciences, Universidad de Concepción, Concepción, Chile

Abstract

Altered expression and function of lectin-like oxidized low-density lipoprotein receptor-1 (LOX-1) has been associated with several diseases such as endothelial dysfunction, atherosclerosis and obesity. In these pathologies, oxLDL/LOX-1 activates signaling pathways that promote cell proliferation, cell motility and angiogenesis. Recent studies have indicated that *olr*1 mRNA is over-expressed in stage III and IV of human prostatic adenocarcinomas. However, the function of LOX-1 in prostate cancer angiogenesis remains to be determined. Our aim was to analyze the contribution of oxLDL and LOX-1 to tumor angiogenesis using C4-2 prostate cancer cells. We analyzed the expression of pro-angiogenic molecules and angiogenesis on prostate cancer tumor xenografts, using prostate cancer cell models with overexpression or knockdown of LOX-1 receptor. Our results demonstrate that the activation of LOX-1 using oxLDL increases cell proliferation, and the expression of the pro-angiogenic molecules VEGF, MMP-2, and MMP-9 in a dose-dependent manner. Noticeably, these effects were prevented in the C4-2 prostate cancer model when LOX-1 expression was knocked down. The angiogenic effect of LOX-1 activated with oxLDL was further demonstrated using the aortic ring assay and the xenograft model of tumor growth on chorioallantoic membrane of chicken embryos. Consequently, we propose that LOX-1 activation by oxLDL is an important event that enhances tumor angiogenesis in human prostate cancer cells.

Editor: Salvatore V. Pizzo, Duke University Medical Center, United States of America

Funding: This research was supported by Fondecyt Grant 1121159, Conicyt, Chile. The funders had no role in study design, data collection and analysis, decision to publish, or preparation of the manuscript.

Competing Interests: The authors have declared that no competing interests exist.

* Email: jotoledo@udec.cl

Introduction

Lectin-like oxidized low-density lipoprotein receptor-1 (LOX-1) is a member of the scavenger receptor family [1], which mediates the recognition and internalization of oxidized LDL (ox-LDL) [2]. LOX-1 is mainly expressed in endothelial cells, although this receptor can also be found in many other cell types such as monocytes, cardiomiocytes, adipocytes, platelets, macrophages and vascular smooth muscle cells [3]. The altered expression and function of LOX-1 receptor has been associated with diseases such as endothelial dysfunction, atherosclerosis, obesity, and recently also with tumor development [4–6]. The activation of LOX-1 by oxLDL in human endothelial cells induces expression of adhesion molecules; pro inflammatory signaling pathways; and pro-angiogenic proteins, such as metalloproteinase-2 and 9 (MMP-2 and MMP-9), angiotensin II (Ang II) and vascular endothelial growth factor (VEGF) [7–10]. Angiogenesis is a physiological process, which determines the formation of new blood vessels from preexisting vessels [11]. It is considered a normal phenomenon during embryonic development, growth of the organism and wound healing [12]. However, the angiogenesis is also a

fundamental process for the development and progression of several types of tumors [13]. Tumor angiogenesis is regulated by the balance between pro- and anti-angiogenic molecules released by tumor cells and tumor stromal cells such as fibroblasts and macrophages, which determine the switch-on of tumor angiogenesis [14,15]. The gene expression in tumor angiogenesis is further regulated in response to several stimuli, including hypoxia, oxidative stress and inflammation. In this connection between stimuli and pro-angiogenic protein expression, VEGF has been identified as a major factor in tumor angiogenesis [16,17]. Hypoxia, cytokine secretion and oxidative stress in tumor cells increase the expression of VEGF, thus inducing tumor angiogenesis [18].

LOX-1 has been suggested as a possible link between obesity, dyslipidemia, and cancer [19]. Consistently, clinical conditions of obesity and atherosclerosis have been associated to tumor progression and metastasis in prostate cancer [20–22]. Patients diagnosed with metabolic syndrome, chronic inflammatory diseases and autoimmune conditions showed a high incidence and aggressiveness in tumor development [23]. Indeed, recent studies have shown an increased expression of LOX-1 in human prostate adenocarcinomas at stages III and IV [5], which require new vascularization and angiogenesis for local invasion. However, the specific effect of LOX-1 in tumor angiogenesis has not yet been described.

This work demonstrates that LOX-1 and its activation using oxLDL induce tumor angiogenesis and stimulate cell proliferation in prostate cancer cells. Specifically, we demonstrate that the activation of LOX-1 using oxLDL promotes cell proliferation, and the expression of pro-angiogenic molecules VEGF, MMP-2, and MMP-9 in a dose-dependent manner. Notably, these effects were prevented in the C4-2 prostate cancer model when LOX-1 expression was knocked down. Furthermore, the angiogenic effect of LOX-1 activated by oxLDL was demonstrated using the aortic ring assay and the xenograft model of tumor growth on chorioallantoic membranes (CAM) of chicken embryos. Therefore, we propose that LOX-1 activation by oxLDL is a relevant activation pathway required for the angiogenic enhancement of tumor development of human prostate cancer cells.

Results

Generation of prostate cancer cell lines overexpressing LOX-1 and shRNA against olr1

The C4-2 prostate cancer cell lines were transduced with the lentiviral expression vector LvCW-LOX-1, encoding the *olr1* gene under the control of the cytomegalovirus promoter (CMVP), and isolated using the limiting dilution cloning method. Overexpression of LOX-1 in C4-2 cells was determined using real-time PCR, immunoblotting, and immunofluorescence. Seven different clones with LOX-1 overexpression were obtained, out of these, 3 clones were selected after Western blot experiments and analyzed using real-time PCR (Fig. 1A and D). The selected cell clone C4-2/LOX-1(+) (clone 5) had an 1.2×10^3 fold expression over basal LOX-1 mRNA levels of the native C4-2 cell line or the C4-2/GFP overexpression control. In addition, LOX-1 overexpression in this clone was immunolocalized in the cell membrane using confocal microscopy (Fig. 1F). To determine whether overexpression mediated by lentiviral particles had an effect on the expression of LOX-1, an overexpression control (C4-2/GFP cells) was generated. We did not observed significant changes in the expression of LOX-1 in this control compared with the native C4-2 cell line (Fig. 1C and F).

The LOX-1 knockdown in C4-2 cells was achieved using a shRNA against the mRNA encoded by the *olr1* gene. C4-2 cells were transduced with lentiviral vectors for the expression of each shRNA (LvW-U6/*olr1*) sequence against *olr1* under the control of the U6 promoter. The transduced cells were isolated using the limiting dilution cloning method, and LOX-1 down-expression was analyzed using real-time PCR, immunoblotting, and immunofluorescence (Fig. 1). Two different shRNA sequences, shRNA-A and shRNA-B, were analyzed. Three different clones of shRNA-A and shRNA-B LOX-1 knockdown were obtained. The selected shRNA-B clone decreased LOX-1 expression by 98%, compared with basal LOX-1 mRNA levels of the native C4-2 cell line or the C4-2/LvEmpty knockdown control cell line (Fig. 1B–E). Furthermore, the down-expression of LOX-1 in this clone was verified by immunohistochemistry (Fig. 1F). To determine whether the knockdown mediated by lentiviral particles had an effect on the expression of LOX-1 a knockdown control (C4-2/LvEmpty) was generated. We did not observe significant changes in the expression of LOX-1 in this control compared with the native C4-2 cell line (Fig. 1C and F).

The prostate cancer cell models obtained, namely C4-2/LOX-1(+) [clone 5], C4-2/LOX-1(−) [clone shRNA-B1] and native C4-

2 cell line, were used as models in all assays performed in this work.

oxLDL has not cytotoxicity effects in prostate cancer cell models

Starting from the oxidation of native LDL from normolipemic patient we obtained a fraction of medium level oxidized LDL (oxLDL) which was checked by generation of conjugated dienes and sodium borate buffer electrophoresis in 1% agarose (Fig. 2A). To determine whether the oxLDL obtained had some cytotoxic effect we incubated the prostate cancer cell models with oxLDL (25 to 150 µg/mL) during 12 hours. Our results showed no cytotoxic effects of oxLDL on any of the prostate cell models for the range of concentrations assayed (Fig. 2B). However, we observed a significant increase in cell proliferation of C4-2, C4-2/GFP, C4-2/LvEmpty and C4-2/LOX-1(+) cellular models for all oxLDL concentrations used, compared to the same untreated prostate cancer cell models. Moreover, a significant increase in cell proliferation was observed in C4-2/LOX-1(+) compared with the C4-2, or the overexpression and knockdown controls for all oxLDL concentrations analyzed. However, the proliferative effect was totally prevented in the C4-2/LOX-1(−) cell model, over all concentrations analyzed (Fig. 2B).

The oxLDL ligand increases the expression of pro-angiogenic markers

The prostate cancer C4-2 cell line was incubated with increasing concentrations of oxLDL (25, 50, 100 µg/mL) during 12 hours, and the expression of the pro-angiogenic markers VEGF, MMP-2 and MMP-9 was analyzed using real-time PCR. Our results showed a significant increase in the expression of VEGF, MMP-2 and MMP-9, proportional to the oxLDL concentrations used, with a respective 3.5-, 2.5-, and 3-fold increase, when 100 µg/mL of oxLDL was used. Moreover, LOX-1 expression was also proportionally increased with the concentrations of oxLDL used, showing a 3-fold increase at 100 µg/mL (Fig. 3).

Increased expression of pro-angiogenic markers in prostate cancer cells requires activation of LOX-1 by oxLDL

The prostate cancer cells models C4-2/LOX-1(−) and C4-2/LOX-1(+) were incubated with 100 µg/mL oxLDL during 12 hours, and expression of the pro-angiogenic markers (VEGF, MMP-2 and, MMP-9) was analyzed. Expression of VEGF, MMP-2 and, MMP-9 in the C4-2 cell line incubated with oxLDL increased significantly (2-, 2-, and 2.5-fold, respectively), compared with untreated C4-2 cells (Fig. 4A). Interestingly, the expression of pro-angiogenic markers induced by oxLDL, was prevented in the C4-2/LOX-1(−) prostate cancer cell model. On the other hand, the stimulation of C4-2/LOX-1(+) with oxLDL significantly increased the expression of all pro-angiogenic markers analyzed (VEGF and MMP-2, 2-fold; MMP-9 3-fold), compared with untreated C4-2 cells. The expression of VEGF, MMP-2, and MMP-9 in C4-2/LOX-1(+) cells was also significantly increased (1.6-, 1.5-, and 1.4-fold, respectively), even in the absence of oxLDL stimulation, and decreased by 20%, 50%, and 20% in C4-2/LOX-1(−) cells, compared with the endogenous expression in the C4-2 cell line without oxLDL stimulation (Fig. 4A).

The conditioned media from prostate cancer cell models incubated with oxLDL [100 µg/mL] were collected and concentrated. Later VEGF expression was evaluated by immunoblotting, and the activity of MMP-2 and MMP-9 was analyzed by

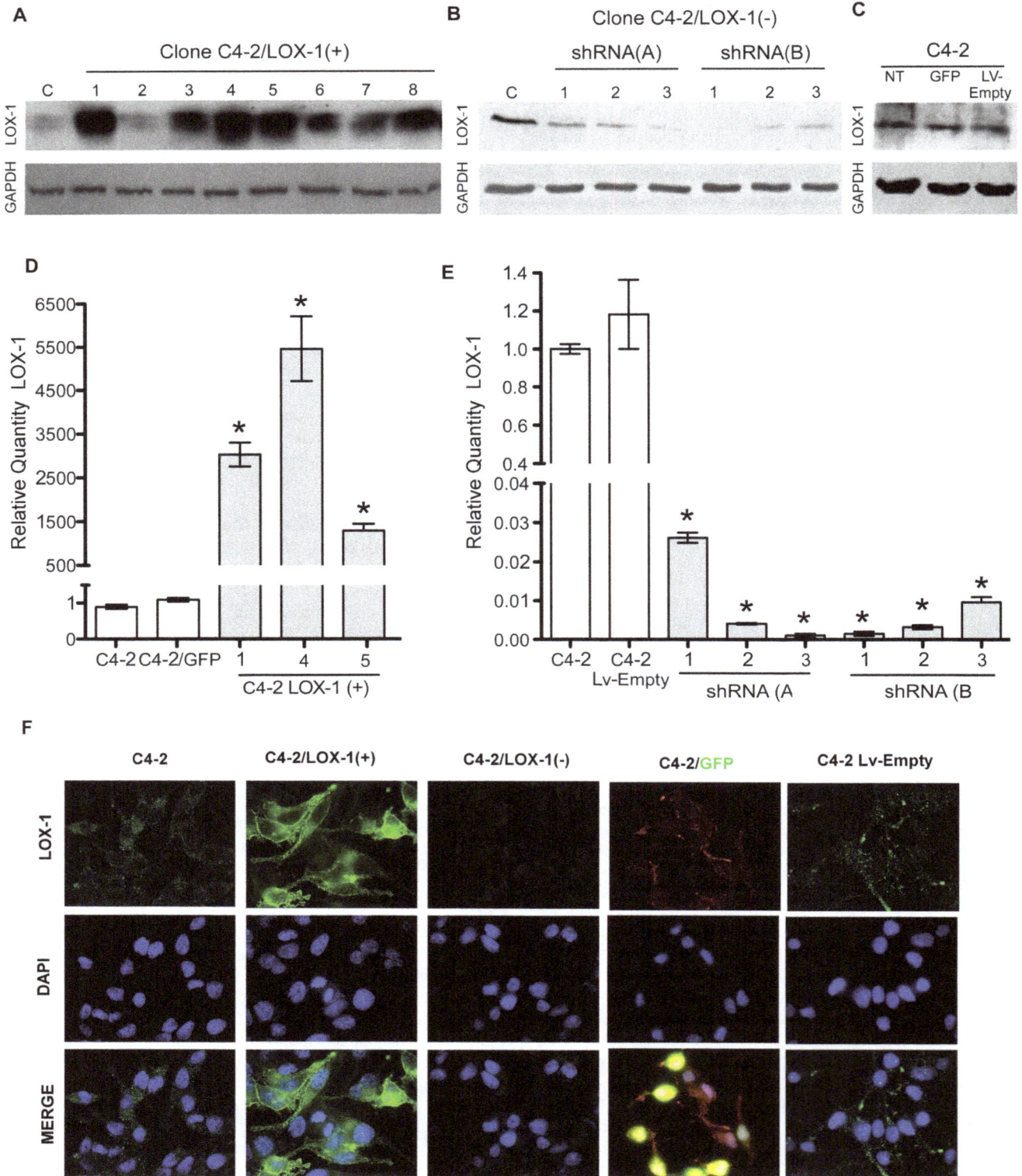

Figure 1. Generation of stable prostate cancer cell lines with LOX-1 over-expression and shRNA against *olr1*. A) Western blot for LOX-1 (40 kDa) expression in human CaP clones with overexpression of LOX-1. **B)** Western blot for LOX-1 (40 kDa) expression in human prostate cancer cell clones with LOX-1 knockdown **C)** Real-time PCR for LOX-1 expression in three clones with overexpression of LOX-1. **D)** Real-time PCR for LOX-1 expression was determined in three clones that express shRNA/LOX-1(A), and three clones that express shRNA/LOX-1(B). The data represent the means ± S.D. of three independent experiments performed in triplicate, and statistically analyzed using one-way analysis of variance and Dunnett's post-test; (***$p \leq 0.001$, **$p \leq 0.01$, *$p \leq 0.05$).

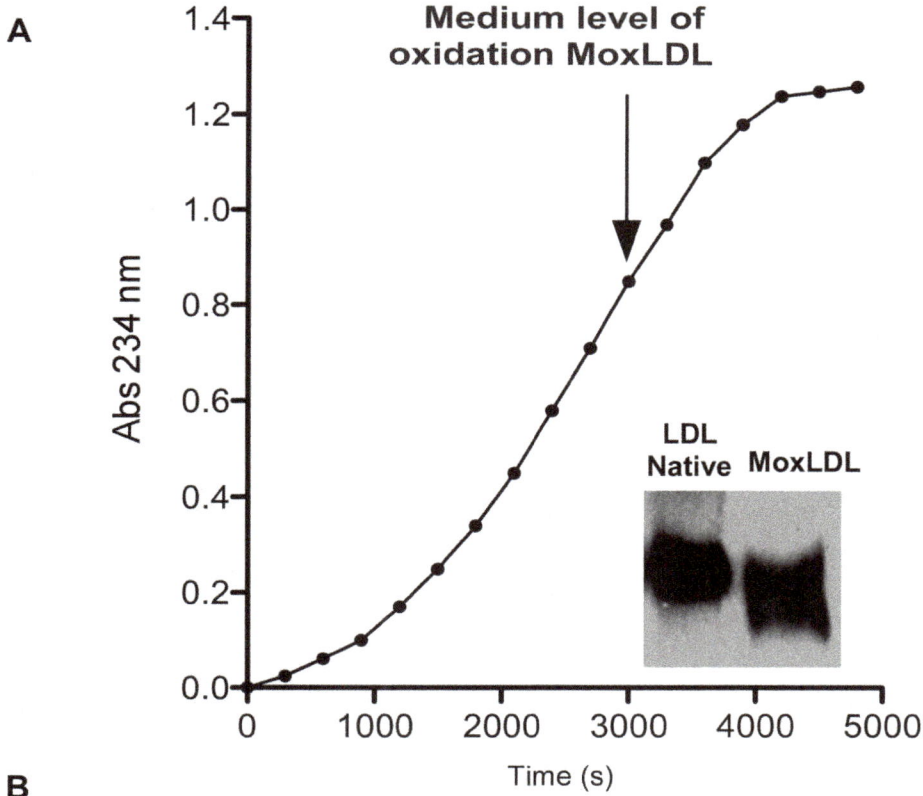

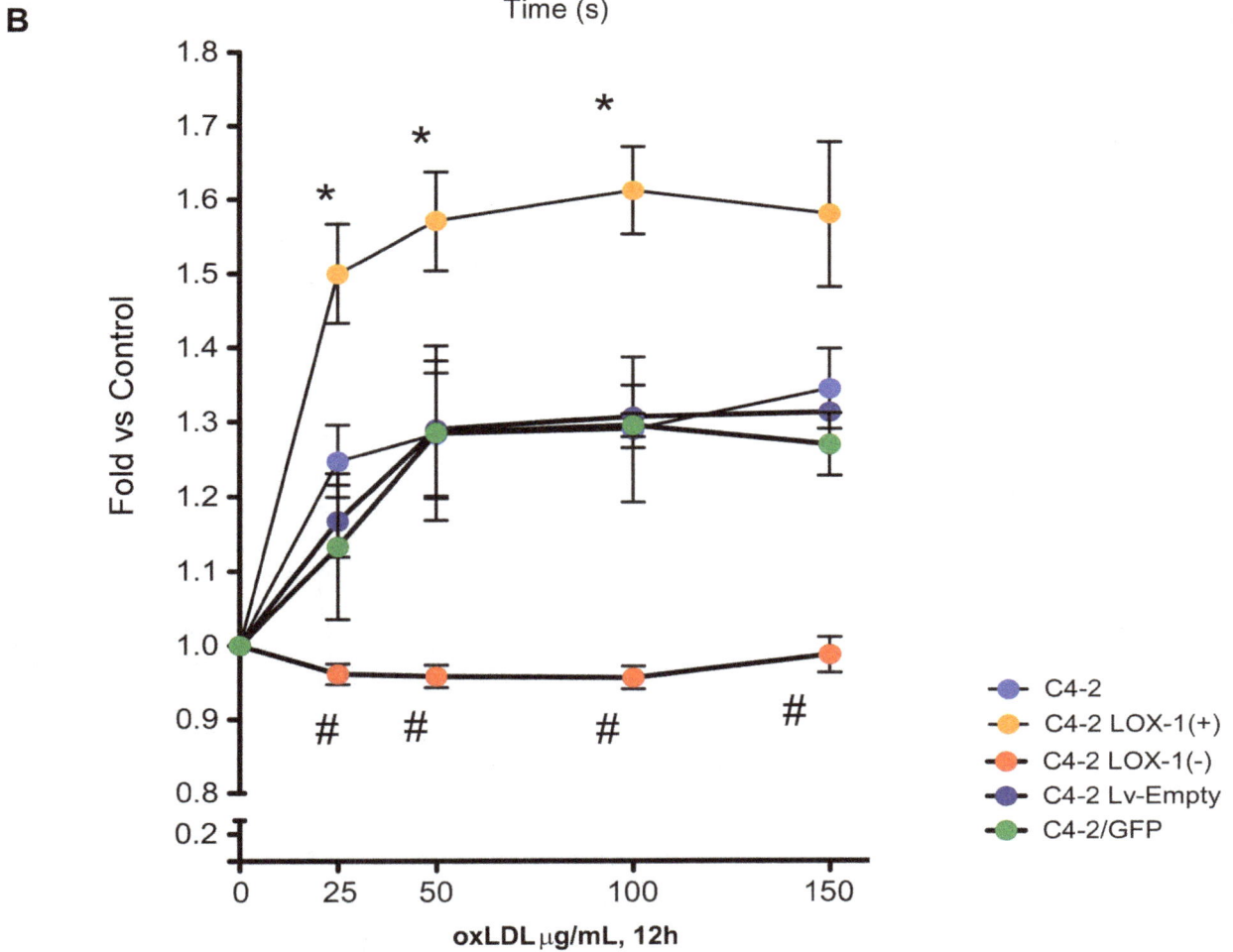

Figure 2. oxLDL characterization and citotoxicity assay. A) oxLDL obtained from human plasma was oxidized with 7 uM of $CuSO_4$, monitored by spectrophotometry at λ 243 nm and electrophoresed in 1% agarose gels with sodium borate buffer. **B)** Cytotoxicity assay of prostate cancer cell models treated with 25, 50, and 100 µg/mL oxLDL during 12 hours. The data represent the means $\pm$ S.D. of three independent experiments performed in triplicate and statistically analyzed using one-way ANOVA and Dunnett's post-test (* or # $p \leq 0.05$).

zymography. Our results indicted that VEGF expression was increased in C4-2 cells incubated with oxLDL, when comparing with C4-2 cells without oxLDL, whereas the expression of VEGF was prevented in C4-2/LOX-1(–) cells incubated with oxLDL [100 µg/mL]. Moreover, VEGF expression was increased in C4-2/LOX-1(+) cells with o without oxLDL treatment (Fig. 3B). Analysis of metalloproteinase activity showed an increment in the gelatinase activity of MMP-2 and MMP-9 in the conditioned medium from C4-2 cells incubated with oxLDL, and was prevented in conditioned medium from C4-2/LOX-1(–) cells incubated with oxLDL. Furthermore, LOX-1 overexpression in C4-2/LOX-1(+) cells showed an increased activity of MMP-2 and MMP-9 with or without oxLDL stimulation (Fig. 4C).

Activation of LOX-1 by oxLDL promotes the generation of sprout in mouse aortic rings

We analyzed C4-2 model cells incubated with oxLDL to determine whether the generation of endothelial sprouts could be stimulated in the aortic ring assay by the differential secretion of pro-angiogenic markers. The C4-2, C4-2/LOX-1(–) and C4-2/LOX-1(+) cell models were incubated with 100 µg/mL of oxLDL during 12 hours, and the conditioned media was collected, concentrated and used for the treatment of mouse aortic rings.

The stimulation of aortic rings with conditioned media from C4-2 and C4-2/LOX-1(+) cells treated with oxLDL significantly enhanced the generation of sprouts compared to the untreated C4-2 cell line. However, the differences between aortic ring sprout generation using conditioned media from C4-2/LOX-1(–) with or without oxLDL stimulation, were not significant. Thus, over-expression of LOX-1 promoted sprouts generation with or without oxLDL stimulation (Fig. 5A).

Activation of LOX-1 by oxLDL promotes angiogenesis in prostate cancer cell xenografts on chorioallantoic membrane of chicken embryos

For angiogenesis studies on chorioallantoic membrane (CAM) of chicken embryos, prostate cancer cell clones C4-2, C4-2/LOX-1(–), and C4-2 LOX-1(+) were pre-incubated with oxLDL 100 µg/mL for 2 hours. Approximately 1×10^6 cells were then inoculated on CAM of 10-days-old chicken embryos. Five days after inoculation, tumors were extracted from the CAMs and the extent of tumor vascularization was analyzed. C4-2 cells pre-incubated with oxLDL showed a significant increase of tumor vascularization compared with the untreated C4-2 cells. Further, LOX-1 overexpression in C4-2/LOX-1(+) cells also showed an increased tumor vascularization when the cells were incubated with or without oxLDL compared to the untreated C4-2 cells. Notably, C4-2/LOX-1(–) cells treated with oxLDL did not show significant variations in tumor vascularization, compared with both C4-2 and C4-2/LOX-1(–) untreated cells (Fig. 5B).

The *olr1* gene is overexpressed in public array datasets from metastatic prostate cancer

With the aim to determine if the observed effects on tumor angiogenesis mediated by oxLDL/LOX-1 in C4-2 prostate cancer cells had any clinical relevance in patients, we used NCBI Gene Expression Omnibus (GEO) database to determine the expression of *olr1* receptor in the GDS2545 dataset, which has different stages of prostate cancer progression. This data allows the comparative analysis of human metastatic prostate tumors, primary prostate tumors and normal donor tissue. In this context, the expression of *olr-1* was found to be significantly increased in primary prostate tumors and metastatic prostate tumors compared with normal prostate tissue (Fig. 6).

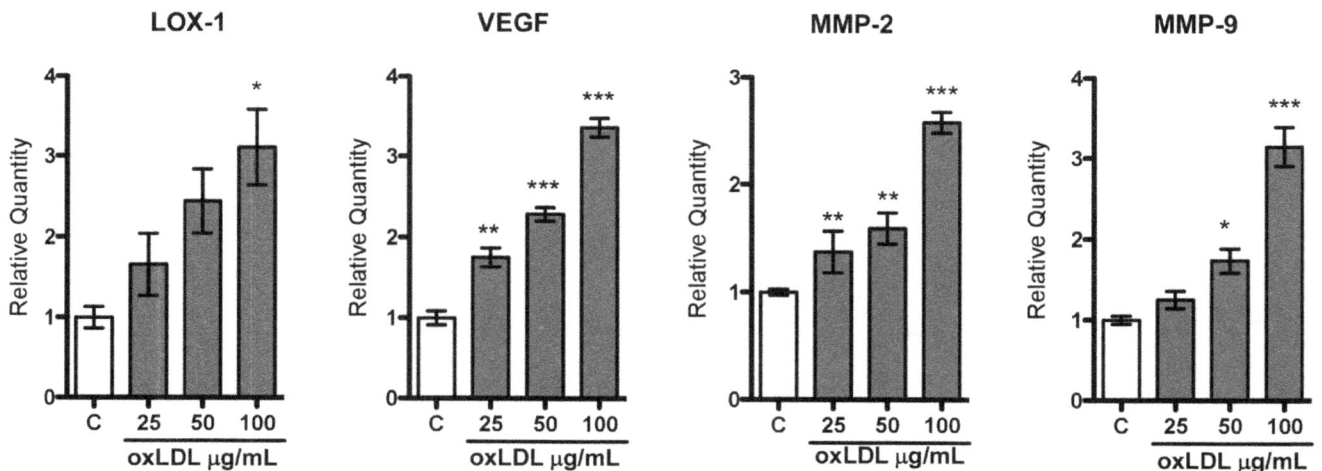

Figure 3. The oxLDL ligand increases the expression of pro-angiogenic markers. Relative quantification of LOX-1, VEGF, MMP-2, and MMP-9 expression was performed using real-time PCR in human prostate cancer cell line C4-2 incubated with increasing concentration of oxLDL (25, 50, 100 µg/mL) for 12 hours. The data represent mean $\pm$ S.D. of three independent experiments performed in triplicate, and statistically analyzed using one-way analysis of variance and Dunnet post-test; (***$p \leq 0.001$, **$p \leq 0.01$, *$p \leq 0.05$).

A

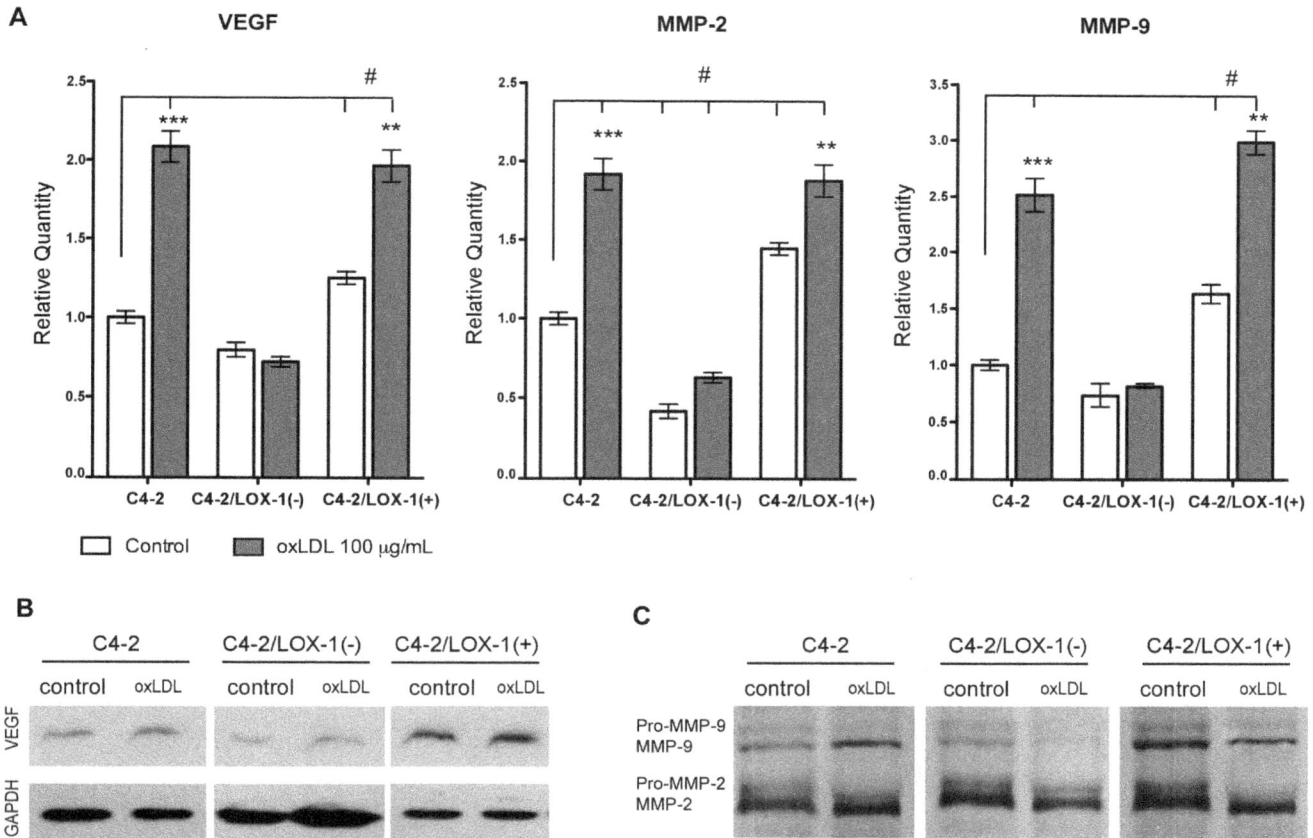

Figure 4. Activation of LOX-1 by oxLDL increases the expression of pro-angiogenic markers. C4-2, C4-2/LOX-1(−), and C4-2 LOX-1(+) human prostate cancer cell models were incubated in the with or without oxLDL [100 µg/mL] for 12 hours. **A)** Relative quantification of VEGF, MMP-2, and MMP-9 expression was analyzed using real-time PCR. The data represent the means ± S.D. of three independent experiments performed in triplicate and statistically analyzed using one-way analysis of variance and Dunnet post-test; (***$p \leq 0.001$, **$p \leq 0.01$, *$p \leq 0.05$). **B)** Western blot for VEGF expression (30 kDa). **C)** Zymogram for MMP-2 (72 kDa pro-form; 64 kDa active-form) and MMP-9 (92 kDa pro-form; 84 kDa active-form) activities in conditioned medium.

Discussion

In this work we demonstrate, for the first time, the role of the LOX-1 receptor and its activation using oxLDL, on the proliferation and angiogenesis of human C4-2 prostate cancer cells. Specifically, we demonstrate that an increase in oxLDL concentrations promoted cell proliferation and significantly and proportionally increases the expression of the pro-angiogenic markers VEGF, and the metalloproteinases MMP-2 and MMP-9. In addition, cellular stimulation of LOX-1 with oxLDL also increased the expression of the LOX-1 receptor, generating a positive feedback-loop of LOX-1 expression.

The association of LOX-1 and oxLDL with diseases, such as endothelial dysfunction, atherosclerosis, acute myocardial infarction, stroke, diabetes, hypertension, metabolic syndrome and obesity, has been extensively studied [3,5,24]. Obesity, itself, has also been associated as an important risk factor for atherosclerosis, type 2 diabetes mellitus and cancer, as well as other diseases [25]. Clinical studies suggest an association between high serum oxLDL concentrations and an increased risk of developing colon cancer [26]. Furthermore, oxLDL concentrations have also been shown to increase in obese patients [27].

Consistent with these findings, previous reports had shown that obesity is associated with an increased risk for developing highly malignant and metastatic prostate cancer [21,28]. Moreover, in

the Transgenic Adenocarcinoma of the Mouse Prostate (TRAMP) mouse model, feeding of the mice with an hypercaloric diet, increases the histological grade of the prostate tumors, the number of metastases, tumor mass, and the degree of vascularization, as compared to TRAMP mice fed with normal diet [29].

There is a special relevance in the relationship between cholesterol and prostate cancer, because androgen and other steroid hormones are synthesized from cholesterol, and are fundamental in the development and maintenance of prostate cancer [30]. Under physiological conditions androgens are involved in the acquisition of secondary sexual characteristics, growth and normal development of the prostate. However, they have also been associated with tumor progression in prostate cancer [31]. Thus, many of the prostate cancers refractory to androgen deprivation, increase cholesterol uptake, which is the primary substrate for androgen synthesis [31,32]. In this respect, the major source of cholesterol for tumor cells is LDL, which is mainly endocyted by the LDL receptors (LDLR) [33,34]. However, we consider that the oxidant and pro-inflammatory tumor microenvironment rich in ROS [35] could be promoting LDL modification by lipoperoxidation [36], avoiding the recognition by LDLR and favoring its uptake by scavenger receptors of oxLDL. According to this, we analyzed the expression of scavengers receptors for modified lipoproteins and the expression

A

B

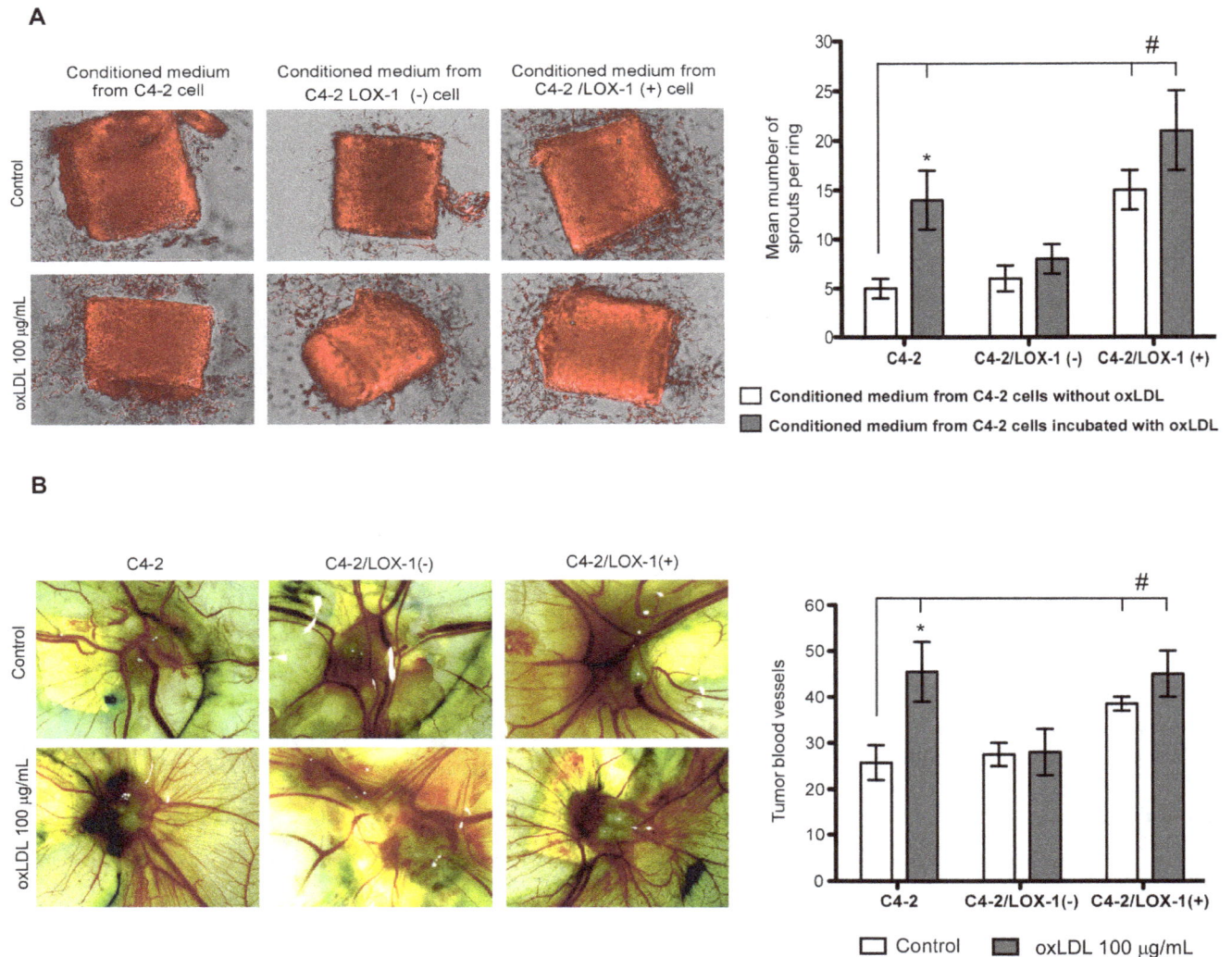

Figure 5. The activation of LOX-1 using oxLDL promotes the generation of sprouts in mouse aortic ring assays. A). Microphotography of mouse aortic rings and quantification of sprouts per ring incubated with conditioned medium from prostate cancer C4-2, C4-2/LOX-1(–), and C4-2 LOX-1(+) cells previously stimulated with or without oxLDL [100 µg/mL]. **B)** LOX-1 activation by oxLDL promotes tumor angiogenesis in CaP xenograft models on chorioallantoic membrane of chicken embryos. Microphotography and quantification of tumor blood vessels in xenografts of C4-2, C4-2/LOX-1(–), and C4-2 LOX-1(+) cells, previously incubated with or without oxLDL [100 µg/mL], in chorioallantoic membranes of 10-days-old chicken embryos. The data represent the means ± S.D. of three independent experiments performed in triplicate, and was statistically analyzed using one-way analysis of variance with Dunnett's post-test (***$p \leq 0.001$, **$p \leq 0.01$, *$p \leq 0.05$).

of the LDL receptor in the GDS2545 dataset, obtained from the public database (GEO profile) [37]. Therein, we observed a significant increase in the expression of the scavenger receptors *olr1, scarf* and *scarb1* in primary tumors and metastasis of prostate cancer, and a significant increase in the expression of the *CD36* and *olr1* receptor in prostate cancer metastasis compared to normal prostate tissue. Interestingly, the expression of LDLR showed a significant decrease in its expression in tumor metastasis and no significant difference was observed between primary prostate tumors and normal prostate tissue (data not shown).

Considering this, high concentrations of circulating LDL in obese patients with prostate cancer could contribute to tumor progression through LOX-1 activation by oxidation modified LDL (oxLDL) generated in the oxidant microenvironment, present in the prostate tumor stroma. In this respect, we generated a medium level oxidized LDL, which should be representative of

the oxLDL present in the tumor microenvironment. Our results demonstrated that the oxLDL used in this study has no cytotoxic effect in any of the C4-2 prostate cancer cells models assayed. In this regard, it has been reported that oxLDL has a differential cytotoxic effect depending on the cell type. Cancer cells lines K562/AO2 (Leukemia) and EC9706 (esophageal carcinoma) treated with oxLDL present a higher rate of cell viability compared whit non-tumor cells such as HUVEC (Human umbilical vein endothelial cells) [38].

Interestingly, we observed a significant increase in cell proliferation of the C4-2, C4-2/GFP, C4-2/LvEmpty and C4-2/LOX-1(+) cellular models, over the whole range of oxLDL concentrations assayed compared to the untreated cell lines. Also, the C4-2/LOX-1(+) cell model showed a higher proliferation compared with the control cells models C4-2, C4-2/GFP, and C4-2/LvEmpty, for all concentrations assayed. However, the prolif-

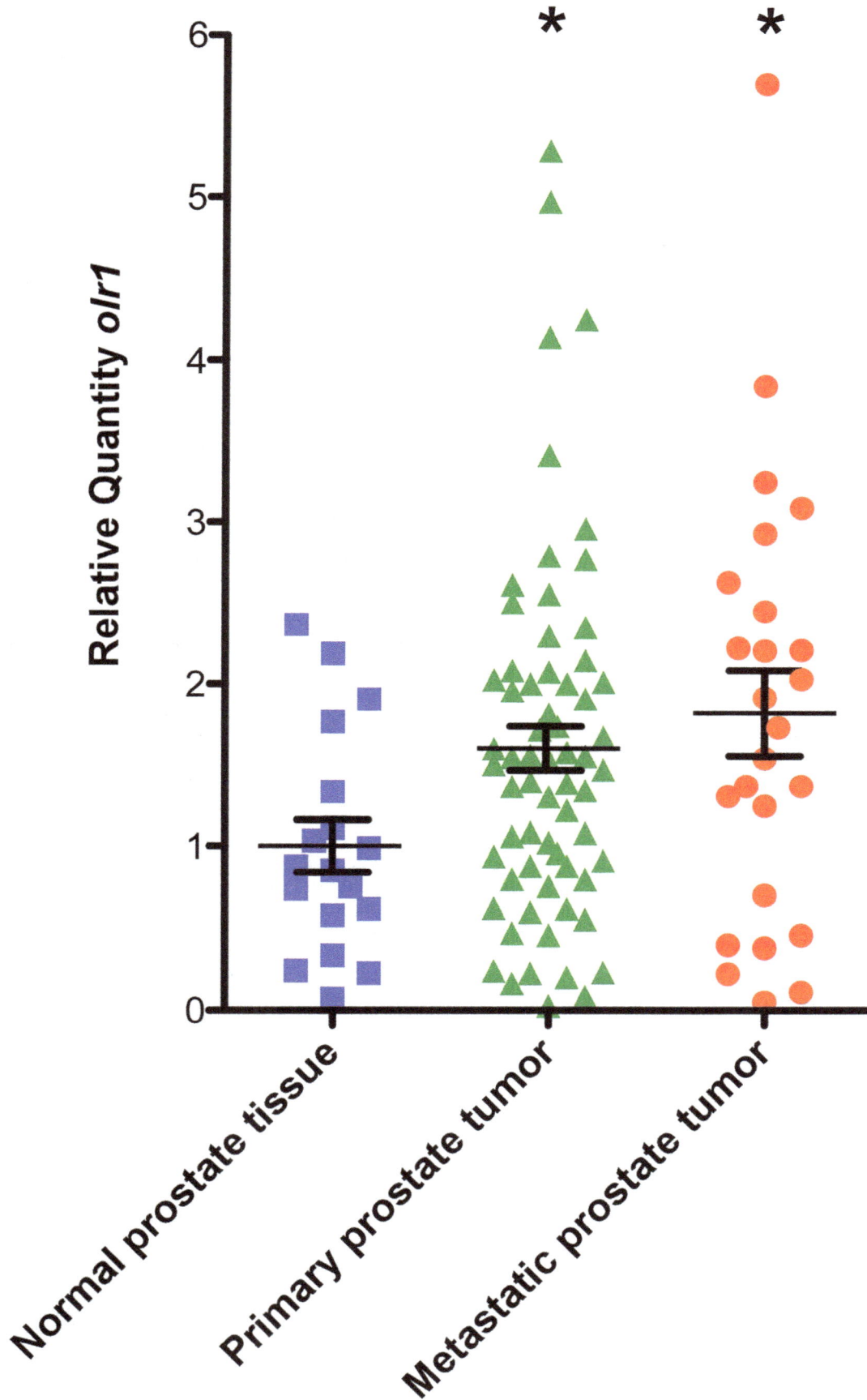

Figure 6. Analysis of *olr1* expression in prostate cancer progression using public databases arrays. The expression of *olr1* at different stages of prostate cancer tumor progression was determined using the public database GDS2545 at the NCBI Gene Expression Omnibus (GEO). The data represent the means ± S.E. of human normal donor tissue n = 17, primary prostate tumors n = 64 and metastatic prostate tumors n = 50, which were statistically analyzed using a *t* test (*p≤0.05).

erative effect of oxLDL was prevented in the C4-2/LOX-1(−) cell model, indicating that this effect is closely related to the activation of the LOX-1 receptor by oxLDL. In this sense, the proliferative effect promoted by oxLDL/LOX-1 has been described in muscle cells, endothelial cells and recently in breast cancer cells through activation pathways that involve p38 (MAPK), p44/42 MAPK, and NF-kB [6,39]. However, the proliferative effects on prostate cancer cells had not yet been described.

In vitro studies have shown that oxLDL stimulation of human umbilical vein endothelial cells (HUVECs) activates the expression of the LOX-1 receptor, generating an overexpression of adhesion molecules, inflammatory proteins, and the MMP-2 and MMP-9 metalloproteinases, [8,40,41]. Furthermore, endothelial cells from bovine aorta treated with ox-LDL promote capillary formation regulated by LOX-1, and the activation of NADPH oxidase/MAPKinase/NF-kappa B, with an increase in VEGF expression [9,42]. Our results demonstrated that the expression of VEGF, and the activation of MMP-2 and MMP-9, is closely mediated by oxLDL/LOX-1 in C4-2 prostate cancer cell line.

We also confirm, using the aortic ring assay and the chicken embryo CAM xenograft model, that the increase of VEGF, MMP-2 and MMP-9 expression mediated by LOX-1/oxLDL has a tumoral angiogenic effect both *in vivo* and *ex vivo* on C4-2 prostate cancer cells models. This is consistent with previous *ex vivo* studies, where pro-angiogenic factors like angiotensin II did not induce capillary sprout formation in aortic rings isolated from *olr-1 KO* mice [10]. Likewise, the ablation of the *olr-1* gene markedly decreased the choroidal neovascularization in murine models of laser-induced injury [43]. Signaling induced by oxLDL/LOX-1 could have a critical role in the process of tumor angiogenesis because microvessel density is an important prognostic indicator in prostate cancer, and is associated with clinical stage, progression, metastasis, and prostate cancer survival [44,45].

In conclusion, we demonstrate a direct relationship between obesity factors, such as LOX-1/oxLDL and the enhancement of expression of proliferation and pro-angiogenic markers, which have a biological effect in tumor angiogenesis *ex vivo* and *in vivo* in C4-2 prostate cancer cells models. Hence, we suggest that LOX-1 could be an essential regulator in prostate cancer cells, with the ability to enhance tumor angiogenesis towards malignancy and metastasis in obese patients.

Materials and Methods

Cell culture

Human C4-2 prostate cancer [46,47] and HEK-293 FT cells were grown in RPMI 1640 and DMEM medium respectively, supplemented with 2 mM of L-glutamine (Hyclone), 10% fetal bovine serum (FBS) and 1% penicillin streptomycin (GIBCO).

Animals

Male BALB/c mice were obtained from Harlan Winkelmann GmbH (Borchen, Germany) and housed under controlled and sterile ambient conditions. Four mice (8–12 weeks old) were used for the experiments.

Eggs of *Gallus gallus domesticus* were obtained from ISP (Instituto de Salud Pública, Chile), were washed with a 7 μM copper sulfate solution to prevent fungal contamination, and were

incubated at 37.5°C and 80% of relative humidity for 10 days. The eggs were flipped periodically with an automatic dual turner (GQF Hova-bator Manufacturing Co. USA) to prevent adhesion and rupture of the CAM from the eggshell. Embryos inoculated with the C4-2 cells models were incubated at 37.5°C, 80% humidity and 5% CO$_2$ for 5 days.

All the studies involving experimentation with animals were in accordance with the guidelines and recommendations of the NIH Guide for the Care and Use of Laboratory Animals (current edition) and followed the policies indicated in the Chilean Biosafety Manual of Conicyt (National Agency for Science and Technology). The experimental protocols were drafted by the authors and approved by the Institutional Ethics Committee. In all cases, supervision of veterinary authorities from the School of Biological Sciences, Universidad de Concepción, Chile, was guaranteed. When mice were used for experimentation, they were housed in individual rooms and appropriate feeding, water supply and health monitoring was permanently provided. Animals euthanized were humanly handled. They were subjected to initial anesthetization and potassium chloride injection intravenously to avoid suffering.

ox-LDL preparation

Blood samples (20 mL) were obtained from four volunteers, who signed a written consent. This protocol was approved by Ethics Committee of the Universidad de Concepción, Chile. Human LDL (1.019 to 1.063 g/mL) was isolated from the blood plasma of healthy human subjects by sequential ultracentrifugation at 4°C. LDL was dialyzed against filtered (0.45-μm) LDL buffer (150 mmol/L NaCl; 0.24 mmol/L EDTA; pH 7.4), changed thrice, for 36 hours at 4°C. After extensive dialysis against PBS, with 3 changes, for 36 hours at 4°C, oxidized LDL was prepared by incubating purified LDL with 7 μM CuSO$_4$ for 3 hours at 37°C. Modification of LDL was monitored by spectrophotometry through the generation of conjugated dienes at λ 243 nm, and then an electrophoresis in 1% agarose gel in sodium borate buffer was realized to determine the change in the electrophoretic migration of oxLDL compared with LDL. The gel was stained with 0.25% Coomassie Blue R-250, during 2 hours, and destained during 4 hours using 5% MeOH, 7.5% HOAC, 87.5% H$_2$O. The bands of LDL and oxLDL were analyzed with the Odyssey CLX instrument (LI-COR, EEUU).

Cytotoxicity evaluation

The prostate cancer cell models were incubated with 25, 50, and 100 μg/mL oxLDL during 12 hours. After that, the medium was removed, the cultures were washed with phosphate-buffered saline, and cell viability was measured incubating the cultures with 10 mg/ml of 3-(4,5-dimethylthiazol-2-yl)-2,5-diphenyl tetrazolium bromide (MTT) at 37°C for 30 min, and measuring absorbance at 570 nm in solubilized cells using a UV-visible SPECTROstar *Nano* spectrometer (BMG LABTECH, Germany).

Lentiviral vectors that express orl-1 or shRNA against olr1

The human LOX-1 sequence was sub-cloned into the lentiviral pLCW vector, generating the pLCW-LOX-1 construct. Further, a sequence coding for GFP was inserted in the pLCW vector, generating the pLGW plasmid.

To generate the pLU6W plasmid, the cytomegalovirus promoter (CMVP) was removed from the pLCW lentiviral vector, and in its place, an U6 promoter obtained from the retroviral plasmid pGFP-V-RS was inserted. The codifying shRNA sequences were purchased as oligos of 65 bases (IDT, Coralville, USA) and phosphorylated with polynucleotide kinase PNK (New Englad Biolabs, UK). For annealing, oligos were incubated at 95°C for 5 minutes, and left at 25°C during 1 hour. Hybridization of the shRNAs was analyzed by electrophoresis in 2% agarose gels. The double strand codifying shRNA sequences were cloned using *Xma*I and *Xho*I restriction sites into pLU6W, generating the pLU6W/shRNAolr1 (A and B variants).

Lentiviral vector production

Production of lentiviral particles was performed by co-transfection of HEK-293FT cells with the constructs generated (pLCW-LOX-1, pLGW, pLU6W or pLU6W/shRNA*olr1*,) and three helper plasmids: pLP1, pLP2 and pLP/VSVG (ViraPowerTM Lentiviral Expression System, Invitrogen-Life Technologies, USA). Forty-eight hours post-transfection, the culture media were collected, centrifuged at 3000 rpm for 10 minutes, and the supernatants filtered through 0.45 μm pore size membranes (Millipore). Later, the lentiviral particles (Lv-LOX-1, Lv-GFP, Lv-shRNA/*olr1* and Lv-Empty [derived from pLU6W plasmid]) were concentrated by ultracentrifugation at 25000 rpm (SW28 rotor) for 90 minutes. The supernatant was removed and the pellet was resuspended in 100 μL of culture medium. Finally, the lentiviral particles were collected, aliquoted and stored at −80°C until used.

Stable cell line generation for over-expression or knockdown of LOX-1

C4-2 cells were seeded into 96-well plates and cultured up to 80% confluence. Then, the cells were incubated with the lentiviral vectors Lv-LOX-1, Lv-GFP, Lv-shRNA/*olr1* or Lv-Empty, during 12 hours. After incubation, the culture medium was removed, and fresh RPMI medium supplemented with 10% FBS was added to the cells, which were cultured until confluence. The transduced cells, with each of the lentiviral vectors, were seeded into 96 wells by serial micro-dilution down to 1 cell per well. The cultures were maintained with RPMI-10% FBS to reach 100% confluence. Stable cell pools were established for [C4-2/LOX-1(+), C4-2/GFP, C4-2/LOX-1(−) and C4-2/Lv-Empty], and LOX-1 over-expression or knockdown was verified by Western blot, real-time PCR and immunohistochemistry.

Real-Time PCR

Total RNA was purified using TRIZOL (Sigma, USA). The PCR reaction was performed with the commercial kit KAPA SYBR FAST qPCR and the equipment for Stratagene MX3000P real-time PCR. The qPCR was performed using RNA as template, the primers were ordered from Integrated DNA Technologies (Coralville, USA), LOX-1 (sense 5′-AGATCCAGACTGT-GAAGGACCAGC-3′ and antisense 5′-CAGGCACCACCATG-GAGAGTAAAG-3′), VEGF (sense 5′-CTGCTCTACCTCCAC-CATGC-3 and antisense 5′-AGCTGCGCTGATAGACATCC-3′), MMP-2 (sense 5′-CCTATCTCAGGGTTAAAAGAGAG-3′

and antisense 5′-GCACAAACAGGTTGCAGCTC-3′), MMP9 (sense 5′-ACGCACGACGTCTTCCAGTA-3′ and antisense 5′-TTGGTCCACCTGGTTCAACTC-3′) and GAPDH (sense 5′-ACCCCTTCATTGACCTCAAC-3′ and antisense 5′-ATGA-CAAGCTTCCCGTTCTC-3′). The results were analyzed as CT relative quantification. The comparative threshold cycles values were normalized for GAPDH reference gene.

Immunodetection

Western blot and immunostaining were performed using standard protocols. Anti-LOX-1 polyclonal antibody was purchased from R&D Systems Inc. (Minneapolis, MN, USA), anti-VEGF and anti-GAPDH antibodies were obtained from Santa Cruz Biotechnology (Santa Cruz, CA, USA). Anti-mouse IgG/HPR and anti-goat IgG/HPR secondary antibodies, used for Western blot assays were obtained from DAKO (California, USA). Anti-goat IgG/TEXAS-RED and anti-goat IgG/FITC secondary antibodies, used for immunofluorescence were also obtained from DAKO (California, USA).

Aortic ring assays

Conditioned medium obtained from C4-2, C4-2/LOX-1(+), and C4-2/LOX-1(−) cell models incubated with or without oxLDL [100 μg/mL] for 12 hours were collected and concentrated 10 fold. Mouse aortic rings were grown on type I collagen matrix, incubated with a mix of Opti-MEM culture medium and concentrated conditioned medium in a 10:1 ratio. Opti-MEM/conditioned medium were changed daily during 5 days. Aortic rings were then fixed with 4% paraformaldehyde, stained with phalloidin-Texas-Red and analyzed by confocal microscopy (Olympus IX81, Japan).

Xenografts of prostate cancer cell models with overexpression or knockdown of LOX-1 on chorioallantoic membranes of chicken embryos

C4-2, C4-2/LOX-1(+), and C4-2/LOX-1(−) prostate cancer cells were pre-incubated with oxLDL [100 μg/mL] for 2 hours, and 1×10^6 cells were inoculated on chorioallantoic membranes (CAM) of 10-days-old chicken embryos. Five days post-inoculation, the tumors were extracted from the CAM and the extent of tumor vascularization was determined by quantifying blood vessels area [48,49], using the SZX16 Olympus stereoscope and the ImageJ software.

Statistical analysis

Data are presented as means with standard deviations (sd). Statistical analyses were performed with Graphpad Prism v5.0 software. Multiple comparisons were analyzed by one-way ANOVA with Dunnett's post test. A p value<0.05 was considered to be significant.

Author Contributions

Conceived and designed the experiments: IGC JRT. Performed the experiments: IGC RPC NCP FAS SPJ EAF NAG. Analyzed the data: IGC JRT FAZ VAO LIL. Contributed reagents/materials/analysis tools: OS SAO JCV. Wrote the paper: IGC JRT SAO JCV FSR.

References

1. Yamada Y, Doi T, Hamakubo T, Kodama T (1998) Scavenger receptor family proteins: roles for atherosclerosis, host defence and disorders of the central nervous system. Cell Mol Life Sci 54: 628–640.

2. Sawamura T, Kume N, Aoyama T, Moriwaki H, Hoshikawa H, et al. (1997) An endothelial receptor for oxidized low-density lipoprotein. Nature 386: 73–77.

3. Chen XP, Du GH (2007) Lectin-like oxidized low-density lipoprotein receptor-1: protein, ligands, expression and pathophysiological significance. Chin Med - J (Engl) 120: 421–426.

4. Chen M, Masaki T, Sawamura T (2002) LOX-1, the receptor for oxidized low-density lipoprotein identified from endothelial cells: implications in endothelial dysfunction and atherosclerosis. Pharmacol Ther 95: 89–100.

5. Hirsch HA, Iliopoulos D, Joshi A, Zhang Y, Jaeger SA, et al. (2010) A transcriptional signature and common gene networks link cancer with lipid metabolism and diverse human diseases. Cancer Cell 17: 348–361.

6. Khaidakov M, Mehta JL (2012) Oxidized LDL triggers pro-oncogenic signaling in human breast mammary epithelial cells partly via stimulation of MiR-21. PLoS One 7: e46973.

7. Sugimoto K, Ishibashi T, Sawamura T, Inoue N, Kamioka M, et al. (2009) LOX-1-MT1-MMP axis is crucial for RhoA and Rac1 activation induced by oxidized low-density lipoprotein in endothelial cells. Cardiovasc Res 84: 127–136.

8. Garbin U, Fratta Pasini A, Stranieri C, Manfro S, Mozzini C, et al. (2008) Effects of nebivolol on endothelial gene expression during oxidative stress in human umbilical vein endothelial cells. Mediators Inflamm 2008: 367590.

9. Dandapat A, Hu C, Sun L, Mehta JL (2007) Small concentrations of oxLDL induce capillary tube formation from endothelial cells via LOX-1-dependent redox-sensitive pathway. Arterioscler Thromb Vasc Biol 27: 2435–2442.

10. Hu C, Dandapat A, Mehta JL (2007) Angiotensin II induces capillary formation from endothelial cells via the LOX-1 dependent redox-sensitive pathway. Hypertension 50: 952–957.

11. Yancopoulos GD, Davis S, Gale NW, Rudge JS, Wiegand SJ, et al. (2000) Vascular-specific growth factors and blood vessel formation. Nature 407: 242–248.

12. DiPietro LA (2013) Angiogenesis and scar formation in healing wounds. Curr Opin Rheumatol 25: 87–91.

13. Bergers G, Benjamin LE (2003) Tumorigenesis and the angiogenic switch. Nat Rev Cancer 3: 401–410.

14. Baeriswyl V, Christofori G (2009) The angiogenic switch in carcinogenesis. Semin Cancer Biol 19: 329–337.

15. Moserle L, Casanovas O (2012) Anti-angiogenesis and metastasis: a tumour and stromal cell alliance. J Intern Med.

16. Hoeben A, Landuyt B, Highley MS, Wildiers H, Van Oosterom AT, et al. (2004) Vascular endothelial growth factor and angiogenesis. Pharmacol Rev 56: 549–580.

17. Kapoor P, Deshmukh R (2012) VEGF: A critical driver for angiogenesis and subsequent tumor growth: An IHC study. J Oral Maxillofac Pathol 16: 330–337.

18. Tzeng HE, Tsai CH, Chang ZL, Su CM, Wang SW, et al. (2013) Interleukin-6 induces vascular endothelial growth factor expression and promotes angiogenesis through apoptosis signal-regulating kinase 1 in human osteosarcoma. Biochem Pharmacol 85: 531–540.

19. Khaidakov M, Mitra S, Kang BY, Wang X, Kadlubar S, et al. (2011) Oxidized LDL receptor 1 (OLR1) as a possible link between obesity, dyslipidemia and cancer. PLoS One 6: e20277.

20. Pettersson A, Lis RT, Meisner A, Flavin R, Stack EC, et al. (2013) Modification of the Association Between Obesity and Lethal Prostate Cancer by TMPRSS2: ERG. J Natl Cancer Inst 105: 1881–1890.

21. Park J, Cho SY, Lee SB, Son H, Jeong H (2013) Obesity is associated with higher risk of prostate cancer detection in a Korean biopsy population. BJU Int.

22. Golabek T, Bukowczan J, Chlosta P, Powroznik J, Dobruch J, et al. (2013) Obesity and Prostate Cancer Incidence and Mortality: A Systematic Review of Prospective Cohort Studies. Urol Int.

23. LeRoith D, Novosyadlyy R, Gallagher EJ, Lann D, Vijayakumar A, et al. (2008) Obesity and type 2 diabetes are associated with an increased risk of developing cancer and a worse prognosis; epidemiological and mechanistic evidence. Exp Clin Endocrinol Diabetes 116 Suppl 1: S4–6.

24. Yoshimoto R, Fujita Y, Kakino A, Iwamoto S, Takaya T, et al. (2011) The discovery of LOX-1, its ligands and clinical significance. Cardiovasc Drugs Ther 25: 379–391.

25. Hsu IR, Kim SP, Kabir M, Bergman RN (2007) Metabolic syndrome, hyperinsulinemia, and cancer. Am J Clin Nutr 86: s867–871.

26. Pischon T, Nothlings U, Boeing H (2008) Obesity and cancer. Proc Nutr Soc 67: 128–145.

27. Norris AL, Steinberger J, Steffen LM, Metzig AM, Schwarzenberg SJ, et al. (2011) Circulating oxidized LDL and inflammation in extreme pediatric obesity. Obesity (Silver Spring) 19: 1415–1419.

28. Tewari R, Rajender S, Natu SM, Goel A, Dalela D, et al. (2013) Significance of obesity markers and adipocytokines in high grade and high stage prostate cancer in North Indian men - a cross-sectional study. Cytokine 63: 130–134.

29. Llaverias G, Danilo C, Wang Y, Witkiewicz AK, Daumer K, et al. (2010) A Western-type diet accelerates tumor progression in an autochthonous mouse model of prostate cancer. Am J Pathol 177: 3180–3191.

30. Pelton K, Freeman MR, Solomon KR (2012) Cholesterol and prostate cancer. Curr Opin Pharmacol 12: 751–759.

31. (2011) Cholesterol and prostate cancer. Harv Mens Health Watch 15: 6–7.

32. Chen Y, Hughes-Fulford M (2001) Human prostate cancer cells lack feedback regulation of low-density lipoprotein receptor and its regulator, SREBP2. Int J Cancer 91: 41–45.

33. Allijn IE, Leong W, Tang J, Gianella A, Mieszawska AJ, et al. (2013) Gold nanocrystal labeling allows low-density lipoprotein imaging from the subcellular to macroscopic level. ACS Nano 7: 9761–9770.

34. Yoshida H, Yokode M, Yamamoto A, Masaki R, Murayama T, et al. (1999) Compensated endocytosis of LDL by hamster cells co-expressing the two distinct mutant LDL receptors defective in endocytosis and ligand binding. J Lipid Res 40: 814–823.

35. Fiaschi T, Chiarugi P (2012) Oxidative stress, tumor microenvironment, and metabolic reprogramming: a diabolic liaison. Int J Cell Biol 2012: 762825.

36. Zeman M, Zak A, Vecka M, Tvrzicka E, Pisarikova A, et al. (2005) [Effect of n-3 polyunsaturated fatty acids on plasma lipid, LDL lipoperoxidation, homocysteine and inflammation indicators in diabetic dyslipidemia treated with statin + fibrate combination]. Cas Lek Cesk 144: 737–741.

37. Chandran UR, Ma C, Dhir R, Bisceglia M, Lyons-Weiler M, et al. (2007) Gene expression profiles of prostate cancer reveal involvement of multiple molecular pathways in the metastatic process. BMC Cancer 7: 64.

38. Li H, Li XX, Ma Q, Cui J (2013) The variability of oxLDL-induced cytotoxicity on different types of cell lines. Cell Biochem Biophys 67: 635–644.

39. Hu C, Dandapat A, Sun L, Khan JA, Liu Y, et al. (2008) Regulation of TGFbeta1-mediated collagen formation by LOX-1: studies based on forced overexpression of TGFbeta1 in wild-type and lox-1 knock-out mouse cardiac fibroblasts. J Biol Chem 283: 10226–10231.

40. Li D, Williams V, Liu L, Chen H, Sawamura T, et al. (2002) LOX-1 inhibition in myocardial ischemia-reperfusion injury: modulation of MMP-1 and inflammation. Am J Physiol Heart Circ Physiol 283: H1795–1801.

41. Dunn S, Vohra RS, Murphy JE, Homer-Vanniasinkam S, Walker JH, et al. (2008) The lectin-like oxidized low-density-lipoprotein receptor: a pro-inflammatory factor in vascular disease. Biochem J 409: 349–355.

42. Kanata S, Akagi M, Nishimura S, Hayakawa S, Yoshida K, et al. (2006) Oxidized LDL binding to LOX-1 upregulates VEGF expression in cultured bovine chondrocytes through activation of PPAR-gamma. Biochem Biophys Res Commun 348: 1003–1010.

43. Inomata Y, Fukushima M, Hara R, Takahashi E, Honjo M, et al. (2009) Suppression of choroidal neovascularization in lectin-like oxidized low-density lipoprotein receptor type 1-deficient mice. Invest Ophthalmol Vis Sci 50: 3970–3976.

44. Weidner N, Carroll PR, Flax J, Blumenfeld W, Folkman J (1993) Tumor angiogenesis correlates with metastasis in invasive prostate carcinoma. Am J Pathol 143: 401–409.

45. Lissbrant IF, Stattin P, Damber JE, Bergh A (1997) Vascular density is a predictor of cancer-specific survival in prostatic carcinoma. Prostate 33: 38–45.

46. Wu HC, Hsieh JT, Gleave ME, Brown NM, Pathak S, et al. (1994) Derivation of androgen-independent human LNCaP prostatic cancer cell sublines: role of bone stromal cells. Int J Cancer 57: 406–412.

47. Thalmann GN, Anezinis PE, Chang SM, Zhau HE, Kim EE, et al. (1994) Androgen-independent cancer progression and bone metastasis in the LNCaP model of human prostate cancer. Cancer Res 54: 2577–2581.

48. Ribatti D (2008) The chick embryo chorioallantoic membrane in the study of tumor angiogenesis. Rom J Morphol Embryol 49: 131–135.

49. Durupt F, Koppers-Lalic D, Balme B, Budel L, Terrier O, et al. (2012) The chicken chorioallantoic membrane tumor assay as model for qualitative testing of oncolytic adenoviruses. Cancer Gene Ther 19: 58–68.

17

KCTD10 Is Involved in the Cardiovascular System and Notch Signaling during Early Embryonic Development

Kaiqun Ren[1,2,3,9], Jing Yuan[1,9], Manjun Yang[1,9], Xiang Gao[2], Xiaofeng Ding[1], Jianlin Zhou[1], Xingwang Hu[1], Jianguo Cao[3], Xiyun Deng[3], Shuanglin Xiang[1]*, Jian Zhang[1]*

1 Key Laboratory of Protein Chemistry and Developmental Biology of State Education Ministry of China, College of Life Science, Hunan Normal University, Changsha, P. R. China, 2 Model Animal Research Center, MOE Key Laboratory of Model Animal for Disease Research, Medical School, Nanjing University, Nanjing, P.R. China, 3 College of Medicine, Hunan Normal University, Changsha, P. R. China

Abstract

As a member of the polymerase delta-interacting protein 1 (PDIP1) gene family, potassium channel tetramerisation domain-containing 10 (KCTD10) interacts with proliferating cell nuclear antigen (PCNA) and polymerase δ, participates in DNA repair, DNA replication and cell-cycle control. In order to further investigate the physiological functions of KCTD10, we generated the KCTD10 knockout mice. The heterozygous KCTD10$^{+/-}$ mice were viable and fertile, while the homozygous KCTD10$^{-/-}$ mice showed delayed growth from E9.0, and died at approximately E10.5, which displayed severe defects in angiogenesis and heart development. Further study showed that VEGF induced the expression of KCTD10 in a time- and dose-dependent manner. Quantitative real-time PCR and western blotting results revealed that several key members in Notch signaling were up-regulated either in KCTD10-deficient embryos or in KCTD10-silenced HUVECs. Meanwhile, the endogenous immunoprecipitation (IP) analysis showed that KCTD10 interacted with Cullin3 and Notch1 simultaneously, by which mediating Notch1 proteolytic degradation. Our studies suggest that KCTD10 plays crucial roles in embryonic angiogenesis and heart development in mammalians by negatively regulating the Notch signaling pathway.

Editor: Robert W. Dettman, Northwestern University, United States of America

Funding: This work was supported by the 973 project of Ministry of Science and Technique of China (No. 2010CB529900), the Cooperative Innovation Center of Engineering and New Products for Developmental Biology of Hunan Province (No. 20134486), the program for excellent talents in Hunan Normal University (No. ET13107), and the Construct Program of the Key Discipline of Basic Medicine in Hunan Province. The funders had no role in study design, data collection and analysis, decision to publish, or preparation of the manuscript.

Competing Interests: The authors have declared that no competing interests exist.

* Email: xshlin@hunnu.edu.cn (SX); Zhangjian@hunnu.edu.cn (JZ)

9 These authors contributed equally to this work.

Introduction

KCTD10 is a member of the polymerase delta-interacting protein 1 (PDIP1) gene family [1], which consists of 3 members, PDIP1, KCTD10 and TNFAIP1 [2–5]. All the three members contain a conserved BTB/POZ domain, a potassium channel tetramerisation (K-tetra) domain (a relative of BTB/POZ domain) at the N-terminus, and a proliferating cell nuclear antigen (PCNA)-binding motif at the C-terminus [1,4]. KCTD10 is inducible by TNF-α, interacts with PCNA and the small subunit (p50) of DNA polymerase δ [3]. In A549 lung adenocarcinama cells, knockdown of KCTD10 decreases PCNA expression [6]. Promoter analysis showed that KCTD10 can be regulated positively by SP1 and negatively by AP-2 transcription factors [5]. In a recent study, KCTD10 was reported to be regulated by a novel transcription factor ETV1 which is unique to gastrointestinal stromal tumors (GISTs), and RNAi-mediated silencing of KCTD10 increased cell invasion, suggesting that KCTD10 function as a tumor suppressor protein [7]. However, the exact functions of KCTD10 in mammalian development remain unclear. Reports showed that KCTD10 was highly expressed in human heart, skeletal muscle, and placenta, and may regulate the development of neural tube, neuroepithelium and the dorsal root ganglion in mammals [8], suggesting that this protein may play important roles in tissue development [3,6].

Formation of the vascular system is one of the earliest and most important events during embryogenesis in mammals. Among the early stages of vascular development in both the mammalian embryo and its extra-embryonic membranes, endothelial cell precursors differentiate and coalesce into a network of homogeneously sized primitive blood vessels in a process termed vasculogenesis [9]. This primary vascular plexus is then remodeled by the process of angiogenesis, which involves the sprouting, branching, splitting, and differential growth of vessels in the primary plexus to form both the large and small vessels of the mature vascular system [9,10]. In the mesoderm, cardiovascular system arises, pluripotent hemangioblast cells give rise to the blood islands, meanwhile the peripheral cells differentiate into endothelial cells (ECs) which later form the capillaries [11]. The vasculogenesis and angiogenesis begin at E8.5 in mouse embryonic development. As blood vessels are essential for the transport of fluids, gases, nutrients, and signaling molecules between placenta and embryos, many genes' mutation related to angiogenesis causes embryonic delay or embryonic lethality between E8.5 and E11.5.

One of the most important pathways that control the vascular differentiation is Notch signaling, which is critically involved in many cellular processes including cell proliferation, survival, apoptosis, migration, invasion, angiogenesis, and metastasis [12]. Functional studies showed that Notch signaling is crucial for the angiogenic growth in mice, fish, and human. In mice, the absence of Notch signaling results in defective yolk sac vascular remodeling and aberrant formation of arterial-venous circuits in the embryos, that often leads to embryonic death [13]. There are four different Notch receptors in mammals, referred to as Notch1, Notch2, Notch3, and Notch4. Both Notch1 and Notch4 display prominent arterial expression [13]. Mice with a dual Notch1 and Notch4 deletion show severe defects in angiogenesis: the uniform vessel networks initially form in the yolk sac but fail to properly remodel into large vessels and small capillaries [14,15]. Notch2 is highly expressed in the heart myocardium [16]. Mice homozygous for the Notch2 mutation died perinatally from defects in heart development including pericardial edema and myocardial wall atrophy [17]. Notch3 is associated with CADASIL (Cerebral Autosomal Dominant Arteriopathy with Subcortical Infarcts and Leukoencephalopathy), which is a rare autosomal dominant genetic disease characterized by recurrent stroke, migraine headaches, cognitive deficits, and psychiatric symptoms [18]. In mammals, Hey and Hes represent the main Notch signal transducers during development [19]. The combined loss of Hey1 and Hey2 leads to a lethality vascular defect that affects the placenta, yolk sac, and embryo itself, which has been attributed to impaired arterial fate determination and maturation [20].

In this study, we found the KCTD10-deficient mouse embryos showed delayed growth from E9.0, and died at approximately E10.5 due to angiogenesis defects, heart and neuron developmental failure. Further research showed that the key members in Notch signaling, such as Dll4, Notch1 and Notch4 were upregulated in KCTD10-deficient mice. Molecular biology studies showed that KCTD10 negatively regulated Notch signaling by mediating Notch1 proteolytic degradation.

Materials and Methods

Mice

Mice of C57BL/6J, 129P strains were obtained from the Jackson Laboratory (Bar Harbor, ME). Mice were maintained on a normal 12 h/12 h light/dark cycle with regular mouse chow and water ad libitum at an AAALAC accredited specific pathogen-free facility. Animal welfare and experimental procedures were carried out strictly in accordance with the care and use of laboratory animals (National Research Council, 1996). All the animals were well regulated and animal ethics were approved in this research. All animal experiments were performed in accordance with the institutional guidelines of the Model Animal Research Center, Nanjing University, and Hunan Normal University. The University Committee on Animal Care of Nanjing University and Hunan Normal University approved the experimental protocols.

Generation of KCTD10$^{-/-}$ mice

We used the standard BAC (Bacterial Artificial Clone) retrieval method to construct the *Kctd10* flox allele [21]. Briefly, a 9.6-kb DNA fragment containing the targeting region was retrieved from the BAC containing the whole genomic DNA sequence of *Kctd10*. The first loxP site was inserted into intron 2, and the second loxP together with neomycin-resistant gene flanked by FRT sites were inserted into intron 3. The construct was electroporated into 129 derived R1 embryonic stem (ES) cells. [22]. Targeted ES cell clones were identified by PCR and southern blotting. Chimeric mice were generated by microinjection of the positive ES cells into

C57BL/6J strain blastocysts. Genetic transmission was confirmed by backcrossing the chimera to C57BL/6J mice. As previously described [23], the Neo-cassette was removed by mating to FLP-ER transgenic mice (129S4/SvJaeSor-Gt(ROSA)26-Sortm1(FLP1)Dym/J, the Jackson Laboratory). To get the allele deletion of *Kctd10*, the floxed mice were crossed to EIIA-Cre (FVB/N-Tg(EIIa-cre)C5379Lmgd/J) transgenic mice (The Jackson Laboratory, Bar Harbor, ME, stock number #003314) [24] to remove the genomic DNA fragment between the two loxP sites that includes the 2nd exon of *Kctd10*. Then we back-crossed the positive pups onto C57BL/6J mice to obtain heterozygous KCTD10$^{+/-}$ mice. The homozygous KCTD10$^{-/-}$ embryos were obtained by inter-cross of KCTD10$^{+/-}$. The genotyping of the pups were identified by PCR analysis, all the genotyping primers and estimated size of PCR products are shown in Table 1.

Plasmid construction

We amplified the coding sequence of mouse KCTD10 cDNA (GenBank Accession No. NM_026145) from mouse brain cDNA library using indicated primers as shown in Table 1. HA-KCTD10 was generated by inserting the above mouse KCTD10 cDNA into the plasmid pCMV-HA (Clontech). For KCTD10 RNA probe synthesis that used in situ hybridization, the probe fragment was digested by EcoR I from the plasmid HA-KCTD10 and inserted into the pBluescript II SK vector. Positive clones were verified by restriction enzyme digestion and sequencing. HA-cullin3 was kindly provided by Dr. Yue Xiong (University of North Carolina at Chapel Hill).

Cell culture, siRNA transfection, VEGF induction and western blotting

HUVECs (human umbilical vessel endothelial cells, Clonetics, Inc.) were grown in modified MCDB 131 medium supplemented with 12 mg/mL bovine brain extracts (BBE), 0.01 mg/mL human epidermal growth factor (hEGF), 1 mg/mL hydrocortisone, 2% FBS and 50 mg/mL gentamycin (as recommended by the HUVEC culture protocol of Clonetics). Cells were transfected with KCTD10 siRNA or negative control siRNA as detailed in Table 1 by Lipofectamine 2000 (Invitrogen) according to the manufacturer's instructions. Cells were harvested 24 h post-transfection.

HUVECs were treated with 10 ng/mL VEGF-A$_{165}$ (Sigma) for the indicated time (0, 30, 45, 60, 90 and 120 min), or treated with different concentrations (0, 5, 10 ng/mL). After treatment, the cells were harvested and lysed in RIPA buffer (50 mM Tris-HCl (pH 7.2), 150 mM NaCl, 1% (v/v) Triton X-100, 1% (w/v) sodium deoxycholate, 0.1% (w/v) SDS and protease inhibitors) for protein extraction. Sample proteins were separated on 10% SDS-PAGE gel and transferred onto a PVDF membrane (Bio-Rad, Richmond, CA). Then the membrane was detected by rabbit polyclonal anti- KCTD10 (Nanjing Chuanbo Biotech Co., Ltd.), anti-Notch1 (Santa Cruze, sc-9170), anti-Notch4 (Santa Cruze, sc-5594), anti-Jag1 (Santa Cruze, sc-8303), or anti-Fringe (Santa Cruze, sc-100756), anti-NICD (CST, 2421S) antibodies separately.

Semiquantitative and real-time RT-PCR

Total RNAs from embryos at different points were isolated using Trizol reagent (Invitrogen, Carlsbad, CA). Subsequently, the first cDNA strand was synthesized according to the manufacturer's protocol (Qiagen, Valencia, CA). The mRNA levels of KCTD10, Dll4, JAG1, Mfng, Hes1, Hey1 and GAPDH were quantified using TaqMan RT-PCR on the ABI Prism 7700 sequence

Table 1. Oligonucleotide primers used in this study and estimated size of PCR products.

Name of primers	Sequences (5' to 3')
KCTD10 genotyping P1	TATCTATGTCCTGTATTGTACCAG
KCTD10 genotyping P2	CAGGAGCGGAAGATAACACCAAA
KCTD10 genotyping P3	CGGGAGTGTAGGAACTAGGCTGAA
KCTD10 5-prob-F	CTGCATTGAGCGAGCTGGGTGTT
KCTD10 5-prob-R	CAGACTTTGCTCGATTCCAAGGGTA
KCTD10 3-prob-F	GAAGCCCGCATTTATGAGGAGAC
KCTD10 3-prob-R	CCAACTGCCAAACTAAGTCCTTGA
KCTD10 cDNA clone sense primer	CTCGGAATTCCGATGGAAGAGATGTCAGGAGAC
KCTD10 cDNA clone anti-sense primer R	CTGAGAATTCTCACTGGTGGAGGTGGGC
KCTD10 siRNA sequence	CCAGCAAUUCUGACGACAATTUUGUCGUCAGAAUUGCUGGTA
KCTD10 siRNA NC sequence	GGGCCGGAAGAUUGCUGAAUUUCAGCAAUCUUCCGGCCCTG
KCTD10 sense for IHC	GCAACTGAGTCCAGCTAGGG
KCTD10 antisense for IHC	TGTGAGCCCTTAGTGTGCAG
Dll4 sense	GGAACCTTCTCACTCAACATCC
Dll4 antisense	CTCGTCTGTTCGCCAAATCT
JAG1 sense	TCTCTGACCCCTGCCATAAC
JAG1 antisense	TTGAATCCATTCACCAGATCC
Mfng sense	CACCCTCAGCTACGGTGTCT
Mfng antisense	GGGTGTGCTGGGTAGAGGA
Hes1 sense	ACACCGGACAAACCAAAGAC
Hes1 antisense	CGCCTGTTCTCCATGATAGG
Hey1 sense	CATGAAGAGAGCTCACCCAGA
Hey1 antisense	CGCCGAACTCAAGTTTCC
GAPDH sense	ACCACAGTCCATGCCATCAC
GAPDH antisense	TCCACCACCCTGTTGCTGTA
KCTD10 siRNA	CCAGCAAUUCUGACGACAATTUUGUCGUCAGAAUUGCUGGTA
KCTD10 nc siRNA	CCGUGAAGUUGCUCUACAAUUUGUAGAGCAACUUCACGGCT
Name of primers	Estimated size of PCR products
KCTD10 genotyping P1	WT allele: 4 kb
KCTD10 genotyping P2	KCTD10$^{+/-}$: 670 bp+306 bp
KCTD10 genotyping P3	KCTD10$^{-/-}$: 306 bp

The oligonucleotide sequences used in this study are listed in the upper table. The oligonucleotide primers were used to genotype the mice, to obtain genomic fragments of Kctd10. The estimated sizes of PCR products obtained during genotyping the mice are indicated in the lower table.

detection platform. Cycle threshold (Ct) was determined in the exponential phase of the amplification curve. Human GAPDH was used as the internal control. The $\Delta\Delta$Ct method was used to calculate fold changes in mRNA levels between controls and treated samples.

Histology and immunostaining

Embryos were fixed in 4% paraformaldehyde (Sigma) and embedded in paraffin (Sigma). Then the embryos were cut into sections of 6-μm thickness, and stained with hematoxylin and eosin (H&E, Sigma) or analyzed by immunohistochemistry using polyclonal goat anti-mouse KCTD10 antibody according to the manufacturer's instructions.

For whole-mount staining of blood vessels, embryos or yolk sacs were fixed in 4% paraformaldehyde, then blocked in PBS containing 3% milk and 0.3% triton X-100, and incubated with rat monoclonal antibody against mouse PECAM-1 (BD Pharmingen) overnight at 4°C. Alexa 594-conjugated antibody (Molecular

Probes, Eugene, OR) was used as a secondary antibody. After intermittent washing, the samples were mounted and analyzed under a Leica DMZRB microscope.

For staining of cryosections, tissues were fixed in 4% paraformaldehyde for 2 h on ice, incubated in 20% sucrose/PBS overnight and embedded in O.C.T. compound (Tissue-Tek, Sakura Finetek USA, Inc., Torrance, CA). Sections were then incubated with primary antibodies that diluted in PBS with 1% (v/v) normal goat serum for 1 h and with the secondary antibodies under the same conditions. The primary antibodies used were anti-KCTD10 or anti-PECAM-1antibodies as mentioned above, while the secondary antibodies were Alexa 594 goat anti-rat and Alexa 488 goat anti-Rabbit antibodies (Molecular Probes). Hoechst 33258 (Sigma) was used to stain the nucleus. The slides were mounted with 50% glycerol in PBS and images were acquired under a fluorescence microscope (Leica).

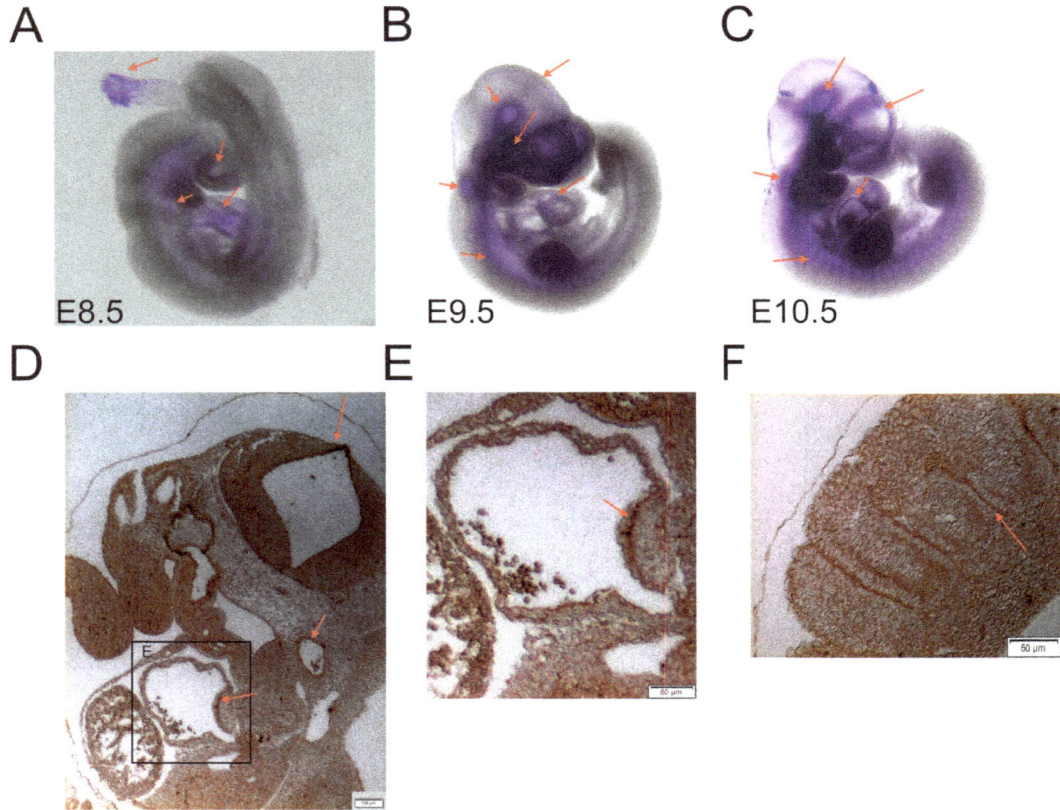

Figure 1. KCTD10 is expressed during the early phase of mouse development. (A–C), whole mount in situ hybridization analysis indicates KCTD10 is mainly expressed in the heart, brain, dorsal aorta and umbilical vein during the early stages of mouse development. (D–F), immunohistochemistry of paraffin sectioned E9.5 embryos exhibited strong KCTD10 mRNA signals in the neuroepithelium of the brain, dorsal aorta, heart and the boundaries of somites.

Whole mount in situ hybridization

Embryos were fixed and processed according to the previously published protocols [25] with the following modifications: Endogenous peroxidases were quenched with 6% H_2O_2 for 2 h prior to proteinase K digestion and hybridization. Hybridization was performed for 40 h at 63°C in 5× SSC (pH 4.5), 50% formamide, 5 mM EDTA, 50 μg/mL yeast tRNA, 0.2% Tween 20, 0.5% CHAPS, and 100 μg/mL heparin. Color was developed with the NBT/BCIP substrate. Embryos were post-fixed and photographed in 50% glycerol in PBS.

Results

KCTD10 is expressed during the early phase of mouse development

It was previously demonstrated that KCTD10 is predominately expressed in the lung, followed by the heart and testis in the rat [3]. Other groups cloned KCTD10 from a human aorta cDNA library, and their data showed a high level of KCTD10 expression in adult human heart, skeletal muscle and placenta [6]. In order to explore the functions of KCTD10 during mouse early embryogenesis, whole-mount in situ hybridization was used to determine the temporal expression of KCTD10. Embryos were collected and stained from embryonic day of 8.5. At E8.5, when embryos completed the "turning" process that included development of onset of heart and blood vessels, KCTD10 mRNA signals mainly appeared in the heart, brain, dorsal aorta and umbilical vein

(Fig. 1A). While at E9.5 and E10.5, strong KCTD10 signals were detected in the brain neuroepithelium, the optic vessel, otic vesicle, only weak signals were observed in the heart and the dorsal aorta (DA) (Figs. 1B, C). In addition, sections of the brain neuroepithelium, dorsal aorta and heart of E9.5 embryos showed KCTD10 mRNA signals (Figs. 1D, E). In addition, in situ hybridization and immunohistochemistry results indicated that KCTD10 was also expressed in the somite boundaries (Figs. 1B, C and F). Thus, mouse KCTD10 was mainly expressed in the dorsal aorta and heart at E8.5, and strongly expressed in brain neuroepithelium, optic vessel, and otic vesicle at E9.5 in embryos. These results indicate that KCTD10 might play crucial roles during the mouse angiogenesis and neurogenesis in early embryogenesis.

Deletion of KCTD10 is associated with embryonic lethality and growth retardation

The gene *Kctd10* consists of seven exons, and encodes a 35 kD protein. The *Kctd10* targeting constructs were designed to delete endogenous exon 2, which resulted in KCTD10 loss of function of KCTD10 (Fig. 2A). The positive ES cells and knockout mice were confirmed by Southern blotting (Figs. 2B, C and D), genotyping (Fig. 2E), RT-PCR (Fig. 2F) and western blotting (Fig. 2G) analysis. The heterozygous KCTD10$^{+/-}$ mice were viable and fertile, but there were no homozygous KCTD10$^{-/-}$ mice among the off-springs. We dissected the embryos from E8.5 to E14.5, and found no detectable differences between littermates at E8.5. While at E9.5, some embryos showed developmental delay. Genotyping

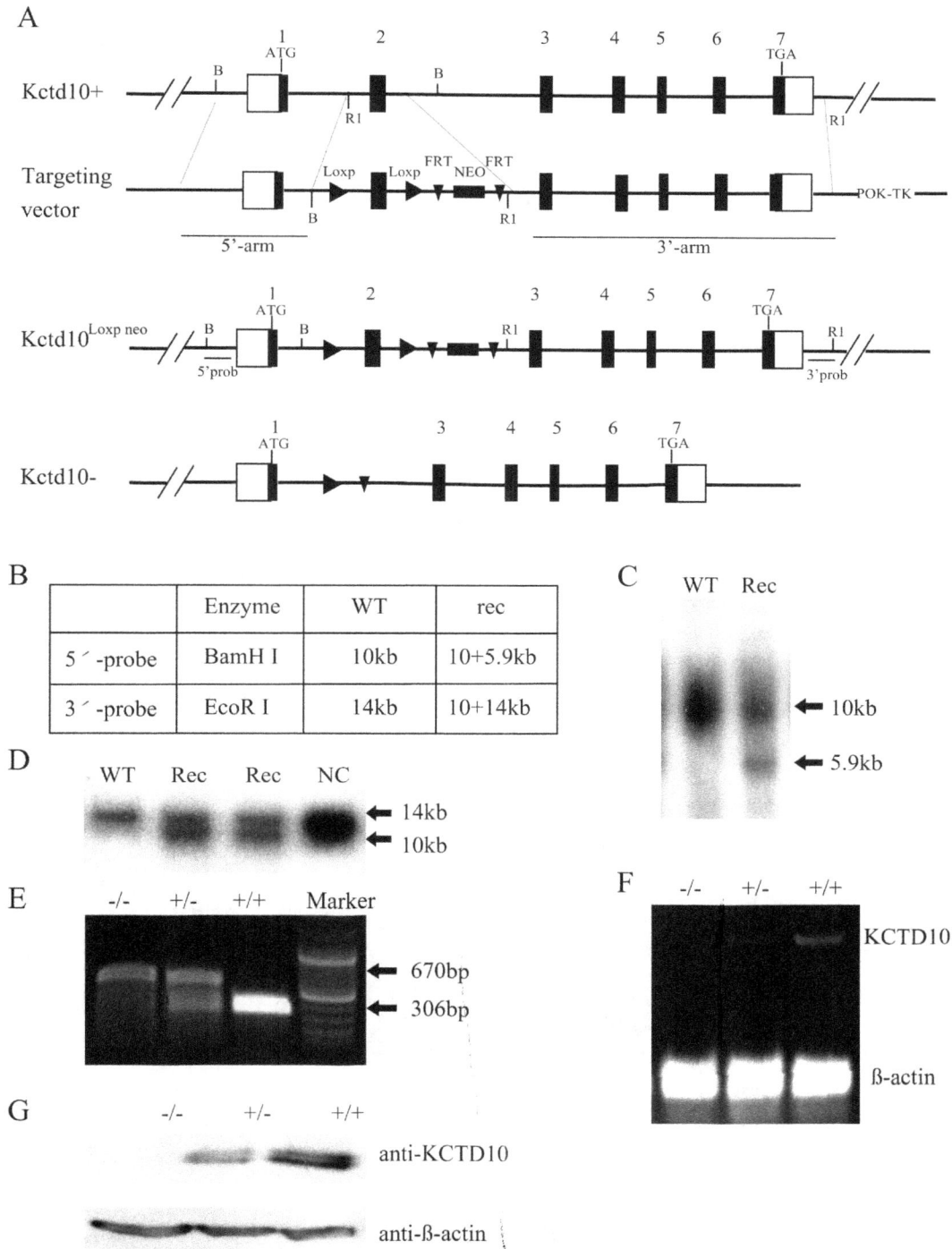

Figure 2. Generation of KCTD10$^{-/-}$ mice. (A), the genomic DNA of *Kctd10* gene includes 7 exons and 6 introns. The genetic manipulation of *Kctd10* was designed to delete exon 2, the first loxP was inserted into intron 2, and the second loxP together with neomycin-resistant gene flanked by FRT sites was inserted into intron 3. (B–D), Gene disruption was confirmed using Southern blotting in positive ES cells. (E), Genotyping strategy of the mutant mouse, there is only a 670 bp band in KCTD10$^{-/-}$ mice, two bands (670 bp and 306 bp) in the KCTD10$^{+/-}$ mice, and only a 306 bp in the wild type mice. (F–G), RT-PCR and western blotting results indicate that the deletion is successful. (F), embryos with the same genotype were collected, and total RNA was extracted separately, reverse transcribed into cDNA and real-time PCR was performed to determine the KCTD10 mRNA levels. (G), embryos with the same genotype were collected, and total protein was extracted separately and immunoblotted by anti-KCTD10 antibody.

analysis revealed that these embryos were homozygous KCTD10$^{-/-}$ mice. Further analysis indicated that the mutant embryos showed developmental delay from E9.5, exhibited severe morphological abnormalities, and died between E10.5 and E11.5.

Table 2. statistical of abnormal embryos at E9.5–E14.5.

	Normal	Abnormal	Ratio
E9.5–E10.5	156/197	41/197	20.81%
	Normal	**Dead**	**Ratio**
E11.5–E12.5	57/73	16/73	21.92%
	Normal	**Reabsorbed**	**Ratio**
E13.5–E14.5	55/70	15/70	27.27%
	Normal	**Abnormal**	**Ratio**
Total	268/340	72/340	21.18%

The ratio of mutants was about 25% (Table 2), which is consistent with the Mendel's principles of inheritance.

KCTD10 deficient embryos show angiogenic defects

When we isolated E10.5 embryos, we found the vitelline circulation on the yolk sac of KCTD10$^{-/-}$ embryos was absent compared to that in wild type embryos (Fig. 3A). These embryos were severely retarded (Fig. 3B) and the pericardial space was enlarged (white arrows in Fig. 3A), indicating embryonic circulation defects. We then visualized the vascular network of mutant embryos and littermates by staining with an antibody against platelet endothelial cell adhesion molecule-1 (PECAM-1), a specific marker for vascular endothelial cells [26]. In the mutant yolk sac, the primary vascular plexus appeared to form normally, indicating no apparent defects in vasculogenesis in the mutants. But the caliber of the major vitelline arteries and the arterial branching were reduced (Fig. 3C), suggesting that the primary vascular plexus failed to remodel and form blood vessels in the mature yolk sac. In addition, reduced tip cell formation was also observed in the abnormal yolk sac (Fig. 3D). Vascular defects were

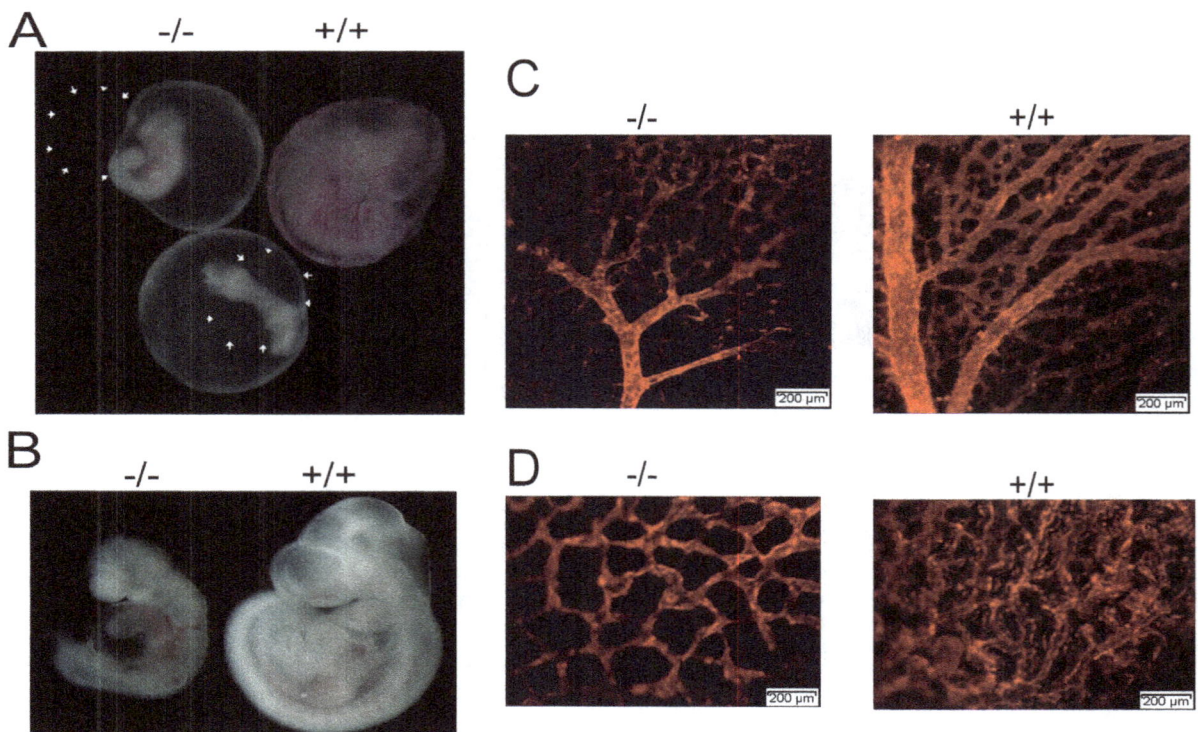

Figure 3. KCTD10-deficient embryos show angiogenesis defects. (A), embryos at E9.5 were dissected, and were taken photos under the stereomicroscope before the yolk sacs were split. The white arrowhead indicates the enlarged pericardial space. (B), embryos of (A) were been split the yolk sac and taken photos under the stereomicroscope, showing the underdeveloped of KCTD10$^{-/-}$ mice. (C, D), PECAM-1 immunostaining of the yolk sacs, showing angiogenesis defects(C) and tip cells (D) in KCTD10$^{-/-}$ mice.

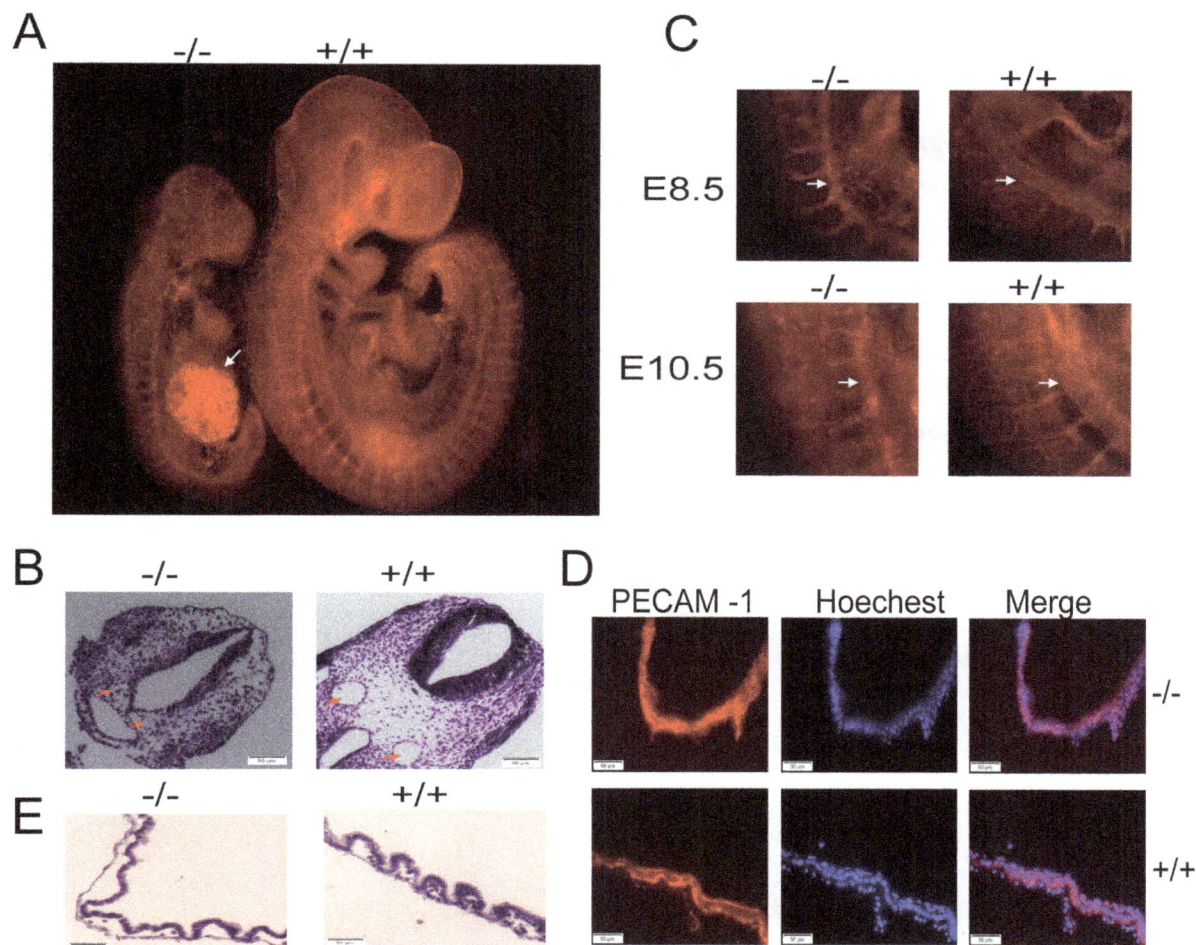

Figure 4. Angiogenesis defects is the direct cause for embryonic lethality in KCTD10$^{-/-}$ embryos. (A), the wild type (+/+) and mutant (−/−) embryos at E10.5 were stained using PECAM-1. (B), HE staining of E10.5 embryos. The red arrow indicates the abnormal dorsal aorta in the KCTD10$^{-/-}$ embryos. (C), wild type (+/+) and mutant (−/−) embryos at E8.5 and E10.5 were stained using PECAM-1, showing the changes of dorsal aorta (DA) development. (D), the yolk sacs at E10.5 were isolated and fixed, frozen sectioned, and immunostained using PECAM-1. The yolk sac showed disorganized in the KCTD10$^{-/-}$ embryos.(E), yolk sacs were dissected from the wild type (+/+) and mutant (−/−) embryos at E10.5 and paraffin sectioned, and then stained using Hemotoxylin/eosin. Enlarged lacunae between the endodermal and mesodermal layers in the mutant (−/−) embryos were observed.

also seen in the KCTD10$^{-/-}$ embryos, among the 60% of the KCTD10$^{-/-}$ embryos, the umbilical artery (UA) became a big ball that was strongly stained by PECAM-1 (white arrow in Fig. 4A). In all of the KCTD10$^{-/-}$ embryos, the internal carotid artery (ICA), dorsal aorta (DA), arterial branches, and cardinal veins were disorganized and much thinner than those in the wild types. All these findings were confirmed by hematoxylin and eosin (H&E) staining on cross-sections. As shown in Fig. 4B, the dorsal aorta was abnormal or even missing in some severe phenotypes. We compared the dorsal aorta between E8.5 and E10.5 embryos that were immunostained by PECAM-1 (Fig. 4C). At E10.5, the dorsal aorta showed no growth in mutant embryos compared to that in E8.5 embryos (white arrows in Fig. 4C), which further confirmed the conclusion that angiogenesis defects is the direct cause for embryonic lethality. In the PECAM-1 immunostained yolk sac frozen sections, we found that the endothelial cells of the yolk sac were poorly organized in the homozygotes KCTD10$^{-/-}$ compared to those in wild type embryos (Fig. 4D). H&E staining of E10.5 yolk sac sections revealed that the abnormal yolk sac

vascular surface was due to the formation of dramatically enlarged endothelial-lined lacunae between the endoderm and mesoderm layers (Fig. 4E).

KCTD10 deficient embryos show heart defects

The disruption of KCTD10 in mice caused heart developmental failure. As described above, the mutant embryos had a dramatically enlarged pericardial edema, which was different from that in wild type littermates (Fig. 3A, B). To characterize the defects in detail, the KCTD10$^{-/-}$ and wild type embryos were sectioned and H&E stained for histological analysis. The mutant embryos showed extended pericardial edema, and the myocardial wall was relatively thinner compared with that in the wild type embryos (Fig. 5A, red arrows). In addition, KCTD10$^{-/-}$ embryos exhibited defects in cardiac valve formation. An obvious atrioventricular valve (AVV) presented in the wild type embryos, but showed defects in the KCTD10$^{-/-}$ embryonic heart (Fig. 5B, red arrow heads). Thus, KCTD10 loss of function leads to heart defects during the early embryonic development.

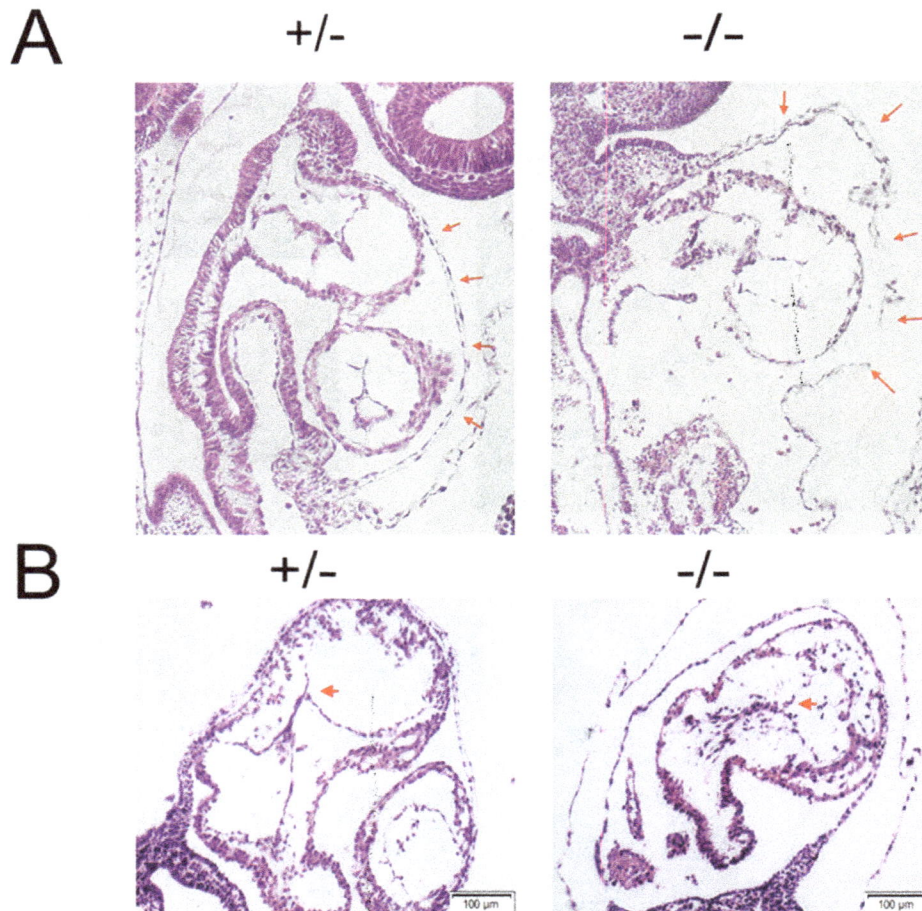

Figure 5. KCTD10-deficient embryos show heart defects. (A), embryos with almost the same somites were cut longitudinally in paraffin, and stained using Hemotoxylin/eosin. The red arrows show the enlarged pericardial edema in mutant embryos. (B), embryos with almost the same somites were cut athwartships in paraffin, and the red arrowheads show the atrioventricular valve defects in the KCTD10$^{-/-}$ embryos.

KCTD10 is induced by VEGF in a dose- and time-dependent manner

Vascular endothelial growth factor (VEGF) plays a critical role in angiogenesis. Most of the factors that affect embryonic vascular maturation are downstream targets of VEGF. Based on the defects in angiogenesis and heart development in KCTD10 deficient embryos, we investigated whether KCTD10 was regulated by VEGF. As described in the Materials and Methods, HUVECs were treated by VEGF-A$_{165}$ at a concentration of 10 ng/mL for different time durations (0, 30, 45, 60, 90, 120 min), the protein levels of KCTD10 were upregulated (Fig. 6A) in a time-dependent manner. As shown in Fig. 6B, the expression of KCTD10 increased when the dose of VEGF was added (0, 5, 10 ng/mL). In order to confirm the results, immunofluorescence staining was performed and enhanced protein levels of KCTD10 were detected (Fig. 6C) after treatment. The total RNA of HUVECs were extracted after 10 ng/mL VEGF treatment for indicated time, RT-PCR analysis showed the mRNA levels of KCTD10 increased(Fig. 6D). These results demonstrated that KCTD10 is time- and dose- dependently regulated by VEGF.

KCTD10 negatively regulates Notch signaling

The phenotype of KCTD10$^{-/-}$ embryos described above were highly similar to that in Dll4$^{+/-}$ mice [27], Notch1/4 mutant mice

[15] and Hey1/Hey2 double knockout mice [20]. Therefore, we asked whether the disruption of KCTD10 affects the Notch signaling pathway. The total RNAs of embryos were extracted and quantitative real-time PCR (Q-RT-PCR) analysis were performed. As shown in Fig. 7A, the mRNA levels of Dll4, Fringe, Hey1, and TNFR1 robustly increased in the homozygous KCTD10$^{-/-}$ mouse embryos, whereas the mRNA levels of TNFR2 decreased. The mRNA levels of Jagged1 and Hes1 did not change. Dll4 up-regulation was further confirmed by semi-quantitative reverse transcription PCR (Figs. 7B, C). These data demonstrated that Dll4 is possibly involved in the KCTD10 disruption-mediated vascular defects.

Furthermore, the protein levels of Notch1, Notch4, Fringe, and Jagged1 were measured by western blotting. As shown in Fig. 7D, compared to the wild types, the protein levels of Notch1, Notch4, and Fringe were up-regulated in homozygous KCTD10$^{-/-}$ embryos, while Jagged1 showed no change, which were consistent with the Q-PCR results. In addition, the protein levels of Notch1 and Fringe were also up-regulated in KCTD10 knockdown HUVECs (Fig. 7E). All these data support the hypothesis that the disruption of KCTD10 results in Dll4 up-regulation, followed by the activation of Notch signaling.

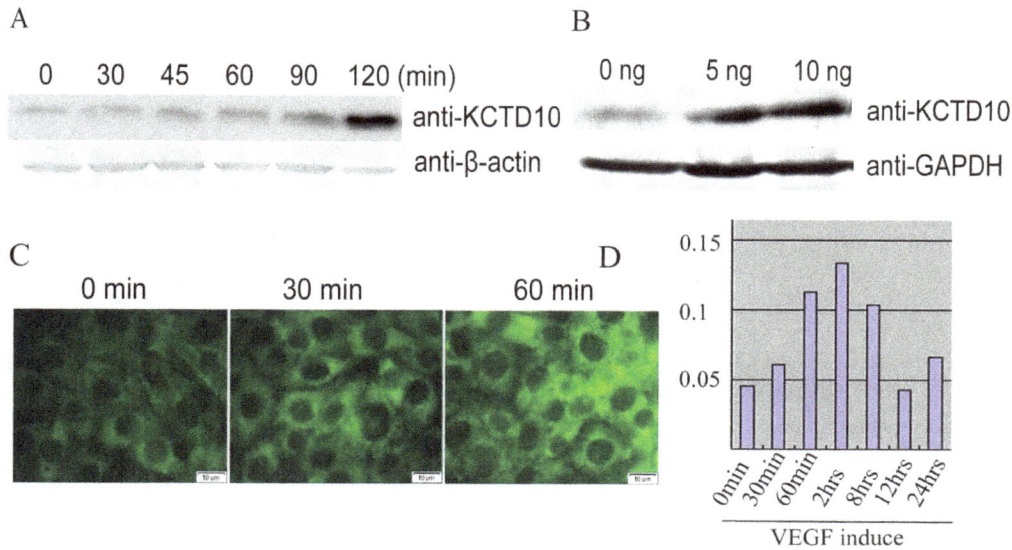

Figure 6. KCTD10 is induced by VEGF in a dose- and time-dependent manner. (A), HUVECs were incubated with 10 ng/mL VEGF for 0 min, 30 min, 45 min, 60 min, 90 min and 120 min, the cell extractions were subjected to SDS-PAGE, and immunoblotted with polyclonal antibody against KCTD10 and β-actin separately. (B), HUVECs were incubated with 0, 5, 10 ng/mL VEGF for 120 min, the cell extractions were subjected to SDS-PAGE, and immune-blotted with polyclonal antibody against KCTD10 and β-actin separately. (C), HUVECs were incubated with 10 ng/mL VEGF for 0 min, 30 min, and 60 min, and the cells were fixed and immune-stained polyclonal antibody against KCTD10. (D), HUVECs were treated with 10 ng/mL VEGF for indicated time, and the total RNA of the cells were extracted, RT-PCR analysis showing the mRNA levels of KCTD10.

KCTD10 interacts with Notch1 and mediates its proteolytic degradation by Cullin3

As KCTD10 contains a conserved BTB/POZ domain and a potassium channel tetramerisation (K-tetra) domain (a relative of BTB/POZ domain) at the N-terminus. The BTB domain was known to be a highly conserved protein-protein interaction motif in multiple species. BTB-domain-containing proteins have been reported to act as substrate-specific adaptors for multimeric cullin3 ligase reactions by recruiting proteins for ubiquitination and mediating subsequent degradation of the substrates [28–32]. We

then asked whether KCTD10 induces the Notch degradation. In our study, HUVEC lysates were immunoprecipitated by rabbit polyclonal antibody against Notch1 or a negative control IgG, and the immunoprecipitates were detected by mouse monoclonal anti-cullin3 and polyclonal anti-KCTD10 antibodies, respectively. As shown in Fig. 8A, KCTD10 and cullin3 exist simultaneously in the Notch1 immune complex, but the preimmune IgG did not show any reactivity in blots. To further confirm the results, HUVECs were transfected with HA-cullin3, and the cell lysates were immunoprecipitated by antibodies against Notch1, NICD,

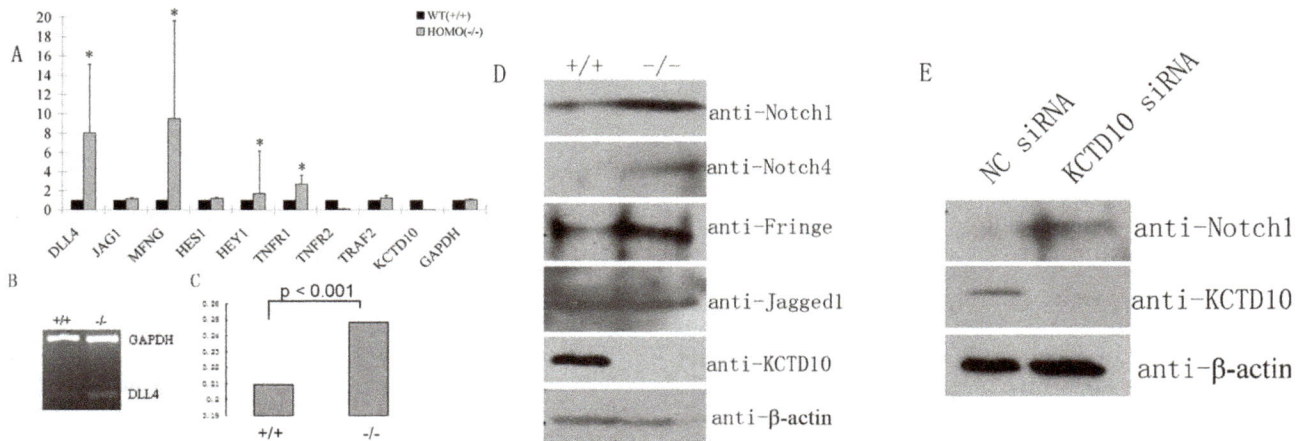

Figure 7. KCTD10 negatively regulates Notch signaling. (A), total RNA was extracted from the mutant embryos that have the same number of somites. Quantitative real-time PCR results showed the mRNA levels of indicated gene in KCTD10$^{-/-}$ embryos and in wild type embryos. (B), Semi-quantitative real-time PCR analysis confirmed the mRNA changes of Dll4. (C), Densitometric analysis of the Dll4/GAPDH ratio in (B). (D), the total proteins were extracted from KCTD10$^{-/-}$ embryos and wild type embryos, western blotting analysis showed the protein changes of Notch signaling in KCTD10$^{-/-}$ embryos. (E), HUVECs were transfected with KCTD10 siRNAs and negative control siRNAs, the cell lysates were subjected to SDS-PAGE and detected by the indicated antibodies.

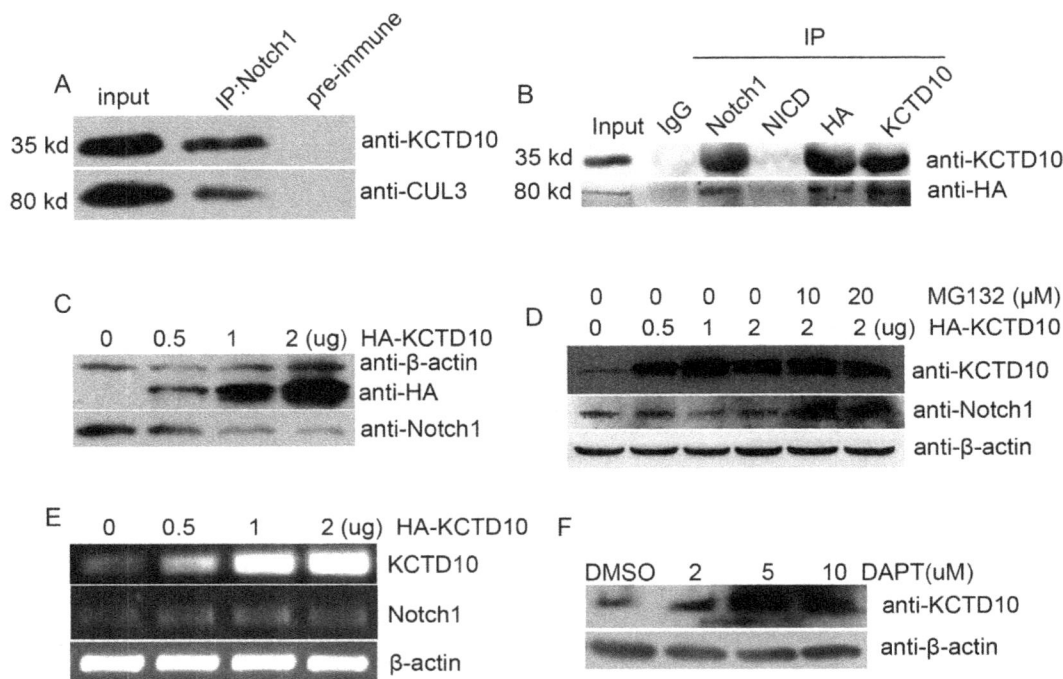

Figure 8. KCTD10 may mediate Notch1 proteolytic degradation by Cullin3. (A), total proteins were extracted from KCTD10$^{-/-}$ embryos and in wild type embryos, endogenous immunoprecipitation was performed to show KCTD10 and cullin3 exist in the immune complex of Notch1 simultaneously. However, rabbit preimmune IgG did not recognize any target protein. (B), HUVECs were transfected with HA-cullin3 and harvested 24 h after transfection, the cell lysate were immunoprecipitated by the antibodis against Notch1, NICD, HA, and KCTD10. The precipitated protein were separated by 10% SDS-PAGE and immunoblotted with anti-HA and anti-KCTD10 antibody. (C, D), HUVECs were transfected with an increasing amount of pCMV-HA-KCTD10 (0, 0.5, 1, 2 μg) and treated with MG132 (D), and harvested 8 h after transfection. Cell lysates were prepared and separated using 10% SDS-PAGE electrophoresis. A single blot membrane was cut into strips based on molecular weight and incubated with anti-KCTD10, anti-Notch1 (Santa), and β-actin antibodies to detect the KCTD10, Notch1 and β-actin protein levels, respectively. (E), HUVECs were transfected with an increasing amount of pCMV-HA-KCTD10 (0, 0.5, 1, 2 μg), the total RNA were extracted and the mRNA levels of KCTD10 and Notch1 were detected. (F), HUVECs were treated by increasing amount of DAPT for 2 h, and the KCTD10 and β-actin protein levels were detected using Western blotting.

HA, and KCTD10, immunoblotted by anti-HA and anti-KCTD10 antibody, Notch1 existed in the immune complexes of HA-cullin3 and KCTD10 and KCTD10 existed in the immune complexes of HA-cullin3. But in the immune complex of NICD (intracellular domains of Notch1), we failed to detect either KCTD10 or cullin3 (Fig. 8B). These results further confirmed the interaction between Notch1, KCTD10 and cullin3. We next wondered whether Notch1 proteins levels were affected by KCTD10. To this end, HUVECs were transfected with increasing amounts of pCMV-HA-KCTD10 (0, 0.5, 1, 2 μg). Western blotting results showed that the endogenous Notch1 protein decreased while the amounts of pCMV-HA-KCTD10 increased (Fig. 8C, D), suggesting that KCTD10 disrupted the protein stability of Notch1. Furthermore, MG132 treatment attenuated the changes(Fig. 8D), and the mRNA levels of Notch1 did not affected by KCTD10 (Fig. 8E), indicating proteolytic degradation of Notch1by KCTD10. We then blocked Notch signaling activation by DAPT, which is a γ-secretase inhibitor in HUVECs [27]. Western blotting analysis showed that the KCTD10 protein levels increased as the DAPT concentration increased (Fig. 8F), suggesting that KCTD10 mediated the γ-secretase of proteolytic processing of Notch1.

In summary, KCTD10 interacts with Notch1 and Cullin3 simultaneously, and decreases the Notch1 protein stability, which indicates that KCTD10 may regulate Notch1 proteolytic degradation by interacting with cullin3.

Discussion

Recently, there are publications showed that KCTD10 plays critical roles for heart development in zebrafish [33,34]. Here we explored whether KCTD10 plays critical roles in mammalian development. Like all other members in PDIP1 gene family, KCTD10 contains a BTB/POZ domain at the N-terminals, which is a highly conserved protein-protein interacting domain found in many essential transcription regulators that are involved in various developmental processes, and is important for homeostasis, cell differentiation, and even oncogenesis [35–37]. The BTB domain is the key functional domain that directly inhibits endothelial cell tube formation and reduces VEGF expression, another BTB domain protein, PLZF, was reported to inhibit endothelial cell angiogenesis in HUVECs [38]. VEGF is known as the most critical molecule controlling blood vessel morphogenesis. In our study, western blotting, RT-PCR and immunofluorescence showed that KCTD10 is VEGF-inducible in a time- and dose-dependent manner, suggesting KCTD10 might be regulated by a VEGF feed-back loop. Notch signaling is known to be the downstream target of VEGF, and Dll4 expression is induced in response to VEGF [39]. Dll4 is the specific mammalian endothelial ligand for autocrine endothelial Notch signaling, and is required in a dosage-sensitive manner for normal arterial patterning in development [27]. Dll4 inhibits the angiogenic response of adjacent ECs to VEGF stimulation by mediating

Notch signaling. Reduction of the Dll4 protein level or blocking of Notch signaling blocking enhances the formation of tip cells, resulting in dramatically increased sprouting, branching and fusion of endothelial tubes [27,39–43]. Heterozygous deletion of Dll4 results in prominent albeit variable defects in artery, and the down-regulation of Notch downstream target genes [44]. In our study, we deleted the 2nd exon of mouse KCTD10, which destroyed the BTB domain and caused loss of function of this gene. A homozygous deletion of KCTD10 in mice caused embryonic lethality because of cardiovascular defects, accompanied by elevated Dll4 levels and activated Fringe, Hey1, and TNFR1 in Notch signaling. These results are consistent with previous research that KCTD10 is TNF-α inducible [4], but the detailed mechanisms need to be further explored.

The Notch signaling pathway is a critical component of vascular formation and morphogenesis in both development and pathology. It was reported that Notch was required for endocardial differentiation and formation of the primordial cardiac valve during the cardiac valve development [45,46]. In a normal embryo, Notch signaling induces endocardial expression of the transcriptional repressor Snail, and in turn, represses VE-cadherin expression, allowing the epithelial-to-mesenchyme transformation (EMT), followed by the formation of the valvular primordium [46]. Abrogation of Notch signaling in mouse or zebrafish blocks EMT [47]. The Notch downstream target gene Hey was shown to control cardiomyocyte differentiation and EMT in endocardial cells [48]. It is possible that deletion of KCTD10 increases Notch1 and then up-regulates Hey1, resulting in a thinner myocardium and EMT defects in the homozygous KCTD10$^{-/-}$ embryos.

Notch receptors are expressed on the cell surface as heterodimeric proteins. They are composed of an extracellular domain containing up to 36 EGF-like repeats followed by 3 cysteine rich LIN repeats and an intracellular domain containing multiple protein-protein interaction domains. Notch signaling is triggered upon ligand-receptor interaction, which induces two sequential proteolytic cleavages. The first cleavage is in the extracellular domain, and is mediated by metalloproteases of the ADAM family; the second cleavage is within the transmembrane domain, and it is mediated by presenilin (PS) γ-secretase activity. The secondary cleavage allows the release and translocation of Notch intracellular domain (NICD) into the nucleus [49]. Consistent with reports that the KCTD10 BTB/POZ domain mediates protein-protein interactions and is involved in proteolysis mediated by Cullin3 [11,31,50–52], we revealed that KCTD10 interacts with Cullin3 and Notch1 simultaneously, and the γ-secretase-specific inhibitor DAPT [27] regulates the KCTD10 protein level. The possible mechanism is that KCTD10 mediates the second proteolytic cleavage and transfers the NICD into the nucleus. Thus, KCTD10 deletion causes Notch1 accumulation, which stimulated more Dll4, and leads to disruption of angiogenesis.

In summary, we generated KCTD10 knockout mice by disrupting exon 2, leading to loss of function of KCTD10. This study provided evidence that KCTD10 plays important roles in embryonic angiogenesis during mammalian development, cardiovascular development, and negative regulation of Notch signaling. Thus, KCTD10 is one of the most important factors in regulating embryonic development and angiogenesis.

Acknowledgments

We thank Prof. Yang Zhong-zhou (Nanjing University) and Prof. Wu Xiushan (Hunan Normal University) for their kind suggestions.

Author Contributions

Conceived and designed the experiments: SX J. Zhang. Performed the experiments: KR JY MY. Analyzed the data: KR JY MY XG X. Ding J. Zhou XH JC X. Deng. Contributed reagents/materials/analysis tools: JY MY XG X. Ding J. Zhou XH JC X. Deng. Wrote the paper: KR.

References

1. He H, Tan CK, Downey KM, So AG (2001) A tumor necrosis factor alpha- and interleukin 6-inducible protein that interacts with the small subunit of DNA polymerase delta and proliferating cell nuclear antigen. Proc Natl Acad Sci U S A 98: 11979–11984.

2. Zhou J, Hu X, Xiong X, Liu X, Liu Y, et al. (2005) Cloning of two rat PDIP1 related genes and their interactions with proliferating cell nuclear antigen. J Exp Zool A Comp Exp Biol 303: 227–240.

3. Zhou J, Ren K, Liu X, Xiong X, Hu X, et al. (2005) A novel PDIP1-related protein, KCTD10, that interacts with proliferating cell nuclear antigen and DNA polymerase delta. Biochim Biophys Acta 1729: 200–203.

4. Zhou J, Fan C, Zhong Y, Liu Y, Liu M, et al. (2005) Genomic organization, promoter characterization and roles of Sp1 and AP-2 in the basal transcription of mouse PDIP1 gene. FEBS Lett 579: 1715–1722.

5. Liu R, Zhou A, Ren D, He A, Hu X, et al. (2009) Transcription factor specificity protein 1 (SP1) and activating protein 2alpha (AP-2alpha) regulate expression of human KCTD10 gene by binding to proximal region of promoter. FEBS J 276: 1114–1124.

6. Wang Y, Zheng Y, Luo F, Fan X, Chen J, et al. (2009) KCTD10 interacts with proliferating cell nuclear antigen and its down-regulation could inhibit cell proliferation. J Cell Biochem 106: 409–413.

7. Kubota D, Yoshida A, Tsuda H, Suehara Y, Okubo T, et al. (2013) Gene expression network analysis of ETV1 reveals KCTD10 as a novel prognostic biomarker in gastrointestinal stromal tumor. PLoS One 8: e73896.

8. Sun JK, Zhang B, Zhang J, Zhou JL (2007) [Preparation of mouse KCTD10 antibody and expression analysis of KCTD10 in neuroepithelium of neural tube and dorsal root ganglion]. Sheng Wu Gong Cheng Xue Bao 23: 1011–1016.

9. Carmeliet P, Ferreira V, Breier G, Pollefeyt S, Kieckens L, et al. (1996) Abnormal blood vessel development and lethality in embryos lacking a single VEGF allele. Nature 380: 435–439.

10. Gale NW, Yancopoulos GD (1999) Growth factors acting via endothelial cell-specific receptor tyrosine kinases: VEGFs, angiopoietins, and ephrins in vascular development. Genes Dev 13: 1055–1066.

11. Sekhar KR, Rachakonda G, Freeman ML (2010) Cysteine-based regulation of the CUL3 adaptor protein Keap1. Toxicol Appl Pharmacol 244: 21–26.

12. Zhou W, Wang G, Guo S (2013) Regulation of angiogenesis via Notch signaling in breast cancer and cancer stem cells. Biochim Biophys Acta.

13. Shawber CJ, Kitajewski J (2004) Notch function in the vasculature: insights from zebrafish, mouse and man. Bioessays 26: 225–234.

14. Swiatek PJ, Lindsell CE, del Amo FF, Weinmaster G, Gridley T (1994) Notch1 is essential for postimplantation development in mice. Genes Dev 8: 707–719.

15. Krebs LT, Xue Y, Norton CR, Shutter JR, Maguire M, et al. (2000) Notch signaling is essential for vascular morphogenesis in mice. Genes Dev 14: 1343–1352.

16. Thurston G, Gale NW (2004) Vascular endothelial growth factor and other signaling pathways in developmental and pathologic angiogenesis. Int J Hematol 80: 7–20.

17. McCright B, Gao X, Shen L, Lozier J, Lan Y, et al. (2001) Defects in development of the kidney, heart and eye vasculature in mice homozygous for a hypomorphic Notch2 mutation. Development 128: 491–502.

18. Delibas S, Guven H, Comoglu SS (2009) A case report about CADASIL: mutation in the NOTCH 3 receptor. Acta Neurol Taiwan 18: 262–266.

19. Iso T, Kedes L, Hamamori Y (2003) HES and HERP families: multiple effectors of the Notch signaling pathway. J Cell Physiol 194: 237–255.

20. Fischer A, Schumacher N, Maier M, Sendtner M, Gessler M (2004) The Notch target genes Hey1 and Hey2 are required for embryonic vascular development. Genes Dev 18: 901–911.

21. Liu P, Jenkins NA, Copeland NG (2003) A highly efficient recombineering-based method for generating conditional knockout mutations. Genome Res 13: 476–484.

22. Nagy A, Rossant J, Nagy R, Abramow-Newerly W, Roder JC (1993) Derivation of completely cell culture-derived mice from early-passage embryonic stem cells. Proc Natl Acad Sci U S A 90: 8424–8428.

23. Farley FW, Soriano P, Steffen LS, Dymecki SM (2000) Widespread recombinase expression using FLPeR (flipper) mice. Genesis 28: 106–110.

24. Lakso M, Pichel JG, Gorman JR, Sauer B, Okamoto Y, et al. (1996) Efficient in vivo manipulation of mouse genomic sequences at the zygote stage. Proc Natl Acad Sci U S A 93: 5860–5865.

25. Henrique D, Adam J, Myat A, Chitnis A, Lewis J, et al. (1995) Expression of a Delta homologue in prospective neurons in the chick. Nature 375: 787–790.

26. Baldwin HS, Shen HM, Yan HC, DeLisser HM, Chung A, et al. (1994) Platelet endothelial cell adhesion molecule-1 (PECAM-1/CD31): alternatively spliced,

functionally distinct isoforms expressed during mammalian cardiovascular development. Development 120: 2539–2553.

27. Suchting S, Freitas C, le Noble F, Benedito R, Breant C, et al. (2007) The Notch ligand Delta-like 4 negatively regulates endothelial tip cell formation and vessel branching. Proc Natl Acad Sci U S A 104: 3225–3230.

28. Bayon Y, Trinidad AG, de la Puerta ML, Del Carmen Rodriguez M, Bogetz J, et al. (2008) KCTD5, a putative substrate adaptor for cullin3 ubiquitin ligases. FEBS J 275: 3900–3910.

29. Furukawa M, He YJ, Borchers C, Xiong Y (2003) Targeting of protein ubiquitination by BTB-Cullin 3-Roc1 ubiquitin ligases. Nat Cell Biol 5: 1001–1007.

30. Geyer R, Wee S, Anderson S, Yates J, Wolf DA (2003) BTB/POZ domain proteins are putative substrate adaptors for cullin 3 ubiquitin ligases. Mol Cell 12: 783–790.

31. Pintard L, Willems A, Peter M (2004) Cullin-based ubiquitin ligases: Cul3-BTB complexes join the family. EMBO J 23: 1681–1687.

32. Xu L, Wei Y, Reboul J, Vaglio P, Shin TH, et al. (2003) BTB proteins are substrate-specific adaptors in an SCF-like modular ubiquitin ligase containing CUL-3. Nature 425: 316–321.

33. Hu X, Gan S, Xie G, Li L, Chen C, et al. (2014) KCTD10 is critical for heart and blood vessel development of zebrafish. Acta Biochim Biophys Sin (Shanghai).

34. Tong X, Zu Y, Li Z, Li W, Ying L, et al. (2014) Kctd10 regulates heart morphogenesis by repressing the transcriptional activity of Tbx5a in zebrafish. Nat Commun 5: 3153.

35. Chang CC, Ye BH, Chaganti RS, Dalla-Favera R (1996) BCL-6, a POZ/zinc-finger protein, is a sequence-specific transcriptional repressor. Proc Natl Acad Sci U S A 93: 6947–6952.

36. Shaffer AL, Yu X, He Y, Boldrick J, Chan EP, et al. (2000) BCL-6 represses genes that function in lymphocyte differentiation, inflammation, and cell cycle control. Immunity 13: 199–212.

37. Zollman S, Godt D, Prive GG, Couderc JL, Laski FA (1994) The BTB domain, found primarily in zinc finger proteins, defines an evolutionarily conserved family that includes several developmentally regulated genes in Drosophila. Proc Natl Acad Sci U S A 91: 10717–10721.

38. Rho SB, Choi K, Park K, Lee JH (2010) Inhibition of angiogenesis by the BTB domain of promyelocytic leukemia zinc finger protein. Cancer Lett 294: 49–56.

39. Lobov IB, Renard RA, Papadopoulos N, Gale NW, Thurston G, et al. (2007) Delta-like ligand 4 (Dll4) is induced by VEGF as a negative regulator of angiogenic sprouting. Proc Natl Acad Sci U S A 104: 3219–3224.

40. Noguera-Troise I, Daly C, Papadopoulos NJ, Coetzee S, Boland P, et al. (2006) Blockade of Dll4 inhibits tumour growth by promoting non-productive angiogenesis. Nature 444: 1032–1037.

41. Sainson RC, Aoto J, Nakatsu MN, Holderfield M, Conn E, et al. (2005) Cell-autonomous notch signaling regulates endothelial cell branching and proliferation during vascular tubulogenesis. FASEB J 19: 1027–1029.

42. Hellstrom M, Phng LK, Hofmann JJ, Wallgard E, Coultas L, et al. (2007) Dll4 signalling through Notch1 regulates formation of tip cells during angiogenesis. Nature 445: 776–780.

43. Ridgway J, Zhang G, Wu Y, Stawicki S, Liang WC, et al. (2006) Inhibition of Dll4 signalling inhibits tumour growth by deregulating angiogenesis. Nature 444: 1083–1087.

44. Gale NW, Dominguez MG, Noguera I, Pan L, Hughes V, et al. (2004) Haploinsufficiency of delta-like 4 ligand results in embryonic lethality due to major defects in arterial and vascular development. Proc Natl Acad Sci U S A 101: 15949–15954.

45. Jain R, Rentschler S, Epstein JA (2010) Notch and cardiac outflow tract development. Ann N Y Acad Sci 1188: 184–190.

46. Timmerman LA, Grego-Bessa J, Raya A, Bertran E, Perez-Pomares JM, et al. (2004) Notch promotes epithelial-mesenchymal transition during cardiac development and oncogenic transformation. Genes Dev 18: 99–115.

47. Chaffer CL, Thompson EW, Williams ED (2007) Mesenchymal to epithelial transition in development and disease. Cells Tissues Organs 185: 7–19.

48. Kokubo H, Tomita-Miyagawa S, Hamada Y, Saga Y (2007) Hesr1 and Hesr2 regulate atrioventricular boundary formation in the developing heart through the repression of Tbx2. Development 134: 747–755.

49. Boucher J, Gridley T, Liaw L (2012) Molecular pathways of notch signaling in vascular smooth muscle cells. Front Physiol 3: 81.

50. Marshall J, Blair LA, Singer JD (2011) BTB-Kelch proteins and ubiquitination of kainate receptors. Adv Exp Med Biol 717: 115–125.

51. Willems AR, Schwab M, Tyers M (2004) A hitchhiker's guide to the cullin ubiquitin ligases: SCF and its kin. Biochim Biophys Acta 1695: 133–170.

52. Jiang J (2006) Regulation of Hh/Gli signaling by dual ubiquitin pathways. Cell Cycle 5: 2457–2463.

18

Dimethyloxalylglycine Prevents Bone Loss in Ovariectomized C57BL/6J Mice through Enhanced Angiogenesis and Osteogenesis

Jia Peng[1]⁹, Zuo Gui Lai[1,2]⁹, Zhang Lian Fang[1,3], Shen Xing[1], Kang Hui[1], Chen Hao[1], Qi Jin[1], Zhou Qi[1], Wang Jin Shen[1], Qian Nian Dong[1], Zhou Han Bing[1], Deng Lian Fu[1]*

1 Shanghai Institute of Traumatology and Orthopaedics, Shanghai Key Laboratory for Prevention and Treatment of Bone and Joint Diseases with Integrated Chinese-Western Medicine, Ruijin Hospital, Jiao Tong University School of Medicine, Shanghai, China, 2 Department of Orthopaedics, Qian Fo Shan Hospital, Shang Dong University, Ji Nan, China, 3 Department of Orthopaedics, The First Affiliated Hospital of Soochow University, Suzhou, China

Abstract

Hypoxia-inducible factor 1-α (HIF-1α) plays a critical role in angiogenesis-osteogenesis coupling during bone development and bone regeneration. Previous studies have shown that 17β-estradiol activates the HIF-1α signaling pathway and that mice with conditional activation of the HIF-1α signaling pathway in osteoblasts are protected from ovariectomy (OVX)-induced bone loss. In addition, it has been shown that hypoxia facilitates the osteogenic differentiation of mesenchymal stem cells (MSCs) and modulates Wnt/β-catenin signaling. Therefore, we hypothesized that activation of the HIF-1α signaling pathway by hypoxia-mimicking agents would prevent bone loss due to estrogen deficiency. In this study, we confirmed the effect of dimethyloxalylglycine (DMOG), a hypoxia-mimicking agent, on the HIF-1α signaling pathway and investigated the effect of DMOG on MSC osteogenic differentiation and the Wnt/β-catenin signaling pathway. We then investigated the effect of DMOG treatment on OVX-induced bone loss. Female C57BL/6J mice were divided into sham, OVX, OVX+L-DMOG (5 mg/kg/day), and OVX+H-DMOG (20 mg/kg/day) groups. At sacrifice, static and dynamic bone histomorphometry were performed with micro computed tomography (micro-CT) and undecalcified sections, respectively. Bone strength was assessed with the three-point bending test, and femur vessels were reconstructed and analyzed by micro-CT. Serum vascular endothelial growth factor (VEGF), osteocalcin, and C-terminal telopeptides of collagen type(CTX) were measured by ELISA. Tartrate-resistant acid phosphatase staining was used to assess osteoclast formation. Alterations in the HIF-1α and Wnt/β-catenin signaling pathways in the bone were detected by western blot. Our results showed that DMOG activated the HIF-1α signaling pathway, which further activated the Wnt/β-catenin signaling pathway and enhanced MSC osteogenic differentiation. The micro-CT results showed that DMOG treatment improved trabecular bone density and restored the bone microarchitecture and blood vessels in OVX mice. Bone strength was also partly restored in DMOG-treated OVX mice. Dynamic bone histomorphometric analysis of the femur metaphysic revealed that DMOG increased the mineralizing surface, mineral apposition rate, and bone formation rate. The serum levels of VEGF and osteocalcin were higher in DMOG-treated OVX mice. However, there were no significant differences in serum CTX or in the number of tartrate-resistant acid phosphatase-stained cells between DMOG-treated OVX mice and OVX mice. Western blot results showed that DMOG administration partly rescued the decrease in HIF-1α and β-catenin expression following ovariectomy. Collectively, these results indicate that DMOG prevents bone loss due to ovariectomy in C57BL/6J mice by enhancing angiogenesis and osteogenesis, which are associated with activated HIF-1α and Wnt/β-catenin signaling pathways.

Editor: Rajeev Samant, University of Alabama at Birmingham, United States of America

Funding: Deng Lian Fu received funds from Natural Science Foundation of China (No. 81371958, 81061160510), the Basic Key Project of Science and Technology Commission of Shanghai Municipality (12JC1408200), and the Scientific and Technological Support Program in Biological Medicine of Science and Technology Commission of Shanghai Municipality (13431900702) http://www.nsfc.gov.cn/ http://www.stcsm.gov.cn/. The funders had no role in study design, data collection and analysis, decision to publish, or preparation of the manuscript.

Competing Interests: The authors have declared that no competing interests exist.

* Email: china_boneres@163.com

⁹ These authors contributed equally to this work.

Introduction

Osteoporosis is a disorder characterized by increased bone fragility, low bone mass, and a consequent increase in fracture risk [1]. Fragility fractures resulting from osteoporosis are the main cause of disablement and death among elderly women. These events lead to the consumption of enormous amounts of medical resources and produce heavy economic burdens [2]. Therefore, using current understanding of disease pathogenesis to develop effective drugs for the prevention and treatment of postmenopausal osteoporosis is vital.

The skeleton is a highly vascularized tissue in which bone remodeling is tightly coupled with angiogenesis. The vasculature supplies nutrients, oxygen, and mesenchymal stem cells (MSCs), which are necessary elements for bone formation, and may direct new bone formation by providing a scaffold for bone-forming cells [3]. Although the main cause of postmenopausal osteoporosis is estrogen deficiency, accumulating evidence from studies in cells, animals, and patients suggests that the local blood supply or decreased angiogenesis contributes to estrogen deficiency-induced osteoporosis [4–11].

Angiogenesis depends on hypoxic stimuli and vascular endothelial growth factor (VEGF) production. The hypoxia-inducible factor-α (HIF-α) pathway is the central regulator of the adaptive response to low oxygen levels. The pathway regulates angiogenic genes (e.g., *VEGF, angiopoietins*). The HIF family comprises three α subunits, HIF-1α, HIF-2α, and HIF-3α. HIF-α is an oxygen-labile protein that forms a heterodimeric complex with the HIF-β subunit, which is constitutively expressed [12]. Under normoxic conditions, HIF-α is hydroxylated at a proline residue by prolyl hydroxylases (PHDs), which need oxygen, iron, and 2-oxyglutarate as cofactors. When hydroxylated, HIF-α is bound by von Hippel-Lindau protein (pVHL), an E3 ubiquitin ligase, and is then degraded by the proteasome. Under hypoxic conditions, prolyl hydroxylation of HIF-α is inhibited, and HIF-α accumulates in the nucleus, where it heterodimerizes with the HIF-β subunit and transactivates HIF responsive genes [13–15]. The HIF pathway can be activated under normoxic conditions by small molecule inhibitors of PHDs that interfere with the required PHD cofactors by acting as iron chelators (e.g., desferrioxamine (DFO)) or 2-oxyglutarate analogues (e.g., dimethyloxalylglycine (DMOG)) [14,16].

Importantly, the HIF-α pathway plays a critical role in angiogenesis-osteogenesis coupling. Clemens *et al.* showed that activation of the HIF-α pathway in mature osteoblasts in developing bone increased bone modeling and the effect was largely attributed to enhanced VEGF-mediated bone vessel formation [17]. Similar results were reported by Giaccia *et al.*, who generated mice in which HIF-α was overstabilized in osteoprogenitor cells. The mice exhibited excessive accumulation of trabecular bone in the long bone and increased vascularization [18]. Striking and progressive accumulation of cancellous bone with increased microvascular density and bone formation was also observed in mice lacking *Vhl* in osteochondral progenitor cells [19]. Moreover, the HIF-1α pathway was activated during bone repair and could be manipulated genetically and pharmacologically to accelerate bone regeneration [16,20]. Consistent with the "promoting osteogenesis by enhancing angiogenesis" theory, HIF-1α pathway activators (DMOG, DFO) or mesenchymal stem cells overexpressing HIF-1α have been shown to improve fracture and bone defect healing [21–31].

The HIF-α signaling pathway might be involved in the pathogenesis of estrogen deficiency-induced osteoporosis. Our group reported that bone density, bone vessels, and bone formation were lower in *Hif1a* conditional knockout (KO) ovariectomized(OVX) mice than in wild-type OVX mice [32]. Moreover, the expression of HIF-α and VEGF decreased in OVX mice but not in *Vhl* KO OVX mice. In addition, *Vhl* KO OVX mice, which showed increased angiogenesis and osteogenesis due to activation of the HIF-α pathway, were protected from OVX-induced bone loss [33]. It has been suggested that 17β-estradiol increases HIF-1α and VEGF protein levels and partially stimulates human mesenchymal stem cell (hMSC) proliferation via HIF-1α activation [34]. These data are consistent with the findings of Yen *et al.*, who demonstrated that diosgenin, which has estrogenic

effects, induces HIF-1 activation and angiogenesis through the src kinase, p38 MAPK, and Akt signaling pathways in osteoblasts [35]. Hence, decreased stimulation of the HIF-1α pathway and angiogenesis might be important factors contributing to estrogen deficiency-induced bone loss. Therefore, activation of the HIF-1α pathway might be a new approach to osteoporosis treatment.

In addition to affecting angiogenesis, hypoxia and hypoxia-mimicking agents increase osteogenesis and modulate Wnt/β-catenin signaling [36]. Hypoxia promotes the proliferation of MSCs and accelerates their differentiation [37,38]. Similarly, overexpression of HIF-1α in MSCs upregulates the mRNA and protein expression of osteogenic markers *in vitro* [24,25,39]. *In vivo* studies using transgenic mice have provided strong evidence that activation of HIF-1α signaling in osteochondral progenitor cells or osteoprogenitor cells increases osteoblast proliferation and differentiation [18,19]. Treatment of MSCs/ osteoblasts with DFO also increases osteogenic marker expression, the effect was attributed to activation of the Wnt/β-catenin signaling pathways [40,41]. Two different groups have proposed that DMOG not only improves the angiogenic capacity of MSCs, but also enhances their osteogenic differentiation, though the exact mechanism has not been fully elucidated [21,30]. Considering that reduced osteogenesis of MSCs in postmenopausal women is a causative mechanism for osteoporosis, it is reasonable to promote osteogenesis by activation of the Wnt/β-catenin pathway [42]. Therefore, Wnt/β-catenin pathway stimulation might be a useful approach to osteoporosis treatment [43,44].

In light of their dual role in angiogenesis and osteogenesis, hypoxia-mimicking agents have tremendous potential for inhibiting bone loss. Supporting this notion, two recent studies have shown that activation of HIF-1α signaling by DFO or inactivation of *Vhl* in osteochondral progenitor cells in a tamoxifen-inducible manner prevented age-induced bone loss [19,45]. However, iron overload has been regarded as a risk factor for postmenopausal osteoporosis [46,47]. To exclude the effect of "iron chelation" on the skeleton, we treated OVX mice with DMOG, a cell-permeable prolyl-4-hydroxylase inhibitor that stabilizes HIF-1α under normal oxygen tension by suppressing PHD-mediated HIF-1α degradation [14,16]. DMOG has shown promise as a therapeutic agent for bone defect healing, neuronal protection, diabetic wound healing, renal protection, and prevention of flap necrosis [21,30,48–55].

The present study was designed to assess the effect of DMOG on the skeleton of OVX mice by evaluating bone mass, bone microarchitecture, bone biomechanics, and bone turnover. Furthermore, the mechanism by which DMOG alters the HIF-1α and Wnt/β-catenin pathways was investigated.

Materials and Methods

Reagents and chemicals

All fine chemicals, including DMOG, tetracycline, dexamethasone, ascorbic acid, β-glycerophosphate, alizarin red S (ARS), 17β-estradiol, L-glutamine, paraformaldehyde, ethylenediaminetetraacetic acid (EDTA), 3-(5′-hydroxymethyl-2′-furyl)-1-benzyl indazole (YC-1),and the tartrate-resistant acid phosphatase staining kit (Leukocyte Acid Phosphatase Assay kit), were purchased from Sigma-Aldrich (St. Louis, MO, USA). Dulbecco's modified Eagle's medium (DMEM), fetal bovine serum (FBS), trypsin, penicillin-streptomycin, and TRIzol were purchased from Life Technologies (Gaithersburg, MD, USA). The mouse monoclonal antibodies for HIF-1α and VEGF were purchased from Novus Biologicals (Littleton, CO, USA). The mouse monoclonal antibody for β-catenin was obtained from R&D Systems (Minneapolis, MN, USA), and the mouse monoclonal antibody for β-actin was purchased from Anbo Biotechnology (San Francisco, CA, USA). The rabbit monoclonal antibody for T-cell factor 1 (TCF-1) was from Bioworld Technology, Inc. (St. Louis Park, MN, USA). The lymphoid enhancer-binding factor 1 (LEF-1) polyclonal antibody was obtained from Proteintech Group, Inc. (Chicago, IL, USA). The mouse monoclonal antibody for TATA-binding protein (TBP) was purchased from Abcam (Cambridge, UK). The goat anti-mouse and goat anti-rabbit secondary antibodies conjugated with horseradish peroxidase were purchased from Santa Cruz Biotechnology (Santa Cruz, CA, USA). The VEGF ELISA kit was purchased from R&D Systems (Minneapolis, MN, USA), the osteocalcin ELISA kit was from Biomedical Technologies, Inc. (Ward Hill, MA, USA), and the C-terminal telopeptides of collagen type(CTX) ELISA kit was from Immunodiagnostic Systems (Tyne&Wear, UK). The silicon rubber solution was purchased from Flow Tech (Microfil MV-122; Carver, MA, USA). The primers were synthesized by Invitrogen (Shanghai, China). The RevertAid First Strand cDNA Synthesis Kit was purchased from Thermo Fisher Scientific (Ottawa, Canada). SYBR Premix Ex Taq was purchased from TaKaRa Biotechnology (Dalian, China). The alkaline phosphatase staining (ALP) staining kit was purchased from Shanghai Rainbow Biotechnology (Shanghai, China). The BCA protein assay kit was purchased from Beyotime (Nantong, China). The eECL Western blot kit was obtained from CWBIO (Beijing, China).

Cell culture and treatment

Murine mesenchymal C3H10T1/2 clone 8 cells were obtained from the American Type Culture Collection (Rockville, MD, USA). The cells were cultured in DMEM supplemented with 10% FBS, 50 U/ml penicillin, 50 mg/ml streptomycin, and 4 mM L-glutamine. Cultures were incubated in a humidified incubator at 37°C and 5% CO_2. The cells were passaged every 3–4 days. The cells were then plated in 6-well plates at 1×10^5 cells per well. After 24 hours, the cells were treated with the indicated concentrations of 17β-estradiol, DMOG, or DMOG+YC-1. For the hypoxia experiments, the cells were transferred into humidified incubators at 37°C with 5% CO_2, and the oxygen tension was reduced to 1% using supplemental N_2. In order to confirm the effect of DMOG on HIF-1α signaling pathway, the indicated treatment lasted 24 hours. For the experiment about exploration of DMOG on the differentiation of MSCs, the cells were cultured in osteogenic differentiation medium for 7 days. When treatment finished, the cells were collected for western blotting and quantitative real-time PCR analysis. The culture medium was collected for the measurement of VEGF by ELISA.

Quantitative real-time PCR for mRNA analysis

Total RNA from cells or bone samples were extracted using TRIzol reagent. In order to extract RNA from tibias, the tibias were grounded into pellets after the treatment with liquid nitrogen. cDNA was synthesized using 1 μg of RNA and a RevertAid First Strand cDNA Synthesis Kit. Gene expression was detected with real-time PCR using a SYBR Green qPCR kit and an ABI Step One Plus Real-Time PCR System. The primers used were listed in Table 1.

Western blot analysis

After cells or bone samples were lysed, the protein concentrations were measured using a BCA protein assay kit. Each protein sample (40 g) was subjected to SDS electrophoresis and electroblotted onto a polyvinylidene difluoride membrane (0.45 μm; Millipore, Bedford, MA, USA). Afterwards, the membranes were blocked with 5% non-fat dry milk in Tris-buffered saline with

Tween 20 (TBST) for 1 hour. The membranes were probed with primary anti-HIF-1α (1:500), anti-TCF-1 (1:500), anti-LEF-1 (1:1000), anti-β-catenin (1:500), anti-TBP (1:2000), or anti-β-actin (1:5000) antibodies at 4°C overnight. The membranes were then washed three times with TBST and incubated for 1 hour with HRP-conjugated secondary antibodies (1:5000). The antigen-antibody complexes were visualized using the enhanced chemiluminescence detection system as recommended by the manufacturer.

Alkaline phosphatase staining and alizarin red staining

C3H10T1/2 cells were seeded onto 6-well plates at 1×10^5 cells per well. After the cells reached confluence, the medium was changed to osteogenesis differentiation medium containing 10^{-7} M dexamethasone, 0.15 mM ascorbate-2-phosphate, and 2 mM β-glycerophosphate. The cells were cultured for 14 or 21 days and then subjected to ALP or ARS staining. The procedures were conducted according to established protocols. Briefly, the cells were washed with PBS (pH 7.4) three times and fixed with 4% paraformaldehyde (pH 7.4, dissolved in PBS) for 15 min. The cells were then stained with ALP reagent or 0.2% ARS solution for 30 min at 37°C, after which the cells were washed with deionized water three times. The ALP reagent was prepared according to the manufacturer's instructions.

Animal models

All animal care and experimental procedures were approved by the Institutional Animal Ethics Committee of Shanghai Ruijin Hospital (ethical approval number: 138). Two-month-old female C57BL/6J mice were obtained from Shanghai SLAC Laboratory Animal Co., Ltd (Shanghai, China). The mice were housed five per cage and were maintained under a strict 12-h light:12-h dark cycle at 22°C with standard food pellets and free access to tap water. After a 2-week adaptation, ten-weeks-old mice were randomly divided into four groups as follows: sham group (ovary intact+vehicle (normal saline) i.p.), OVX group (OVX+vehicle), OVX+L-DMOG group (OVX+5 mg/kg/day DMOG i.p.), and OVX+H-DMOG group (OVX+20 mg/kg/day DMOG i.p.). The ovariectomy was performed in a surgery room exposed to ultraviolet radiation overnight. After anesthetization, the bilateral ovaries were exposed and removed from OVX animals; in the sham animals, the ovaries were exposed but left intact. After surgery, each mouse received an i.p. injection of gentamicin (1000 U) for three successive days. In order to confirm the successful establishment of OVX model, the femoral BMD of 8 mice were measured by *in vitro* micro computed tomography (micro-CT) before the surgery, and the BMD of another 8 mice were assessed one month later. The mice were sacrificed by anesthetic overdose. The uterus of each mouse was isolated and weighed. The body weight of each mouse was recorded. The femurs were collected for micro-CT, histological analyses and mechanical test. The left tibia of each mouse was used for PCR analysis, and the right tibia was used for western blot analysis.

Analysis of micro-CT scans

The distal metaphysic right femur were scanned with a high-resolution (8 μm) micro-CT scanner (GE eXplore Locus SP) to evaluate bone mass, geometry, and trabecular microarchitecture. The parameters computed from these data included bone mineral density (BMD), bone volume/tissue volume (BV/TV), trabecular thickness (Tb.Th), trabecular number (Tb.N), and trabecular separation (Tb.Sp).

Table 1. Premiers for Real-time PCR analysis.

Gene	Forward Premier	Reverse Premier
VEGF	5'-GGCTCTGAAACCATGAACTTTCT-3'	5'-GCAGTAGCTGCGCTGGTAGAC-3'
β-catenin	5'-GGAAAGCAAGCTCATCATTCT-3'	5'-AGTGCCTGCATCCACCCA-3'
Runx-2	5'-GTGTCACTGCGCTGAAGAGG-3'	5'-GACCAACCGAGTCATTTAAGGC-3'
Osterix	5'-ACCAGGTCCAGGCAACAC-3'	5'-GCAGTCGCAGGTAGAACG-3'
ALP	5'-ACGAGATGCCACCAGAGG-3'	5'-AGTTCAGTVCGGTTCCAG-3'
Osteocalcin	5'-TGCTCACTCTGCTGACCCTG-3'	5'-TTATTGCCCTCCTGCTTG-3'
RANKL	5'-CGTACCTGCGGACTATCTTCA-3'	5'-CTTGGACACCTGGACGCTAA-3'
OPG	5'-CATCGAAAGCACCCTGTA-3'	5'-CACTCAGCCAATTCGGTAT-3'
β-actin	5'-CCCTGTATGCCTCTGGTC-3'	5'-GTCTTTACGGATGTCAACG-3'

Mechanical testing

The femora from the mice were wrapped in medical gauze saturated with normal saline and stored at 4°C for use the next day. Before testing, the samples were brought to room temperature for 1 hour. The three-point bending test of the left femur was carried out using an Instron 5569 materials testing machine (Instron Inc., Norwood, MA, USA). The femur was placed posterior side down between two supports, which were 6 mm apart. A load was applied at the mid-span, which bent the bone about the anteroposterior axis. Load-displacement curves were recorded at a crosshead speed of 1 mm/s.

Imaging of femoral blood vessels

Specimens were prepared as previously reported [33]. Briefly, after the mice were euthanized, the thoracic cavity was opened, and the inferior vena cava was dissected and flushed with 0.9% normal saline containing heparin sodium (100 U/ml) to remove the blood from the vessels. Afterwards, the vasculature was perfused with 10% neutral buffered formalin. The vasculature was then injected with 5 ml of silicone rubber compound. Sufficient perfusion was defined as a yellow color change in the lower limbs and liver. The specimens were stored at 4°C overnight, after which the femora were dissected and fixed in 4% paraformaldehyde for an additional 48 hours. The femora were then decalcified in 10% EDTA for four weeks. Images were obtained with a high-resolution (isotropic voxel size of 16 μm) micro-CT imaging system. A threshold of 100 was chosen, and the vessel volume within a region of 5 mm beginning from the distal end of the femur was evaluated.

Histological preparation and tartrate-resistant acid phosphatase staining

The specimens were decalcified in 10% EDTA for four weeks, and the EDTA solution was changed twice a week. The bones were then dehydrated in a graded series of ethanol washes from 70%–100% before embedding the samples in paraffin. Five-micron-thick longitudinal serial sections were cut and mounted on poly-lysine-coated slides. The deparaffinized slides were washed with PBS three times. The slides were then incubated at 37°C for 60 min in the dark in a solution containing sodium nitrite, fast garnet, naphthol AS-BI phosphoric acid, acetate, and tartrate from the Leukocyte Acid Phosphatase Assay kit, according to the manufacturer's instructions. Finally, the nuclei were counterstained with methyl green. Multinucleated cells with three or more nuclei were scored as osteoclasts. The average number of

osteoclasts per mm of bone surface was then calculated for each femur.

Fluorochrome labeling and bone histomorphometry

A double tetracycline (25 mg/kg) label was injected subcutaneously at 10 and 3 days before necropsy. At necropsy, the femora were cleaned of soft tissue and fixed in 70% ethanol. The bones were dehydrated and embedded in methyl methacrylate. Thin frontal sections of the femur (5μm) were cut using a microtome (Leica RM2255). Bone histomorphometric parameters were determined according to the report of the American Society of Bone and Mineral Research Nomenclature Committee [56]. Histomorphometric measurements included single-labeled surface (sLS), double-labeled surface (dLS), and interlabel thickness (IrLTh). These data were used to calculate the mineralizing surface/bone surface ratio (MS/BS), mineral apposition rate (MAR), and bone formation rate (BFR) as follows: MS/BS = (1/2sLS+dLS)/BS(%), MAR = Ir.L.Th/Ir.L.t, and BFR/BS = MAR×MS/BS (m^3/m^2/day).

Enzyme-linked immunosorbent assay

Blood from the mice was collected, and the serum was separated by centrifugation at 3000 rpm for 30 min. Serum VEGF, osteocalcin, and CTX levels were measured by ELISA, following the manufacturers' protocols.

Statistical analysis

The results were expressed as the mean ± SD. All experimental data were analyzed with one-way analysis of variance (ANOVA) followed by Duncan's test. $P < 0.05$ was considered statistically significant.

Results

Effect of 17β-estradiol and DMOG on the HIF-1α signaling pathway

Consistent with previous reports, our western blot analysis showed that 17β-estradiol stabilized HIF-1α under normal oxygen tension (Fig. 1A). Furthermore, 17β-estradiol increased the expression of VEGF protein (control vs. $10^{-9}E_2$ $P = 0.001 < 0.05$, control vs. $10^{-7}E_2$ $P = 0.000 < 0.05$, control vs. $10^{-5}E_2$ $P = 0.000 < 0.05$), the main downstream angiogenic target of the HIF-1α pathway, in a dose-dependent manner (Fig. 1B). Similarly, DMOG enhanced HIF-1α protein expression under normal

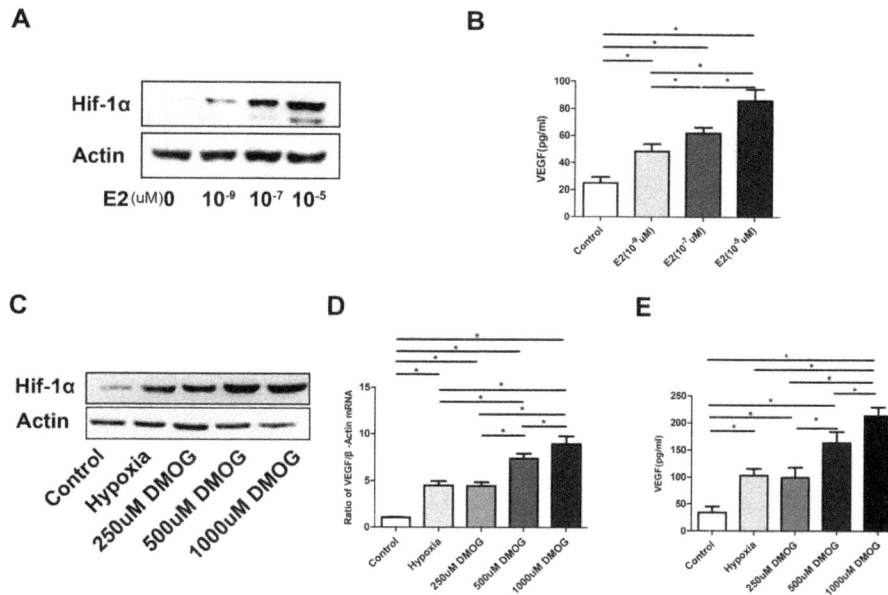

Figure 1. Effect of 17β-estradiol and DMOG on HIF-1α signaling pathway. (A) 17β-estradiol stabilized HIF-1α under normal oxygen pressure. (B) 17β-estradiol upregulated VEGF protein expression. (C) DMOG enhanced HIF-1α protein expression. (D–E) DMOG upregulated VEGF expression at the mRNA and protein levels. $P < 0.05$ for comparisons among the groups designated with an asterisk.

oxygen tension and upregulated VEGF expression at the mRNA and protein levels (Fig. 1C–E).

Effect of DMOG on MSC osteogenic differentiation and the Wnt/β-catenin signaling pathway

ALP and ARS staining showed that DMOG treatment enhanced osteogenic differentiation and calcium deposition (Fig. 2A). Consistent with osteogenesis, RUNX-2 and osterix mRNA levels were increased (RUNX-2 $P = 0.000 < 0.05$, osterix $P = 0.000 < 0.05$) (Fig. 2B). Investigation into the underlying mechanism revealed that DMOG upregulated the levels of β-catenin mRNA and protein ($P = 0.000 < 0.05$) (Fig. 2C). To determine whether the effect of DMOG on Wnt/β-catenin signaling was mediated by HIF-1α signaling, we treated MSCs with YC-1, a widely used HIF-1α inhibitor, along with DMOG and assessed the nuclear expression of β-catenin and the downstream effectors LEF-1 and TCF-1. DMOG stimulated HIF-1α protein expression, and YC-1 inhibited the effect of DMOG on HIF-1α. Furthermore, YC-1 attenuated the DMOG-induced increase in nuclear β-catenin, LEF-1, and TCF-1 protein expression (Fig. 2D).

Confirmation of the OVX model

OVX increased body weight by approximately 6% when compared to sham treatment (Sham vs. OVX $P = 0.049 < 0.05$). However, DMOG treatment did not affect the OVX-induced body weight gain (OVX+L-DMOG vs. OVX $P = 0.868 > 0.05$, OVX+H-DMOG vs. OVX $P = 1.000 > 0.05$) (Fig. S1A). The efficacy of OVX was confirmed by changes in uterine and BMD. The average uterine weights in each group were 0.11137 ± 0.0120 g (sham), 0.0319 ± 0.0079 g (OVX), 0.0337 ± 0.079 g (OVX+L-DMOG), and 0.0326 ± 0.0078 g (OVX+H-DMOG) ($P < 0.0001$) (Fig. S1B,C). Before ovariectomy, the BMD of mice was 365.41 ± 18.43 mg/cm^3, and OVX made the BMD of mice decrease to 281.26 ± 29.61 mg/cm^3 ($P < 0.0001$) (Fig. S1D).

The effect of DMOG on BMD, bone microarchitecture, and vessels

To characterize the effects of treatment on the trabecular bone compartments, the distal metaphysic of the femoral bone was evaluated with micro-CT imaging (Table. 2). With regard to trabecular bone alterations, OVX mice showed remarkable reductions in BMD, BV/TV, Tb.N, and Tb.Th, as well as increased Tb.Sp (OVX vs. Sham: BMD $P = 0.000 < 0.05$, BV/TV $P = 0.000 < 0.05$, Tb.N $P = 0.000 < 0.05$, Tb.Th $P = 0.005 < 0.05$, Tb.Sp $P = 0.000 < 0.05$). DMOG treatment, especially at high doses, improved the trabecular microarchitecture and increased BMD (OVX vs. OVX+L-DMOG: BMD $P = 0.025 < 0.05$, BV/TV $P = 0.184 > 0.05$, Tb.N $P = 0.019 < 0.05$, Tb.Th $P = 0.94 > 0.05$, Tb.Sp $P = 0.191 > 0.05$; OVX vs. OVX+H-DMOG: BMD $P = 0.000 < 0.05$, BV/TV $P = 0.000 < 0.05$, Tb.N $P = 0.000 < 0.05$, Tb.Th $P = 0.047 < 0.05$, Tb.Sp $P = 0.016 < 0.05$) (Fig. 3A). Micro-fil-perfused femora were analyzed with micro-CT to assess vascularity. The number of blood vessels in the femur was lower 4 weeks after OVX ($P = 0.000 < 0.05$). However, DMOG treatment led to a dose-dependent increase in femur vessel volume relative to that in the OVX group (OVX vs. OVX+L-DMOG $P = 0.045 < 0.05$, OVX vs. OVX+H-DMOG $P = 0.000 < 0.05$), although differences among the DMOG-treated groups and the sham group were evident (Sham vs. OVX+L-DMOG $P = 0.000 < 0.05$, Sham vs. OVX+H-DMOG $P = 0.009 < 0.05$) (Fig. 3B).

Bone mechanical strength examination

The three-point bending test was used to evaluate bone strength (Table. 3). The femurs of the OVX mice exhibited decreases in ultimate stress, ultimate load, energy to failure, and modulus, all of which reflected a decline in bone strength following OVX (Sham vs. OVX: ultimate stress $P = 0.000 < 0.05$, ultimate load $P = 0.000 < 0.05$, energy to failure $P = 0.000 < 0.05$, modulus $P = 0.000 < 0.05$). DMOG treatment improved ultimate stress, ultimate load, energy to failure, and modulus (OVX vs. OVX+L-DMOG: ultimate stress $P = 0.010 < 0.05$, ultimate load

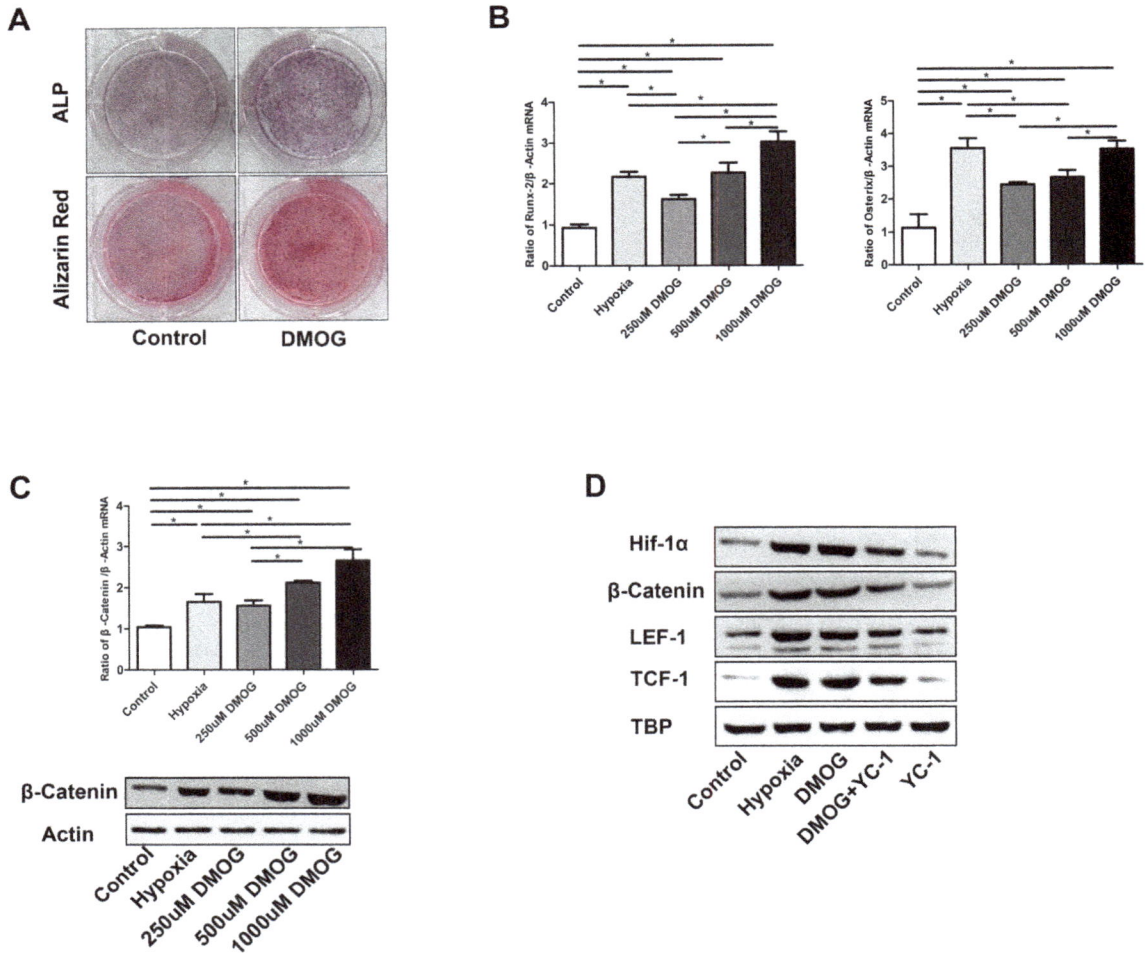

Figure 2. Effect of DMOG on MSC osteogenic differentiation and Wnt/β-catenin signaling. (A) ALP and alizarin red S staining. (B) DMOG promoted RUNX-2 and osterix mRNA expression. (C) DMOG increased β-catenin mRNA and protein expression. (D) DMOG increased nuclear β-catenin, LEF-1, TCF-1, and HIF-1α protein expression. These effects were attenuated by YC-1. $P < 0.05$ for comparisons among the groups designated with an asterisk.

$P = 0.005 < 0.05$, energy to failure $P = 0.024 < 0.05$, modulus $P = 0.051 > 0.05$; OVX vs. OVX+H-DMOG ultimate stress $P = 0.000 < 0.05$, ultimate load $P = 0.000 < 0.05$, energy to failure $P = 0.001 < 0.05$, modulus $P = 0.009 < 0.05$).

Serum VEGF, osteocalcin, and CTX levels

The serum level of VEGF, the main angiogenic cytokine upregulated by HIF-1α, was markedly reduced in OVX mice ($P = 0.000 < 0.05$), and DMOG treatment improved VEGF levels in a dose-dependent manner (OVX vs. OVX+L-DMOG $P = 0.003 < 0.05$, OVX vs. OVX+H-DMOG $P = 0.000 < 0.05$).

Table 2. Micro-CT analysis of trabecular BMD, bone microarchitecture and vasculature in the distal femur.

	Sham	OVX	OVX+L-DMOG	OVX+H-DMOG
BMD(mg/cm³)	379.69±24.61[#]	284.46±17.49*	309.10±19.03*[#]	335.62±30.94*[#]
BV/TV(%)	0.1331±0.0061[#]	0.0947±0.0139*	0.1013±0.0105*	0.1143±0.0119*[#]
Tb.N(1/mm)	3.7268±0.2478[#]	2.5724±0.4024*	2.9317±0.2273*[#]	3.3250±0.3884*[#]
Tb.Th(um)	0.0345±0.0013[#]	0.0322±0.0014*	0.0323±0.0109*	0.0339±0.0025[#]
Tb.Sp(um)	0.2351±0.0211[#]	0.3033±0.0379*	0.2854±0.0183*	0.2693±0.0371*[#]
Vessel volume(mm³)	0.4441±0.0396[#]	0.2189±0.0419*	0.2766±0.0243*[#]	0.3529±0.0315*[#]

The groups designated with an asterisk shown significant differences with Sham group (*P<0.05*), the groups designated with a pound sign shown significant differences with OVX group (*P<0.05*).

A

Sham   OVX   OVX+L-DMOG OVX+H-DMOG

B

Sham   OVX

OVX+L-DMOG OVX+H-DMOG

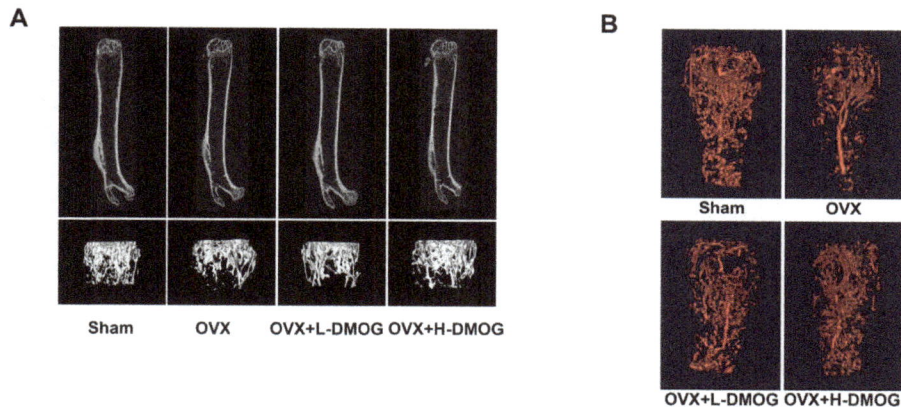

Figure 3. BMD and bone microarchitecture of the trabecular bone in the distal femur. (A) DMOG abrogated the decrease in BMD and the deterioration in bone microarchitecture induced by OVX, as measured by micro-CT. **Morphological analysis of the vasculature within the distal femur from Microfil-perfused mice.** (B) OVX decreased the vessel volume at the distal metaphysic of the femur, while DMOG treatment partly restored vessel volumes.

Serum osteocalcin, a marker for bone formation, was higher in OVX mice than in sham mice, but the difference was not significant ($P = 0.053 > 0.05$). The osteocalcin levels in the DMOG-treated group were significantly higher than those in the OVX group (OVX vs. OVX+L-DMOG $P = 0.008 < 0.05$, OVX vs. OVX+H-DMOG $P = 0.000 < 0.05$). Serum CTX, a marker of bone resorption, was approximately two-fold higher in OVX mice than in sham mice ($P = 0.000 < 0.05$), while DMOG treatment did not affect serum CTX levels (OVX vs. OVX+L-DMOG $P = 0.714 > 0.05$, OVX vs. OVX+H-DMOG $P = 0.770 > 0.05$). All the data were listed in Table 4.

Osteoclast number

Consistent with the results of the serum CTX analysis, the TRAP assay revealed a striking increase in osteoclast number following OVX (5.200 ± 0.836 and 13.200 ± 1.303 in the sham group and OVX group, respectively ($P = 0.000 < 0.05$)). DMOG administration did not noticeably prevent OVX-induced osteoclast formation (12.800 ± 1.643 in the OVX+L-DMOG group and 12.600 ± 2.673 in OVX+H-DMOG group; OVX+L-DMOG vs. the OVX group $P = 1.000 > 0.05$, OVX+H-DMOG vs. the OVX group $P = 0.637 > 0.05$) (Fig. 4A).

Dynamic bone histomorphometry

The dynamic histology of the trabecular bone in the distal femur was compared among the various groups. OVX resulted in significant increases in MS/BS and BFR/BS (Sham vs. OVX: MS/BS $P = 0.000 < 0.05$, BFR/BS $P = 0.004 < 0.05$) and increased

MAR though without statistical difference ($P = 0.057 > 0.05$). H-DMOG treatment further increased MS/BS, MAR, and BFR/BS compared with OVX group (MS/BS $P = 0.000 < 0.05$, MAR $P = 0.001 < 0.05$, BFR/BS $P = 0.000 < 0.05$); and L-DMOG administration increased MAR and BFR/BS (MAR $P = 0.035 < 0.05$, BFR/BS $P = 0.000 < 0.05$) but not MS/BS ($P = 0.061 > 0.05$) compared to OVX group (Fig. 4B).

Alterations in HIF-1α and Wnt/β-catenin signaling in DMOG-treated mice

To illustrate the enhanced angiogenesis and osteogenesis in DMOG-treated mice, we used western blot to detect alterations in HIF-1α and Wnt/β-catenin signaling pathways in collected bone samples (Fig. 5A). As previously highlighted, OVX substantially reduced HIF-1α expression; the reduction in HIF-1α was accompanied by a decrease in VEGF expression. However, in the DMOG-treated group, the expression of HIF-1α and VEGF increased significantly. Moreover, DMOG administration enhanced β-catenin expression relative to expression in the OVX group.

Bone formation and bone resorption markers in DMOG-treated mice

Real-time PCR results for ALP, osteocalcin, RUNX-2, RANKL, OPG, and β-actin expression in each group are shown in Fig. 5B. OVX increased ALP, osteocalcin, and RUNX-2 mRNA levels over those in the sham group, but the difference was not statistically significant (ALP $P = 0.262 > 0.05$, osteocalcin

Table 3. Bone quality of the femur as measured by the three-point bending test.

	Sham	OVX	OVX+L-DMOG	OVX+H-DMOG
Ultimate load(N)	$15.31 \pm 0.85^{\#}$	$11.85 \pm 0.30^*$	$13.14 \pm 0.42^{*\#}$	$14.11 \pm 0.37^{*\#}$
Ultimate stress(Mpa)	$99.41 \pm 7.10^{\#}$	$69.56 \pm 4.88^*$	$80.98 \pm 5.59^{*\#}$	$90.13 \pm 2.37^{*\#}$
Energy to failure(MJ)	$8.69 \pm 0.50^{\#}$	$6.75 \pm 0.24^*$	$7.39 \pm 0.30^{*\#}$	$7.92 \pm 0.31^{*\#}$
Modulus(Mpa)	$4162.65 \pm 377.13^{\#}$	$2910.93 \pm 355.07^*$	$3407.78 \pm 291.51^*$	$3624.83 \pm 255.12^{*\#}$

The groups designated with an asterisk shown significant differences with Sham group ($P<0.05$), the groups designated with a pound sign shown significant differences with OVX group ($P<0.05$).

Table 4. Biochemical markers of bone in serum as measured by ELISA.

	Sham	OVX	OVX+L-DMOG	OVX+H-DMOG
VEGF(pg/ml)	116.37±6.21#	82.37±8.90*	93.13±5.51*#	100.75±5.31*#
Osteoclacin(ng/ml)	68.33±14.22	80.80±18.87	98.32±9.95*#	107.60±10.91*#
CTX(ng/ml)	16.21±1.61	28.01±1.95*	28.46±4.35*	27.65±2.10*

The groups designated with an asterisk shown significant differences with Sham group (*P<0.05*), the groups designated with a pound sign shown significant differences with OVX group (*P<0.05*).

$P = 0.089 > 0.05$, RUNX-2 $P = 0.346 > 0.05$). The osteocalcin mRNA level was higher in the DMOG-treated OVX groups than in the OVX groups (OVX vs. OVX+L-DMOG $P = 0.030 < 0.05$, OVX vs. OVX+H-DMOG $P = 0.000 < 0.05$), and ALP and RUNX-2 mRNA levels were markedly higher in the H-DMOG treated group than in the OVX group (ALP $P = 0.001 < 0.05$, RUNX-2 $P = 0.004 < 0.05$). In OVX mice, RANKL/OPG expression was markedly increased when compared with expression in the sham group ($P = 0.006 < 0.05$). However, DMOG administration did not significantly attenuate the OVX-induced

increase in RANKL/OPG expression (OVX vs. OVX+L-DMOG $P = 0.733 > 0.05$, OVX vs. OVX+H-DMOG $P = 0.984 > 0.05$).

Discussion

In the present study, DMOG improved angiogenesis and osteogenesis *in vitro*. The effects were attributed to activation of the HIF-1α and Wnt/β-catenin signaling pathways, respectively. We investigated whether DMOG ameliorated OVX-induced osteoporosis in mice. Our results showed that DMOG improved BMD, trabecular microarchitecture, and bone strength in OVX mice. In addition, DMOG treatment partly restored the blood

A

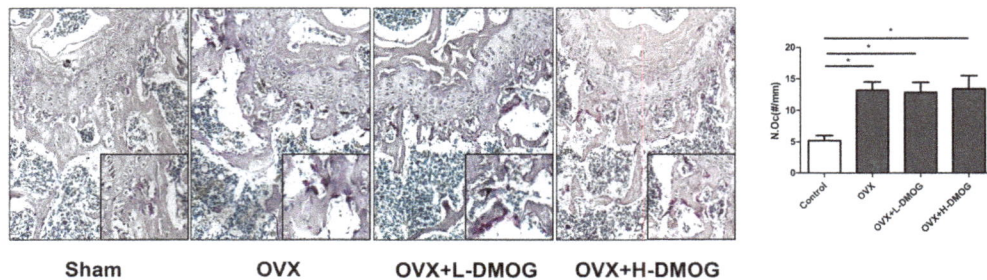

B

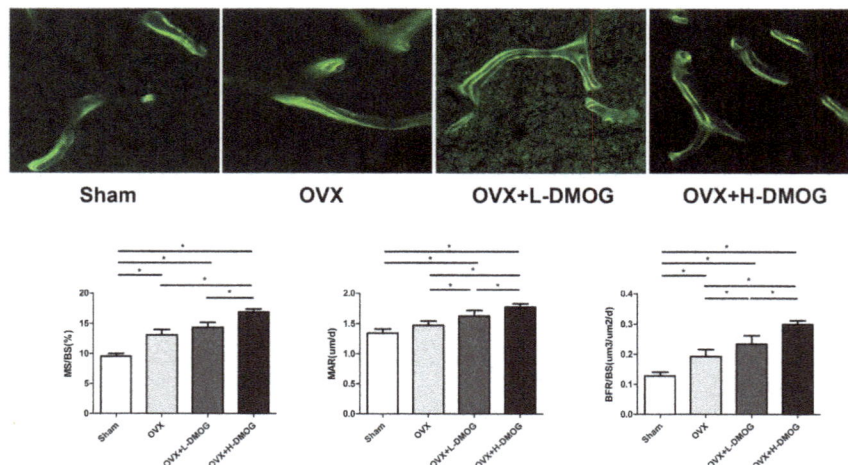

Figure 4. Osteoclast numbers assayed by tartrate-resistant acid phosphatase staining of femoral sections. (A)Osteoclast counting results showed that DMOG treatment had no obvious effect on OVX-enhanced osteoclast formation. Original magnification, ×100. **Dynamic bone formation illustrated by double tetracycline labeling.** (B) DMOG administration promoted bone formation, as evidenced by improved MS/BS, MAR, and BFR/BS. Original magnification, ×200. *P<0.05* for comparisons among the groups designated with an asterisk.

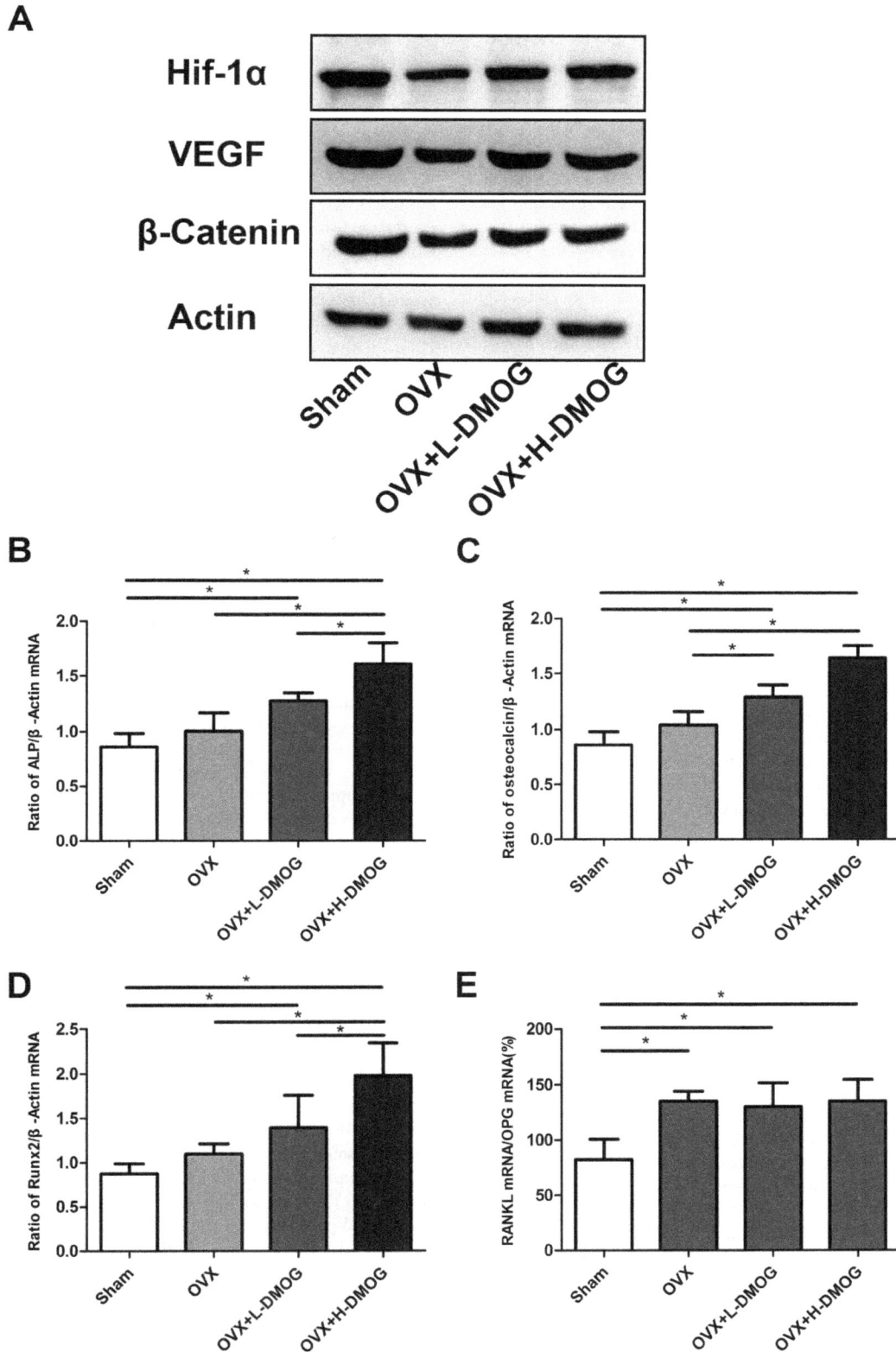

Figure 5. HIF-1α, VEGF, and β-catenin expression in bone samples detected by western blot. (A) HIF-1α, VEGF, and β-catenin expression was lower in OVX mice than in sham mice. However, DMOG treatment increased HIF-1α, VEGF, and β-catenin expression relative to expression in the OVX group. Effects of DMOG administration on tibial ALP, osteocalcin, RUNX-2, and RANKL/OPG mRNA expression in OVX mice assessed by real-time PCR. (B) ALP/β-actin ratio. (C) Osteocalcin/β-actin ratio. (D) RUNX-2/β-actin ratio. (E) RANKL/OPG/β-actin ratio. $P < 0.05$ for comparisons among the groups designated with an asterisk.

vessels of OVX mice. Enhanced osteogenesis might underlie these improvements, as indicated by the acceleration in MS/BS, BFR/BS, and MAR; the increase in serum osteocalcin; and the upregulation of tibial ALP, osteocalcin, and RUNX-2 mRNA. In addition, significant remediation of angiogenesis resulting from increases in VEGF also led to improved bone health in OVX mice.

Stimuli other than hypoxia also cause HIF-1α to accumulate in normoxic cells. For example, growth factors such as insulin-like growth factor can induce HIF-1α synthesis through activation of the PI3 K/Akt/mTOR signal transduction pathway [57,58]. Here, we found that 17β-estradiol stabilized HIF-1α under normal oxygen tension and increased VEGF protein expression, consistent with previous reports [34,35]. This phenomenon explains our previous finding that OVX decreased HIF-1α and VEGF expression in osteoblasts [33]. Impaired regulation of HIF-1α is also observed in other pathological processes, such as the development of diabetic wounds, and stabilization of HIF-1α is pivotal for reversing these pathological processes [59]. Mice in which HIF-1α signaling was activated developed extremely dense, heavily vascularized bones, and these mice were protected from OVX or age-induced bone loss [19,33]. More importantly, age-related bone loss has been prevented by administration of DFO, a hypoxia-mimicking agent [45]. Therefore, stabilization of HIF-1α by a hypoxia-mimicking agent might also help prevent estrogen deficiency-induced bone loss. Another widely used hypoxia-mimicking agent, DMOG, modulated VEGF mRNA and protein levels, which were mainly associated with activated HIF-1α under normal oxygen pressure [14,16,20].

In addition to its angiogenic effects, DMOG also has potent osteogenic effects. Enhanced osteogenic differentiation of DMOG-treated MSCs was demonstrated by ALP staining and calcium deposition, which are early and late stage osteogenic markers, respectively. To characterize the underlying molecular mechanism, alterations in the mRNA levels of RUNX-2 and osterix, essential transcription factors for the differentiation of osteoblasts from MSCs [60], were assessed. Our results and those of two recent studies indicate that DMOG upregulates RUNX-2 and osterix mRNA expression [21,30]. These results were supported by the finding that osteogenesis was enhanced in MSCs expressing a constitutively active form of HIF-1α [24,25,39]. Osteoblastic differentiation is predominantly regulated by the Wnt/β-catenin signaling pathway. Wnt binds to Frizzled receptors and their co-receptors, low-density lipoprotein receptor-related proteins (LRP5/6), to stabilize cytosolic β-catenin. β-Catenin then enters the nucleus and stimulates the transcription of Wnt target genes [61]. A reduction in serum β-catenin might contribute to the pathogenesis of postmenopausal osteoporosis [62]. In our studies, DMOG upregulated β-catenin mRNA and protein expression in a dose-dependent manner. Our findings are consistent with those of other groups, which showed that hypoxia and hypoxia mimetics, such as DFO, increase Wnt/β-catenin signaling in MSCs and osteoblasts [40,41]. As for the relationship between HIF-1α signaling and Wnt/β-catenin signaling, a previous study showed that HIF-1α modulated Wnt/β-catenin signaling in embryonic stem cells [36]. Our studies showed that this phenomenon occurs in MSCs. DMOG increased the expression of nuclear β-catenin and the downstream effectors LEF-1 and TCF-1. The effects were abrogated by the HIF-1α signaling inhibitor YC-1 [63–66]. These results suggest that the effect of DMOG on Wnt/β-catenin signaling is mediated by HIF-1α signaling.

In view of the dual role of DMOG in angiogenesis and osteogenesis, we hypothesized that DMOG would attenuate bone loss in OVX mice. As expected, DMOG administration increased the BMD of the trabecular bone. In addition to the BMD, the bone microarchitecture is a critical factor commonly associated with bone quality. Our results showed that BV/TV, Tb.N, Tb.Th, and Tb.Sp, the four fundamental indices of trabecular architecture as determined by the American Society for Bone and Mineral Research, were partly restored to differing extents by DMOG treatment, especially in the H-DMOG-treated group [67]. Because both bone mineral density and microarchitecture, two important factors that determine bone quality, improved significantly, we tested bone strength using the three-point bending test, which showed that DMOG treatment partly rescued the decline in bone mechanical strength due to OVX. These findings strongly suggest that DMOG prevents bone loss and improves bone quality in OVX mice.

Given that angiogenesis and osteogenesis are closely coupled, multiple studies have investigated the role of angiogenesis in the pathogenesis of osteoporosis. Accumulating evidence from studies in cells, animals, and patients indicates that low estrogen levels contribute to fewer vessels or decreases in angiogenic factors, resulting in the progression of osteoporosis [4–11]. Our current study supports this idea. OVX decreased the femoral vessel volumes of OVX mice, but femoral vessel volumes were partly restored in the DMOG-treated groups. The alteration in bone vessel volumes was in accordance with that of bone parameters. Furthermore, the restoration of bone vessel volume was coincident with the increased expression of HIF-1α and VEGF in bone samples. VEGF, the best known and most critical angiogenic factor, induces vessel formation and regulates the balance between osteogenic and adipogenic differentiation in MSCs. Mice with VEGF deficiency in osteoblastic precursor cells exhibited an osteoporosis-like phenotype characterized by reduced bone mass and increased bone marrow fat content [68]. Hence, normalization of low VEGF levels in postmenopausal women might be of critical significance.

Compared with antiresorptive drugs, which excessively reduce bone turnover and result in inadequate microdamage repair, drugs targeted towards impaired bone formation might be better suited to the rehabilitation of osteoporotic bone [69]. Our in vivo data, including serum osteocalcin, real-time PCR, and dynamic bone histomorphometry results, indicated that DMOG administration further increased osteogenesis in OVX mice [60]. These results are consistent with findings that inactivation of Vhl in osteochondral progenitor cells or osteoprogenitor cells increases the proliferation and differentiation of osteoblast lineage cells in vivo [18,19]. Furthermore, the expression of osteoprogenitor and osteoblast markers, including osterix, bone γ-carboxyglutamate protein, and integrin-binding sialoprotein, increased in the long bone of DFO-treated aged mice [45]. The enhanced differentiation of osteoblasts was probably attributed to elevated β-catenin protein expression, which was confirmed by westernblot. In addition to the regulation of the Wnt/β-catenin pathway by HIF-1α signaling, demonstrated in vitro in this study, the increased level of VEGF might be another pivotal factor for β-catenin accumulation [70]. Although it has been suggested that activation of the Wnt/β-catenin pathway decreases bone resorption, we did not detect a significant alteration in bone resorption following DMOG treatment, as shown by the serum CTX levels and the osteoclast numbers in the femur [71,72].

There were several limitations to this study: 1) the BMD and microarchitecture of the lumbar vertebra were not assessed; 2) it would be better if the treatment lasts longer time.

Conclusions

The results of present study demonstrate that DMOG treatment prevents bone loss, rescues bone microarchitecture deterioration, and restores bone strength in OVX mice. The effects might result from enhanced angiogenesis and osteogenesis. Following DMOG administration, new vessel formation, induced by angiogenic factors, would supply the bone with oxygen, nutrients, and a variety of cells, especially MSCs. Activation of the Wnt/β-catenin signaling pathway would enhance the osteogenic differentiation of MSCs and promote bone formation. To the best of our knowledge, this is the first report to describe the use and dual role of DMOG in the treatment of OVX-induced osteoporosis. DMOG may be a new strategy for the treatment of postmenopausal osteoporosis.

Supporting Information

Figure S1 Body weight, uterus weight, representative picture of uterus in each group and BMD alterations before and after OVX. (A) OVX significantly increased body weight of mice in OVX, OVX+L-DMOG and OVX+H-DMOG groups compared to Sham group. (B) OVX significantly decreased the uterus weight. (C) Representative picture of uterus in each group. (D) OVX obviously decreased the BMD of mice. $P<0.05$ for comparisons among the groups designated with an asterisk. (TIF)

Acknowledgments

This work was supported by the Natural Science Foundation of China (No. 81371958, 81061160510), the Basic Key Project of Science and Technology Commission of Shanghai Municipality (12JC1408200), and the Scientific and Technological Support Program in Biological Medicine of Science and Technology Commission of Shanghai Municipality (13431900702).

Author Contributions

Conceived and designed the experiments: JP ZGL DLF. Performed the experiments: JP ZGL ZLF KH CH SX QJ ZQ WJS QND ZHB. Analyzed the data: JP DLF. Contributed reagents/materials/analysis tools: QND WJS. Contributed to the writing of the manuscript: JP DLF ZGL.

References

1. Kanis JA (1994) Assessment of fracture risk and its application to screening for postmenopausal osteoporosis: synopsis of a WHO report. WHO Study Group. Osteoporos Int 4: 368–381.
2. Qu B, Ma Y, Yan M, Wu HH, Fan L, et al. (2014) The economic burden of fracture patients with osteoporosis in western China. Osteoporos Int. 25: 1853–1860.
3. Brandi ML, Collin-Osdoby P (2006) Vascular biology and the skeleton. J Bone Miner Res 21: 183–192.
4. Mekraldi S, Lafage-Proust MH, Bloomfield S, Alexandre C, Vico L (2003) Changes in vasoactive factors associated with altered vessel morphology in the tibial metaphysis during ovariectomy-induced bone loss in rats. Bone 32: 630–641.
5. Ding WG, Wei ZX, Liu JB (2011) Reduced local blood supply to the tibial metaphysis is associated with ovariectomy-induced osteoporosis in mice. Connect Tissue Res 52: 25–29.
6. Vogt MT, Cauley JA, Kuller LH, Nevitt MC (1997) Bone mineral density and blood flow to the lower extremities: the study of osteoporotic fractures. J Bone Miner Res 12: 283–289.
7. Griffith JF, Wang YX, Zhou H, Kwong WH, Wong WT, et al. (2010) Reduced bone perfusion in osteoporosis: likely causes in an ovariectomy rat model. Radiology 254: 739–746.
8. Shih TT, Liu HC, Chang CJ, Wei SY, Shen LC, et al. (2004) Correlation of MR lumbar spine bone marrow perfusion with bone mineral density in female subjects. Radiology 233: 121–128.
9. Senel K, Baykal T, Seferoglu B, Altas EU, Baygutalp F, et al. (2013) Circulating vascular endothelial growth factor concentrations in patients with postmenopausal osteoporosis. Arch Med Sci 9: 709–712.
10. Mueller MD, Vigne JL, Minchenko A, Lebovic DI, Leitman DC, et al. (2000) Regulation of vascular endothelial growth factor (VEGF) gene transcription by estrogen receptors alpha and beta. Proc Natl Acad Sci U S A 97: 10972–10977.
11. Pufe T, Claassen H, Scholz-Ahrens KE, Varoga D, Drescher W, et al. (2007) Influence of estradiol on vascular endothelial growth factor expression in bone: a study in Gottingen miniature pigs and human osteoblasts. Calcif Tissue Int 80: 184–191.
12. Min JH, Yang H, Ivan M, Gertler F, Kaelin WG Jr, et al. (2002) Structure of an HIF-1alpha -pVHL complex: hydroxyproline recognition in signaling. Science 296: 1886–1889.
13. Maxwell PH, Wiesener MS, Chang GW, Clifford SC, Vaux EC, et al. (1999) The tumour suppressor protein VHL targets hypoxia-inducible factors for oxygen-dependent proteolysis. Nature 399: 271–275.
14. Jaakkola P, Mole DR, Tian YM, Wilson MI, Gielbert J, et al. (2001) Targeting of HIF-alpha to the von Hippel-Lindau ubiquitylation complex by O2-regulated prolyl hydroxylation. Science 292: 468–472.
15. Ohh M, Park CW, Ivan M, Hoffman MA, Kim TY, et al. (2000) Ubiquitination of hypoxia-inducible factor requires direct binding to the beta-domain of the von Hippel-Lindau protein. Nat Cell Biol 2: 423–427.
16. Shen X, Wan C, Ramaswamy G, Mavalli M, Wang Y, et al. (2009) Prolyl hydroxylase inhibitors increase neoangiogenesis and callus formation following femur fracture in mice. J Orthop Res 27: 1298–1305.
17. Wang Y, Wan C, Deng L, Liu X, Cao X, et al. (2007) The hypoxia-inducible factor alpha pathway couples angiogenesis to osteogenesis during skeletal development. J Clin Invest 117: 1616–1626.
18. Rankin EB, Wu C, Khatri R, Wilson TL, Andersen R, et al. (2012) The HIF signaling pathway in osteoblasts directly modulates erythropoiesis through the production of EPO. Cell 149: 63–74.
19. Weng T, Xie Y, Huang J, Luo F, Yi L, et al. (2014) Inactivation of Vhl in osteochondral progenitor cells causes high bone mass phenotype and protects against age-related bone loss in adult mice. J Bone Miner Res 29: 820–829.
20. Wan C, Gilbert SR, Wang Y, Cao X, Shen X, et al. (2008) Activation of the hypoxia-inducible factor-1alpha pathway accelerates bone regeneration. Proc Natl Acad Sci U S A 105: 686–691.
21. Wu C, Zhou Y, Chang J, Xiao Y (2013) Delivery of dimethyloxalyl glycine in mesoporous bioactive glass scaffolds to improve angiogenesis and osteogenesis of human bone marrow stromal cells. Acta Biomater 9: 9159–9168.
22. Fan W, Crawford R, Xiao Y (2010) Enhancing in vivo vascularized bone formation by cobalt chloride-treated bone marrow stromal cells in a tissue engineered periosteum model. Biomaterials 31: 3580–3589.
23. Wu C, Zhou Y, Fan W, Han P, Chang J, et al. (2012) Hypoxia-mimicking mesoporous bioactive glass scaffolds with controllable cobalt ion release for bone tissue engineering. Biomaterials 33: 2076–2085.
24. Zou D, Zhang Z, He J, Zhang K, Ye D, et al. (2012) Blood vessel formation in the tissue-engineered bone with the constitutively active form of HIF-1alpha mediated BMSCs. Biomaterials 33: 2097–2108.
25. Zou D, Zhang Z, He J, Zhu S, Wang S, et al. (2011) Repairing critical-sized calvarial defects with BMSCs modified by a constitutively active form of hypoxia-inducible factor-1alpha and a phosphate cement scaffold. Biomaterials 32: 9707–9718.
26. Donneys A, Weiss DM, Deshpande SS, Ahsan S, Tchanque-Fossuo CN, et al. (2013) Localized deferoxamine injection augments vascularity and improves bony union in pathologic fracture healing after radiotherapy. Bone 52: 318–325.
27. Farberg AS, Jing XL, Monson LA, Donneys A, Tchanque-Fossuo CN, et al. (2012) Deferoxamine reverses radiation induced hypovascularity during bone regeneration and repair in the murine mandible. Bone 50: 1184–1187.
28. Zhang W, Li G, Deng R, Deng L, Qiu S (2012) New bone formation in a true bone ceramic scaffold loaded with desferrioxamine in the treatment of segmental bone defect: a preliminary study. J Orthop Sci 17: 289–298.
29. Stewart R, Goldstein J, Eberhardt A, Chu GT, Gilbert S (2011) Increasing vascularity to improve healing of a segmental defect of the rat femur. J Orthop Trauma 25: 472–476.
30. Ding H, Gao YS, Wang Y, Hu C, Sun Y, et al. (2014) Dimethyloxaloylglycine Increases the Bone Healing Capacity of Adipose-Derived Stem Cells by Promoting Osteogenic Differentiation and Angiogenic Potential. Stem Cells Dev. 23: 990–1000.
31. Grewal BS, Keller B, Weinhold P, Dahners LE (2014) Evaluating effects of deferoxamine in a rat tibia critical bone defect model. J Orthop 11: 5–9.
32. Liu XD, Deng LF, Wang J, Qi J, Zhou Q, et al. (2007) [The regulation of hypoxia inducible factor-1alpha on osteoblast function in postmenopausal osteoporosis]. Zhonghua Wai Ke Za Zhi 45: 1274–1278.
33. Zhao Q, Shen X, Zhang W, Zhu G, Qi J, et al. (2012) Mice with increased angiogenesis and osteogenesis due to conditional activation of HIF pathway in osteoblasts are protected from ovariectomy induced bone loss. Bone 50: 763–770.
34. Yun SP, Lee MY, Ryu JM, Song CH, Han HJ (2009) Role of HIF-1alpha and VEGF in human mesenchymal stem cell proliferation by 17beta-estradiol: involvement of PKC, PI3K/Akt, and MAPKs. Am J Physiol Cell Physiol 296: C317–326.

35. Yen ML, Su JL, Chien CL, Tseng KW, Yang CY, et al. (2005) Diosgenin induces hypoxia-inducible factor-1 activation and angiogenesis through estrogen receptor-related phosphatidylinositol 3-kinase/Akt and p38 mitogen-activated protein kinase pathways in osteoblasts. Mol Pharmacol 68: 1061–1073.

36. Mazumdar J, O'Brien WT, Johnson RS, LaManna JC, Chavez JC, et al. (2010) O2 regulates stem cells through Wnt/beta-catenin signalling. Nat Cell Biol 12: 1007–1013.

37. Ren H, Cao Y, Zhao Q, Li J, Zhou C, et al. (2006) Proliferation and differentiation of bone marrow stromal cells under hypoxic conditions. Biochem Biophys Res Commun 347: 12–21.

38. Wagegg M, Gaber T, Lohanatha FL, Hahne M, Strehl C, et al. (2012) Hypoxia promotes osteogenesis but suppresses adipogenesis of human mesenchymal stromal cells in a hypoxia-inducible factor-1 dependent manner. PLoS One 7: e46483.

39. Zou D, Zhang Z, Ye D, Tang A, Deng L, et al. (2011) Repair of critical-sized rat calvarial defects using genetically engineered bone marrow-derived mesenchymal stem cells overexpressing hypoxia-inducible factor-1alpha. Stem Cells 29: 1380–1390.

40. Qu Z-H, Zhang X-L, Tang T-T, Dai K-R (2008) Promotion of osteogenesis through β-catenin signaling by desferrioxamine. Biochem Biophys Res Commun 370: 332–337.

41. Genetos DC, Toupadakis CA, Raheja LF, Wong A, Papanicolaou SE, et al. (2010) Hypoxia decreases sclerostin expression and increases Wnt signaling in osteoblasts. J Cell Biochem 110: 457–467.

42. Bidwell JP, Alvarez MB, Hood M Jr, Childress P (2013) Functional impairment of bone formation in the pathogenesis of osteoporosis: the bone marrow regenerative competence. Curr Osteoporos Rep 11: 117–125.

43. Li L, Yao XL, He XL, Liu XJ, Wu WC, et al. (2013) Role of mechanical strain and estrogen in modulating osteogenic differentiation of mesenchymal stem cells (MSCs) from normal and ovariectomized rats. Cell Mol Biol (Noisy-le-grand) Suppl 59: OL1889–1893.

44. Yang N, Wang G, Hu C, Shi Y, Liao L, et al. (2013) Tumor necrosis factor alpha suppresses the mesenchymal stem cell osteogenesis promoter miR-21 in estrogen deficiency-induced osteoporosis. J Bone Miner Res 28: 559–573.

45. Kusumbe AP, Ramasamy SK, Adams RH (2014) Coupling of angiogenesis and osteogenesis by a specific vessel subtype in bone. Nature 507: 323–328.

46. Jia P, Xu YJ, Zhang ZL, Li K, Li B, et al. (2012) Ferric ion could facilitate osteoclast differentiation and bone resorption through the production of reactive oxygen species. J Orthop Res 30: 1843–1852.

47. Ishii KA, Fumoto T, Iwai K, Takeshita S, Ito M, et al. (2009) Coordination of PGC-1beta and iron uptake in mitochondrial biogenesis and osteoclast activation. Nat Med 15: 259–266.

48. Zhao HX, Wang XL, Wang YH, Wu Y, Li XY, et al. (2010) Attenuation of myocardial injury by postconditioning: role of hypoxia inducible factor-1alpha. Basic Res Cardiol 105: 109–118.

49. Song YR, You SJ, Lee YM, Chin HJ, Chae DW, et al. (2010) Activation of hypoxia-inducible factor attenuates renal injury in rat remnant kidney. Nephrol Dial Transplant 25: 77–85.

50. Takaku M, Tomita S, Kurobe H, Kihira Y, Morimoto A, et al. (2012) Systemic preconditioning by a prolyl hydroxylase inhibitor promotes prevention of skin flap necrosis via HIF-1-induced bone marrow-derived cells. PLoS One 7: e42964.

51. Botusan IR, Sunkari VG, Savu O, Catrina AI, Grunler J, et al. (2008) Stabilization of HIF-1alpha is critical to improve wound healing in diabetic mice. Proc Natl Acad Sci U S A 105: 19426–19431.

52. Rey S, Lee K, Wang CJ, Gupta K, Chen S, et al. (2009) Synergistic effect of HIF-1alpha gene therapy and HIF-1-activated bone marrow-derived angiogenic cells in a mouse model of limb ischemia. Proc Natl Acad Sci U S A 106: 20399–20404.

53. Poynter JA, Manukyan MC, Wang Y, Brewster BD, Herrmann JL, et al. (2011) Systemic pretreatment with dimethyloxalylglycine increases myocardial HIF-1alpha and VEGF production and improves functional recovery after acute ischemia/reperfusion. Surgery 150: 278–283.

54. Patel TH, Kimura H, Weiss CR, Semenza GL, Hofmann LV (2005) Constitutively active HIF-1alpha improves perfusion and arterial remodeling in an endovascular model of limb ischemia. Cardiovasc Res 68: 144–154.

55. Sun Y, Li QF, Zhang Y, Hu R, Jiang H (2013) Isoflurane preconditioning increases survival of rat skin random-pattern flaps by induction of HIF-1alpha expression. Cell Physiol Biochem 31: 579–591.

56. Dempster DW, Compston JE, Drezner MK, Glorieux FH, Kanis JA, et al. (2013) Standardized nomenclature, symbols, and units for bone histomorphometry: a 2012 update of the report of the ASBMR Histomorphometry Nomenclature Committee. J Bone Miner Res 28: 2–17.

57. Zelzer E, Levy Y, Kahana C, Shilo BZ, Rubinstein M, et al. (1998) Insulin induces transcription of target genes through the hypoxia-inducible factor HIF-1alpha/ARNT. EMBO J 17: 5085–5094.

58. Fukuda R, Hirota K, Fan F, Jung YD, Ellis LM, et al. (2002) Insulin-like growth factor 1 induces hypoxia-inducible factor 1-mediated vascular endothelial growth factor expression, which is dependent on MAP kinase and phosphatidylinositol 3-kinase signaling in colon cancer cells. J Biol Chem 277: 38205–38211.

59. Botusan IR, Sunkari VG, Savu O, Catrina AI, Grunler J, et al. (2008) Stabilization of HIF-1 is critical to improve wound healing in diabetic mice. Proceedings of the National Academy of Sciences 105: 19426–19431.

60. Long F (2012) Building strong bones: molecular regulation of the osteoblast lineage. Nat Rev Mol Cell Biol 13: 27–38.

61. Rossini M, Gatti D, Adami S (2013) Involvement of WNT/beta-catenin signaling in the treatment of osteoporosis. Calcif Tissue Int 93: 121–132.

62. Xu XJ, Shen L, Yang YP, Zhu R, Shuai B, et al. (2013) Serum beta -Catenin Levels Associated with the Ratio of RANKL/OPG in Patients with Postmenopausal Osteoporosis. Int J Endocrinol 2013: 534352.

63. Shin DH, Kim JH, Jung YJ, Kim KE, Jeong JM, et al. (2007) Preclinical evaluation of YC-1, a HIF inhibitor, for the prevention of tumor spreading. Cancer Lett 255: 107–116.

64. Liu L, Yu Q, Lin J, Lai X, Cao W, et al. (2011) Hypoxia-inducible factor-1alpha is essential for hypoxia-induced mesenchymal stem cell mobilization into the peripheral blood. Stem Cells Dev 20: 1961–1971.

65. van de Wetering M, Cavallo R, Dooijes D, van Beest M, van Es J, et al. (1997) Armadillo coactivates transcription driven by the product of the Drosophila segment polarity gene dTCF. Cell 88: 789–799.

66. Reya T, Clevers H (2005) Wnt signalling in stem cells and cancer. Nature 434: 843–850.

67. Bouxsein ML, Boyd SK, Christiansen BA, Guldberg RE, Jepsen KJ, et al. (2010) Guidelines for assessment of bone microstructure in rodents using micro-computed tomography. J Bone Miner Res 25: 1468–1486.

68. Liu Y, Berendsen AD, Jia S, Lotinun S, Baron R, et al. (2012) Intracellular VEGF regulates the balance between osteoblast and adipocyte differentiation. J Clin Invest 122: 3101–3113.

69. Chapurlat RD, Delmas PD (2009) Bone microdamage: a clinical perspective. Osteoporos Int 20: 1299–1308.

70. Maes C, Goossens S, Bartunkova S, Drogat B, Coenegrachts L, et al. (2010) Increased skeletal VEGF enhances beta-catenin activity and results in excessively ossified bones. EMBO J 29: 424–441.

71. Henriksen K, Tanko LB, Qvist P, Delmas PD, Christiansen C, et al. (2007) Assessment of osteoclast number and function: application in the development of new and improved treatment modalities for bone diseases. Osteoporos Int 18: 681–685.

72. Spencer GJ, Utting JC, Etheridge SL, Arnett TR, Genever PG (2006) Wnt signalling in osteoblasts regulates expression of the receptor activator of NFkappaB ligand and inhibits osteoclastogenesis in vitro. J Cell Sci 119: 1283–1296.

Permissions

List of Contributors

Zhili Wen
Department of Infectious Disease, Nanchang University Medical School, Nanchang, Jiangxi, China

Wei Huang
Department of Pathology and Lab Medicine, University of Cincinnati
Medical Center, Cincinnati, Ohio, United States of America

Yuliang Feng
Department of Pathology and Lab Medicine, University of Cincinnati
Medical Center, Cincinnati, Ohio, United States of America

Wenfeng Cai
Department of Pathology and Lab Medicine, University of Cincinnati
Medical Center, Cincinnati, Ohio, United States of America

Yuhua Wang
Department of Pathology and Lab Medicine, University of Cincinnati
Medical Center, Cincinnati, Ohio, United States of America

Xiaohong Wang
Department of Pharmacology and Cell Biophysics, University of Cincinnati Medical Center, Cincinnati, Ohio, United States of America,

Jialiang Liang
Department of Pathology and Lab Medicine, University of Cincinnati
Medical Center, Cincinnati, Ohio, United States of America

Mashhood Wani
Department of Pathology and Lab Medicine, University of Cincinnati
Medical Center, Cincinnati, Ohio, United States of America

Jing Chen
Department of Environmental Health, University of Cincinnati Medical Center, Cincinnati, Ohio, United States of America,

Pin Zhu
Guangdong Cardiovascular Institute, Guangdong Academy of Medical Sciences, Guangzhou, Guandong, People's Republic of China

Ji-Mei Chen
Guangdong Cardiovascular Institute, Guangdong Academy of Medical Sciences, Guangzhou, Guandong, People's Republic of China

Ronald W. Millard
Department of Pharmacology and Cell Biophysics, University of Cincinnati Medical Center, Cincinnati, Ohio, United States of America

Guo-Chang Fan
Department of Pharmacology and Cell Biophysics, University of Cincinnati Medical Center, Cincinnati, Ohio, United States of America

Yigang Wang
Department of Pathology and Lab Medicine, University of Cincinnati Medical Center, Cincinnati, Ohio, United States of America

Guo-Hua Dai
Affiliated Hospital of Shandong University of Traditional Chinese Medicine, Jinan, China

Pei-Ze Ma
Shandong University of Traditional Chinese Medicine, Jinan, China

Xian-Bo Song
Shandong University of Traditional Chinese Medicine, Jinan, China

Ning Liu
Shandong University of Traditional Chinese Medicine, Jinan, China

Tong Zhang
Affiliated Hospital of Shandong University of Traditional Chinese Medicine, Jinan, China

Bo Wu
Affiliated Hospital of Shandong University of Traditional Chinese Medicine, Jinan, China

Beverly L. Falcon
Department of Cancer Angiogenesis, Eli Lilly and Company, Lilly Corporate Center, Indianapolis, Indiana, United States of America

Michelle Swearingen
Department of Cancer Angiogenesis, Eli Lilly and Company, Lilly Corporate Center, Indianapolis, Indiana, United States of America

Wendy H. Gough
Department of Quantitative Biology, Eli Lilly and Company, Lilly Corporate Center, Indianapolis, Indiana, United States of America

Linda Lee
Department of Cancer Angiogenesis, Eli Lilly and Company, Lilly Corporate Center, Indianapolis, Indiana, United States of America

Robert Foreman
Department of In Vivo Pharmacology, Eli Lilly and Company, Lilly Corporate
Center, Indianapolis, Indiana, United States of America

Mark Uhlik
Department of Cancer Angiogenesis, Eli Lilly and Company, Lilly Corporate Center, Indianapolis, Indiana, United States of America

Jeff C. Hanson
Department of Informatics Capabilities, Eli Lilly and Company, Lilly Corporate Center, Indianapolis, Indiana, United States of America

Jonathan A. Lee
Department of Quantitative Biology, Eli Lilly and Company, Lilly Corporate Center, Indianapolis, Indiana, United States of America

Don B. McClure
Department of BioTDR, Eli Lilly and Company, Lilly Corporate Center, Indianapolis, Indiana, United States of America

Sudhakar Chintharlapalli
Department of Cancer Angiogenesis, Eli Lilly and Company, Lilly Corporate Center, Indianapolis, Indiana, United States of America

Amy J. Naylor
Rheumatology Research Group, Centre for Translational Inflammation Research, University of Birmingham, Birmingham, West Midlands, United Kingdom

Helen M. McGettrick
Systems Science for Health, University of Birmingham, Birmingham, West Midlands, United Kingdom

William D. Maynard
Rheumatology Research Group, Centre for Translational Inflammation Research, University of Birmingham, Birmingham, West Midlands, United Kingdom

Philippa May
Rheumatology Research Group, Centre for Translational Inflammation Research, University of Birmingham, Birmingham, West Midlands, United Kingdom

Francesca Barone
Rheumatology Research Group, Centre for Translational Inflammation Research, University of Birmingham, Birmingham, West Midlands, United Kingdom

Adam P. Croft
Rheumatology Research Group, Centre for Translational Inflammation Research, University of Birmingham, Birmingham, West Midlands, United Kingdom

Stuart Egginton
Faculty of Biological Sciences, University of Leeds, Leeds, West Yorkshire

Christopher D. Buckley
Rheumatology Research Group, Centre for Translational Inflammation Research, University of Birmingham, Birmingham, West Midlands, United Kingdom
Systems Science for Health, University of Birmingham, Birmingham, West Midlands, United Kingdom

Xiao Qiong Liu
Key Laboratory of Cardiovascular Remodeling and Function Research, Shandong University Qilu Hospital, Jinan, Shandong, China
Department of Traditional Chinese Medicine, Shandong University Qilu Hospital, Jinan, Shandong, China

Yang Mao
Key Laboratory of Cardiovascular Remodeling and Function Research, Shandong University Qilu Hospital, Jinan, Shandong, China

Bo Wang
Department of Traditional Chinese Medicine, Shandong University Qilu Hospital, Jinan, Shandong, China

Xiao Ting Lu
Key Laboratory of Cardiovascular Remodeling and Function Research, Shandong University Qilu Hospital, Jinan, Shandong, China

Wen Wu Bai
Key Laboratory of Cardiovascular Remodeling and Function Research, Shandong University Qilu Hospital, Jinan, Shandong, China
Department of Traditional Chinese Medicine, Shandong University Qilu Hospital, Jinan, Shandong, China

Yuan Yuan Sun
Key Laboratory of Cardiovascular Remodeling and Function Research, Shandong University Qilu Hospital, Jinan, Shandong, China
Department of Traditional Chinese Medicine, Shandong University Qilu Hospital, Jinan, Shandong, China

Yan Liu
Key Laboratory of Cardiovascular Remodeling and Function Research, Shandong University Qilu Hospital, Jinan, Shandong, China

Hong Mei Liu
Department of Endodontics, Jinan Stomatologic Hospital, Jinan, Shandong, China

Lei Zhang
Key Laboratory of Cardiovascular Remodeling and Function Research, Shandong University Qilu Hospital, Jinan, Shandong, China

Yu Xia Zhao
Department of Traditional Chinese Medicine, Shandong University Qilu Hospital, Jinan, Shandong, China

Yun Zhang
Key Laboratory of Cardiovascular Remodeling and Function Research, Shandong University Qilu Hospital, Jinan, Shandong, China

Lei Qi
Department of Thoracic Surgery, Qi Lu Hospital, Shandong University, Jinan, Shandong Province, China

Feng Zhu
Department of Thoracic Surgery, Shan dong Provincial Chest Hospital, Jinan, Shandong Province, China

Shu-hai Li
Department of Thoracic Surgery, Qi Lu Hospital, Shandong University, Jinan, Shandong Province, China

Li-bo Si
Department of Thoracic Surgery, Qi Lu Hospital, Shandong University, Jinan, Shandong Province, China

Li-kuan Hu
Department of Thoracic Surgery, Qi Lu Hospital, Shandong University, Jinan, Shandong Province, China

Hui Tian
Department of Thoracic Surgery, Qi Lu Hospital, Shandong University, Jinan, Shandong Province, China

J. Kowshik
Department of Biochemistry and Biotechnology, Faculty of Science, Annamalai University, Annamalainagar, Tamil Nadu, India

Abdul Basit Baba
Department of Biochemistry and Biotechnology, Faculty of Science, Annamalai University, Annamalainagar, Tamil Nadu, India

Hemant Giri
Laboratory of Vascular Biology, Department of Biotechnology, Indian Institute of Technology Madras, Chennai, Tami Nadu, India

G. Deepak Reddy
Medicinal Chemistry Research Division, Vishnu Institute of Pharmaceutical Education and Research, Narsapur, India

Madhulika Dixit
Laboratory of Vascular Biology, Department of Biotechnology, Indian Institute of Technology Madras, Chennai, Tami Nadu, India

Siddavaram Nagini
Department of Biochemistry and Biotechnology, Faculty of Science, Annamalai University, Annamalainagar, Tamil Nadu, India

Ian M. Packham
Centre for Cardiovascular Sciences, School of Clinical and Experimental Medicine, College of Medical and Dental Sciences, University of Birmingham, Edgbaston, Birmingham, United Kingdom

Steve P. Watson
Centre for Cardiovascular Sciences, School of Clinical and Experimental Medicine, College of Medical and Dental Sciences, University of Birmingham, Edgbaston, Birmingham, United Kingdom

Roy Bicknell
Centre for Cardiovascular Sciences, School of Immunity and Infection, College of Medical and Dental Sciences, University of Birmingham, Edgbaston, Birmingham, United Kingdom

Stuart Egginton
Centre for Cardiovascular Sciences, School of Clinical and Experimental Medicine, College of Medical and Dental Sciences, University of Birmingham, Edgbaston, Birmingham, United Kingdom
School of Biomedical Sciences, Faculty of Biological Sciences, University of Leeds, Leeds, United Kingdom

Saptak Banerjee, Tithi Ghosh, Subhasis Barik, Arnab Das, Sarbari Ghosh, Avishek Bhuniya, Anamika Bose and Rathindranath Baral
Department of Immunoregulation and Immunodiagnostics, Chittaranjan National Cancer Institute (CNCI), Kolkata, India

Heng Zeng, Lanfang Li and Jian-Xiong Chen
Department of Pharmacology and Toxicology, University of Mississippi Medical Center, Jackson, Mississippi, United States of America

Kaori Suenaga
Department of Vascular Biology, Institute of Development, Aging, and Cancer, Tohoku University, Aoba-ku, Sendai, Miyagi, Japan
Department of Obstetrics & Gynecology, Tohoku University School of Medicine, Aoba-ku, Sendai, Miyagi, Japan

Shuji Kitahara
Department of Anatomy and Developmental Biology, Tokyo Women's Medical University, Shinjuku-ku, Tokyo, Japan

Yasuhiro Suzuki
Department of Vascular Biology, Institute of Development, Aging, and Cancer, Tohoku University, Aoba-ku, Sendai, Miyagi, Japan

Miho Kobayashi
Department of Vascular Biology, Institute of Development, Aging, and Cancer, Tohoku University, Aoba-ku, Sendai, Miyagi, Japan

Sachiko Horie
Department of Vascular Biology, Institute of Development, Aging, and Cancer, Tohoku University, Aoba-ku, Sendai, Miyagi, Japan

Junichi Sugawara
Department of Obstetrics & Gynecology, Tohoku University School of Medicine, Aoba-ku, Sendai, Miyagi, Japan
Tohoku Medical Megabank Organization, Tohoku University, Aobaku, Sendai, Miyagi, Japan

Nobuo Yaegashi
Department of Obstetrics & Gynecology, Tohoku University School of Medicine, Aoba-ku, Sendai, Miyagi, Japan
Tohoku Medical Megabank Organization, Tohoku University, Aobaku, Sendai, Miyagi, Japan

Yasufumi Sato
Department of Vascular Biology, Institute of Development, Aging, and Cancer, Tohoku University, Aoba-ku, Sendai, Miyagi, Japan

John Gounarides, Jennifer S. Cobb, Jing Zhou, Frank Cook, Xuemei Yang, Chang Rao, Hong Yin
Analytical Sciences, Novartis Institutes for Biomedical Research, Cambridge, MA, United States of America

Erik Meredith and Muneto Mogi
Global Discovery Chemistry, Novartis Institutes for Biomedical Research, Cambridge, MA, United States of America

Qian Huang and YongYao Xu
Developmental and Metabolic Pathways, Novartis Institutes for Biomedical Research, Cambridge, MA, United States of America

Karen Anderson, Andrea De Erkenez, Sha-Mei Liao,Maura Crowley, Natasha Buchanan, Stephen Poor, Yubin Qiu, Elizabeth Fassbender, Siyuan Shen, Amber Woolfenden, Amy Jensen, Rosemarie Cepeda, Bijan Etemad-Gilbertson, Shelby Giza, Bruce Jaffee and Sassan Azarian
Ophthalmology, Novartis Institutes for Biomedical Research, Cambridge, MA, United States of America

Christine Weinl, Heidemarie Riehle, Christine Stritt, and Alfred Nordheim
Department of Molecular Biology, Interfaculty Institute for Cell Biology, University of Tuebingen, Tuebingen, Germany

Christine Wasylyk, Michel J. Roux and Bohdan Wasylyk
Institut de Génétique et de Biologie Mol éculaireet Cellulaire, Illkirch, France
Centre National de la Recherche Scientifique, Illkirch, France
Institut National de la Santé et de la Recherche Médicale, Illkirch, France
Université de Strasbourg, Illkirch, France

Marina Garcia Garrido, Vithiyanjali Sothilingam, Susanne C. Beck, Mathias W. Seeliger
Division of Ocular Neurodegeneration, Centre for Ophthalmology, Institute for Ophthalmic Research, University of Tu¨ bingen, Tu¨ bingen, Germany

Ju-Geng Lai
Institute of Molecular and Genomic Medicine, National Health Research Institutes, Zhunan Town, Miaoli, Taiwan, ROC

Su-Mei Tsai
Institute of Molecular and Genomic Medicine, National Health Research Institutes, Zhunan Town, Miaoli, Taiwan, ROC

Hsiao-Chen Tu
Institute of Molecular and Genomic Medicine, National Health Research Institutes, Zhunan Town, Miaoli, Taiwan, ROC
Institute of Biotechnology, National Tsing Hua University, Hsinchu, Taiwan, ROC

Wen-Chuan Chen
Institute of Molecular and Genomic Medicine, National Health Research Institutes, Zhunan Town, Miaoli, Taiwan, ROC

Fong-Ji Kou
Institute of Molecular and Genomic Medicine, National Health Research Institutes, Zhunan Town, Miaoli, Taiwan, ROC

Jeng-Wei Lu
Institute of Molecular and Genomic Medicine, National Health Research Institutes, Zhunan Town, Miaoli, Taiwan, ROC

Horng-Dar Wang
Institute of Biotechnology, National Tsing Hua University, Hsinchu, Taiwan, ROC

Chou-Long Huang
Departments of Medicine, University of Texas Southwestern Medical Center, Dallas, Texas, United States of America

Chiou-Hwa Yuh
Institute of Molecular and Genomic Medicine, National Health Research Institutes, Zhunan Town, Miaoli, Taiwan, ROC
College of Life Science and Institute of Bioinformatics and Structural Biology, National Tsing-Hua University, Hsinchu, Taiwan, ROC
Department of Biological Science and Technology, National Chiao Tung University, Hsinchu, Taiwan, ROC
College of Medicine, Kaohsiung Medical University, Kaohsiung, Taiwan, ROC

Chih-Wei Chou, You-Lin Zhuo, Zhe-Yu Jiang and Yi-Wen Liu
Department of Life Science, Tunghai University, Taichung, Taiwan

Iván González-Chavarría, Rita P. Cerr, Natalie P. Parra, Felipe A. Sandoval , Silvana P. Jiménez, Edelmira A. Fernandez, Nicolas A. Gutié rrez, Federico S. Rodriguez, Jorge R. Toledo and Juan C. Vera
Biotechnology and Biopharmaceuticals Laboratory, Department of Pathophysiology, School of Biological Sciences, Universidad de Concepció n, Concepció n, Chile

Felipe A. Zu ñ iga and Liliana I. Lamperti
Department of Clinical Biochemistry and Immunology, School of Pharmacy, Universidad de Concepció n, Concepció n, Chile

Valeska A. Omazábal
Department of Basic Sciences, Faculty of Medicine, Universidad Cató lica de la Santísima Concepció n, Concepció n, Chile

Sergio A. Onate
Translational Research Unit, School of Medicine, Universidad de Concepció n, Concepció n, Chile

Oliberto Sánchez
Department of Pharmacology, School of Biological Sciences, Universidad de Concepció n, Concepció n, Chile

Kaiqun Ren
Key Laboratory of Protein Chemistry and Developmental Biology of State Education Ministry of China, College of Life Science, Hunan Normal University, Changsha, P. R. China
Model Animal Research Center, MOE Key Laboratory of Model Animal for Disease Research, Medical School, Nanjing University, Nanjing, P.R. China
College of Medicine, Hunan Normal University, Changsha, P. R. China

Jing Yuan
Key Laboratory of Protein Chemistry and Developmental Biology of State Education Ministry of China, College of Life Science, Hunan Normal University, Changsha, P. R. China

Manjun Yang
Key Laboratory of Protein Chemistry and Developmental Biology of State Education Ministry of China, College of Life Science, Hunan Normal University, Changsha, P. R. China

Xiang Gao
Model Animal Research Center, MOE Key Laboratory of Model Animal for Disease Research, Medical School, Nanjing University, Nanjing, P.R. China

Xiaofeng Ding
Key Laboratory of Protein Chemistry and Developmental Biology of State Education Ministry of China, College of Life Science, Hunan Normal University, Changsha, P. R. China

Jianlin Zhou
Key Laboratory of Protein Chemistry and Developmental Biology of State Education Ministry of China, College of Life Science, Hunan Normal University, Changsha, P. R. China

Xingwang Hu
Key Laboratory of Protein Chemistry and Developmental Biology of State Education Ministry of China, College of Life Science, Hunan Normal University, Changsha, P. R. China

Jianguo Cao
College of Medicine, Hunan Normal University, Changsha, P. R. China

Xiyun Deng
College of Medicine, Hunan Normal University, Changsha, P. R. China

Shuanglin Xiang
Key Laboratory of Protein Chemistry and Developmental Biology of State Education Ministry of China, College of Life Science, Hunan Normal University, Changsha, P. R. China

Jian Zhang
Key Laboratory of Protein Chemistry and Developmental Biology of State Education Ministry of China, College of Life Science, Hunan Normal University, Changsha, P. R. China

Jia Peng
Shanghai Institute of Traumatology and Orthopaedics, Shanghai Key Laboratory for Prevention and Treatment of Bone and Joint Diseases with Integrated Chinese- Western Medicine, Ruijin Hospital, Jiao Tong University School of Medicine, Shanghai, China

Zuo Gui Lai
Shanghai Institute of Traumatology and Orthopaedics, Shanghai Key Laboratory for Prevention and Treatment of Bone and Joint Diseases with Integrated Chinese- Western Medicine, Ruijin Hospital, Jiao Tong University School of Medicine, Shanghai, China
Department of Orthopaedics, Qian Fo Shan Hospital, Shang Dong University, Ji Nan, China

Zhang Lian Fang
Shanghai Institute of Traumatology and Orthopaedics, Shanghai Key Laboratory for Prevention and Treatment of Bone and Joint Diseases with Integrated Chinese- Western Medicine, Ruijin Hospital, Jiao Tong University School of Medicine, Shanghai, China
Department of Orthopaedics, The First Affiliated Hospital of Soochow University, Suzhou, China

Shen Xing
Shanghai Institute of Traumatology and Orthopaedics, Shanghai Key Laboratory for Prevention and Treatment of Bone and Joint Diseases with Integrated Chinese- Western Medicine, Ruijin Hospital, Jiao Tong University School of Medicine, Shanghai, China

Kang Hui
Shanghai Institute of Traumatology and Orthopaedics, Shanghai Key Laboratory for Prevention and Treatment of Bone and Joint Diseases with Integrated Chinese-Western Medicine, Ruijin Hospital, Jiao Tong University School of Medicine, Shanghai, China

Chen Hao
Shanghai Institute of Traumatology and Orthopaedics, Shanghai Key Laboratory for Prevention and Treatment of Bone and Joint Diseases with Integrated Chinese-Western Medicine, Ruijin Hospital, Jiao Tong University School of Medicine, Shanghai, China

Qi Jin
Shanghai Institute of Traumatology and Orthopaedics, Shanghai Key Laboratory for Prevention and Treatment of Bone and Joint Diseases with Integrated Chinese-Western Medicine, Ruijin Hospital, Jiao Tong University School of Medicine, Shanghai, China

Zhou Qi
Shanghai Institute of Traumatology and Orthopaedics, Shanghai Key Laboratory for Prevention and Treatment of Bone and Joint Diseases with Integrated Chinese- Western Medicine, Ruijin Hospital, Jiao Tong University School of Medicine, Shanghai, China

Wang Jin Shen
Shanghai Institute of Traumatology and Orthopaedics, Shanghai Key Laboratory for Prevention and Treatment of Bone and Joint Diseases with Integrated Chinese-Western Medicine, Ruijin Hospital, Jiao Tong University School of Medicine, Shanghai, China

Qian Nian Dong
Shanghai Institute of Traumatology and Orthopaedics, Shanghai Key Laboratory for Prevention and Treatment of Bone and Joint Diseases with Integrated Chinese-Western Medicine, Ruijin Hospital, Jiao Tong University School of Medicine, Shanghai, China

Zhou Han Bing
Shanghai Institute of Traumatology and Orthopaedics, Shanghai Key Laboratory for Prevention and Treatment of Bone and Joint Diseases with Integrated Chinese-Western Medicine, Ruijin Hospital, Jiao Tong University School of Medicine, Shanghai, China

Deng Lian Fu
Shanghai Institute of Traumatology and Orthopaedics, Shanghai Key Laboratory for Prevention and Treatment of Bone and Joint Diseases with Integrated Chinese-Western Medicine, Ruijin Hospital, Jiao Tong University School of Medicine, Shanghai, China

Index